Ancestral Diets and Nutrition

Ancestral Diets and Nutrition

Christopher Cumo

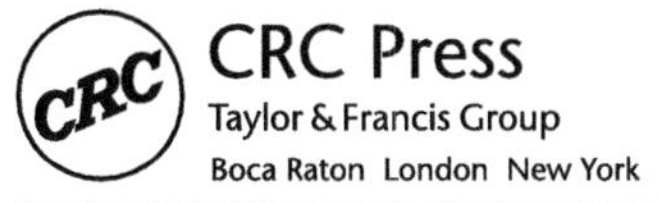

CRC Press is an imprint of the
Taylor & Francis Group, an **informa** business

First edition published 2021
by CRC Press
6000 Broken Sound Parkway NW, Suite 300, Boca Raton, FL 33487-2742

and by CRC Press
2 Park Square, Milton Park, Abingdon, Oxon, OX14 4RN

CRC Press is an imprint of Taylor & Francis Group, LLC

ISBN: 9780367235987 (pbk)
ISBN: 9780367236090 (hbk)
ISBN: 9780429280719 (ebk)

Typeset in Times
by codeMantra

Contents

List of Figures

List of Tables

List of Graphs

Preface

This book originated in the happy courtship of the remarkable woman who is now my wife. During this time, she shared with me her interest in food, nutrition, and health. Much of her information came from journalism and best-selling books. Because so many opinions conflicted, she found herself switching from one regimen to another without coming any closer to knowing what foods were healthiest. Such a scenario created bewilderment and dissatisfaction, sentiments common to many Americans who want the greatest vitality without knowing quite how to proceed.

The fact that diet, nutrition, and health are at the core biological matters led me to plan a book on the interrelatedness among these topics partly to combat what may be perceived as a denial of physicality that goes back to the foundations of civilization. British mathematician and philosopher Alfred North Whitehead's (1861–1947) description of Western philosophy as "a series of footnotes to Plato" applies to how we understand ourselves in the most fundamental ways.[1] At the root of this understanding is the conviction that a person is not just a body because cognition produces ideas that cannot always be tied to something tangible. For example, someone might ponder the notion of infinity even though everything he experiences is finite. If ideas emanate from beyond the physical, then we must have some metaphysical faculty—the intellect for our purposes—that generates these concepts and is separate from the body, itself a chemical machine and thus unambiguously physical.

Greek philosopher Plato (c. 427–c. 347 BCE) emphasized the separation between body and intellect—using a term usually translated as "soul"—forcefully enough to create duality between the two. Perhaps nowhere was his ability to engage this topic on greater display than in *Phaedo* (c. 360 BCE), an account of his mentor Socrates' (469–399 BCE) execution. Plato, stating his absence on this day, signaled that *Phaedo* was a literary creation because he was not present to transcribe the discussion among Socrates and his friends.[2] Because Plato could not have reproduced Socrates' words, the dialogue's ideas—though Socrates may have outlined some of them—likely belonged to his pupil.[3]

Facing his end, Socrates' thoughts probably turned to death, a circumstance that Plato used to define death as the moment when body and soul parted.[4] The soul's liberation from the body resembled an inmate's release from prison.[5] Equation of body and prison devalued the body, an appraisal Plato pursued by emphasizing it as an impediment to knowledge. The soul apprehends truth only "when it is completely by itself and says good-bye to the body, and so far as possible has no dealings with it, when it reaches out and grasps that which really is."[6] This language elevates the intellect at the body's expense. "For whenever the soul tries to examine anything in company with the body, it is plain that it is deceived by it."[7] If the body causes error by impeding the intellect, then only intellect merits trust. The body is a danger and a detour from reality.

German philosopher Friedrich Wilhelm Nietzsche (1844–1900) warned against this dualism, in *The Birth of Tragedy* (1872) contrasting Socrates' excessive intellectualism with "well-being," "overflowing health," and "*abundance* of existence."[8] In *On the Genealogy of Morals* (1887), Nietzsche rejected any attempt to "downgrade physicality."[9] His perspective deserves consideration in a world where too many people retain Plato's disinterest in the body without ever having thumbed through his dialogues. Technology reinforces this attitude because we no longer depend on brawn as premodern peoples did. Today the body occupies a car or elevator, which does the work of moving from one location to another. The body crouches in a chair before a computer monitor, a stance a person adopts several hours each day without any conscious attention to the body and its ceaseless chemical activities. The body has become an extension of inanimate technology rather than a source of kinetic energy and volition.

Disinterest can become distrust of the body, a wariness evident in discomfort with overt sexuality. Although less obvious, distrust may manifest in intrusiveness. Without my soliciting their opinion, neighbors and acquaintances have expressed dismay that I dig my garden with a spade every spring and autumn when the job would be much easier with a rototiller. One neighbor, settling his deceased mother's estate, offered me hers, assuring me that once I tried it, I would discard my spade. Such appeals disconcert me, especially because I should not have to justify my preference for hand tools. After all, I have never tried to dissuade someone from using gasoline, or electric, gadgets or to convince him to trade his automobile for a bicycle, as I have. Nonetheless, the academic dean at the university where I once taught labeled me "weird" for bicycling to campus. This comment, coming from a man otherwise progressive on economic and social issues, demonstrates the limits of tolerance for physicality in a world in which technology trumps it. These circumstances compel the inference that modernity defines exertion as abnormal.

This book rejects such nonsense, which has devolved into mental and physical atrophy. The following pages attempt to evaluate foods' healthfulness in an effort to reclaim corporeality and the vitality that everyone claims to want but that many people believe eludes them in some way. This evaluation amasses data from prehistory and history by examining what past peoples ate and how healthy or ill they were. The first chapter describes this method and its limitations. Chapter 2 delineates the nutrients and their chemistry. Chapter 3 traces the evolution of pre-human and human diets. Chapters 4 through 9 cover the principal protein sources: meat, fish, poultry, dairy, legumes, and nuts in that order. Chapters 10 through 12 examine edibles that are often in the news: fat, sweeteners, and grains, again in that sequence. Chapter 13 investigates the chief roots and tubers. Chapters 14 and 15 treat fruits and vegetables, respectively, and the last chapter highlights this book's findings in hopes that readers integrate them into the daily routine.

NOTES

1 Robert S. Brumbaugh, *The Philosophers of Greece* (Albany: State University of New York Press, 1981), 133.
2 Plato, *Phaedo*, in *Great Dialogues of Plato*, trans. W. H. D. Rouse (New York and Scarborough, Ontario: New American Library, 1956), 462.
3 F. M. Cornford, *Before and After Socrates* (Cambridge, UK: Cambridge University Press, 1932), 54-56, 75-77.
4 Plato, 467.
5 Ibid., 470.
6 Ibid., 468.
7 Ibid.
8 Friedrich Nietzsche, *The Birth of Tragedy*, trans. Douglas Smith (Oxford and New York: Oxford University Press, 2000), 3-4.
9 Friedrich Nietzsche, *On the Genealogy of Morals*, trans. Walter Kaufmann and R. J. Hollingdale (New York: Vintage Books, 1969), 118.

Acknowledgments

This is my second book for CRC Press, and the second time I have had the privilege of working with Senior Editor Randy Brehm. Her professionalism and responsiveness to queries eased my job. Thanks are also due to her editorial assistants Laura Piedrahita and Julia Tanner for answering many questions. At the Stark County District Library, Jacquelyn Szakacs helped me borrow books and articles from distant libraries.

The greatest thanks go to my wife Dietra, whose curiosity about nutrition and health spurred me to write this book. She read every draft, and her suggestions along the way helped me appreciate the need to detail concepts in straightforward language. She typed the tables and graphs, saving me time in the hectic months before deadline. Finally, I thank my daughters Francesca and Allie for their love. This world would be bleak without them.

Author

Christopher Cumo is a historian with interests in the natural sciences and agriculture. He seeks in some small way to illuminate how biology has shaped history. This is his ninth book and second with CRC Press. Besides writing books, he has edited a three-volume encyclopedia and contributed articles and reviews to journals, entries to encyclopedias, and articles and short fiction to magazines.

1 Introduction and Method

1.1 THE STATUS QUO

1.1.1 Problems amid Prosperity

Skillful writers and thinkers are adept at tunneling below a society's flowers to find the roots of discontent. In the *Manifesto of the Communist Party* (1848), the *Communist Manifesto* for short, German economists Karl Marx (1818–1883) and Friedrich Engels (1820–1895) dug beneath the plentitude of mass production to demonstrate that factory owners exploited workers.[1] Closer to home, African-American sociologist William Edward Burghardt (W. E. B.) Du Bois (1868–1963) punctured the façade of American complacency in 1910 by creating *The Crisis*, the flagship magazine of the National Association for the Advancement of Colored People (NAACP).[2] The name captured the reality of racism and discrimination in a nation rhetorically committed to equality and justice.

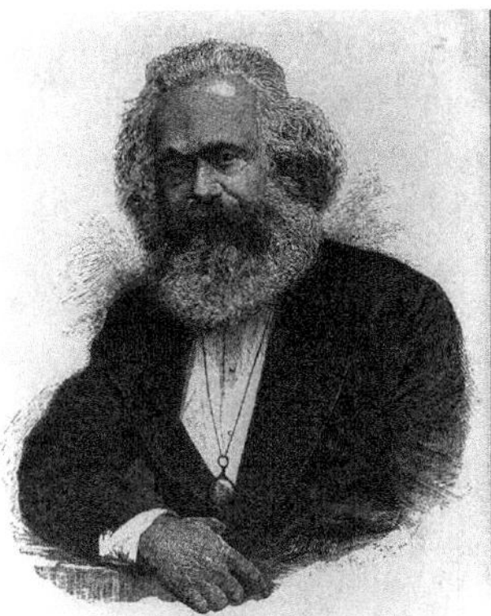

FIGURE 1.1 Karl Marx. (Photo courtesy of Library of Congress. https://www.loc.gov/pictures/item/2004672075/.)

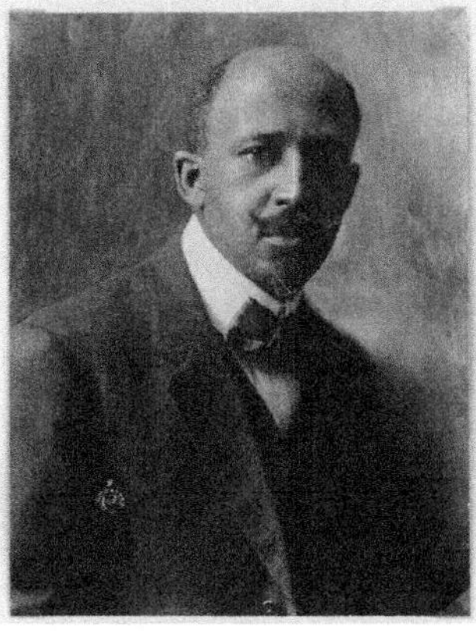

FIGURE 1.2 W. E. B. Du Bois. (Photo courtesy of Library of Congress. https://www.loc.gov/pictures/item/2003681451/.)

These problems remain while we confront new ones amid the foliage of optimism. Cause for celebration is evident in the fact that the tree of longevity appears no longer to be a shrub. If ancient and medieval peoples were lucky to reach age forty, a girl born today in Hong Kong can expect to approach ninety.[3] Yet for all this advancement, critics fear that humanity has stepped off the path toward progress. For example, American anthropologist Robert Jurmain and coauthors challenged the belief that we are living longer and better, remarking in 2014 that "our evolved biology may not be well matched with our contemporary lives, thus resulting in poorer health and shorter lives than those of even our recent ancestors."[4]

Such concern may be justified given widespread complaints about fatigue, overwork, insomnia, stress, tension, and kindred conditions. Diagnoses of heart disease, cancers, type 2 diabetes and other metabolic disorders, obesity, depression, anxiety, and related ailments mar quality of life for millions and possibly billions of sufferers worldwide. The magnitude of these problems is difficult to grasp at least partly because mental health issues are underreported given the stigma attached to them. People are fortunate to live longer than their remote ancestors, a circumstance explored in later chapters, but happiness and vitality may be as elusive as ever.

1.1.2 Belief That Diet Is at the Root of Modern Ailments

Physicians, academics, the media, and writers are sounding the alarm against these diseases and modernity's general malaise, proposing a variety of solutions. Attention has turned to diet and nutrition given the conviction that food is central to who we are and how we live. After all, Greek physician Hippocrates (c. 460–c. 375 BCE)—medicine's putative founder, though several authors wrote his texts—is thought to have equated food with health some 2,400 years ago.[5] Since then, medicine—at least its less intrusive manifestations—has developed from a belief that foods play a pivotal role in restoring and maintaining vigor, though doctors bemoan spending too much time treating symptoms rather than modifying diet and lifestyle to attack problems.[6] Summarizing the creed that foods heal, American nutritionist Thomas Colin Campbell (b. 1934) wrote in 2013 that "nutrition is the master key to human health."[7]

Discussion of health requires its definition despite American demographer S. Ryan Johansson and American anthropologists Douglas Owsley and Stephen Le's assertions that it is a vague, fluid concept.[8] In their view, societal expectations generate and modify its definitions. In contrast, this book promotes a single definition in arguing that health is more than absence of disease. It is vitality, vigor, fitness, or whatever other language conveys capacity for exertion. For example, healthy people do not take an elevator or escalator for fear that a flight of stairs will wind them. They spade rather than rototill the flower beds and garden and cut grass on foot, not seated on a riding mower. Examples need not be multiplied to demonstrate that health, far from being ideation, must measurably improve life by endowing people with capacity for work. In practice, health is more verb than noun in necessitating action.

Emphasis on diet and nutrition is even more important than the foregoing has indicated given medicine's limits. The era of "magic bullets"—the appellation applied to antibiotics—appears to have ended. Perhaps this outcome is desirable because humanity never enjoyed a time when suffering could be banished simply by consuming a pill. Such belief is wishful and counterproductive because it perpetuates the illusion that vitality is the default rather than a status that must be earned. We must acknowledge that restoration and maintenance of health require relentless commitment to hard work and a realization that simple answers and shortcuts solve nothing.

The desire for a quick fix has created a cottage industry of books and articles that purport a magic-bullets approach to diet and nutrition. Authors, posing as renegades who combat the food industry, government, and hidebound medical authorities, offer a seductive message: by supplanting dangerous foods with a list of safe options and supplements, health is once more attainable.[9] These authors claim to have discovered which foods are harmful and which are beneficial, news that they alone suppose themselves to possess. Such information must therefore come as a revelation. Apart from them, medical and health practitioners toil in ignorance, unable or unwilling to grasp the truth.

1.1.3 Hunter-Gatherers as Models of Sound Nutrition and Health

These authors and many others offer humanity's hunter-gatherer predecessors as models of sound nutrition, an approach that should be sensible given that most of our evolution unfolded during a lengthy apprenticeship as plant collectors, scavengers, hunters, and fishers. By one estimate, hunter-gatherers constituted 90 percent of everyone who ever lived.[10] "A conviction has been growing among some observers that contemporary human health could be substantially improved if we would just emulate our hunter-gatherer ancestors in dietary matters," wrote American historian Kenneth Franklin Kiple (1939–2016) in 2000.[11] Agriculture and animal husbandry, occupying only the last 10,000 years of our tenure on Earth, are novelties. Taking an evolutionary approach—Chapter 3's subject—Jurmain and colleagues remarked that "diets for many people are mismatched with the nutrients required for healthy bodies."[12]

Although this book agrees that modern diets often undermine rather than enhance vitality, concentration on the remote past suffers from inability to pinpoint a hunter-gather diet because no one group of foods can typify such vast stretches of time and place. Geography, climate, technology, and time all shaped diet such that people ate what the environment supplied in season. No less problematic is popular writers' failure to connect prehistoric diet with daily life. This obliviousness allows them to ignore unpleasant realities. For example, Paraguay's preagricultural Ache (see Chapter 4), who consumed about 2,700 calories per day, nonetheless lived by the creed that "If you are hungry, don't think about it."[13] Those who scraped by with less were even hungrier.

Moreover, Ache hunters labored seven hours per day in pursuit of game, and women shouldered the burden of collecting plants and childcare.[14] Neither sex could resort to automobiles, airplanes, vacuum cleaners, daycare centers, supermarkets, or another contrivance that saved time and effort. They did not have treats like chocolate, ice cream, twinkies, or apple (*Malus domestica*) pie. Comfort, convenience, and instant gratification define modern life to an extent that prohibits most people from appreciating hunter-gatherers' tribulations. This book stops short of advocating a return to primitivism while acknowledging, as popular literature does not, that achievement and maintenance of health require self-denial, restraint, exertion, and willingness to endure discomfort. Athlete, outdoorsman, and twenty-sixth U.S. President Theodore Roosevelt (1858–1919) encapsulated these traits by urging Americans to lead "the strenuous life."[15]

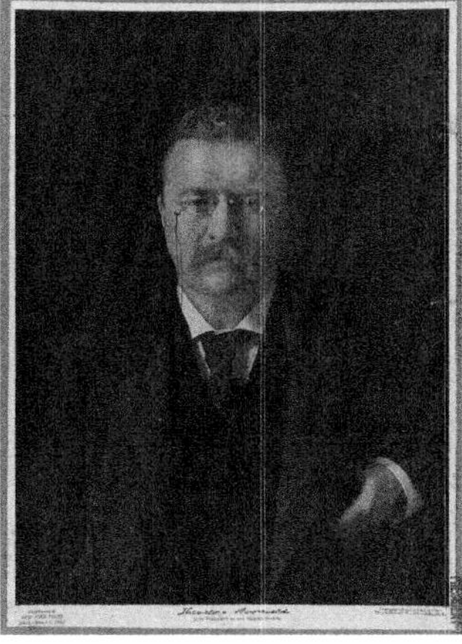

FIGURE 1.3 Theodore Roosevelt. (Photo courtesy of Library of Congress. https://www.loc.gov/pictures/item/2013645476/.)

The foregoing indicates that hunter-gatherers are imperfect models. Attempts to link them to us depend on the existence of a hunter-gather diet that may be contrasted to ours. But no single diet characterizes either the remote past or today. Then, now, and as noted above and elsewhere, humans have eaten many foods, making arbitrary the selection of a paleo diet that must be superior to ours. Even were it possible to identify an authentic prehistoric diet, its advocates would need to contrast it with what followed. This contrast is couched as preagricultural diet versus agricultural, but the boundary between the two is more difficult to fix than popular writers admit. For example, these authors—treated in Chapter 3—identify grains as unhealthy because humans ate them only upon making the terrible decision to farm.

This assertion is untrue. Chapter 12 notes that southwestern Asians harvested wild barley (*Hordeum spontaneum*) and wheat (*Triticum* species) at least 12,500 years before agriculture's invention there.[16] The gradual transition from harvesting wild plants to domesticating them typified the movement toward farming worldwide. Humans ate wild versions of beans (*Phaseolus vulgaris, P. lunatus, P. acutifolius*, and *P. coccineus*), peas (*Pisum sativum*), chickpeas (*Cicer arientinum*), lentils (*Lens culinaris*), soybeans (*Glycine max*), rice (*Oryza sativa, O. glaberrima*, and related species), millet (species in the tribe Eragrostideae), sorghum (*Sorghum* species), and many other plants before domesticating them. To cite another example, preagricultural New Guineans chewed the pith of sugarcane (*Saccharum officinarum*) stems long before the plant's domestication. In other words, no sharp distinction separates the putatively healthy diets before farming from the supposedly debilitating fare afterward.

Even were it possible to create such contrasts, hunter-gatherers cannot be models for modernity given differences in lifestyle as well as diets. Elsewhere this book emphasizes that hunter-gatherers were more active than we are. Machines like automobiles allow us to use the internal combustion engine rather than muscles to accomplish tasks like moving from one spot to another. For all of prehistory and most of history, people had to walk to get anywhere. Because we lead different lives than hunter-gatherers and because popular writers admit that diet and lifestyle are inextricably linked, the reality that we are inactive compared to hunter-gatherers implies that we should eat less, and possibly different, foods than they did. Emulation of preagricultural diets should benefit us only to the extent that we mimic hunter-gatherers. We must jettison not merely bread but automobiles and kindred gadgets if we are to regain the vitality that popular authors insist typified them but not us. Perceptive students of hunter-gatherers concede that moderns must exert themselves to recapture hunter-gatherer physicality.[17]

Despite the chasm between preagricultural peoples and us, popular writers assume that deviation from hunter-gatherer diets must be harmful. Such thinking harkens back to antiquity when change was feared as misfortune's harbinger. Aversion to innovation seems strange today given its expectation and acceptance. For example, consumers are eager to buy the newest computers, cell phones, and other technologies. To cite another example, clothing is an innovation; yet no scientist or scholar insists that it must harm us because garments cause their wearers to deviate from the natural state of nakedness. To be sure, excessive coverage of the body deprives it of sunlight necessary to synthesize vitamin D and is deleterious absent supplementation, but clothes are not innately hazardous. As a last example, we do not reject the automobile, discussed elsewhere, because it is a novelty antithetical to hunter-gatherer lifeways.

Attribution of supposed hunter-gatherer superiority to diet, lifestyle, or another environmental factor is inadequate explanation of the differences between them and us. For example, American nutritionist and exercise physiologist Loren Cordain (b. 1950) identified the muscularity and fitness evident in photographs of hunter-gatherers as evidence that their diets were better than ours.[18] But this supremacy, real or imaginary, must have a hereditary component. In 1993—the last year surveyed—the Ache, mentioned earlier, suffered 12 percent mortality from birth to age one.[19] Practicing infanticide, parents killed weak or deformed newborns.[20] The old or ailing who could not keep pace with the hunt were left to die, buried alive, or incinerated to quicken their demise. Accidents, violence, insects, arachnids, jaguars, snakes, and natural disasters killed unfortunates. Such dynamics presumably operate less in the modern world. These differences suggest that the Ache and nature culled weaklings whereas modern societies preserve them. Such selection pressures may produce sturdiness absent in modern populations.

Perhaps the worst flaw in popular accounts of hunter-gatherer diets is failure to link them with definite health outcomes. The attempt to eat like preagricultural peoples may enhance vitality, but espousal of such diets should acknowledge, as implied above, that diseases, parasites, rodents, insects, predators, and early deaths marred the remote past. Without this understanding, diet and nutrition books enter a fantasy world of speculation and generalities. The rest of this book situates the context of daily life as indispensable to an examination of diet, nutrition, and health.

1.1.4 The Search for Enlightened Dietary and Nutritional Advice

At another conceptual level, modern dietary advice depends on the premise that an elite few can attain enlightenment while the rest of us grope in the dark. The contrast between light and darkness harkens back to Greek philosopher Plato (c. 427–c. 347 BCE). The preface criticized his devaluation of the body. In the *Republic* (c. 380 BCE), he described humanity as imprisoned in a dim cave.[21] One man freed himself, struggled up and out of the cave, and saw the sun's light. Now possessing truth, he returned to the others in hopes of convincing them.

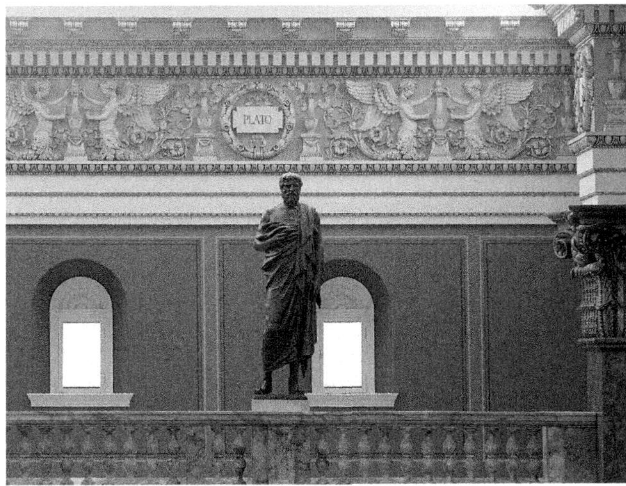

FIGURE 1.4 Plato. (Photo courtesy of Library of Congress. https://www.loc.gov/pictures/item/2007684417/.)

The problem with the current state of diet and nutrition, however, is that too many people profess enlightenment, as endless claims and counterclaims enshroud each other in shadow. The advocates of meat consumption clash with those who favor a plant-based diet. Fat was once bad, but today its cheerleaders elevate it above carbohydrates. A generation ago carbohydrates were integral to a sensible diet. Today they are suspect; sucrose—$C_{12}H_{22}O_{11}$, commonly known as sugar—and high fructose corn syrup (HFCS), both carbohydrates defined in Chapter 2 and discussed in Chapter 11, are demonized as among the worst edibles a person can ingest. Nutritionists often tout the benefits of vitamins and minerals, though the recommended dietary allowances (RDA) are in dispute and have changed over time.[22] For example, attention has focused on the benefits of vitamin D, raising its public profile; yet controversy rages over whether absorption is best and safest from food, supplements, or sunshine.

1.1.5 Dietary Types

The result is an avalanche of opinions. "Plant-based diets are all the buzz in the nutrition world," wrote American dietician Stephanie Green in 2016.[23] The observation that those who favor plants tend to be healthier than meat eaters stimulated this interest.[24] This camp is vegetarianism, an ancient approach to food. Tradition counts Greek mathematician and philosopher Pythagoras (c. 570–c. 495 BCE) and Greek philosopher Empedocles (c. 495–c. 435 BCE) among its practitioners.[25]

Vegetarianism need not be a choice. Throughout history, economic inequalities reserved animal products for elites. Commoners, unable to afford meat, subsisted on plants. American historian of medicine James Clifton Whorton (b. 1942) remarked that "Human populations often have been obliged to subsist on an all-vegetable diet because of a poverty or scarcity of animal foods."[26] As late as the last century, Spain's rural poor ate no meat.[27] Focusing on antiquity, British classicist Peter David Arthur Garnsey (b. 1938) noted animal products' dearth in the Mediterranean basin.[28] Chapter 4 demonstrates that ancient Egypt's masses seldom ate meat. Even though they lived near the Nile River, little evidence supports the notion that they ate fish. Chapter 4 indicates, however, that elites were another matter.

As an alternative to meat-based diets, vegetarianism varies in stringency. Ovo-lacto vegetarians, the largest subset, eat dairy and eggs.[29] Lacto adherents consume dairy but not eggs whereas ovo devotees are the reverse. Those who eschew all animal products are vegans. Even honey is suspect because honeybees (*Apis mellifera*) make it.

As noted, some who claim to be vegetarians nonetheless consume butter, eggs, cheese, or some combination of them. Their allegiance to plant foods may be questioned. A step removed from this group are pescatarians, who eat seafood—Chapter 5's topic—but no other flesh. Fish's uniqueness may derive from religion. Catholic and Orthodox faiths have long permitted it but not meat on Fridays during Lent, the forty weekdays between Ash Wednesday and Easter. The distinction between these foods appears to originate in the gospels, which transformed fish into a symbol for Jesus. The four canonical accounts state that he fed thousands by multiplying two fish and some bread.[30] The gospel of Luke indicates that the apostles Simon (Peter), James, and John joined him after he directed the netting of so many fish that their boat was in danger of sinking, an episode termed the "miraculous catch."[31] The last canonical gospel, John might have consulted its predecessors to learn these stories. John retells the miraculous catch, placing it after Jesus' resurrection.[32] A second post-resurrection story has Jesus prove his body's corporeality by eating fish.[33] Doubtless, fish's adequacy for Jesus and the apostles recommended it for all Christians. Whatever fish's merits, pescatarianism deviates from veganism and related forms of vegetarianism.

Variants of plant diets include those that tout fruits, Chapter 14's subject. Known as fruitarianism or frugivory, this approach need not restrict consumption to dessert fruits because the botanical definition of a fruit encompasses all structures, developing from the ovary after pollination, that hold seeds. Anyone who has grown tomatoes (*Solanum esculentum*) in the garden has witnessed fruit production. Maturing from a flower's ovary, tomatoes are fruits rather than vegetables despite an 1893 U.S. Supreme Court decision, discussed in Chapter 14, to the contrary.[34] Other foods usually deemed vegetables qualify for inclusion within fruitarianism. Although the garden pea (*Pisum sativum*)—a subject of Chapter 8—is a seed, it develops in pods. Because they bear seeds and develop from the flower, the pods are fruits. This logic applies to other seed legumes, though consumption of pods and seeds rather than just seeds is necessary to satisfy the definition of fruit. Some nuts (see Chapter 9), peppers (*Capsicum* species), eggplants (*Solanum melongena*), pumpkins (*Cucurbita pepo*) and other squashes (*Cucurbita* species), olives (*Olea europaea*), and cucumbers (*Cucumis sativus*) are also fruits and so permissible for consumption among fruitarians.

Some who promote fruits perceive them as low calorie, an imprecise designation given absence of consensus about what constitutes low, medium, or high. Nonetheless, Table 1.1 shows that apples, strawberries (*Fragaria x ananassa*), grapefruit (*Citrus paradisi*), oranges (*Citrus sinensis* and *C. aurantium*), blueberries (*Vaccinium angustifolium, Vaccinium corymbosum*, and related species), cranberries (*Vaccinium oxycoccos* and related species), raspberries (*Rubus idaeus*), papaya (*Carica papaya*), watermelon (*Citrullus lanatus*), peaches (*Prunus persica*), nectarines (*Prunus persica var. nucipersica*), tomatoes, eggplants, and cantaloupes (*Cucumis melo*) may qualify, all under 65 calories per 100 grams (3.5 ounces) fresh.[35] Chapter 2 extends treatment of the calorie to

TABLE 1.1
Calories in Low Calorie Fruits 100 g

Fruit	Calories
Tomatoes	18
Grapefruits	19
Eggplants	26
Watermelons	29
Oranges	32
Cantaloupes	35
Peaches	25
Strawberries	35
Nectarines	42
Papaya	42
Apples	50
Raspberries	53
Blueberries	60

additional foods. Others deem fruits capable of removing toxins that the body accumulates from pollution, pesticides, and foods full of preservatives.[36] Cleansing may include consumption of fruit or vegetable juices. This practice may accomplish little given that the liver and kidneys continually remove wastes.

Other options promote plant foods and permit animal products. The dietary approaches to stop hypertension (DASH) emphasizes fruits, vegetables, whole grains, unsaturated fats, nuts, and seeds.[37] Protein should come from low-fat dairy and lean meats, fish, and poultry. Adherents should eliminate meat from two meals and eat under five egg yolks per week. The American Heart Association's therapeutic lifestyle changes (TLC) diet is similar in omitting high-fat foods.[38] Another alternative, the Ornish diet limits fat—Chapter 10's subject—to 10 percent of calories to counteract heart disease.[39] It recommends whole grains, vegetables, and fruits and restricts animal products to nonfat dairy and egg whites. Campbell affirmed the 10 percent ceiling on fats and advocated consumption of vegetables, fruits, nuts, beans and other seed legumes, and whole grains.[40] Wary of animal products, he faulted the appetite for meat with overpopulating Earth with cattle (*Bos taurus*), whose flatulence exacerbates global warming and climate change.[41]

Chapter 10 indicates that aversion to fat is not universal. The Atkins and keto diets cause the body to metabolize fats, a process known as ketosis, by restricting carbohydrates. Ketosis produces ketones, which have the formula $(CH_2)_{\#}O$, where # is a positive integer. Although ketones harm the body in excess, such diets remain trendy. "I'm going to rescue you from a lifetime of trying to avoid eating fat and cholesterol and prove how these delicious ingredients preserve the highest functioning of your brain," wrote American neurologist David Perlmutter (b. 1954) in 2018.[42] He asserted without evidence that evolution shaped humans to derive 75 percent of calories from fat—a claim scrutinized in Chapter 10—and that cravings for it prove its worth.[43] Readers might test this logic by noting that cravings for nicotine do not demonstrate that tobacco benefits smokers. Chapter 10 examines claims for and against fatty foods.

Perlmutter decried grains, a stance evident in *Wheat Belly* (2011), in which American cardiologist William R. Davis (b. 1957) faulted modern bread wheat (*Triticum aestivum*) for causing overeating and obesity.[44] Chapter 12 examines these criticisms. American cardiac surgeon Steven Gundry expanded this assault in 2017 to include most plants. He asserted that evolution armed them with lectin proteins to deter animals, including humans, from eating them.[45] Evolution, therefore, designed plants to make people ill and overweight. Several chapters critique Gundry's claims.

These putative dangers leave animal products as the alternative. Despite its name, the grapefruit diet has little interest in fruits, instead advocating consumption of eggs, bacon and other meats, and salads drenched in oils. The accent is on protein and fat. Wary of too much fat, the paleo diet champions protein in the form of lean meats including game, fish, eggs, nuts, and seeds. Chapter 9 demonstrates that most nuts contain abundant fat. Chapters 3 and 10 question the extent to which such a diet fed preagricultural peoples and, if so, whether it can be duplicated today. Lean sources of protein characterize the South Beach diet, named after an upscale part of Miami, Florida. Carbohydrates may come from vegetables and fruits.

Endorsement of animal products also comes by the circuitous route of attacking gluten, a group of over one hundred proteins in wheat (*Triticum monococcum*, *T. dicoccon*, *T. aestivum*, and *T. durum*), rye (*Secale cereale*), barley (*Hordeum vulgare*), and triticale (*Triticale hexaploide*).[46] Although oats (*Avena sativa*) lack gluten, they may acquire it if processed at a facility that handles other grains. For this reason, those who eschew gluten must avoid most breads, pastas, and other grain products. Lacking gluten, animal products are safe options. The Celiac Disease Foundation in Woodland Hills, California, includes meat, poultry, or seafood daily in a week's sample menu.[47]

Meat unites the Atkins, keto, grapefruit, paleo, and South Beach formulations and is permissible outside vegan, vegetarian, fruitarian, and pescatarian strongholds. Chapter 4 examines meat's effects on health through time and space. This chapter notes that it is more than food. Like fish in religious contexts, meat functions as a symbol in anthropological circles. Since the 1920s, anthropologists have sought humanity's origins in the pursuit and consumption of meat.[48] It is thought to have inspired hunting and, with it, communal organization and hierarchy. Meat's partisans believe that it fixed gender roles, giving men status and establishing women as helpmates. The quest for big game supposedly permeated men's genome, galvanizing them millennia later to undertake the safari. Meat is hypothesized to have provided the nutrients and calories that enlarged the brain during the last 2 million years. Summarizing its importance, American anthropologist Henry Bunn wrote in 2007 that "meat made us human."[49]

1.1.6 Absence of Consensus

The existence of and contradictions implicit in so many diets create bewilderment. Dutch physiologist Fred Brouns, nutritionist Vincent van Buul, and British botanist Peter Shewry expressed frustration with the transitory fads that buffet people eager to regain a trim figure and vitality. Responding to Davis' *Wheat Belly* in 2013, they wrote that after "discussions on the roles of fat, fructose, high fructose corn syrup and added sugar in foods, it seems that it is now the turn of wheat to take the blame for obesity."[50]

Other authors appear to revel in uncertainty, aware that baffled readers may be ready to believe nearly anything. "Suppose…I told you that everything you thought you knew about your diet, your health, and your weight is wrong," wrote Gundry as prelude to his claims of nutritional expertise.[51] The current tumult forces those interested in diet and nutrition to penetrate a forest in search of a path beneath a profusion of vegetation, all the while wondering whether the trail exists.

This thicket of contradictions, conflicts, and ignorance ensnares us in ambiguities that invite comparison with prescientific periods of inquiry. In *The Structure of Scientific Revolutions* (1962), American physicist and philosopher of science Thomas Samuel Kuhn (1922–1996) articulated the absence of consensus during such times.[52] Without a model of how some aspect of the universe works, prescientific eras produce division. Bereft of a uniform vision of reality, intellectuals cannot agree on the issues that merit study or the questions that must be answered. The investigation of diet and nutrition may not suffer all these ills, though the status quo exhibits the fuzziness of a prescientific age in inability to supply definitive guidelines about what to eat.

But despair may be premature. Sometimes a problem thought intractable resists solution because of a conceptual roadblock. So long as people adhere to wrong ideas, progress is impossible. Consider pellagra, a serious disease into the twentieth century. The fact that it caused dermatitis (rash) and skin sores initially prompted belief that pellagra—Italian for "rough skin"—was a skin ailment.[53] Thinking in these terms, physicians were unable to cure the disease. Rather, treatments often worsened symptoms.[54] The discovery of the first vitamins in the early twentieth century, however, created a new conceptual framework for reexamining pellagra. A focus on diet led to corn (*Zea mays*) as the culprit. The body cannot absorb vitamin B_3 (niacin or nicotinic acid), the amino acid tryptophan, iron, and several other nutrients from corn that has not been soaked in an alkaline solution, notes Chapter 12. Malabsorption, especially of B_3, causes pellagra. In other words, only when medicine reconceptualized pellagra as a nutritional deficiency rather than a type of dermatitis could it be cured.

The contradictions that riddle today's study of nutrition are more fundamental because they stem from both conceptual shortsightedness and inability to approach diet with the method likely to yield the most relevant evidence. Pride makes us susceptible to narcissism. We are a species that celebrates brainpower, using cognition to separate us from all other life. Both Greek philosopher Aristotle (384–322 BCE) and Swedish naturalist Carl von Linne (1707–1778)—known in Latin as Carolus Linnaeus—made rationality our defining feature.[55]

Such smugness exposes us to errors, perhaps the most seductive being reification: the tendency to act as though ideas express concrete aspects of reality. In other words, to reify means to make an idea into a noun and to believe that that noun exists. For example, long ago people bundled notions of various types of perfection into the being commonly known as God and worshipped it. Such reification may be appropriate. On the other hand, I can visualize a $20 bill in my mind, noting every detail with camera-like fidelity. But if I have no money, this imaginary greenback will not buy lunch for me or anyone else.

The problem with reification is our insistence that the nouns we invent are almost always more than mental exercises. Nouns like medicine, biology, geology, economics, sociology, psychology, and many more have come to stand for real fields of knowledge complete with boundaries between them. Safe within their disciplinary citadels, historians seldom consult biologists, who avoid sociologists as though knowledge comes only in discrete packets. Such partitioning may be necessary to enable everyone from student to researcher to focus on a single topic rather than dabble in too many areas. But balkanization of knowledge is unreal and perilous when it binds knowledge in straightjackets. Such compartmentalization did not exist for Plato, for example, who never tried to confine knowledge within narrow limits.

Many scholars understand this danger and work to weaken or eliminate barriers by cooperating with one another to build bridges between disciplines. Such interdisciplinary approaches can yield powerful insights. For example, anthropologists and historians are using the science of climate change to generate fresh insights into the rise and fall of civilizations and empires. Work along these lines strengthens ties among the humanities, social sciences, and natural sciences, benefitting everyone who is curious about the momentous developments that have shaped our world.

The conceptual problem with diet and nutrition, then, stems from reluctance to abandon artificial categories and boundaries and instead embrace an interdisciplinary mindset. This is not to say that diet and nutrition are never contemplated from multiple perspectives; but even so, much research concentrates on their clinical aspects. For example, the clinician can tell us that a gram of sucrose or another sugar has 3.6 calories.[56] For the sake of completeness, the dietician's calorie—sometimes rendered Calorie—is really the kilocalorie of physics. A kilocalorie, hereinafter simply calorie, has the energy to raise the temperature of 1 kilogram of water 1 degree Celsius. This information is useful because it is precise. The claim that pizza has lots of calories, for example, tells us much less than the statement that a slice—100 grams for the sake of illustration—of cheese pizza has 300 calories. Such information becomes meaningful when quantification is expanded throughout the exigencies of daily existence. For example, someone who requires 2,000 calories to maintain body mass understands that 300 calories furnish almost one-seventh the total.

Meaningful as these numbers are, they fall short of satisfying health-conscious consumers' desire to know what to eat and how much and what to avoid. It is natural, for example, to ponder what 300 calories of pizza supply beyond energy. The next chapter enlarges this discourse to include carbohydrates, fats, proteins, minerals, vitamins, phytochemicals, and water. These components are essential to understanding the nutritional differences among foods, but they cannot prescribe what to eat and what to eschew in an absolute sense because diet and lifestyle are intertwined. That is, generalizations, when pushed too far, gloss over the fact that lifestyle, and the diet necessary to fuel it, can vary markedly among people. Researchers are right to use clinical trials in their search for answers, though such investigations are not always able to tease apart contributions of diet and lifestyle to health. More can be done upon removal of the conceptual barrier that confines diet and nutrition largely to the laboratory.

1.2 AN ALTERNATIVE TO THE STATUS QUO: A PREHISTORICAL AND HISTORICAL APPROACH TO DIET AND NUTRITION

Preoccupation with lab and clinic hinders us from seeing diet and nutrition from the best vantage point. Anyone who wants to survey the landscape will ascend the highest spot from which to see the largest expanse of territory. Applying this metaphor to our predicament, diet and nutrition may be evaluated from a perspective that allows their tracking over not just one set of clinical trials from a single generation of participants but rather over the vast expanse of humanity's tenure on Earth. To put the matter plainly, what is needed is an examination of diet and nutrition from a historical perspective.

Returning to this introduction's beginning, Marx, Engels, and Du Bois were penetrating writers and thinkers partly because they knew how to frame their arguments in historical terms. In the *Communist Manifesto*, for example, Marx and Engels introduced the notion of class conflict not as an abstraction but as a historical reality that pitted "Freeman and slave, patrician and plebian, lord and serf, guild-master and journeyman, in a word; oppressor and oppressed."[57]

Narrated in this way, history has power that can be harnessed to investigate problems, in our case the relationship among diet, nutrition, and health. Part of this power derives from history's ability to illuminate how economic and social inequalities made food a weapon against the poor, whose diets paled beside the wealthy's extravagances. Since antiquity, sumptuous feasts have reinforced the divide between elites and commoners. Not only are the masses unwelcome at these gatherings, but they cannot afford to put even a fraction of the smorgasbord on their table. Hunger and privation concretize their inferiority. In this context, food magnifies a society's hierarchy. In the Pacific Northwest, for example, shortages prompted Chinook elites to confiscate the poor's food.[58] When disease destroyed Ireland's potato crop in the 1840s, the masses starved while well-fed officials debated, delayed, and never moved much beyond laissez-faire inaction.[59]

Attention to inequalities emphasizes that a prehistorical and historical approach to diet illuminates ordinary people's lives. Such a perspective makes the study of history more useful than myopic fascination with the wealthy, who have always been a privileged minority that illustrate little about societies beyond greed, materialism, selfishness, ostentation, and arrogance. Frustrated with insularity, French entomologist and naturalist Jean Henri Casimir Fabre (1823–1915) lamented that history "knows the names of the kings' bastards but cannot tell us the origin of wheat."[60] Aligning with Fabre's sentiment, this book seeks to gauge the health of those who ate bread, porridge, and similar victuals. Caviar consumers must find affirmation elsewhere.

Historical investigation of diet and nutrition, or any phenomenon, teaches the necessity of attending to people and events. Because these specifics are unique in time and place, details matter, a circumstance that discomforts even historians. Studying for a doctorate in history, attorney, scholar, university president, and twenty-eighth U.S. President Thomas Woodrow Wilson (1856–1924) complained about memorizing "one or two thousand minute particulars of the quarrels of nobody knows who with an obscure governor for nobody knows what. Just think of all that energy wasted!"[61] To be sure, trivia is worthless, but facts are essential in constructing and evaluating hypotheses about prehistory and history.

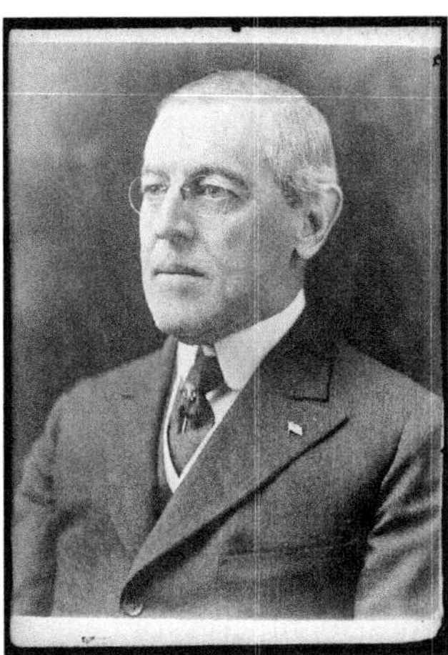

FIGURE 1.5 Woodrow Wilson. (Photo courtesy of Library of Congress. https://www.loc.gov/pictures/item/2017668637/.)

History's attention on specifics is valuable as a check against imprudent generalizations. Humans' penchant for generalization expresses the search for absolutes. The natural sciences model this approach by seeking laws that apply under all circumstances, thereby ordering the universe. For example, the force of gravity is a universal that operates throughout the cosmos. All matter is subject to it. In 1915, German physicist Albert Einstein (1879–1955) determined in his general theory of relativity that even light experiences gravity—really the curvature of space—when it nears an enormous mass.[62] Readers should note that scientists are usually skeptical about a new law, demanding repeated verification before accepting it. In this instance, an eclipse in 1919 allowed physicists to confirm general relativity, elevating Einstein to international prominence. Even then, he did not receive the Nobel Prize in physics until 1922, an award that omitted general relativity.[63] The theory was still too novel to persuade the entire physics community.

Skepticism requires willingness to question ideas and demand evidence before accepting generalities. These qualities are in shortage given humans' tendency to construct and believe absolutes that hold for all times and places. Such simplifications are seductive because they make the world seem predictable. The danger of this approach stems partly from reality's tendency to be messy and sometimes counterintuitive. For example, Earth orbits the sun even though our senses tell us otherwise. Another peril lies in the fact that absolutes are easy to craft and seem so natural that they are difficult to detect. Dietary and nutritional advice contains such formulations, most of which pass unnoticed and are accepted as true. For example, a nutritional tenet holds that some fats are "healthy." In *Grain Brain* (2018), Perlmutter called attention to them by bolding their letters and urging that they be "consumed liberally".[64]

The problem with this language is obvious by analogy. Let us substitute antibiotics for fats under the supposition that Augmentin, or any other brand, is a healthful antibiotic. The term "healthful" is meant to convey belief that Augmentin benefits those who ingest it. If Augmentin is a boon in an absolute sense, then everyone should profit from consuming it. Yet such action may be unwise. Anyone allergic to Augmentin should not take it. Moreover, it confers no benefit to someone suffering from anything other than a bacterial infection. It is useless, therefore, against influenza, yellow fever, rubella, rabies, hepatitis, the common cold, or another viral infection. That is, circumstances condition use of Augmentin or another antibiotic.

This stipulation applies to fat, which is not universally healthful but instead depends on particulars. Returning to the example of Augmentin, someone allergic to it would suffer from its ingestion. A parallel is bile acid malabsorption (BAM) or fat intolerance, which is less our focus than the imperatives of daily existence. Worldwide, many people live amid plentiful food. Abundance reduces but does not eradicate hunger and starvation. That said, the real dangers are overconsumption, overweight, obesity, and related maladies. This predicament prompts concern over fat, healthy or otherwise. Being the most caloric edible, fat exacerbates rather than ameliorates overconsumption and its perils, just as overuse of antibiotics increases rather than reduces the hazards of bacterial infections over the long term. On the other hand, where food is scarce, fat supplies badly needed energy. As in the case of antibiotics, therefore, circumstances dictate the healthfulness or unhealthiness of fat or any other commodity. Treating foods throughout time and place, this book underscores the conviction that their worth is contingent on context. Throughout this discussion, readers should not conflate fat with fatty acids. Chapter 2 defines fatty acids, noting that the body must consume omega 3 and omega 6 fatty acids because it cannot manufacture them, a fact that makes them essential.

Concerns about overweight and obesity, evident throughout this book, require definitions for context. Health practitioners define obesity in terms of body mass index (BMI): a person's mass (kilograms) divided by height (meters) squared (kg/m^2). Numbers at or above thirty for an adult signify obesity.[65] The World Health Organization (WHO) defines childhood obesity as a statistical measure calculated in standard deviations above the median. Standard deviation quantifies a number's degree of departure from the norm. In this case, the WHO equates norm with median because what is the midpoint may be thought average or typical. The WHO considers children under age five obese whose BMI is at least three standard deviations above the median. Children between ages five and nineteen are obese if their BMI is two standard deviations over the median. BMI between the norm and obesity is defined as overweight. Because the abdomen accumulates fat, Harvard University's School of Public Health defined women with waist circumferences over 89 centimeters (35 inches) and men with circumferences above 101.6 centimeters (40 inches) as obese.[66] A third definition specified overweight as 10 to 19 percent—and obesity as at least 20 percent—over the norm.[67]

Returning to history's uses and keeping in mind its value in guarding against gratuitous generalities, foods may be traced throughout the past to determine vitality at various times and places. In the vernacular, the word "history" means any period before the present. Scholars, however, restrict the term to roughly the last 5,000 years because they rely on written documents to understand the past and writing was invented around 3300 BCE.[68] Earlier times are prehistory.

1.2.1 Types and Interpretation of Evidence

Any attempt to evaluate diet must investigate both prehistory and history if it is to be relevant. Yet no account of diet can be comprehensive because of gaps in our knowledge. Where evidence is scant or absent, diet cannot be reconstructed. But the situation is not hopeless. Although no one can hope to know what everyone who ever lived ate, this limitation does not justify despair. At a minimum, diet may be inferred from three sources, preferably in combination so that one line of evidence can reinforce the others: skeletons and their teeth, middens (trash heaps), and coprolites (fossilized feces).

Skeletons and teeth, particularly when abundant and from numerous age ranges, reveal much about growth, height, and nutritional deficiencies. When pathogens and parasites can be ruled out, subnormal growth usually signals inadequate nutrition. Stunting is most apparent in childhood when growth is normally rapid, making juvenile skeletons invaluable markers of undernutrition, which this book defines as insufficient calories, nutrients, or both. In premodern societies, children were most vulnerable to undernourishment at weaning, when they transitioned from mother's milk to solids of lesser quality. Later chapters indicate that children who died between ages two and five tended to manifest undernutrition severe enough to have killed them. In other cases, they succumbed to contagion or parasitism.

When nutrients are adequate in adulthood, the body may grow to average heights, compensating for childhood deficiencies. Undernutrition evokes images of emaciation. Genesis recounted a dream of "gaunt cows" and "ears of grain, thin and blasted by the east wind."[69] Orthodox Christian icons depict slender ascetics on the path toward sainthood. Insufficient calories, protein, vitamins, and minerals arrest growth. Too few nutrients thin enamel, a condition known as hypoplasia and evident in skeletons with intact teeth. As noted above, the body may compensate for childhood deficiencies if nourishment is adequate in adulthood. Bones, though not teeth, regain density, forming marks known as Harris lines after British anatomist Henry Albert Harris (1886–1968). These lines, apparent in X-rays of skeletons, memorialize the position of growth plates when nutrition was inadequate, infection or parasitism severe, or their combination stopped growth. Adult skeletons with small head circumferences may reveal food scarcity in childhood. Head and brain normally grow rapidly early in life, but insufficient nourishment arrests growth, preserving dearth into adulthood. Small vertebral width also indicates undernourishment during infancy and childhood.

Skeletons may betray nutritional deficiencies in other ways. Curvature (bowing) of leg bones signals rickets, a condition that Chapter 2 examines. Such deformation reveals paucity of vitamin D, calcium, phosphorus, or their combination. Inadequate calcium or phosphorus implicates diet, but not enough vitamin D indicates sunlight deprivation more than dietary deficiency because the sun's ultraviolet radiation is the chief source of the vitamin. Chapter 2 notes that instances of rickets increased during the industrial revolution, when people moved from countryside to city and from work outdoors to factories. The fact that urbanites were often indoors led researchers to posit that vitamin D deficiency weakened Austrian composers Wolfgang Amadeus Mozart (1756–1791) and Gustav Mahler's (1860–1911) immune system such that they could not fight the infections that killed them.[70]

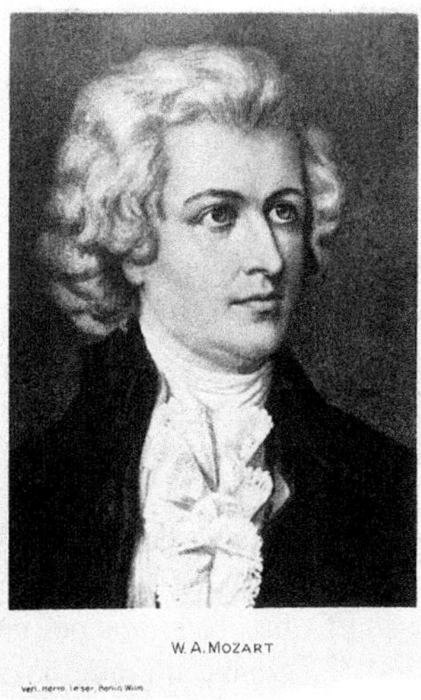

FIGURE 1.6 Wolfgang Amadeus Mozart. (Photo courtesy of Library of Congress. https://www.loc.gov/pictures/item/2016816928/.)

Refocusing on diet, the skull yields evidence of anemia when parietal bones or the roof of eye orbits appears porous or spongy. The first is known as porotic hyperostosis and the second as cribra orbitalia. Absent pathogens or parasites, undernutrition causes these problems. When diet is to blame, porotic hyperostosis or cribra orbitalia may result from iron deficiency, deprivation of vitamin B_9 (folate, folic acid, or pteroylmonoglutamic acid), B_{12} (cobalamin), C, or D, or inadequate iron and B_9 or B_{12}.[71] When iron and B vitamin are involved, neither shortage need be marked to produce the pathologies.

Adequate iron and vitamins may not prevent anemia when foods inhibit absorption. Plants have what is known as non-heme iron, which the body absorbs less than heme iron. Animal products have heme iron, named because it is in hemoglobin and other blood proteins. Moreover, vitamin C paucity, fiber including bran, coffee (*Coffea* species), tea (*Camellia sinensis*), soybean protein, peanuts (*Arachis hypogaea*), and some nuts may cause anemia by hindering iron absorption. Entanglement among diet, pathogens, and parasites is difficult to unravel because many parasites and pathogens deplete iron. The problem of assigning blame is marked at the transition from hunting and gathering to farming and livestock raising when people abandoned nomadism. Dense settlements enabled pathogens, insects, and parasites to multiply. Under these conditions, humans may have evolved anemia as protection against invaders.[72] By rendering iron inaccessible—for example, by storing it in the spleen, liver, and bone marrow—and inducing anemia in the process, the body starved pathogens and parasites that needed the mineral to survive and reproduce.[73] Agricultural societies may therefore exhibit anemia when diet supplies enough iron and vitamins.

Stunting may reveal dearth of calories, protein, vitamin A, or zinc.[74] Chapter 2 details the chemistry and functions of these and other nutrients. Dietary deficiencies characterized the masses, who went hungry more than elites. Obviously, when parasites and diseases cannot be eliminated from consideration, the prudent course is not to speculate about nutrition.

In addition to skeletons and teeth and as in our own times, trash contains bones and other indicators of diet. Feces, what the body did not absorb during digestion, may contain seeds and other items. Beyond these sources, graves indicate diet whenever people buried food with the deceased, but only when these perishables resist decay. As a rule, communities added food and other items to graves whose deceased enjoyed wealth and prestige in life. Conversely, absence identifies commoners. By their nature, therefore, grave goods furnish information about elites, not the masses who populate society and toil to create the luxuries that pamper the fortunate few.

Chemistry reveals additional insights into diet. Information comes from photosynthesis because plants use carbon dioxide (CO_2) differently depending on their origins in temperate regions or the tropics. Temperate plants—for example, potatoes (*Solanum tuberosum*), wheat, rye, barley, oats, lentils, chickpeas, soybeans, and peas—transform the carbon dioxide they absorb into phosphoglyceric acid ($C_3H_7O_7P$), a compound with three carbons, by a pathway known as C_3. All fruit trees and some plants that arose in the tropics—for example, sweet potatoes (*Ipomoea batatas*), tomatoes, and *Phaseolus* beans—are also C_3. In contrast, other tropical plants—for example, sugarcane, corn, millet, and sorghum—use carbon dioxide to make oxaloacetic acid ($C_4H_4O_5$), a four-carbon molecule, by the C_4 pathway. Corn's tropical origins may surprise readers who know it is grown in Canada, but this hardiness resulted from selection by American Indians, who expanded the grass' geography over innumerable generations. C_3 plants represent roughly 85 percent of florae.[75]

C_3 and C_4 pathways use different carbon isotopes. Isotopes of an element have identical chemical properties because the number of protons is constant but different masses because the numbers of neutrons differ. Most carbon, known as ^{12}C, has 12 grams per mole, with a mole being a standard, huge number of atoms (6×10^{23}). These 12 grams, the atomic mass, are the sum of carbon's six protons and six neutrons in its nucleus. Carbon (^{13}C) with seven neutrons has an atomic mass of thirteen, and carbon (^{14}C) with eight neutrons has a mass of fourteen. Of these isotopes, ^{12}C and ^{13}C are stable and far more abundant in nature than ^{14}C. Being unstable ^{14}C decays into nitrogen. Being more numerous, ^{12}C and ^{13}C are available to form molecules, including the carbon dioxide that plants absorb, with other elements. Because C_3 plants absorb more ^{12}C than do C_4 plants, whatever eats more C_3 than C_4 plants fixes more ^{12}C in bones and teeth. Consequently, people who ingest more C_3 than C_4 plants or more animals with this pattern of consumption yield skeletons and teeth with greater ratios of ^{12}C to ^{13}C. Such information, for example, distinguishes barley from millet eaters.

Chemistry has the potential to yield surprises about the past. For example, Chapter 4 notes that in 2014 French Egyptologists and archeologists, using ^{12}C to ^{13}C ratios in bones, teeth, and hair from forty-five mummies, determined that these people, when alive, ate C_3 plants such as barley, wheat, and peas.[76] C_4 plants such as sorghum and millet comprised under 10 percent of their diets.

Their hair had few animal proteins, indicating a largely vegetarian diet. This finding appears to contradict ancient Egyptian literature and art, which document fish's dietary importance. Moreover, Egyptian and Greek literature, notably Greek historian Herodotus' (c. 485–c. 420 BCE) *Histories* (c. 425 BCE), indicates that the wealthy beef, veal, pork, mutton, lamb, chevon, capretto (kid), rabbit (*Oryctologus cuniculus*), gazelle (*Gazella* species), oryx (*Oryx* species), goose (species in the genera *Anser* and *Branta*), duck (species in Anatidae family), quail (*Coturnix coturnix*), pigeon (*Columba livia domestica*), heron (species in subfamily Botaurinae), and pelican (*Pelecanus occidentalis*).[77] These are the people who could afford mummification; yet the forty-five mummies in this study evince vegetarianism rather than carnivory or omnivory. (Herbivores and carnivores are specialists because they feed at a single tropic level whereas humans are omnivores because they feed at two levels by eating plants and animals.) Even more striking were discoveries of numerous pig (*Sus scrofa domesticus*) bones with cut marks that betray butchery and pork consumption. All these data highlight difficulties in investigating the remote past. Not only is evidence elusive, but it sometimes yields paradoxes.

Minerals in bones and teeth supply additional information about diets. Animals, including people, that eat plants ingest more calcium than barium or strontium than do meat eaters. Accordingly, a large ratio of calcium to barium or calcium to strontium in bones and teeth identifies an herbivore or, if not exclusively an herbivore, an animal that favored plants over insects and meat. By contrast, this ratio is smallest in bones and teeth of carnivores and smaller in omnivores that ate more meat and insects than plants.

Such uses of evidence support the view that skeletons, teeth, middens, coprolites, and other measurables supply the raw materials for assessing health. Factors germane to an assessment of health include height, diseases, and longevity. Previous paragraphs acknowledged that interpretation of such data is less straightforward than might be supposed. Chapter 3 notes that agriculture's critics blame it for shortening farmers, stockmen, and the urbanites who consumed their surpluses. Detractors believe that domesticated plants and animals provided less nourishment than their wild counterparts, diminishing heights. There is, however, another explanation. Height reductions are part of a trend toward smallness that began before people farmed.[78] This trend may have resulted from decreases in life's arduousness. Existence may have required less brawn as our ancestors began to use their intellect to secure life's necessities. Given competing interpretations, height may not provide unambiguous information about health when lifestyles and environments differ markedly.

Emphasizing the environment, Bergmann's rule, named after German biologist Carl Georg Lucas Christian Bergmann (1814–1865), states that among individuals within a species, size tends to increase with latitude.[79] This phenomenon is a function of heat radiation. Small individuals have a high ratio of surface area to volume. Another way to achieve this ratio is for the body to be lanky, with long, slender arms and legs. Lots of surface provides ample space for release of heat into the surrounding air. Heat dissipation aids individuals in hot climates near the equator. The reverse is true of large, stocky individuals, whose small surface area relative to volume allows them to retain heat, a benefit in cold climates distant from the equator. Interplay among diet, arduousness of life, and climate complicates attempts to pinpoint diet as determiner of height and size. This uncertainty means that these attributes do not always pinpoint dietary effects on health.

Height and mass are products of evolution in another way. As primates, humans are social animals. In primate societies that foster competition for mates, large males tend to outcompete small ones for access to females. In this system, large males pass more of their genes to the next generation than their smaller competitors whereas females of all sizes are available for mating. Consequently, males are bigger than females. Size differences, known as sexual dimorphism, are conspicuous among baboons (*Papio* species) and mandrills (*Mandrillus sphinx*), whose males are twice the size of females.[80] Male orangutans (*Pongo pygmaeus*, *P. abelii*, and *P. tapanuliensis*) and male mountain gorillas (*Gorilla beringei beringei*) may more than double females in mass.[81] Differences are less pronounced among chimpanzees (*Pan troglodytes*), whose males are about one-third larger than females.[82] By contrast, gibbons (*Hylobates* species) display no dimorphism because, being primarily monogamous, most males have an opportunity to mate irrespective of size.[83] The lineage leading to humanity must have behaved more like gibbons than gorillas because early fossils show little dimorphism.[84] Humans display small differences in size, with men seldom over several centimeters taller than women.

Returning to diseases and diets, an earlier section, treating pellagra, acknowledged that nutritional deficiencies cause some maladies. Chapter 2 expands this discussion by examining night blindness, scurvy, rickets, and anemia. But, as noted, other factors may be involved. For example, parasites that infest the intestines may cause anemia. Where present, infectious diseases may implicate undernutrition, which tends to compromise the immune system.

In this context, Chapter 3 mentions that one of humanity's worst calamities, the Black Death (1347–1351), followed repeated famines that left Europeans too weak to fight diseases.[85] Crowding benefits contagion, which may kill even adequately fed urbanites who live and work near one another. No lone example should be pushed too far, though it is sobering that German composer Johann Sebastian Bach (1685–1750) lost his first wife to an unspecified illness at age thirty-five and ten of his twenty children as youths despite earning enough money to feed them all.[86] Although cause of death was seldom pinpointed in the past, infectious diseases played a greater role than diet in Bach's tragedies. This example fits the pattern that between Neanderthal prehistory and 1900 CE, half of all children died before puberty.[87] Ignorance of these realities distorts the past by overstating health.[88]

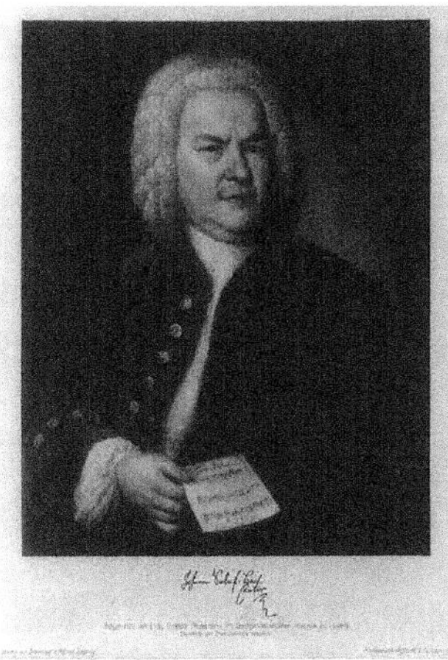

FIGURE 1.7 Johann Sebastian Bach. (Photo courtesy of Library of Congress. https://www.loc.gov/pictures/item/2004671945/.)

Lifespan may be the toughest parameter to interpret because so many variables affect it. For example, American historian Richard Slator Dunn (b. 1928) blamed tropical diseases, undernutrition, overwork, suicide, execution, accidents, and poor medical care for slaves' brief lives in the Caribbean islands in the seventeenth and early eighteenth centuries.[89] Interplay among these factors prevented him from attempting to gauge which was most lethal. The situation is even more complex because recent research indicates that, independent of other variables, poverty shortens life.[90] Moreover, upbringing, marital status, and hereditary factors like gender and ethnicity modify lifespan. This mélange complicates attempts to pinpoint diet and nutrition's roles in longevity.

Additionally, longevity's treatment through calculation of life expectancy, usually at birth (e^0), poses problems. Convention interprets life expectancy as a measure of mortality. This position is intuitive given that death fixes lifespan, allowing its averaging with others' age at death to derive a population's life expectancy at birth or another age. In this scheme, increase signals improvement whereas decrease indicates a population in trouble.

Since the early twenty-first century, however, demographers have emphasized that e^0 reveals more about birthrate than mortality.[91] A high birthrate diminishes e^0 because an increase in births raises the total number of youths, the pool of people subject to early death, and so increases the number of juvenile deaths even when infant mortality—usually defined as deaths before age five—is not enormous. A fertile population therefore tends to yield lower e^0 than a barren one even though an unfruitful group may be under greater distress than its fecund counterpart.

Another problem with treatment of life expectancy is the expectation of progress from short to long lifespans over time. For example, in 1965, American anthropologist Francis Clark Howell (1925–2007) reported lifespans between Neanderthal prehistory and the mid-twentieth century CE, showing an increase of forty years over the roughly 40,000 years that separate these periods.[92]

But this gain is not a trend. The remains of 12,520 people who lived in the Americas between roughly 4000 BCE and 1900 CE reveal the greatest longevity and overall health in the early millennia.[93] Lifespan and health deteriorated with the rise of agriculture and animal husbandry, cities, and governments. An onlooker might hypothesize that the initial period promoted longevity because the first migrants into the Americas were few, and they encountered pristine lands rich in edible plants and animals. Over time, populations increased to the point of devouring food faster than nature could replenish it. Shortages truncated lives.

Yet this view conflicts with the understanding, noted above, that abundant food increases birthrate, a consequence of which is a larger number of deaths during infancy than results from low birthrate, all else being equal. But high infant mortality reduces e^0, giving the impression of short lifespan and abysmal health. This scenario underscores the difficulties in attempting to interpret e^0 and questions the assumption that it increases over time as a function of progress.

The relationship between food and fertility, however, may not be straightforward. British demographers Edward Anthony Wrigley (b. 1931) and Roger Snowden Schofield (1937–2019) stated that birthrate decreases when calories and nutrients fall below subsistence.[94] But above this threshold, nutritional improvements do not boast fertility. Whatever the merits of their argument, Chapters 13 and 14 demonstrate that potatoes and bananas (*Musa x paradisiaca*), respectively, increased birthrates.

At its most basic, discussion of longevity requires knowledge of age at death. Without writing, prehistory yields skeletons, teeth, and other tangibles as the only data. But age upon death cannot be pinpointed from remains, necessitating estimation. In approximating age, physical anthropologists and forensic scientists rely on developmental milestones. In rough terms, the skeleton develops until around age thirty, after which it deteriorates. At birth, the skeleton is least formed, softest, and has over 300 parts that fuse during maturation into the 206 bones of an adult. The rate of fusion is known and may be compared to skeletons in question. After about age thirty, deterioration may be visible as wear at joints. For example, the knees and spine bear the body's mass and may evince osteoarthritis in the femur, tibia, and vertebrae. But because activity as well as age may cause osteoarthritis, its presence cannot pinpoint age at death. The number and type of teeth also provide information about age. The timing and order in which deciduous and adult teeth erupt help dental experts estimate age upon death. For example, absence of wisdom teeth implies death before age eighteen. Teeth develop into a person's mid-twenties, after which severity of wear aids approximation of age at death. An optimistic opinion holds that estimates of children's age at death are accurate within three years, though skeletons of individuals who lived beyond age thirty-five are subject to greater error.[95] In 2001, Austrian historian Walter Scheidel (b. 1966) doubtless spoke for other skeptics in deeming such approximations imprecise.[96]

Remote times yield the least precision because the number and quality of skeletons sometimes formed too small and fragmentary a sample to permit generalizations. In distant eras, countless human remains perished, especially delicate newborn and infant bones that tended to decay quicker than those of adults, creating an illusion of low infant mortality and thereby inflating e^0.[97] E^0 was even more exaggerated whenever people did not inter dead youths.

Despite limitations, the remotest periods furnish unique evidence because, as implied earlier, skeletons and teeth from anatomically modern humans are not the only materials for analysis. *Homo neanderthalensis* (Neanderthals or Neandertals) also buried their dead, a practice that preserved hundreds of partial and complete skeletons for comparison with us. The above markers of development and deterioration allow anthropologists to estimate Neanderthal longevity. Among findings is American anthropologist Erik Trinkaus' (b. 1948) conclusion that Neanderthals lived as long as modern humans during the last 100,000 years.[98]

Prehistory is not alone in interesting demographers. By supplying written records, history presents other materials for determining age at death: government sources like census returns, tombstone inscriptions, and church and hospital records. Some societies furnished additional evidence. For example, ancient Egyptian mummies sometimes had a tag with age at death.[99] But these sources are imperfect because written records tend to memorialize the affluent, ignoring the rest as debris. Like other societies, ancient Egypt harbored biases in favor of elites because only the wealthy could afford mummification such that mummy tags recorded birth and death years of only the rich. Today the wealthy outlive the poor, though this advantage was not automatic earlier, when contagion killed indiscriminately and affluent diets were sometimes worse than commoners' plain viands.[100] For example, Chapter 11 states that Belleville, Canada's prosperous nineteenth-century sucrose consumers had an e^0 of only twenty-one years.[101] Yet wealth correlated with lifespan in the seventeenth and eighteenth centuries Massachusetts.[102]

Written documents tended to underreport deaths during infancy, early childhood, and old age.[103] The deaths that traumatized societies enough to be recorded were those of teens and vigorous adults: people between roughly ages ten and thirty-nine. Furthermore, written records tended to report urban deaths more than rural because governments had more control of city than countryside, allowing bureaucrats to practice demography in municipalities. Mortality is unlikely to have been identical in both because crowding made cities more prone to epidemics than rural districts. Being more prominent than women, men tended to be memorialized upon death in greater numbers. This prejudice exaggerated life expectancy in premodern societies because men did not face the hazards of childbirth that truncated women's lives. Religious status also overstated longevity because monks, priests, and other devout people's age at death was sometimes inflated to imply holiness, a practice as old as Genesis.[104] All these biases introduced errors into computation of life expectancy.

1.2.2 Hypothesis Testing

Whatever the difficulties in interpreting evidence, evaluation of foods as proposed above involves testing hypotheses, a feature of the Scientific Method. The tendency to link hypothesis testing with the natural sciences is inevitable whenever experimentation is invoked. Equation of experimentation and the sciences is unhelpful when clinicians insist that no knowledge is valid apart from what can be verified through experiment. A corollary of this view is the conviction that hypotheses are untestable absent experimentation. For example, study of history may be thought subjective because historians cannot design experiments about the past, whose events are unrepeatable. This rationale fails to consider that hypotheses may be tested in other ways.

History's critics pigeonhole it in the humanities rather than the sciences in the belief that the humanities are inexact and impressionistic, as noted. Such trivialization ignores the fact that history aligns with scientific practices by testing hypotheses. Historians craft and evaluate hypotheses by reviewing the past. For example, history teachers often espouse freedom as a hallmark of the United States. The Declaration of Independence (1776) enumerates liberty (freedom) as a basic right. The Star-Spangled Banner (1814) declares America the "land of the free." The Pledge of Allegiance (1892) celebrates "liberty and justice for all." These proclamations reach back to the origins of the United States given that the Declaration of Independence is a foundational document. In this context, recitation of words and phrases yields the hypothesis that the United States has long been a free society.

This idea is no abstraction insulated from scrutiny. Treated as a hypothesis, it is untrue because slavery was legal when the United States was founded. Statesman and third U.S. President Thomas Jefferson (1743–1826), architect of the Declaration of Independence, owned slaves, as did his distant cousin Francis Scott Key (1779–1843), author of the Star-Spangled Banner. Slavery's abolition in 1865 upon ratification of the Thirteenth Amendment did not end unfree labor. Rather, this amendment permitted "slavery" and "involuntary servitude … as a punishment for crime."[105] Moreover, coercion persisted in sharecropping, peonage, and convict leasing, as the quote implies. These facts contradict the idealism enshrined in traditional interpretations of American history, demonstrating how historians marshal evidence to test assumptions and hypotheses about the past.

This method applies to an evaluation of foods because hypotheses may be fashioned and tested in the same way. Returning to corn, in 2019, the United Nations Food and Agriculture Organization (FAO) in Rome, Italy ranked the grain second worldwide in total harvest, trailing only sugarcane.[106] This magnitude may prompt the supposition that corn must be nourishing to have achieved such prominence. Such reasoning may be refuted by noting that tobacco (*Nicotiana tabacum*) is a world crop despite being noxious. Nonetheless, corn's putative wholesomeness supplies a hypothesis that Chapter 12 tests by evaluating health among prehistoric and historic peoples who subsisted on it.

Foods may be approached through anecdotes that enliven history. Sometimes quirky, these stories populate the past, achieving independent existence even when they seem improbable. Despite their unreliability, peculiar accounts reveal assumptions that may be framed as hypotheses. For example, folklore about World War I includes the case of a man who ate only peanuts.[107] The notion that they sustained him during this time of privation reveals a belief in their healthfulness. Such confidence challenges scientists and scholars to appraise peanuts wherever and whenever they were prominent in diets. Chapter 8 examines peanuts within an inquiry into legumes' contributions to diets, nutrition, and health worldwide.

Readers might note that just one piece of contrary evidence invalidates a hypothesis. A single instance of frailty among corn or peanut eaters that cannot be ascribed to another cause exposes that food as unhealthful. That is, when an environmental factor like food can be isolated as the lone variable, nothing else can explain a health outcome. Admittedly the past, full of complexity, seldom produces situations that allow treatment of only one variable. Nonetheless, evidence that corn, peanuts, or another commodity repeatedly yielded similar outcomes among peoples who lived in various places and at different times permits generalizations about that food's contributions to vigor, feebleness, or a status between these extremes. Despite an ability to illuminate the past in this way, historians cannot confirm a hypothesis so decisively that all doubts vanish because history resembles the natural sciences in employing induction, amassing specifics to support a conclusion. Even aggregation of innumerable particulars does not eliminate the possibility that the next fact to be uncovered might falsify the conclusion to which the others tend.

1.2.3 Limitations of a Prehistorical and Historical Approach to Diet and Nutrition

The forgoing acknowledges the strengths and limitations of historical research. In leveraging the methods of historical analysis, this book concedes the imperfections inherent in the evidence at its disposal. Skeletons and teeth disclose people's status upon death. The dying are always sicker than the living; otherwise they would not have perished, at least not when they did. In this way, skeletons represent the worst outcomes in a population.

Yet skeletons cannot record diseases that kill too quickly to leave traces in bones and teeth. Moreover, absent attempts at trephination, a person's mental health cannot be inferred from bones and teeth. These factors underreport diseases, counteracting the tendency, mentioned earlier, to interpret the presence and number of skeletons as evidence of mass debilitation or illness.

Middens tend to preserve bones and other hard items. Plant remains often decay too quickly to linger in trash, skewing the evidence to overreport meat, fish, and poultry consumption. Yet even where plants are absent from the archeological record, their place in the diet may be inferred from presence of abrasive stones, mortars and pestles, and querns for processing seeds, spades (with bone, stone, or metal blades) and kindred digging implements for extraction of tubers and roots, and other plant gathering and preparation technologies. In the same way, of course, projectile points, blades, bows and arrows, harpoons, fishhooks, nets, and similar artifacts evidence acquisition of meat and fish. Not all technologies are durable. Wooden implements like bows or sticks—whether to extract termites from logs, dig tubers or roots, or probe a hive for honey—deteriorate too readily to retain a place in the archeological record. Other items may escape detection. For example, a slender bone may substitute for a stick, serving the above functions while appearing to be merely another piece of garbage.

Coprolites reveal only what the body did not digest and so indicate nothing on their own about what was assimilated. For example, the body tends to absorb animal proteins, making them uncommon in feces. For this reason, coprolites are poor indicators of meat intake.[108] This limitation does not eliminate such evidence from consideration but instead urges caution.

Examination of the above technologies supplies additional dietary information. As noted, profusion of hunting, fishing, and butchering equipment indicates centrality of meat and fish in the diet. On the other hand, when technologies to access and process plants are numerous, nuts, seeds, roots, tubers, leaves, stems, flowers, and other plant parts must constitute the diet. Comparison of meat to plant acquisition and processing technologies yields a ratio of animals to plants in the diet. Such comparisons are imperfect to the degree that technologies do not persist in the archeological record, but they are valuable, along with other lines of evidence, in helping paint an overall picture of past diets.

Use of historical evidence is weakest whenever past and present are most dissimilar, making comparisons between the two least valid. For example, the trip between Philadelphia, Pennsylvania, and St. Augustine, Florida, can be completed much quicker today than in 1700, but the thought that people must be more energetic today because they travel faster and farther is unwarranted. Such a conclusion is meaningless because it fails to account for differences in transportation between these years. It might be argued that someone who tried to walk part or all the distance in 1700 worked harder, at least as a measure of calories expended, than a person who types on a laptop while sitting in an airplane today.

Yet comparisons of dissimilarities are in vogue in dietary and nutritional circles, as physicians and scientists use hunter-gatherers as models of health, a topic discussed throughout this book. Perlmutter praised their "lean and toned bodies," the result of vigorous activity and no junk foods.[109] Stephen Le and American radiologist Stanley Boyd Eaton (b. 1938) elevated them into archetypes of hearty diets and vigor.[110] These views make sense because almost all our evolution occurred in the context of hunting, fishing, and foraging. Over innumerable millennia, natural selection adapted humans to diets and lifestyles like those of their nomadic ancestors and different from the norm among today's affluent peoples, especially in the developed world.

Chapter 3 notes that the dichotomy between hunter-gatherers and us tends to focus on the divide between preagricultural and agricultural eras. This section and later chapters disagree. The advent of farming and livestock rearing did not enfeeble humans. Egypt's pyramids, China's Great Wall and Grand Canal, Cambodia's Angkor Wat, Easter Island's statues, Mexico's Pyramid of the Sun, Palenque, Calakmul, and Chichen Itza, Guatemala's Tikal, Honduras' Copan, Peru's Machu Picchu, England's Stonehenge, continental Europe's Romanesque and Gothic cathedrals, and other landmarks demonstrate agricultural peoples' capacity for exertion. In an era before machines, armies spread over continents on foot, navies rowed galleys across the sea, and people built roads, bridges, and aqueducts, dug qanats, irrigation works, and similar public works worldwide through brute force, tilled the soil by walking behind plows, terraced hillsides to permit agriculture, broadcast seeds by hand, planted seedlings and saplings with spades, weeded vast hectarages with hoes, and harvested grains with sickle, scythe, or cradle. United Kingdom (UK) pharmacologist Paul Clayton and historian Judith D. Rowbotham (b. 1952) wrote in 2009 that such vigor persisted into the nineteenth century.[111] Not only was work fatiguing, but laborers walked to and from the job.

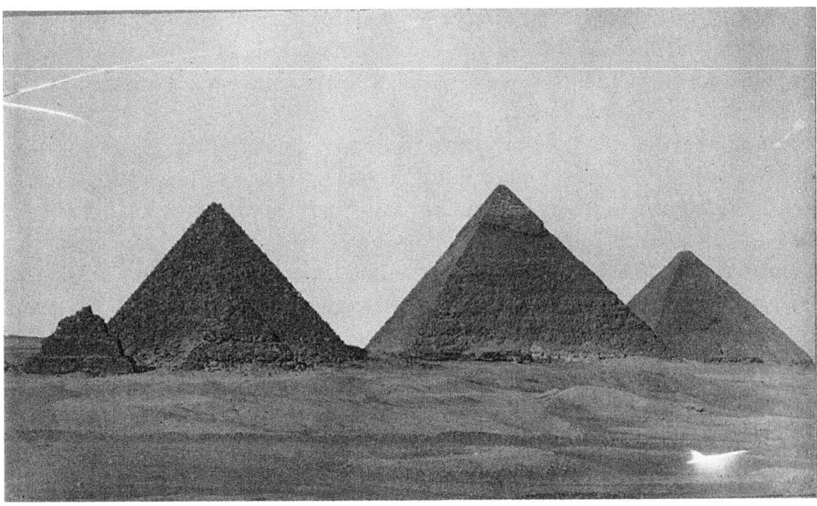

FIGURE 1.8 Egypt's pyramids. (Photo courtesy of Library of Congress. https://www.loc.gov/pictures/item/2016887869/.)

These circumstances lead this book to argue for continuity before and after agriculture's advent. The real chasm, this book maintains, opened in the twentieth century, when the automobile, tractor, bus, airplane, and kindred machines reduced life's drudgery. Accordingly, the real contrast is between pre- and post-automobile ages rather than between hunter-gatherers on one hand and farmers, stockmen, and the urbanites who consumed their surpluses on the other.

Such considerations warn against comparing dissimilarities. As previous examples implied, much has changed over time, complicating attempts to compare past and present. As noted earlier, longevity has increased in recent times. Focus on life's brevity before roughly 1900 CE might prompt the inference that past peoples must have had terrible diets given their early demise. Such a belief is untenable as a generalization. Many factors, pathogens and parasites for example, can shorten lives even when diet is adequate or excellent. In other words, when the issue is lifespan—which an earlier section described as difficult to interpret—a past devoid of vaccines, antibiotics, clean water, pasteurized milk, readily available food, and other advantages cannot be compared easily with a present that offers these benefits.

1.2.4 Examination of the Past on Its Own Terms

Although Chapter 3 expands treatment of differences between past and present, the emphasis here and throughout this book is on examining the past on its own terms. Returning to an earlier topic, anthropologists and economists have determined when and where several groups of Amerindians added corn to diets. The presence of skeletons, middens, and coprolites, as noted permits an assessment of health and its comparison with the vigor of prior generations of hunter-gatherers who did not eat corn. In other words, it is not always necessary or desirable to reference the present in evaluating health. The gulf between past and present does not mean, however, that corn's health effects on early peoples are irrelevant today because this information supplements what nutritionists already know about the grass. For example, they have found its nutrients incomplete, as was mentioned earlier and as Chapter 12 demonstrates, because of deficiencies in amino acids, vitamins, and minerals and because it retards iron absorption from other foods.

This knowledge is important given corn's global reach. The U.S. Department of Agriculture (USDA) estimated that the world produced over 41 billion bushels of corn between October 1, 2017, and September 30, 2018.[112] No other grain supplies as much of the world's food and feed. In this context of enormity, corn's dietary shortfalls become more conspicuous if it can be established that American indigenes who adopted the grain as their primary food ailed more than their ancestors, and others, who did not eat it. In this way, the past can corroborate what is known today as easily as it can challenge the prevailing wisdom.

Use of evidence from Native Americans returns us to prehistory because few of them invented writing. Absence of written records might appear to confine treatment to skeletons, teeth, middens, and coprolites in attempting to evaluate diet, nutrition, and health. But we can do better by using modern hunter-gatherers to represent prehistoric peoples. This approach makes sense given that humans hunted, scavenged, fished, and gathered edibles throughout all but prehistory's last few millennia. Some prehistoric peoples—Australia's aborigines, for example—never transitioned to farming and livestock raising as Europeans define these activities. Use of modern hunter-gatherers as models helps anthropologists assess plants' importance in preagricultural diets, a valuable insight given plant remains' poor preservation at archaeological sites, as noted.

Yet modern hunter-gatherers are imperfect proxies because they occupy marginal areas unsuitable for agriculture or pastoralism. These regions are resource poor by definition and so inappropriate for making comparisons to prehistoric peoples who settled areas rich in edible plants and animals. It is difficult to imagine, for example, that American Indians who lived near rivers in the Pacific Northwest—an area with abundant fish like salmon (*Oncorhynchus* species) most of the year—had to work as hard for food as today's hunters in desolate lands.

Movement from prehistory to history yielded a new source of evidence—written records, which described what and sometimes how much food people ate as well as their health. Such evidence is especially important when the writer expressed surprise at unusual findings. or example, travelers to unfamiliar lands often recorded their observations about what the inhabitants ate and drank. These foreigners carried their prejudices with them, frequently assuming the novelties were substandard in some way. Observations to the contrary were important because they shattered assumptions, requiring the writer, and us as readers, to see these foods in a new light.

Yet, as with other types of evidence, written accounts have shortcomings. The poor, servants, and slaves were too busy working to document their lives. Only elites had the leisure to record their impressions, many of which exhibited the biases inherent in unequal economic, social, and political systems. Historians understand that such documents, being subjective, do not permit accurate reconstruction of bygone events. The partisan and fragmentary nature of written records allows historians, at best, to approximate the past. Such inexactitude cannot hope to satisfy readers who expect mathematical precision.

In all these ways, and despite weaknesses in interpretation, prehistory and history furnish information about which foods promote health and which undermine it. In other words, and as emphasized in the context of hypothesis testing, the past functions as a laboratory in which to gauge various diets. Foods that invigorated peoples, at least in relative terms, at different times and places must have value. On the other hand, readers might wish to reduce or eliminate those that diminished vitality time and again throughout the past.

NOTES

1 Frederick Engels, "Preface," in *Communist Manifesto*, Karl Marx and Friedrich Engels, trans. Samuel Moore (Chicago, IL: Great Books Foundation, 1955), 1; Karl Marx and Friedrich Engels, *Communist Manifesto*, trans. Samuel Moore (Chicago, IL: Great Books Foundation, 1955), 8–14.

2 Kimberly M. Curtis, "Du Bois, W. E. B.," in *Encyclopedia of African American History*, vol. 3, ed. Leslie M. Alexander and Walter C. Rucker (Santa Barbara, CA: ABC-CLIO, 2010), 748.

3 F. Clark Howell, *Early Man* (New York: Time-Life Books, 1965), 174; John P. McKay, Bennett D. Hill, John Buckler, Clare Haru Crowston, Merry E. Wiesner-Hanks, and Joe Perry, *Understanding Western Society: A Brief History* (Boston, MA and New York: Bedford/St. Martin's, 2012), 212; "Life Expectancy at Birth (Male and Female), 1971–2017," *Centre for Health Protection*, last modified January 11, 2019, accessed January 20, 2019, https://www.chp.gov.hk/en/statistics/data/10/27/111.html.

4 Robert Jurmain, Lynn Kilgore, Wenda Trevathan, and Russell L. Ciochon, *Introduction to Physical Anthropology*, 2013–2014 edition (Belmont, CA: Wadsworth Cengage Learning, 2014), 442.
5 John Wilkins, "Medical Literature, Diet, and Health," in *A Companion to Food in the Ancient World*, ed. John Wilkins and Robin Nadeau (Oxford: Wiley Blackwell, 2015), 60.
6 David Perlmutter, *Grain Brain: The Surprising Truth about Wheat, Carbs, and Sugar—Your Brain's Silent Killers*, rev. ed. (New York: Little, Brown Spark, 2018), 33–34, 51–52.
7 T. Colin Campbell, *Whole: Rethinking the Science of Nutrition* (Dallas, TX: BenBella Books, 2013), xii.
8 S. Ryan Johansson and Douglas Owsley, "Welfare History on the Great Plains: Mortality and Skeletal Health, 1650 to 1900," in *The Backbone of History: Health and Nutrition in the Western Hemisphere* (Cambridge, UK: Cambridge University Press, 2002), 547; Stephen Le, *100 Million Years of Food: What Our Ancestors Ate and Why It Matters Today* (New York: Picador, 2016), 58–59.
9 Campbell, 82–83; William Davis, *Wheat Belly: Lose the Wheat, Lose the Weight, and Find Your Path Back to Health* (New York: Rodale, 2011), 114–115.
10 Elizabeth S. Wing, "Animals Used for Food in the Past: As Seen by Their Remains Excavated from Archaeological Sites," in *The Cambridge World History of Food*, vol. 1, ed. Kenneth F. Kiple and Kriemhild Conee Ornelas (Cambridge, UK: Cambridge University Press, 2000), 55.
11 Kenneth F. Kiple, "The Question of Paleolithic Nutrition and Modern Health," in *The Cambridge World History of Food*, vol. 2, ed. Kenneth F. Kiple and Kriemhild Conee Ornelas (Cambridge, UK: Cambridge University Press, 2000), 1704.
12 Jurmain, Kilgore, Trevathan, and Ciochon, 449.
13 Kim Hill and A. Magdalena Hurtado, "The Ache of Paraguay," in *The Cambridge Encyclopedia of Hunters and Gatherers*, ed. Richard B. Lee and Richard Daly (Cambridge, UK: Cambridge University Press, 2002), 93, 95.
14 Ibid.
15 Theodore Roosevelt, "The Strenuous Life," *Speech before the Hamilton Club*, April 10, 1899, accessed February 10, 2019, https://en.wikisource.org/wiki/The_Strenuous_Life.
16 William Rubel, *Bread: A Global History* (London: Reaktion Books, 2011), 11–12.
17 S. Boyd Eaton and Stanley B. Eaton, "Hunter-Gatherers and Human Health," in *The Cambridge Encyclopedia of Hunters and Gatherers*, ed. Richard B. Lee and Richard Daly (Cambridge, UK and New York: Cambridge University Press, 2002), 450, 452, 454–455.
18 Loren Cordain, *The Paleo Diet: Lose Weight and Get Healthy by Eating the Foods You Were Designed to Eat*, rev. ed. (Hoboken, NJ: Wiley, 2011), 6.
19 Kim Hill and A. Magdalena Hurtado, *Ache Life History: The Ecology and Demography of a Foraging People* (New York: Aldine, 1996), 186.
20 Ibid., 156–157.
21 Plato, "Republic," in *The Great Dialogues of Plato*, trans. W. H. D. Rouse (New York and Scarborough, Ontario: New American Library, 1956), 312–315.
22 Alfred E. Harper, "Recommended Dietary Allowances and Dietary Guidance," in *The Cambridge World History of Food*, vol. 2, ed. Kenneth F. Kiple and Kriemhild Conee Ornelas (Cambridge, UK: Cambridge University Press, 2000), 1609–1619.
23 Stephanie Green, *Optimum Nutrition* (New York: Alpha Books, 2016), 254.
24 Ibid., 138–139.
25 Peter Garnsey, *Food and Society in Classical Antiquity* (Cambridge, UK: Cambridge University Press, 1999), 86.
26 James C. Whorton, "Vegetarianism," in *The Cambridge World History of Food*, vol. 2, ed. Kenneth F. Kiple and Kriemhild Conee Ornelas (Cambridge, UK: Cambridge University Press, 2000), 1553.
27 Bob Brier and Hoyt Hobbs, *Ancient Egypt: Everyday Life in the Land of the Nile* (New York: Sterling, 2009), 119.
28 Garnsey, 16.
29 Whorton, 1553.
30 Mark 6:31–44 (New American Bible); Matthew 14:13–21 (New American Bible); Luke 9:12–17 (New American Bible); John 6:1–14 (New American Bible).
31 Luke 5:1–11.
32 John 21:1–14.
33 Luke 24:41–43.
34 Nix v. Hedden, 149 U.S. 304 (1893).

35 "Lowest Calorie Foods," *Health Assist*, 2006–2017, accessed October 2, 2019, http://www.healthassist.net/food/calories-chart.shtml; Allan Borushek, *The CalorieKing Calorie, Fat, and Carbohydrate Counter* (Huntington Beach, CA: Family Health Publications, 2019), 99–101, 159.
36 Green, 259.
37 Ibid., 261–262.
38 Ibid., 259–260.
39 "What Is Ornish Diet?" *U.S. News and World Report*, 2018, accessed January 22, 2019, https://health.usnews.com/best-diet/ornish-diet.
40 Campbell, 7.
41 Ibid., 168.
42 Perlmutter, 84.
43 Ibid., 35, 84.
44 Davis, x.
45 Steven R. Gundry, *The Plant Paradox: The Hidden Dangers in "Healthy" Foods that Cause Disease and Weight Gain* (New York: Harper Wave, 2017), xi.
46 Alina Bradford, "What Is Gluten?" *Live Science*, November 18, 2017, accessed October 2, 2019, https://www.livescience.com/53265-what-is-gluten.html.
47 "7-Day Meal Plan," *Celiac Disease Foundation*, 1998–2018, accessed January 22, 2019, https://celiac.org/eat-gluten-free/meal-plans/7-day-meal-plan.
48 Briana Pobiner, "Meat-Eating among the Earliest Humans," *American Scientist* 104, no. 2 (March-April 2016), https://www.americanscientist.org/article/meat-eating-among-the-earliest-humans; Henry T. Bunn, "Meat Made Us Human," in *Evolution of the Human Diet: The Known, the Unknown, and the Unknowable*, ed. Peter S. Ungar (Oxford and New York: Oxford University Press, 2007), 191.
49 Bunn, 191, 204.
50 Fred J. P. H. Brouns, Vincent J. van Buul, and Peter R. Shewry, "Does Wheat Make Us Fat and Sick?" *Journal of Cereal Science* 58, no. 2 (September 2013): 209–215, https://www.sciencedirect.com/science/article/pii/S0733521013000969#!.
51 Gundry, ix.
52 Thomas S. Kuhn, *The Structure of Scientific Revolutions*, 4th ed. (Chicago, IL and London: University of Chicago Press, 2012), 48.
53 Gail Jarow, *Red Madness: How a Medical Mystery Changed What We Eat* (Honesdale, PA: Calkins Creek, 2014), 20; Karl Y. Guggenheim, *Nutrition and Nutritional Diseases: The Evolution of Concepts* (Lexington, MA and Toronto: D. C. Heath, 1981), 247.
54 Daphne A. Roe and Stephen V. Beck, "Pellagra," in *The Cambridge World History of Food*, vol. 1, ed. Kenneth F. Kiple and Kriemhild Conee Ornelas (Cambridge, UK: Cambridge University Press, 2000), 962–963.
55 Aristotle, *Nicomachean Ethics*, trans. Martin Oswald (Upper Saddle River, NJ: Prentice Hall, 1999), 16–17; Glenn C. Conroy, *Reconstructing Human Origins: A Modern Synthesis* (New York and London: Norton, 1997), 375.
56 Mike Lean and Emilie Combet, *Barasi's Human Nutrition: A Health Perspective*, 3rd ed (Boca Raton, FL: CRC Press, 2017), 314.
57 Marx and Engels, 8.
58 Wayne Suttles, "Coping with Abundance: Subsistence on the Northwest Coast," in *Man the Hunter*, ed. Richard B. Lee and Irven DeVore (Chicago: Aldine, 1968), 59.
59 Cecil Woodham-Smith, "The Great Hunger: Ireland, 1845–1849," in *European Diet from Pre-Industrial to Modern Times*, ed. Elborg Forster and Robert Forster (New York: Harper Torchbooks, 1975), 10–18.
60 Alan L. Mackay, *A Dictionary of Scientific Quotations* (Bristol, UK and Philadelphia: Institute of Physics Publishing, 1991), 88; C. Wayne Smith, *Crop Production: Evolution, History, and Technology* (New York: Wiley, 1995), v.
61 Stephan Thernstrom, *A History of the American People*, vol. 1, to 1877, 2nd ed. (San Diego, CA: Harcourt, Brace, Jovanovich, 1989), vii.
62 Stephen G. Brush, *The History of Modern Science: A Guide to the Second Scientific Revolution, 1800–1950* (Ames: Iowa State University Press, 1988), 288–289.
63 Francoise Balibar, *Einstein: Decoding the Universe*, trans. David J. Baker and Dorie B. Baker (New York: Harry N. Abrams, 2001), 51.
64 Perlmutter, 254.

65 "Overweight and Obesity," *World Health Organization*, February 16, 2018, accessed July 8, 2019, https://www.who.int/news-room/fact-sheets/detail/obesity-and-overweight.
66 "Obesity Definition," *Harvard University*, 2019, accessed April 13, 2019, https://www.hsph.harvard.edu/obesity-prevention-source/obesity-definition.
67 Vishwanath Sardesai, *Introduction to Clinical Nutrition*, 3rd ed. (Boca Raton, FL: CRC Press, 2012), 363.
68 Stephen Bertman, *Handbook to Life in Ancient Mesopotamia* (New York: Facts on File, 2003), 56.
69 Gen. 41:4–6 (New American Bible).
70 Jennifer Welsh, "Mozart's Death Was Written in the Key of (Vitamin) D," *Live Science*, July 6, 2011, accessed February 2, 2019, https://www.livescience.com/14925-mozart-death-vitamin.html.
71 Jerome C. Rose and Melissa Zabecki, "The Commoners of Tell el-Amarna," in *Beyond the Horizon: Studies in Egyptian Art, Archaeology and History in Honour of Barry J. Kemp*, ed. Salima Ikram and Aidan Dodson, vol. 2 (Cairo: Supreme Council of Antiquities, 2009), 415; Clark Spencer Larsen, *Skeletons in Our Closet: Revealing Our Past through Bioarchaeology* (Princeton, NJ and Oxford, UK: Princeton University Press, 2000), 42.
72 Susan Kent, "Iron Deficiency and Anemia of Chronic Disease," in *The Cambridge World History of Food*, vol. 1, ed. Kenneth F. Kiple and Kriemhild Conee Ornelas (Cambridge, UK: Cambridge University Press, 2000), 922.
73 Kiple, 1707.
74 Alan H. Goodman and Debra L. Martin, "Reconstructing Health Profiles from Skeletal Remains," in *The Backbone of History: Health and Nutrition in the Western Hemisphere*, ed. Richard H. Steckel and Jerome C. Rose (Cambridge, UK: Cambridge University Press, 2002), 20.
75 "C_3, C_4 and CAM Plants," *Biology Dictionary*, 2018, accessed January 28, 2019, https://biologydictionary.net/c3-c4-cam-plants.
76 Alexander Hellemans, "What Did Ancient Egyptians Really Eat?" *Inside Science*, May 8, 2014, accessed January 27, 2019, https://www.insidescience.org/news/what-did-ancient-egyptians-really-eat.
77 Barbara Mertz, *Red Land, Black Land: Daily Life in Ancient Egypt* (New York: William Morrow, 1978), 108–109; Don Nardo, *Life in Ancient Egypt* (San Diego: Reference Point Press, 2015), 25.
78 Clark Spencer Larsen, *Our Origins: Discovering Physical Anthropology* (New York and London: Norton, 2008), 360–365.
79 Ibid., 136.
80 Jurmain, Kilgore, Trevathan, and Ciochon, 157, 190.
81 Ibid., 160–161.
82 Ibid., 163.
83 Ibid., 190.
84 Larsen, *Our Origins*, 281.
85 Mortimer Chambers, Raymond Grew, David Herlihy, Theodore K. Rabb, and Isser Woloch, *The Western Experience*, vol. 2, 4th ed. (New York: Knopf, 1987), 395.
86 Joseph Machlis, *The Enjoyment of Music: An Introduction to Perceptive Listening* (New York: Norton, 1955), 423.
87 Edward S. Deevey Jr., "The Human Population," *Scientific American* (September 1, 1960), 202.
88 Garnsey, 43.
89 Richard S. Dunn, *Sugar and Slaves: The Rise of the Planter Class in the English West Indies, 1624–1713* (Chapel Hill: University of North Carolina Press, 1972), 302–317.
90 Peter Dizikes, "New Study Shows Rich, Poor Have Huge Mortality Gap in U.S." *MIT News*, April 11, 2016. http://news.mit.edu/2016/study-rich-poor-huge-mortality-gap-us–0411.
91 Robert McCaa, "Paleodemography of the Americas: From Ancient Times to Colonialism and Beyond," in *The Backbone of History: Health and Nutrition in the Western Hemisphere*, ed. Richard H. Steckel and Jerome C. Rose (Cambridge, UK: Cambridge University Press, 2002), 95–99.
92 Howell, 174.
93 Richard H. Steckel and Jerome C. Rose, "Introduction," in *The Backbone of History: Health and Nutrition in the Western Hemisphere*, ed. Richard H. Steckel and Jerome C. Rose (Cambridge, UK: Cambridge University Press, 2002), 5–6; Richard H. Steckel and Jerome C. Rose, "Patterns of Health in the Western Hemisphere," in *The Backbone of History: Health and Nutrition in the Western Hemisphere*, ed. Richard H. Steckel and Jerome C. Rose (Cambridge, UK: Cambridge University Press, 2002), 563.
94 E. A. Wrigley and R. S. Schofield, *The Population History of England, 1541–1871: A Reconstruction* (Cambridge, UK: Cambridge University Press, 1989), 309.

95 P. Zioupos, A. Williams, G. Christodoulou, and R. Giles, "Determining 'Age at Death' for Forensic Purposes Using Human Bone by a Laboratory-Based Biochemical Analytical Method," *Journal of the Mechanical Behavior of Biomedical Materials* 33 (May 2014): 109. https://dspace.lib.cranfield.ac.uk/bitstream/handle/1826/9951/Determining_%27age_at_death%27_for_forensic_purposes-2014.pdf?sequence=3&isAllowed=y.

96 Walter Scheidel, *Death on the Nile: Disease and the Demography of Roman Egypt* (Leiden, The Netherlands: Brill, 2001), 122–123.

97 Clark Spencer Larsen, "Dietary Reconstruction and Nutritional Assessment of Past Peoples: The Bioanthropological Record," in *The Cambridge World History of Food*, vol. 1, ed. Kenneth F. Kiple and Kriemhild Conee Ornelas (Cambridge, UK: Cambridge University Press, 2000), 28.

98 Erik Trinkaus, "Late Pleistocene Adult Mortality Patterns and Modern Human Establishment," *Proceedings of the National Academy of Sciences* 108, no. 4 (January 25, 2011): 1267–1271, https://www.pnas.org/content/108/4/1267.

99 Scheidel, 10.

100 Dizikes.

101 Shelley R. Saunders, Ann Herring, Larry Sawchuk, Gerry Boyce, Rob Hoppa, and Susan Klepp, "The Health of the Middle Class: The St. Thomas' Anglican Church Cemetery Project," in *The Backbone of History: Health and Nutrition in the Western Hemisphere* (Cambridge, UK: Cambridge University Press, 2002), 146.

102 Jeremy Atack and Peter Passell. *A New Economic View of American History: From Colonial Times to 1940*. 2nd ed. New York and London: Norton, 1994.

103 Scheidel, 30.

104 Gen. 5:4–5:32 (New American Bible).

105 U.S. Const. amend. XIII.

106 Rob Cook, "Top 10 Largest Crops in the World," January 21, 2019, accessed January 22, 2019, http://beef2live.com/story-top-10-largest-crops-world-0-142257.

107 Andrew F. Smith, *Peanuts: The Illustrious History of the Goober Pea* (Urbana, IL and Chicago, IL: University of Illinois Press, 2002), 89.

108 Kristin D. Sobolik, "Dietary Reconstruction as Seen in Coprolites," in *The Cambridge World History of Food*, vol. 1, ed. Kenneth F. Kiple and Kriemhild Conee Ornelas (Cambridge, UK: Cambridge University Press, 2000), 44.

109 Perlmutter, 32.

110 Le, 1–6; S. Boyd Eaton and Stanley B. Eaton III, "Hunter-Gatherers and Human Health," in *The Cambridge Encyclopedia of Hunters and Gatherers*, ed. Richard B. Lee and Richard Daly (Cambridge, UK and New York: Cambridge University Press, 1999), 449–455.

111 Paul Clayton and Judith Rowbotham, "How the Mid-Victorians Worked, Ate and Died," *International Journal of Environmental Research and Public Health* 6, no. 3, March 2009, https://www.ncbi.nlm.nih.gov/pmc/articles/PMC2672390.

112 "Grain: World Markets and Trade," U.S. Department of Agriculture, December 11, 2018, last modified December 21, 2018, accessed January 23, 2019, https://www.fas.usda.gov/data/grain-world-markets-and-trade.

2 Components of Nutrition
Calories, Carbohydrates, Fat, Protein, Minerals, Vitamins, Phytochemicals, and Water

2.1 MACRO- AND MICROLEVEL CONSISTENCY

2.1.1 Expectation and Imperative of Consistency

Last chapter emphasized this study's empiricism. Foods are situated in time and place and their effects on health—measured by fertility, diseases, longevity, height, dental decay, and other factors—observed. Given that this method requires no tabulation of carbohydrates, protein, fat, or any other constituent of food, it may seem peculiar that this chapter focuses on these elements. Yet it is no detour from the main thoroughfare because the natural sciences seek not only to describe reality but also to understand why it functions as our senses indicate.

Suppose an agronomist in a remote area of Nepal identified a previously unstudied plant, whose seeds feed the locals. Upon questioning them, she learned that they have eaten these seeds for many centuries but have never witnessed an instance of cancer. The agronomist convened a press conference to announce the discovery of a healthful food. Seeking additional information, she distributed seeds to a laboratory, which claimed to isolate a carcinogen. At this juncture, other scientists, journalists, and the public would be justified in demanding an explanation. Perhaps the laboratory misidentified the chemical in question. Maybe the seeds harbor the carcinogen in inactive form. Alternatively, the Nepalese may have experienced cases of cancer but misdiagnosed them. The upshot of these conjectures is that people expect scientists to resolve contradictions and paradoxes because such work is within their responsibilities. In other words, nutrition, being a science, must produce consistent results; otherwise no one can have confidence in its method or findings.

Note that the sciences must produce consistency at macro and microlevels. By macrolevel, this book means the system in question. Our focus must be on biology at the macrolevel because nutrition deals with the body, a biological system. The microlevel, on the other hand, is that system's components. In our case, the components are the chemicals and their reactions in the body and the physical laws that govern them. That is, any biological phenomenon should be explicable in chemical and physical terms. In seeking such an explanation, this book affirms that it, when satisfactorily articulated, provides a complete understanding of the phenomenon, a stance known as reductionism. This rationale discomforts people, even scientists who dislike its implication that life is nothing more than an aggregate of chemical reactions.[1] Nevertheless, reductionism is well enough established that the burden of proof rests with those who wish to refute it. That is, if the body is more than the sum of its chemical and physical properties, then someone must specify the extra component.

2.1.2 Investigation of Scurvy as Example of Macro- and Microlevel Consistency

Humanity's long battle against scurvy illustrates how the science of nutrition works at macro – and microlevels. Around 1500 BCE, Egyptians elaborated the disease's symptoms—fatigue worsening over time, pain and sensitivity throughout the body, purple spots on the skin, constipation, swollen gums, and loose teeth—though the connection between food and scurvy developed slowly in the West because physicians focused on supposed imbalances in bodily fluids more than diet.[2] Scurvy reached alarming proportions among sailors as voyages lengthened around 1400 CE, beginning an age of discovery.[3] To remain at sea for long durations, captains provisioned ships with biscuits and other dried foods that resisted spoilage. Paucity of fresh fruits and vegetables, subject to rapid deterioration, was the culprit, a fact that Arabs and Portuguese seem to have understood in the fifteenth century, when they began to experiment with giving sailors *Citrus* fruits.[4] Even this discovery did not galvanize the rest of Europe, perhaps because many Europeans were unfamiliar with the fruits, which are native to tropical Asia, Australia, New Caledonia, and New Guinea. Most of Europe is too far north for lemon (*Citrus limon*), orange (*Citrus sinensis* and *Citrus aurantium*), and lime (*Citrus aurantiifolia*) trees, which cannot tolerate a hard frost. The grapefruit (*Citrus paradisi*) did not then exist but would arise from a chance hybridization in the Caribbean in the eighteenth century.

Yet citrus fruits were not the lone alternatives. Spain and Portugal combatted scurvy by giving sailors pineapple (*Ananas comosus*).[5] Likewise banishing the disease with pineapple, English captain James Cook (1728–1779) also fed his men cabbage (*Brassica oleracea var. capitata*) and other leafy vegetables, yams (*Dioscorea* species), and coconuts (*Cocos nucifera*).[6] He took the additional step of planting pineapples wherever he went in the tropics to ensure an ample supply upon return visits. Potatoes (*Solanum tuberosum*) also protected against scurvy.[7] These findings spurred physicians and scientists to wonder what linked these foods. That is, the macrolevel discovery that many fresh fruits and vegetables prevent scurvy prompted the search for a microlevel understanding that would unite them by identifying the shared component or components that explained these foods' effectiveness.

This understanding came from the emerging science of chemistry, a discipline that sought to identify and describe the behavior of matter's constituents: atoms and molecules. Before the twentieth century, however, the molecules and elements of nutrition (nutrients) included only proteins, carbohydrates, lipids, and minerals.[8] Yet rats languished when fed a diet adequate in these components but absent anything else. The discovery of the first vitamin, a word coined in 1912 and discussed later, opened a new avenue for research, and in 1928, Hungarian biochemist Albert Szent-Gyorgyi (1893–1986) isolated vitamin C, ascorbic acid.[9] Subsequent researchers elucidated its role in helping the body metabolize proteins, carbohydrates, and fats. Its function in collagen synthesis was important in eliminating scurvy's symptoms. Vitamin C's presence in many vegetables and fruits—though coconut is not rich in it—explained their effectiveness against scurvy, providing a microlevel understanding of how these disparate foods combatted the malady.

The imperative of macro- and microlevel consistency, achieved in the previous example, means that this book can hope to persuade readers that certain foods are wholesome only if it is able to identify healthfulness among people who ate them and to explain that vigor in terms of their nutrients. Being the system's outcome, health is the macro quality whereas the nutrients and their functions in the body, all aspects of chemistry, explain that health at the microlevel. Without both levels of analysis, this book would be incomplete. The necessity of appealing to chemistry for an understanding of health and nutrition makes essential an appreciation of the nature and role of calories—derived from carbohydrates, fat, and protein—minerals, vitamins, phytochemicals, and water in the body.

2.2 FOOD AS ENERGY

Reductionism, mentioned above, is compatible with mechanism. Together they view the body as a machine whose parts account for every function. The idea that the body is a machine has roots in ancient Greece, where doctors attempted to understand its workings. Dissections of humans were taboo, but other animals served as models. In the second century CE, Greek anatomist and author Galen (130–210 CE), physician to Roman emperor Marcus Aurelius (121–180 CE), sought an analogy to humans by dissecting and vivisecting monkeys, describing several organs' anatomy and function. Although he made errors, Galen's mechanistic understanding of the body outlived the details of his treatises. This view grew over time, underpinning the physiology of French mathematician, philosopher, and scientist Rene Descartes (1596–1650).[10]

If the body is a machine, then food is its fuel. The connection between food and fuel seems obvious to us because we think in terms of energy, but for most of history, such a concept did not exist. The steam engine's invention in the eighteenth century, however, called for a new type of physics, as scientists and engineers were drawn to its operation. The insight that the steam engine used heat to do work led physicists in the nineteenth century to formalize the word "work" to mean the application of force to move an object. This understanding borrowed from English polymath Isaac Newton (1643–1727), who in the seventeenth century had defined "force" as any action that changed an object's motion. Such changes included direction, speed, or both. Moreover, a force could propel an object from rest into motion or from motion to rest. Newton appreciated that a countervailing force could offset the original force, causing a net effect that perpetuated the status quo.

The definition of work required physicists to scrutinize the application of force. Contrary to idealists' hopes, a machine cannot be constructed that applies force (and so works) forever without any inputs. Something must enable a machine to do work. In the case of the steam engine, it was obvious that heat actuated it. That is, heat boiled water, whose steam rushed through a cylinder to drive a piston. Physicists generalized what heat accomplished by saying that it could do work, using the term "energy" for this capacity. The word owed a debt to Greek philosopher Aristotle (384–322 BCE), who coined *energeia*, a term without an exact English equivalent but that may be understood as "in the act of working." *Energeia*, therefore, is the actuality—rather than mere potentiality—of applying force.

2.2.1 Physics and Chemistry of Energy

While acknowledging a debt to Aristotle, physicists and engineers understood that the modern notion of energy transcended *energeia*. In the nineteenth and twentieth centuries, they partitioned energy into several types. We need not enumerate all. Our concern is one type—chemical—because the body is a machine that derives energy from molecules. This language reminds us that reductionism and mechanism undergird an understanding of life. An important qualification is that these molecules are not energy per se but rather storehouses in which the bonds between atoms contain energy.

The relationship between molecules and energy has informed research since the nineteenth century, occupying the minds of scientists whose stories British chemist Walter Bruno Gratzer (b. 1932) recounted in *Terrors of the Table: The Curious History of Nutrition* (2005). An important nineteenth-century achievement was the generalization of "energy" beyond heat. It was clear, for example, that biological systems depended on more than just heat for energy. That is, organisms are more complex than steam engines.

An example might help concretize the terms "energy" and "work" and their limitations in relation to organisms. A man might cut grass, exerting force to push a lawnmower up a hill so steep that he reaches the point of maximum exertion. No matter how hard he tries, he cannot budge the mower another centimeter. Because the mower is no longer moving, physicists aver that he stopped working the moment he could no longer climb the hill. Cessation of work conflicts with the man's perception of tension in his muscles, perspiration on his brow, and grimace on his face. From his perspective, he has never worked harder. Daily life thus seems to contradict physics' definition of work. The best that can be done is to acknowledge the man's exertions even though they are for naught.

These exertions require energy, the source of which is food, to resurrect the linkage with fuel. Returning to our grass cutter, he might retreat from the yard in exhaustion, prompting an inquiry into the strenuousness of his efforts. He will doubtless feel them to have been extreme, but such an impression, being subjective, tells onlookers little. They want to know how much energy he expended, a query that mandates quantification. Measurement and quantification have been central to the natural sciences since their inception, necessitating definition of fundamental units of measurement that can be manipulated mathematically to yield information. The International System of Units (SI) or metric system, an outgrowth of the French Revolution (1789–1799), defines these units.

We met the calorie—physics' kilocalorie—in the last chapter and will use it throughout this book given its ubiquity among public, food scientists, and nutritionists. Although the previous chapter defined the calorie in metric terms, the SI prefers the joule (J), named after nineteenth-century English physicist and mathematician James Prescott Joule (1818–1889), over the calorie as the unit of energy. The joule builds on an understanding of energy as capacity to do work and work as application of force to move an object. Physicists define force in terms of the newton (N), named to honor Isaac Newton. A newton is the force necessary to accelerate a 1-kilogram (kg) object 1 meter per second squared (m/s^2). That is, someone who pushes a stationary 1-kg ball with a force of 1 N will cause it to move from rest to a speed of 1 m/s after 1 s. Continuation of that force will propel the ball to 2 m/s after the second s, 4 m/s after the third, 16 m/s after the fourth, and so forth. Mindful of this definition, a joule is the energy necessary to exert 1 N of force over 1 m. Nutritionists who use the joule often prefer the kilojoule (kJ) to measure and quantify the large amounts of energy in biological systems.

2.2.2 The Body Uses Chemical Energy

Acknowledging the joule's place in the SI, this book, as noted, follows convention in expressing energy in calories, which are available as carbohydrates, fat, and protein. In the nineteenth century, scientists sought to define these units in chemical terms. Their starting point was the insights of two eighteenth-century French chemists. Many chemists and historians of science regard the more famous of the two, Antoine Lavoisier (1743–1794), as a founder of chemistry and "Father of Nutritional Science."[11] Unquestionably, he did much to emancipate it from alchemy, helping expand the experimental methods of modern science in the process. Among other accomplishments, his experiments demonstrated that plants consist of the elements carbon (C), hydrogen (H), oxygen (O), sulfur (S), and phosphorus (P). To these, his compatriot Claude-Louis Berthellot (1748–1822) added nitrogen (N, not to be confused with newton). He and Lavoisier did not identify all elements in plants, but their contributions were a start. Their work applied to nutrition. In eating plants, people ingest these elements, which nourish them. Put another way, carbon, hydrogen, sulfur, and the rest must give people energy, help them use it, serve as the body's building blocks, or some combination of these possibilities. This insight charged chemists with the task of describing how combinations of these elements, known as molecules, energized the body.

The fact that energy comes from molecules undergirds this chapter. As in the nineteenth century, our focus is on the molecules of energy: carbohydrates, fat, and protein, which later sections examine. Here, brief definitions must suffice. Carbohydrates include sugars and their constructs starch and glycogen. The formula is $C_@(H_2O)_\#$, where @ and # are positive integers. Where @ equals, the ratio of carbon to hydrogen to oxygen simplifies to 1:2:1. The presence of water (H_2O) in this formula occasioned the name "hydrates of carbon," known simply as carbohydrates.

Just as starch and glycogen, both discussed later, are aggregates of sugars, fat, a class of lipids, is constructed from simpler molecules: fatty acids and the alcohol glycerol ($C_3H_8O_3$), also known as glycerin (sometimes spelled glycerine). A fatty acid has a carboxylic acid at one end, which is probably best understood by inspection of its structure:

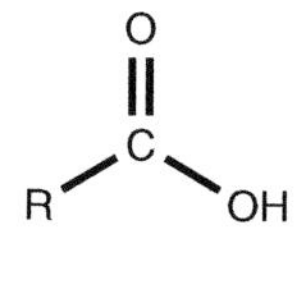

FIGURE 2.1 Carboxylic acid. (Structure from ChemDraw.)

The lines denote bonds, of which carbon forms four. In this diagram, the central carbon accounts for these four with a double bond to oxygen and single bonds each to a hydroxyl group (OH) and R. R denotes a chain with a spine of bonded carbon atoms of unspecified length. In a fatty acid, R almost always has an even number of carbons, typically four to twenty-four. At R's other end in a fatty acid is a methyl group (CH_3), the name taken from methane, a single carbon bonded to four hydrogens (CH_4).

Turning to the alcohol, glycerol has the structure:

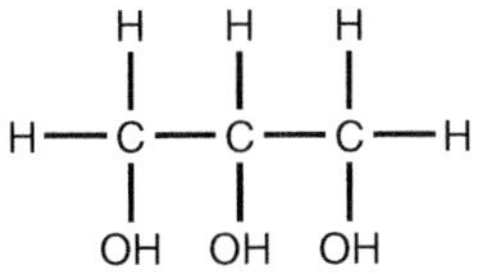

FIGURE 2.2 The alcohol glycerol. (Structure from ChemDraw.)

A fatty acid and glycerol may combine to form a fat molecule as illustrated by the following diagram.

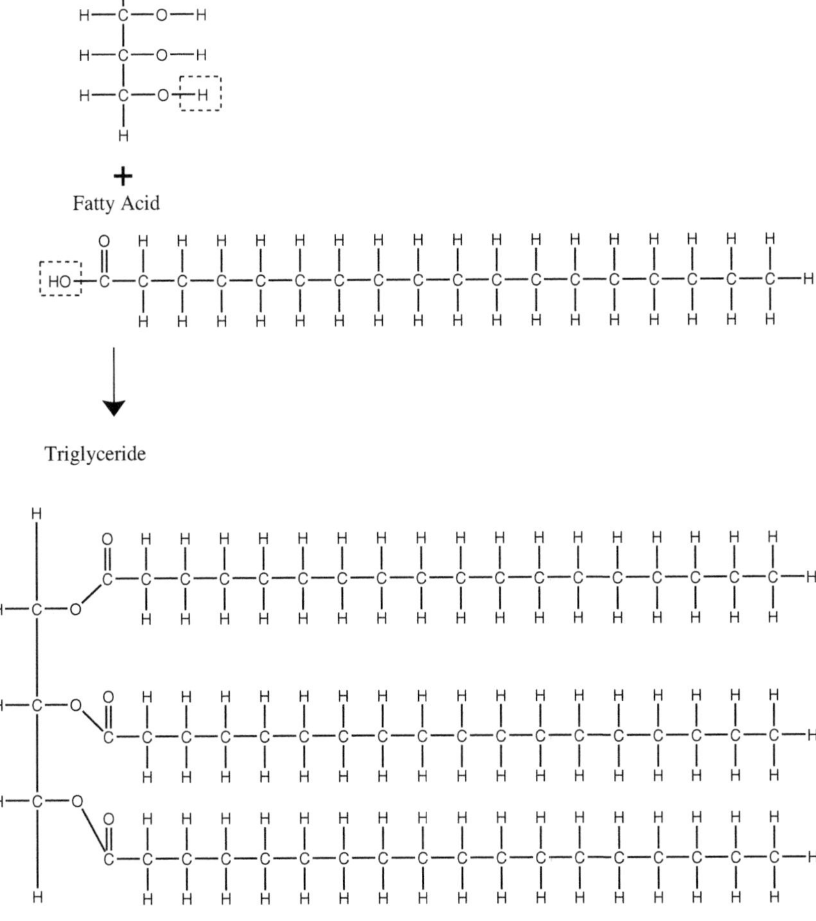

FIGURE 2.3 Formation of triglyceride. (Structure from ChemDraw.)

Note that hydrogen in glycerol and the hydroxyl group in the fatty acid—each within a rectangle in Figure 2.3—play important roles in forming the above fat molecule. Hydrogen has a positive charge (H^+), and the hydroxyl group has a negative charge (OH^-). These opposites attract so that H^+ and OH^- form H_2O. This reaction liberates or releases water and is known as dehydration. The liberation of water leaves the oxygen in glycerol to bond with the carbon that had been part of the terminal carboxylic acid in the fatty acid to form the fat molecule. In this case, the result is a triglyceride (also rendered triacylglycerol or TAG), named after the three-part structure.

Proteins contain nitrogen in an amine (NH_2), taking the form:

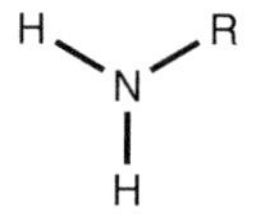

FIGURE 2.4 Amine group. (Structure from ChemDraw.)

This amine combines with a carboxyl group to form:

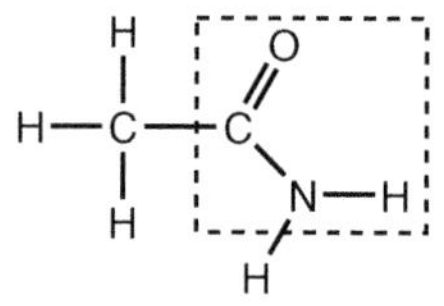

FIGURE 2.5 Example of protein. (Structure from ChemDraw.)

The linkage between carbon and nitrogen, shown within a rectangle for emphasis in Figure 2.5, is a peptide bond and signifies proteins.

Returning to a general discussion of energy, a piece of laboratory equipment known as a bomb calorimeter measures calories in carbohydrates, fat, and protein. Numbers may vary, clustering near 3.6 calories per gram for the sugar glucose ($C_6H_{12}O_6$), 4.1 for starch, 5.6 for protein, and 9.4 for fat.[12] Note that glucose and starch, both carbohydrates, differ by half a calorie per gram, debunking the generalization that all carbohydrates have about 4 calories per gram as too imprecise for comfort. Having the most calories by mass, fat is the richest energy source. Alcohol also has calories but will not receive treatment in order to focus on foods rather than beverages. Admittedly the distinction between food and beverage is somewhat arbitrary. Any nourishment may be classified as food. For this reason, part of Chapter 7 examines milk in the conviction that it qualifies as food and beverage. Carbohydrates, fat, and protein aside, the body requires minerals, vitamins, possibly some phytochemicals, and water, none of which has calories.

A focus on carbohydrates, fat, and protein yields the observation that carbohydrates, despite their status as pariahs, have under half the calories in fat by mass. In fact, the disaccharide sucrose ($C_{12}H_{22}O_{11}$) has just one-third the calories in fat. A dieter who shuns this sugar (see below and Chapter 11) for olive oil (see Chapter 10) in the belief that it is a "healthy fat" but who does not reduce portions risks tripling calories. This switch is questionable from the perspective of mass reduction or maintenance.

From this observation follows the consequence that foods with carbohydrates but little fat tend to have fewer calories than those laden with oil, butter, ghee, margarine, cream, lard, or kindred products (see Chapters 7 and 10 for discussion of dairy and fat, respectively). The emphasis should be on whole foods rather than their processed counterfeits, which usually have plentiful sugars, fat, and salt but few minerals, vitamins, and phytochemicals and little protein.

Tables 2.1 and 2.2 show the difference between low- and high-fat foods. Among low-fat options per 100 grams (3.5 ounces) fresh, celery (*Apium graveolens*) has roughly sixteen calories, cabbage (mentioned earlier) and cucumber (*Cucumis sativus*) eighteen, mushroom (*Agaricus bisporus* and other edible species) and spinach (*Spinacia oleracea*) twenty-three, watermelon (*Citrullus lanatus*) twenty-nine, strawberry (*Fragaria x ananassa*) thirty-five, and carrot (*Daucus carota*) thirty-nine.[13] Even the potato—mentioned above and whose nutrition Chapter 13 discusses—despite its reputation as fattening in some circles, has just seventy-nine calories per 100 grams fresh.[14] Among fatty whole foods per 100 grams fresh, olives (*Olea europaea*) have about 104 calories, avocados (*Persea Americana*) 117, egg yolks 322, pistachios (*Pistacia vera*) and peanuts (*Arachis hypogaea*) 560, cashews (*Anacardium occidentale*) 578, almonds (*Prunus dulcis*) 595, and walnuts (*Juglans* species) 613.[15]

These comparisons should not be construed as justification for eliminating fat from the diet because some whole foods rich in them—egg yolk for example—have many nutrients. Moreover, as a later section emphasizes, the body cannot manufacture all fatty acids, making necessary ingestion of those essential to health. At the same time and as noted abundant fatty foods may make the dieter gain unwanted kilograms, a problem that inactivity compounds.

The amount of energy in foods is not identical to how many calories the body absorbs because digestion is imperfect. As a rule, the body absorbs between 97 and 99 percent of the carbohydrates it ingests, 95 percent of fat, and 92 or 93 percent of protein.[16] Digestibility, like other aspects of nutrition, is subject to revision in the light of new research. For example, U.S. Department of Agriculture (USDA) scientists announced in 2018 that the body absorbs fewer calories from almonds, pistachios, and walnuts—all mentioned in the previous paragraph as caloric foods because of fat content—than

TABLE 2.1
Calories and Fat in Low Fat Foods

Food (100 g)	Fat (g)	Calories
Celery	0	16
Cabbage	0.16	18
Cucumber	0	18
Mushroom	0	23
Spinach	0	23
Watermelon	0	29
Strawberries	0.3	35
Carrot	0	39
Potato	0	79

TABLE 2.2
Calories and Fat in Fatty Foods

Food (100 g)	Fat (g)	Calories
Olives	21.16	104
Avocado	9.8	117
Egg yolks	21.2	322
Pistachios	45.5	560
Peanuts	49.3	560
Cashews	49	578
Almonds	52.5	595
Walnuts	59.5	613

nutritionists previously thought.[17] Additionally, as noted later, little protein is available as energy because the body needs most for muscles.

Humans and other animals must consume food for energy because, Chapter 3 emphasizes, they are heterotrophs, organism that cannot manufacture energy and nutrients, except for vitamin D in the presence of sunlight. Heterotrophs contrast with autotrophs—plants, algae, and photosynthetic bacteria—which use sunlight for energy. Heterotrophs use food to fuel the chemical reactions that sustain life. Absent food's energy, cessation of these reactions causes death. The fact that life requires energy raises the issue of quantification: How much energy does the body need for maintenance, growth, and reproduction? This question is difficult to answer given that several factors influence requirements.

Rather than a rigid amount, Tables 2.3 and 2.4 indicate that the U.S. Department of Health and Human Services (HHS) in Washington, DC recommended that women consume between 1,600 and 2,400 calories daily and men between 2,400 and 3,200.[18] The department's calculations by age and activity represent a curve whereby number of calories increases until roughly age twenty, after which it decreases.

TABLE 2.3
Calorie Requirements for Women from HHS

Age (yr)	Sedentary (cal)	Moderately active (cal)	Active (cal)
2	1,000	1,000	1,000
3	1,000	1,200	1,400
4	1,200	1,400	1,400
5	1,200	1,400	1,600
6	1,200	1,400	1,600
7	1,200	1,600	1,800
8	1,400	1,600	1,800
9	1,400	1,600	1,800
10	1,400	1,800	2,000
11	1,600	1,800	2,000
12	1,600	2,000	2,200
13	1,600	2,000	2,200
14	1,800	2,000	2,400
15	1,800	2,000	2,400
16	1,800	2,000	2,400
17	1,800	2,000	2,400
18	1,800	2,000	2,400
19–20	2,000	2,200	2,400
21–25	2,000	2,200	2,400
26–30	1,800	2,000	2,400
31–35	1,800	2,000	2,200
36–40	1,800	2,000	2,200
41–45	1,800	2,000	2,200
46–50	1,800	2,000	2,200
51–55	1,600	1,800	2,200
56–60	1,600	1,800	2,200
61–65	1,600	1,800	2,000
66–70	1,600	1,800	2,000
71–75	1,600	1,800	2,000
76+	1,600	1,800	2,000

TABLE 2.4
Calorie Requirements for Men from HHS

Age (yr)	Sedentary (cal)	Moderately active (cal)	Active (cal)
2	1,000	1,000	1,000
3	1,000	1,400	1,400
4	1,200	1,400	1,600
5	1,200	1,400	1,600
6	1,400	1,600	1,800
7	1,400	1,600	1,800
8	1,400	1,600	2,000
9	1,600	1,800	2,000
10	1,600	1,800	2,200
11	1,800	2,000	2,200
12	1,800	2,200	2,400
13	2,000	2,200	2,600
14	2,000	2,400	2,800
15	2,200	2,600	3,000
16	2,400	2,800	3,200
17	2,400	2,800	3,200
18	2,400	2,800	3,200
19–20	2,600	2,800	3,000
21–25	2,400	2,800	3,000
26–30	2,400	2,600	3,000
31–35	2,400	2,600	3,000
36–40	2,400	2,600	2,800
41–45	2,200	2,600	2,800
46–50	2,200	2,400	2,800
51–55	2,200	2,400	2,800
56–60	2,200	2,400	2,600
61–65	2,000	2,400	2,600
66–70	2,000	2,200	2,600
71–75	2,000	2,200	2,600
76+	2,000	2,200	2,400

Readers may compare HHS's numbers with those from American nutritionist and microbiologist Anne E. Maczulak in Tables 2.5 and 2.6, though she omitted the category "moderately active."[19]

Science authors and editors Louise Eaton and Kara Rogers estimated women and men's daily calorie requirements between 2,000 and 4,000.[20] Dutch historian Willem Marinus Jongman put daily needs, in Table 2.7, between 2,200 and 2,903 calories for men between ages fifteen and seventy and between 1,883 and 2,400 for women between these years.[21] His numbers for men peaked at age twenty and for women at age fifteen, diminishing thereafter.

Table 2.8's estimates came from British physician and nutritionist Sarah Brewer. Omitting activity, Brewer recommended 2,294–3,155 calories for men between ages fifteen and seventy-five, with intake peaking at age eighteen.[22] Her calories for women between these ages were 1,840–2,462, with the apex at ages seventeen and eighteen.

Calorie requirements vary with activity. Even during deepest sleep, when someone is least active, the body needs energy to circulate blood, breathe, and perform other minimal functions. As the previous paragraph implied, the body's chemical reactions do not cease when a person is inactive,

TABLE 2.5
Calorie Requirements for Women from Maczulak

Age (yr)	Sedentary (cal)	Active (cal)
2–3	1,000	1,400
4–8	1,200	1,800
9–13	1,600	2,200
14–18	1,800	2,400
19–30	2,000	2,400
31–50	1,800	2,200
51+	1,600	2,200

TABLE 2.6
Calorie Requirements for Men from Maczulak

Age (yr)	Sedentary (cal)	Active (cal)
2–3	1,000	1,400
4–8	1,200	2,000
9–13	1,800	2,600
14–18	2,200	3,200
19–30	2,400	3,000
31–50	2,200	3,000
51+	2,000	2,800

TABLE 2.7
Calorie Requirement for Men and Women from Jongman

Age (yr)	Men (cal)	Women (cal)
1	757	700
5	1323	1226
10	1984	1762
15	2700	2400
20	2903	2285
25	2683	2083
30	2683	2083
35	2600	2117
40	2600	2117
45	2600	2117
50	2600	2117
55	2600	2117
60	2600	2117
65	2200	1883
70	2200	1883

TABLE 2.8
Calorie Requirements for Men and Women from Brewer

Age	Men (cals)	Women (cals)
0–2 mo	574	502
3–4 mo	598	550
5–6 mo	622	574
7–12 mo	718	646
1 yr	765	717
2 yr	1,004	932
3 yr	1,171	1,076
4 yr	1,386	1,291
5 yr	1,482	1,362
6 yr	1,577	1,482
7 yr	1,649	1,530
8 yr	1,745	1,625
9 yr	1,840	1,721
10 yr	2,032	1,936
11 yr	2,127	2,032
12 yr	2,247	2,103
13 yr	2,414	2,223
14 yr	2,629	2,342
15 yr	2,820	2,390
16 yr	2,964	2,414
17 yr	3,083	2,462
18 yr	3,155	2,462
19–24 yr	2,772	2,175
25–34 yr	2,749	2,175
35–44 yr	2,629	2,103
55–64 yr	2,581	2,079
65–74 yr	2,342	1,912
75+ yr	2,294	1,840

though they are slower than during exertion. The energy needed to maintain the body during rest, known as basal metabolism (basal metabolic rate or BMR), represents roughly 45–65 percent of daily expenditures.[23] Applying the mean of 55 percent to the HHS figures and assuming equilibrium between energy intake and outlay, BMR should be between 880 and 1,320 calories per day for women and between 1,320 and 1,760 for men.

Activity uses energy, though many factors modify the total. Recalling physics' definitions of work and energy, activity that requires the body to move some distance necessarily burns calories. The amount depends on several variables, mass being one. In the vernacular, the question of heaviness becomes and attempt to fix an object's weight, but weight and mass differ. Weight depends on gravity whereas mass, being the amount of matter, is independent of gravity. That is, mass never varies when the amount of matter is constant, whereas the weight of a static unit of matter changes with the pull of gravity. A 100-pound object on Earth—the pound being the English unit of weight—weighs just 16.5 pounds on the moon, but 100 kilograms, being mass, are 100 kilograms everywhere in the universe. Consistency and conformity to the SI mandate that this book favors mass over weight, though as a courtesy it supplies both, with weight in parentheses and in English units.

Many sports and recreational pursuits, for example, walking, jogging, bicycling, and tennis, require the body to move. Because the body is the load, its mass affects metabolism such that the heavier the mass the more energy is necessary to move it. Distance is also an issue because, all else equal, more energy is needed the greater the distance to be traversed. These factors are evident in daily life. Revisiting the hypothetical grass cutter, his exertions will be more strenuous, and he will burn more calories, the heavier the mower and the larger the yard.

The foregoing acknowledges that variables complicate calculation of calories metabolized per activity, undermining the generality that a walker, for example, burns roughly 60 calories per kilometer (100 calories per mile).[24] Beyond mass, hilliness and ruggedness of terrain, wind, and physiological responses to temperature modify demand for energy. Speed is another consideration, though its effect on metabolism can be exaggerated. At greater velocities, exertions per unit time increase, creating a sensation that the activity burns more calories even when work is constant.

Although calculation of energy metabolized per activity is fraught with difficulties, active people burn many calories. In 2009, United Kingdom (UK) pharmacologist Paul Clayton and historian Judith D. Rowbotham (b. 1952), both introduced in Chapter 1, estimated that the arduousness of life and work about 1850 led British women to burn between 2,750 and 3,500 calories per day and men between 3,000 and 4,500.[25]

Such vigor was not anomalous. On the eve of the potato famine in 1845, Irish men ate as many as 9.5 kilograms (21 pounds) of potatoes daily, though between 4.5 and 6.5 kilograms (10 and 14 pounds) might be safer estimates.[26] Where and when available, other vegetables, cabbage and turnips chief among them, and milk or buttermilk (see Chapter 7) supplemented the diet. Omitting milk and other vegetables yields an upper bound of 7,315 calories daily given a USDA estimate of 770 calories per kilogram of potatoes.[27] Given this number's enormity, a realistic figure may be derived from 4.5 to 6.5 kilograms of potatoes daily, or between 3,465 and 5,005 calories per day. Irish laborers were not overweight, suggesting equilibrium between intake and expenditure. They may therefore have burned between 3,465 and 5,005 calories daily, a range that does not contradict Clayton and Rowbotham's estimates.

2.3 CARBOHYDRATES

2.3.1 Sugars

The previous section noted that simple sugars build complex carbohydrates like starch and glycogen $(C_6H_{10}O_5)_n$, where n is a positive integer. The most basic sugar, glucose (also known as dextrose), is fundamental to life. Through photosynthesis, plants use sunlight to manufacture glucose from carbon dioxide and water according to the reaction

$$6CO_2 + 6H_2O \rightarrow C_6H_{12}O_6 + 6O_2$$

Glucose is a carbohydrate because it fits the formula mentioned in the last section. For completeness, plants construct glucose by taking carbon dioxide (CO_2) from the air and water from the soil. In addition to glucose, photosynthesis produces the oxygen (O_2) necessary for aerobic respiration. Without oxygen, life would consist of only plants and anaerobic microbes. All other organisms, including humans, could not have evolved without the oxygen that plants supply.

Glucose is one of several sugars available in foods. All cannot receive treatment here, but a handful has played important dietary and historical roles. Fructose, along with glucose, is the sugar in honey, high fructose corn syrup (HFCS), and many fruits and vegetables. Fructose has the same formula as glucose but a different structure and a unique metabolic pathway in the body. Chemists categorize the two as isomers because of these properties. Among natural sugars, fructose tastes sweetest. Sweetness is potent in HFCS, examined in Chapter 11, a product of corn starch. In the 1960s, American and Japanese chemists treated corn starch with enzymes to generate corn syrup. Addition of the enzyme xylose isomerase converted some of the resulting glucose into fructose such that HFCS is typically 45 percent glucose and 55 percent fructose, though the latter may be up to 90 percent.[28] By comparison, sucrose, discussed below, is roughly half glucose and half fructose.

Not all the body's organs can metabolize fructose whereas cells throughout the body can metabolize glucose. In the case of fructose, the liver is the primary engine of metabolism, using the sugar to rebuild its store of glycogen. The liver can also use fructose to manufacture a class of fats known as triglycerides, whose structure the last section illustrated. Unlike glucose, the body can metabolize fructose without the hormone and protein insulin. This property allows many diabetics to tolerate fructose better than other sugars. Nonetheless, research implicates fructose in insulin resistance and type 2 diabetes. Additionally, fructose may not prod the brain to signal satiety. Absence of fullness may cause a person to overeat, thereby gaining fat and increasing risk of type 2 diabetes, heart disease, and some cancers.

Among sugars, sucrose has inordinately shaped history. In sugarcane stems and sugar-beet taproot, sucrose has stimulated taste buds since prehistory. Sugarcane fueled the rise of plantations and slavery in the Americas, lands that still grapple with the racism spawned by unequal and unjust economic, social, and political systems. Chemically, sucrose contains molecules of both glucose and fructose, as noted. By mass, sucrose has the same calories (roughly 3.6 per gram) as glucose or fructose and, Chapter 11 notes, has come under scrutiny for undermining health.[29] Like other sugars, sucrose is empty calories, supplying nothing beyond energy. No more helpful is manufacturers' addition of it to processed foods, which have too many sugars and artificial ingredients and too much fat and salt. In such arrangements, sucrose is not the lone villain and attempts to assign it special blame may be misguided (see Chapter 11) given that manufacturers cluster it among allied rubbish, all deserving condemnation.

For completeness, the word "salt" is imprecise because there are many salts, all forming from reactions between acids and bases. Nutritionists and dieticians use the term to mean table salt, the ionic compound sodium chloride (NaCl). It forms a crystal from union of the metal sodium (Na) and the nonmetal chlorine (Cl) in a 1:1 ratio. Such arrangements typify ionic compounds. Although sodium has a dismal reputation among nutritionists, it and chlorine are nutrients. In excess, however, both weaken health. The section on minerals examines them.

The sugar in milk, lactose has the same formula as sucrose; both are disaccharides, though their structures differ. Producing the enzyme lactase, the small intestine digests lactose. People without this enzyme suffer distress upon consuming milk, a phenomenon that Chapter 7 discusses. This condition may exist at birth. In other cases, people can digest lactose as infants only to reduce lactase production with age, impairing milk tolerance. In regions where dairying has a long history—parts of northern Europe, for example—natural selection has equipped most people to produce lactase throughout life and thereby to tolerate milk. Those intolerant need not eschew all dairy products. Being concentrated in milk solids, lactose is largely absent from butter. Separation of curd from whey and removal of the lactose-rich whey from cheese lower the lactose content. Moreover, enzymes that help make many types of cheese break down lactose. A similar process occurs to produce many yogurts.

Chapter 12 mentions that the addition of grains, first harvested as wild plants at least 22,500 years ago, to diets in southwestern Asia and their subsequent spread to many parts of the world introduced humans to the sugar maltose, another disaccharide with the formula $C_{12}H_{22}O_{11}$.[30] The advent of grain cultivation heralded the beginnings of agriculture in southwestern Asia. Among grains, barley (*Hordeum vulgare*) attracted attention as much for making beer as bread. Although ancient peoples were not chemists in any modern sense, they understood how to manipulate barley's maltose content to produce the alcohol ethanol (C_2H_5OH). Through a process known as malting, they soaked seeds in water to hasten germination. Drying these seeds after germination halted growth, stabilizing the amount of maltose for conversion into ethanol.

2.3.2 Starch

Sugars may be stored as starch in plants or as glycogen or fat in animals. Storage holds energy that may be used during lean times in the way that a person might put money in a bank to cover expenses should he lose employment. Sunlight is the ultimate source of energy. Recall that plants use sunlight to manufacture glucose, whose energy fuels their growth and maintenance and whose excess is stored as starch by linking together glucose molecules. The simplest starch molecule, known as amylose, comprises 1,000–600,000 such units.[31] The formula $(C_6H_{10}O_5)_{\#}$, where # is a positive integer, characterizes starch, which is found in plant structures that evolved as energy depots. For example, the edible tubers of the potato plant, being storehouses, hold roughly 87 percent of their carbohydrates as starch.[32] Seeds also tend to have starch to fuel germination. For instance, by mass oats are 45–62 percent starch but under 1 percent sugars.[33]

Due to their structure, not all starches affect the body the same. Being large, straight, and helical, amylose slows digestive enzymes from breaking it apart and is classified as resistant starch. The more amylose food has, the harder it is to digest. Although this characteristic might seem undesirable, foods that resist digestion do not inundate the bloodstream with glucose and so do not cause the pancreas to overproduce insulin. The body needs insulin to metabolize glucose, but too much produced too quickly and too often creates a condition known as insulin insensitivity, whereby cells lose their ability to respond to the hormone. This problem contributes to chronic diseases, notably type 2 diabetes, a malady linked to heart disease, stroke, and kidney disease. In 2017, the U.S. Centers for Disease Control and Prevention (CDC) in Atlanta, Georgia, estimated that 100 million Americans have this kind of diabetes or are on its threshold.[34] In contrast to amylose, the starch amylopectin, although larger, arrays its glucose molecules in branches that digestive enzymes readily dismantle. The more amylopectin in food, the more rapid is digestion, causing the above cascade of perils.

2.3.3 Fiber

Unable to produce enzymes to cleave them, the body cannot digest carbohydrates termed fiber, roughage, or bulk. An example is cellulose, which has the same formula as starch and which plants use to make rigid cell walls. Crucifers, all in the Brassicaceae or Cruciferae family, contain abundant cellulose and include broccoli (*Brassica oleracea var. italica*), kale (*Brassica oleracea var. sabellica*), Brussels sprouts (*Brassica oleracea var. gemmifera*), cauliflower (*Brassica oleracea var. botrytis*), and cabbage (mentioned earlier). Packed with cellulose, these vegetables do not expand the waistline, demonstrating that indigestibility makes fiber a dieter's friend. In addition to controlling mass, fiber-rich foods diminish constipation, the risk of type 2 diabetes, and blood levels of low-density lipoproteins (LDL or "bad cholesterol"), whose properties are discussed later.

Fiber is soluble or insoluble depending on whether it dissolves in water. Soluble fiber, useful against LDL, is in many whole foods, including peas (*Pisum sativum*), beans (*Phaseolus vulgaris, P. lunatus, P. acutifolius*, and *P. coccineus*), oats, citrus fruits, apples (*Malus domestica*), and barley. Insoluble fiber promotes regularity and may be consumed in potatoes, nuts, beans, and wheat (*Triticum monococcum, T. dicoccon, T. aestivum*, and *T. durum*) bran among other foods.

Being a type of carbohydrate, fiber is absent from fat and protein. Consequently, diets rich in these macronutrients tend to lack fiber. Such fare pervades developed countries and affluence everywhere. As incomes rise, people buy meat, eggs, milk, cheese, and other animal products, which crowd plants from the diet. To be sure, animal products contain nutrients but not fiber.

Consider the hamburger, a fast-food staple. The ground beef lacks fiber. The bun has fiber, though the amount may be meager. If made from whole wheat, the bun has roughly 3 grams of fiber per around 50 grams of bread, the standard for a bun.[35] But the fast-food hamburger comes on white bread, which reduces fiber below 1 gram per bun because milling, a process discussed in Chapter 12, strips most of the bran from flour, thereby removing fiber.[36] The consumer might add cheese or bacon to enhance flavor but neither has fiber. Among condiments, 100 grams of mustard have 4 grams of fiber, but the same amount of ketchup or mayonnaise has none.[37] Lettuce (*Lactuca sativa*), tomato (*Solanum esculentum*), and onion (*Allium cepa*) are the most fibrous additions to the hamburger, but what the consumer buys has little roughage. McDonald's counts 3 grams of fiber in its big mac and mushroom and swiss burger, 2 grams in its cheeseburger and bacon smokehouse burger, and 1 gram in its hamburger.[38] McDonald's computes just 6 percent of fiber's daily value (DV) in its hamburger.

Table 2.9 shows that hamburgers deserve no special animus in a world full of low-fiber options. Snacks bulge from supermarket shelves and fill stomachs with little besides fat and sugars. For example, U.S. bakery Hostess Brands' twinkies lack fiber, and ho hos at 85 grams per serving, cupcakes at 45 grams, and ding dongs at 72 grams have 1 gram of it.[39] Being sucrose or HFCS and water, soft drinks and related beverages lack roughage. Depending on the brand, ice cream and chocolate may have some, but in small quantities. Dunkin' Donuts lists a single glazed jelly donut at 1 gram of fiber.[40] Kellogg's tallies under 1 gram of fiber in one brown sugar cinnamon pop tart.[41] These and kindred items are prevalent not because the food industry is particularly malevolent but because consumers demand them. Chapter 3 treats flavor preferences and cravings from an evolutionary perspective.

By contrast, Table 2.10 indicates that whole plant foods tend to have fiber.[42]

TABLE 2.9
Fiber in Processed Foods

Manufacturer	Product (100 g)	Fiber (g)
McDonald's	Big mac	1.38
McDonald's	Mushroom and swiss	1.4
McDonald's	Cheeseburger	1.75
McDonald's	Bacon smokehouse burger	N/A
McDonald's	Hamburger	1
Hostess	Twinkie	0
Hostess	Ho Ho	1.18
Hostess	Cup cake	2.2
Hostess	Ding dong	1.39
Hostess	Soft drink	0
Dunkin Donuts	Glazed jelly donut	1
Kellogg	Brown sugar cinnamon pop tart	<2

TABLE 2.10
Fiber in Whole Foods

Whole Food (100 g)	Fiber (g)
Dried apricots	18
Prunes	13
Dried figs	8
Oatmeal	7
Kidney beans	7
Whole grain bread	7
Mixed nuts	6
Peas	5
Dried dates	4
Whole grain pasta	4

2.3.4 Glycemic Index

Scientists use the glycemic index (GI), a scale between zero and 100, to quantify carbohydrates' digestibility. Recall that sugars are easily digested, enter the bloodstream rapidly, and spike insulin production. Glucose provokes the fastest increase, signified by a value of 100. At the opposite pole, fiber does not raise insulin production and so rates zero. That is, numerical values correlate with insulin production such that the nearer a food comes to 100, the more it elevates the hormone. The Glycemic Index Foundation in New South Wales, Australia, ranks foods as low (under 46), medium (between 46 and 59), or high (more than 59) and cautions against consumption of foods medium or high on the index.[43] These categories are not absolute because not all scientists partition numbers the same way.

2.3.5 Glycogen

Like plants, animals store sugars, as noted, converting them into glycogen or fat. Like starch and cellulose in plants, animals construct glycogen from glucose molecules. Such duplication is unsurprising because these aggregates serve similar purposes in plants and animals and because all life shares a common evolutionary heritage such that the more closely related are two organisms the greater tends to be their chemistry. Muscles and the liver store glycogen but not in quantity, the body holding only about 1 percent of mass as it.[44] Despite such parsimony, glycogen is important. Evolution equipped people to draw upon it for a burst of energy. In crises, the body prepares for battle or retreat, metabolizing glycogen, as well as fatty acids, in expectation of strenuous exertions. Muscles and the brain prefer to draw energy from the glucose in glycogen.[45] Physical activity, including athletics and vigorous recreation, demands carbohydrates. Even endurance athletes metabolize carbohydrates over fat. To be sure, the body burns fat during exertions but only by increasing the demand for oxygen over that required for carbohydrates.

2.3.6 Other Functions of Carbohydrates

Beyond being energy, carbohydrates enable the body to synthesize the molecule of heredity, deoxyribonucleic acid (DNA), and its messenger, ribose nucleic acid (RNA). No cell can exist much less function without them. As with DNA and RNA manufacture, glucose allows the body to make the monosaccharide glucuronic acid, which increases wastes' solubility in urine or bile. Glucose, fructose, and the sugar galactose help the body form protective mucus. Through various pathways, carbohydrates increase cells' efficiency and aid in creating humans' four blood types.

2.3.7 Carbohydrate Critics

Carbohydrates' importance has not spared them criticism, a topic that Chapters 10 and 11 also treat. An earlier paragraph implicated sugars in type 2 diabetes, but hostility goes farther. Nutritionists, dieticians, researchers, and physicians who left the 1980s low-fat bandwagon disparage carbohydrates. Several of the most strident critics have written best-selling books with trade publishers. The dust jacket to American neurologist David Perlmutter's (b. 1954) 2018 edition of *Grain Brain* boasts "more than 1 million copies in print." He targeted carbohydrates and gluten, a complex of over one hundred proteins in some grains, which makes dough sticky, elastic, and able to rise during baking. Because grains have starch and sugars, animus toward gluten provides ammunition against carbohydrates, which Perlmutter characterized as unnatural because the body supposedly prefers to metabolize fat for energy.[46] Carbohydrates' putative unnaturalness predisposes the body to several ailments, including overweight and obesity. He blamed the food industry, especially breakfast cereal companies, for deceiving Americans about carbohydrates. Profits trump health in a case where capitalism devours the masses.

Perlmutter is not a lone voice in the wilderness. Losing more than 14 kilograms (30 pounds) each by cutting carbohydrates, mother Laura Childs and daughter Veronica Childs faulted them for causing an "obesity epidemic" in *The Complete Low Carb, High Fat, No Hunger Diet* (2014).[47] Carbohydrates cause overeating and fatness because they are addictive, prodding the brain to release pleasurable chemicals like neurotransmitter serotonin, believed American dietitian Sandra Woodruff.[48] In the crusade against carbohydrates, American cardiac surgeon Steven R. Gundry excoriated dessert fruits: "The next time you ask for a fruit salad as a 'healthy' breakfast, I suggest that instead you order a bowl of Skittles candy. Go ahead—it's the same poisonous stuff."[49] Readers must decide whether hyperbole enlightens or frightens.

2.4 FAT

2.4.1 Plants and Animals Store Energy Differently

As a rule, animals differ from plants in having extra options for storing energy. The previous section emphasized the body's limited capacity to stockpile energy as glycogen. Beyond this threshold, the body stores energy as fat, whose structure as earlier section described. Although some plants have fat as oils, these lipids seem to be less reserve energy than enticements to tempt animals to eat fatty seeds, which may pass through the digestive tract and be excreted, a phenomenon that Chapter 14 applies to fruits. Excretion deposits them on the ground, which dung fertilizes for seedlings' growth. The previous section—citing peanuts, cashews, walnuts, pistachios, and almonds as examples—noted that some seeds have many calories because of high oil content. Chapters 3 and 10 examine fat, permitting brief treatment here.

2.4.2 Lipids, Fat, and Oil

The previous paragraph introduced fat in the context of lipids and oils. Nutritionists and dieticians think of these as nested categories, the largest being lipids, inside of which is fat, which, in turn, contains oils. But chemists reject this type of nesting, instead defining lipids as the largest category, which houses both fat and oils as separate classes. In this scheme, fats are solid at room temperature, roughly 20 degrees Celsius (68 degrees Fahrenheit), whereas oils are liquid.[50] This book follows nutritional convention in considering oils a type of fat, a simplification that permits treatment of all macronutrients that are neither carbohydrates nor protein as fat. Food labels follow this scheme, dividing macronutrients into fat, carbohydrate, and protein in that order, as shown in the sample.

Original Label

Nutrition Facts
Serving Size 2/3 cup (55g)
Servings Per Container About 8

Amount Per Serving	
Calories 230	Calories from Fat 72
	% Daily Value*
Total Fat 8g	**12%**
Saturated Fat 1g	**5%**
Trans Fat 0g	
Cholesterol 0mg	**0%**
Sodium 160mg	**7%**
Total Carbohydrate 37g	**12%**
Dietary Fiber 4g	**16%**
Sugars 12g	
Protein 3g	
Vitamin A	10%
Vitamin C	8%
Calcium	20%
Iron	45%

* Percent Daily Values are based on a 2,000 calorie diet. Your daily value may be higher or lower depending on your calorie needs.

	Calories:	2,000	2,500
Total Fat	Less than	65g	80g
Sat Fat	Less than	20g	25g
Cholesterol	Less than	300mg	300mg
Sodium	Less than	2,400mg	2,400mg
Total Carbohydrate		300g	375g
Dietary Fiber		25g	30g

New Label

Nutrition Facts
8 servings per container
Serving size 2/3 cup (55g)

Amount per serving	
Calories	**230**
	% Daily Value*
Total Fat 8g	**10%**
Saturated Fat 1g	**5%**
Trans Fat 0g	
Cholesterol 0mg	**0%**
Sodium 160mg	**7%**
Total Carbohydrate 37g	**13%**
Dietary Fiber 4g	**14%**
Total Sugars 12g	
Includes 10g Added Sugars	**20%**
Protein 3g	
Vitamin D 2mcg	10%
Calcium 260mg	20%
Iron 8mg	45%
Potassium 235mg	6%

* The % Daily Value (DV) tells you how much a nutrient in a serving of food contributes to a daily diet. 2,000 calories a day is used for general nutrition advice.

FIGURE 2.6 Food label courtesy of FDA. (FDA public-domain statement https://www.fda.gov/about-fda/about-website/website-policies.)

2.4.3 Saturated Fat

This label introduces the principle of saturation. A saturated fat has carbon atoms forming single bonds, as in the following diagram.

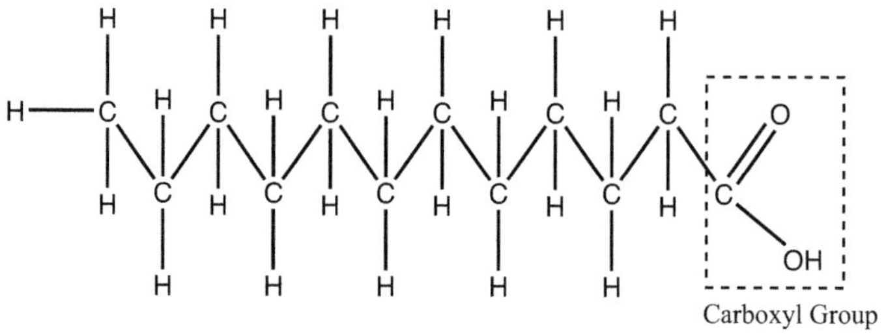

Carboxyl Group

FIGURE 2.7 Example of saturated fat. (Structure from ChemDraw.)

Ignoring the carboxyl group mentioned earlier and within a rectangle in Figure 2.7, each carbon forms two bonds with hydrogen atoms and the other two with adjacent carbons. Aside from the carboxyl group, no carbon has a double bond with another atom.

2.4.4 Unsaturated Fat

In contrast to saturation, unsaturated fats have at least one carbon outside the carboxyl group with a double bond. When only one carbon, excluding the carboxyl group, is involved, the result is a monounsaturated fat. Unsaturated fats with more than one such carbon are polyunsaturated. Comparison of saturated, monounsaturated, and polyunsaturated fats yields the following diagram, whose arrows highlight double bonds apart from the carboxyl group.

Butyric Acid - Saturated Fatty Acid

Oleic Acid - Monounsaturated Fatty Acid

Linoleic Acid - Polyunsaturated Fatty Acid

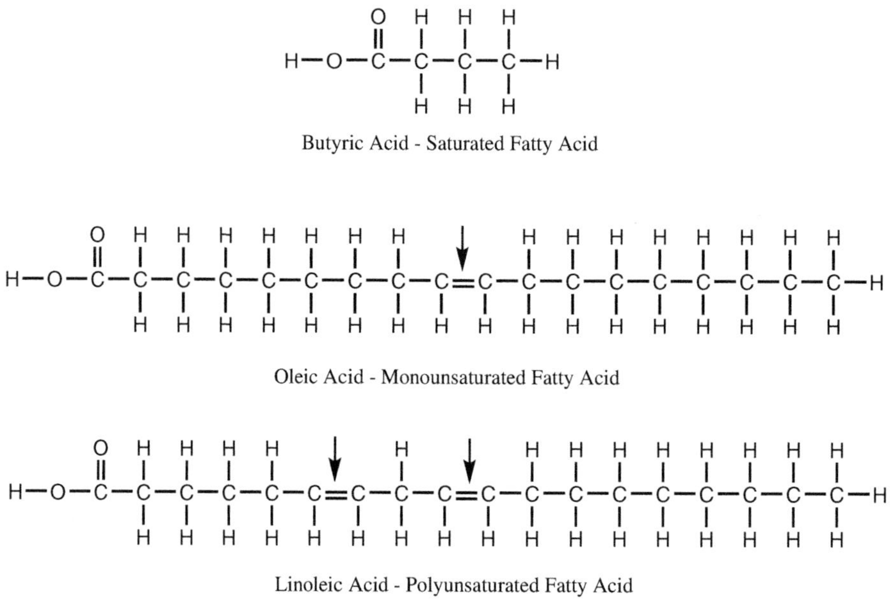

FIGURE 2.8 Comparison of saturated, monounsaturated, and polyunsaturated fatty acids. (Structure from ChemDraw.)

Unsaturated fats promote health better than saturated ones, though the food industry prefers the latter in processed food because they lengthen shelf life and supply textures that consumers favor.[51] Conversion of unsaturated fats into saturated, a process known as hydrogenation, creates foods that increase the risk of heart disease. Attention has focused on partial hydrogenation, which yields trans fats, a configuration uncommon in nature. The U.S. Food and Drug Administration (FDA) in 2015 declared them unsafe, requiring their elimination from foods by January 1, 2020.[52]

2.4.5 Lipids and Organic Solvents

Returning to the concept of nesting and to lipids, the observation that oil and water do not mix applies to all lipids, which dissolve not in water but in alcohols, gasoline, diesel, ether, chloroform, and other organic solvents. Lipids include oils, steroids (notably cholesterol), wax, and the fatty acids mentioned earlier. Oils, the smallest class, are triglycerides, whose structure a previous section illustrated. Their texture and consistency are greasy and thick.

2.4.6 Fat: The Energy Densest Macronutrient

An earlier section described fat as concentrated energy. In general terms, the body derives energy from breaking chemical bonds, a process that may be thought the reverse of photosynthesis, mentioned earlier, whereby plants store energy from sunlight in bonds. Humans and other animals break these bonds through oxidation, a reaction that requires oxygen. Because the body uses more oxygen to break bonds in fat molecules than in carbohydrate or protein molecules, it derives the most energy from fat.

The place of fat in the diet receives treatment from an evolutionary perspective in Chapter 3 and from the vantage point of prehistory and history in Chapter 10. This chapter confines commentary to the observation that throughout the past, food tended to be scarce rather than plentiful. This condition made fat important because it is energy dense. Amid modernity's abundance, however, fatty foods provide too many calories. Of course, excess of any food—excepting the spartan fare of celery, cabbage, cucumber, strawberries, mushrooms, and other austerities mentioned earlier—presents this danger.

2.4.7 Uses of Fat besides Energy

This caveat aside, fat provides more than energy. All the body's cells use fatty acids to construct their membranes, without which no cell can function. The membrane separates animal cells (plant cells have a wall) from their surroundings, preserving their integrity. The membrane's indispensability and the cell's antiquity as the basic unit in microbes, plants, and animals imply that fatty acids are among the earliest organic molecules as life's precursors. Fats are important to the central nervous system (CNS), where they form neural membranes and the myelin sheath that surrounds each neuron's axon. Made of neurons, the brain is roughly 70 percent fat.[53] Cognition, a hallmark of humanity, would be impossible without it.

Fat is the storage medium for the fat-soluble vitamins, which receive treatment later. Its role as storehouse is crucial in another context. Earlier was noted the body's meager ability to store energy as glycogen. As noted, only about 1 percent of body mass is glycogen whereas roughly 25 percent is fat, stored in a type of tissue known as adipose, which holds most of the body's reserve energy.[54] Each adipose cell, known as an adipocyte, harbors a fat droplet. The body retains primarily triglycerides in adipose, possibly an adaptation to the reality that they constitute around 95 percent of edible fats.[55] More than a reserve, adipose insulates the body—an asset in cold but not in heat—cushions organs and helps transmit signals between cells (extracellular) and within a cell (intracellular).

2.4.8 Cholesterol and Its Regulation

Among fats, attention focuses on cholesterol, mentioned earlier, as contributor to heart disease. In this context, medical practitioners distinguish between good and bad cholesterol. This language causes confusion because "good cholesterol" is more than cholesterol—also having protein, triglycerides, and phospholipids (a lipid with phosphorus)—and is known as high-density lipoproteins (HDL).[56] Doctors praise HDL for removing excess cholesterol from the blood whereas low-density lipoproteins (LDL)—having different ratios of the same components—are deemed bad because they carry cholesterol to cells. Cells depend on LDL for it, though problems arise when LDL bring too much. Criticisms of cholesterol should not discount its role in manufacturing cell membranes, acids that help digest food, vitamin D from sunlight, and five types of steroid hormones: progestins, glucocorticoids, mineralocorticoids, estrogens, and androgens, all of which the body requires.

2.4.9 Essential Fatty Acids

The body also needs fatty acids it cannot manufacture: omega-3 and omega-6, both polyunsaturated. Chemists number fatty acids to identify them, analogous to urban planners who number addresses and streets. By convention, chemists begin at the carboxyl group, whose carbon atom is designated alpha to honor the Greek alphabet's first letter. The last carbon, at the methyl end, is omega, the Greek alphabet's last letter. Attending to the methyl (omega) end, nutritionists note the position of the first double bond. For example, an omega-3 fatty acid has its first double bond three carbons from omega. Chapters 3 and 10 treat the nutritional roles and dietary composition of fatty acids, especially omega-3 and omega-6.

2.4.10 Fatty Foods

The body derives fat from foods. Earlier sections mentioned several fatty foods. To this list may be added meat given that livestock fatten as they approach market mass. Sausages, pepperoni, salami, and similar items have abundant fat. Oily fishes include sardine (*Sardina pilchardus*), herring (*Clupea harengus*), anchovy (commercial species are in the genus *Engraulis*), salmon (*Oncorhynchus* species), tuna (*Thunnus thynnus* and *T. albacares*), trout (*Oncorhynchus mykiss*), swordfish (*Xiphias gladius*), and mackerel (*Scomber scombrus*). Dairy products are another option, milk fat having hundreds of fatty acids. Butter, cream, and ghee are primarily fat. Many cheeses, ice creams, and some yogurts have plentiful fat. An ingredient in chocolate, theobroma oil in cacao (*Theobroma cacao*) seeds' cocoa butter has saturated fat, much of it as triglycerides. Nutritionists and dieticians debate the merits of chocolate and cocoa butter. Manufacturers add fat to many processed foods. For example, a serving of Hostess twinkie (77 grams) has 8 grams of fat, most coming from tallow (beef fat).[57] More than one-quarter of its calories are fat. Carbohydrates supply the rest. Another food with processed ingredients, pizza combines cheeses, meats, and vegetable oils, providing more fat and calories than might be desirable. People add fat to foods through frying. In an era of abundance, fat is too plentiful. Chapters 3 and 10 examine fatty foods in diets over time and space.

As noted, fatty foods—nuts were cited as examples—are caloric because fat is energy dense. For this reason, dieters may want to minimize them, though not all promote obesity. Mentioned above, oily fishes are not awash in calories. For example, 100 grams of salmon have 4 grams of fat and 139 calories.[58] These numbers contrast salmon with twinkies, 100 grams of which provides roughly 9 grams of fat and 200 calories. This contrast extends to the big mac, introduced earlier, 100 grams of which supplies about 12 grams of fat and 225 calories.[59] These differences reinforce the fact that not all sustenance is equal. Indeed, readers might doubt that twinkies and similar junk merit designation as sustenance. In addition to Chapters 3 and 10, those on meat (Chapter 4), fish (Chapter 5), dairy (Chapter 7), and nuts (Chapter 9) illuminate fatty foods' health effects.

2.5 PROTEIN

2.5.1 Importance of Protein

Protein, whose structure was illustrated earlier, joins carbohydrates and fat as the third macronutrient. Like carbohydrates and fat, the body can metabolize protein for energy, though not ideally in large quantities. When carbohydrate and fat intake is adequate, the body derives only about 2 percent of energy from protein. In the nineteenth century, a formative period in nutrition, protein was inconspicuous as energy. In 1842, German nobleman and professor Justus von Liebig (1803–1873), a pioneer in nutritional and agricultural chemistry, announced that the body's energy came entirely from carbohydrates and fat, though protein was far from inconsequential.[60] He esteemed it muscles' basic unit. Moreover, protein contained nitrogen, which he considered the primary nutrient for all plants and animals. Although his ideas combined fact and falsehood, Liebig's renown deterred criticism. His work and that of others elevated protein, a word that derived from the Greek *protos*, meaning "first" such that protein has priority among nutrients. Such thinking, whose implications Chapter 4 explores, made meat and other protein-rich foods dietary cornerstones. The nineteenth-century mania for protein led the USDA in the 1890s to counsel men to consume over 110 grams (3.9 ounces) daily.[61]

2.5.2 Recommended Protein Intake

Current recommendations vary, with estimates between 0.3 and 1.2 grams of protein per kilogram (2.2 pounds) of body mass.[62] Variations result from different methods of calculation, which in turn depend on divergent assumptions about digestive efficiency and protein loss through excretion and other processes. At a minimum, age, sex, and dietary quality shape protein requirements. Bodybuilders and athletes who prize strength have long championed protein-rich foods.

The 1890s USDA recommendation may be expressed in grams per kilogram of body mass for an average American man alive then. An absolute is elusive, though the USDA published ranges that vary by height and age. From 1885 to 1900, men averaged between 64 and 89 kilograms (140 and 195 pounds).[63] A recommendation of 110 grams of protein daily translated into 1.7 grams per kilogram of body mass for a 64-kilogram man and just over 1.2 grams per kilogram for an 89-kilogram man. These numbers show that 1890s' advice exceeded the current maximum.

2.5.3 Protein Quantity versus Quality

Preoccupation with numbers may ignore more salient issues. The tussle over how much protein to consume might be compared to a debate over the amount of air to breathe. If it is full of soot and other pollutants, a person should inhale as little as possible and move to a pristine area. In a similar vein, nutritional quality is at least as crucial as quantity because not all proteins are identical. Their components, amino acids, determine quality. Amino acids are fundamental molecules with amine and carboxyl groups, both defined earlier. The body can manufacture from other compounds at least half the twenty amino acids that comprise all life.[64] But it cannot make eight to ten, depending on whom the reader consults, which the diet must supply, and which are therefore essential.[65] In addition, premature newborns and adults with liver damage may require amino acids that are normally unessential.[66]

2.5.4 Protein Sources

Animal products like meat, poultry, eggs, fish, and dairy have all essential amino acids and are regarded complete sources. Some plants are in this category, including potatoes despite seldom being valued in this capacity. As noted, Irish laborers subsisted on them. Chapter 13 examines potato eaters' healthfulness in prehistory and history. This section restricts commentary to the observation that the tuber sustained commoners because of adequate amino acids and other nutrients. Another food seldom linked with amino acids is mushrooms, which also have all essentials.

Traditionally esteemed for protein and amino acids have been legumes and nuts. Chapters 8 and 9 focus on their roles in diet and nutrition, leaving this section to note that, excepting soybeans (*Glycine max*), neither supplies all essential amino acids.[67] Another incomplete source is grains, treated in Chapter 12. They have some protein and amino acids, though taste buds sometimes counter the need for protein and other nutrients. For example, the types of wheat desirable for pastries, cookies, and similar items have starch at the expense of nutrients, including protein. Seeds, root and tuber crops, and kindred foods employ zero-sum properties. Increases in starch diminish space for proteins, vitamins, minerals, phytochemicals, and water. Of course, concentration on protein or appeal to a single criterion provides insufficient breadth for evaluating foods because those deficient in one nutrient may have others.

2.5.5 Inequalities and Protein Intake

Protein quality and quantity require more than an impartial selection of foods. Economic, social, racial, and political inequalities have dietary and nutritional consequences. Developing nations' poor and minorities often cannot afford the complete proteins available in animal products. Later chapters emphasize the pervasiveness of inequalities throughout time and place and their nutritional effects. In modernity as in the past, consumption of meat and allied foods has risen with incomes. This trend yields more and better protein for elites but only by threatening others and the environment as cropland is converted into pasture and as innumerable cattle emit staggering amounts of greenhouse gas methane.

2.5.6 Protein's Roles in the Body

Clamor for animal products cannot be ignored given protein's roles in the body. After water, it is the body's most abundant constituent at roughly 16 percent total mass.[68] Of this amount, about 43 percent is muscle, 16 percent blood, and 15 percent skin, with smaller quantities in other structures. Of the body's proteins, four are most numerous: collagen in skin, tendons, ligaments, and muscles; hemoglobin in blood; and myosin and actin in muscles. Beyond them, every cell in the body has proteins because of genes. DNA, mentioned earlier and present in a cell's nucleus and mitochondria, comprises genes and contains large molecules known as nucleotide bases. Through the intermediary RNA, also mentioned previously, a sequence of three nucleotide bases (codon) directs production of one amino acid outside the nucleus, an area known as the cytoplasm. The order of these bases defines an amino acid. In the cytoplasm, structures known as ribosomes assemble amino acids into proteins.

Proteins perform crucial functions. For example, insulin, mentioned earlier and having fifty-one amino acids, is the hormone that tells cells to admit glucose.[69] In this way, insulin regulates the amounts of glucose inside and outside cells. Insulin also regulates glucose by telling the liver to store excess for release when the sugar becomes scarce in blood. Heme proteins, defined by the presence of iron (Fe), shuttle molecules and electrons throughout the body. Hemoglobin, a component of red blood cells, brings oxygen to cells and removes carbon dioxide for transport to the lungs. Carbon dioxide is a greenhouse gas, though human respiration emits little compared to factories and automobiles. The protein keratin helps form hair and skin. Proteins known as enzymes catalyze the body's reactions. For example, enzymes pepsin and trypsin aid protein digestion by catalyzing cleavage of amino acid peptide bonds, mentioned earlier. Integral to the immune system, proteins that combat pathogens are known as antibodies. Attention has focused on the protein interferon, which targets viruses.

2.6 MINERALS

2.6.1 Need for Minerals

Liebig believed that the macronutrients carbohydrates, fats, and proteins supplied all the body needed for health. Not only was this supposition wrong, but his research helped lay the groundwork for exposing this error. In his role as agricultural chemist, Liebig focused on another nutritional triad, emphasizing that the elements nitrogen, potassium, and phosphorus were plants' most important constituents. Earlier was noted nitrogen's role in amino acids and proteins. Potassium and phosphorus, however, need not be part of organic molecules and are known as minerals, another class of animal nutrient.

2.6.2 Characteristics of Minerals

Minerals differ from carbohydrates, fats, proteins, and phytochemicals (discussed in a later section) in being inorganic compounds. They are solid at room temperature and occur as crystals or other regular structures in rocks, soils (which contain pulverized rocks), meteorites, and dust. From soils, minerals enter roots, thereafter ascending trophic levels to become ubiquitous across flora and fauna and essential to life. Crystalline structure is evident in sodium chloride, mentioned previously and discussed in this section. Nutritionists and dieticians focus on elements within minerals. Having atoms of a single type, each element is unique in nature and a fundamental unit of matter. Shown below, the Periodic Table organizes the elements.

Of the table's 118 elements, ninety-four occur in nature. All heavier than plutonium (Pu) are artificial, being derived in the laboratory.

Left of the zigzag line known as the staircase are metals, notable in electrons' ability to move through them. To the right are nonmetals, which resist electron flow. For completeness, elements on the staircase have characteristics of metals and nonmetals, do not neatly fit either category, and are known as metalloids. Most mineral elements are metals. The major minerals are sodium, calcium, potassium, phosphorus, and magnesium. Necessary in smaller amounts are the minor minerals: manganese, iron, zinc, iodine, fluorine, selenium, copper, chromium, cobalt, and molybdenum. Of these, only fluorine is a nonmetal. Although many nutritionists and dieticians do not consider chlorine a mineral, it appears to fulfill the criteria. It too is a nonmetal. Being in the column (group) of the Periodic Table known as the halogens, fluorine and chlorine share properties. The body needs chlorine as the electrolyte chloride and to make hydrochloric acid, which aids digestion.

2.6.3 Sodium, Chlorine, and Table Salt

These functions may seem incongruous with chlorine's presence in table salt, a villain to nutritionists and dieticians. Salt's other element, sodium, was noted as another mineral. Sodium is in bones, where its function is unknown. Like chlorine, sodium becomes an electrolyte in the body. Sodium and chlorine's roles made salt indispensable to people in hot climates because sweating depletes electrolytes. For this reason, American kinesiologists J. Luke Pryor and Deanna M. Dempsey in 2015 encouraged athletes who perspired heavily to salt food.[70]

Salt's dangers stem from overconsumption. In the body, it ionizes into sodium cations (Na^+) and chloride anions (Cl^-). In this state, attention focuses on sodium's role in raising blood pressure by increasing the density of cations in blood relative to the corresponding density within cells. Through a process known as osmosis, water from cells enters blood to equalize cation density. The heart must work hard to pump this blood, full of extra water, elevating blood pressure. Furthermore, the kidneys must labor to excrete excess sodium. Research also implicates chloride in high blood pressure.[71]

2.6.4 Minerals Interact with Other Nutrients

Exhaustive treatment of minerals is unnecessary. Instead emphasis is on their interactions with other nutrients. In this regard, the relationship between calcium and vitamin D has received study.

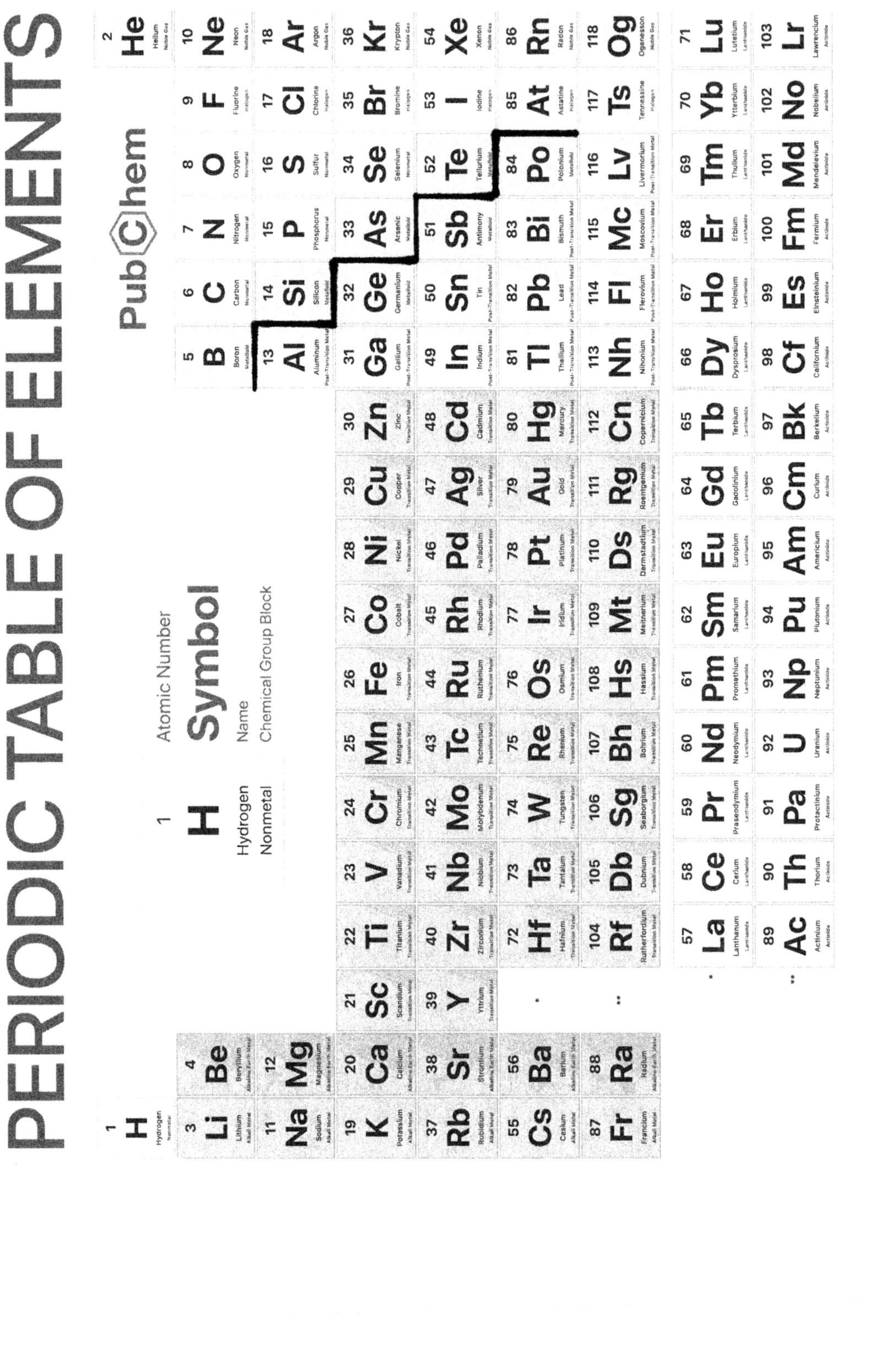

FIGURE 2.9 Periodic Table of the elements. (Adapted from National Institutes of Health [NIH].)

Chapter 1 mentioned vitamin D as an example of a nutrient under scientific, medical, and journalistic scrutiny. The interplay between calcium and vitamin D is wide ranging, affecting bones, teeth, the immune system, muscles including the heart, metabolism, the respiratory system, and retention and activity of phosphorus, magnesium, iron, selenium, copper, and zinc. None of these dynamics was apparent in the eighteenth century, when the rise of factories in Europe and North America lured people from countryside to city and from outdoors to indoors, increasing the number of children with rickets, a condition whereby weak leg bones bow under the upper body's mass.[72] An ailment related to rickets—osteomalacia—afflicted adults. These problems arose because existence indoors deprived skin of sunlight and the concomitant ability to manufacture vitamin D.

Only in the twentieth century did scientists discover this vitamin and begin to understand how it, calcium, and phosphorus prevented and cured rickets and osteomalacia.[73] Bones and teeth require vitamin D to retain calcium, whose absorption improves in the presence of phosphorus and magnesium. Too much phosphorus, however, hinders bones and teeth from absorbing calcium, and too much calcium weakens the body's absorption of phosphorus, zinc, and iron. Calcium also affects the body's uptake of selenium and copper. Magnesium helps regulate vitamin D by reducing excess, increasing dearth, and thereby improving calcium absorption.[74] This list need not be lengthened to underscore the complexity of relationships among minerals and between minerals and vitamins.

2.6.5 Sources of Minerals

A balanced diet gives the body adequate minerals. Nuts, particularly almonds and cashews, provide calcium, copper, iron, selenium, zinc, phosphorus, and magnesium. Seed legumes, notably beans, soybeans, chickpeas (*Cicer arietinum*), and lentils (*Lens culinaris*), supply copper, iron, potassium, phosphorus, zinc, and magnesium. Salmon, tuna, and mackerel have calcium, magnesium, selenium, potassium, and phosphorus. Oysters (species in genera *Crassostrea* and *Ostrea*), mussels (*Mytilus edulis*), clams (*Mercenaria mercenaria* and other edible species), scallops (*Placopecten magellanicus* and other edible species), and other shellfish deliver copper, iron, selenium, phosphorus, and zinc. Seeds from sunflower (*Helianthus annuus*), pumpkin (*Cucurbita pepo*) and other squashes (*Cucurbita* species), and flax (*Linum usitatissimum*) contain copper, iron, phosphorus, selenium, and zinc. Mushrooms have copper, potassium, selenium, and zinc. Milk and yogurt contribute calcium, magnesium, potassium, and phosphorus whereas cheeses tend to be high in calcium, copper, and phosphorus. Spinach, kale, Swiss chard (*Beta vulgaris subsp. vulgaris*), turnip greens (*Brassica rapa ssp. rapa*), and other dark green leafy vegetables contain calcium, copper, iron, potassium, magnesium, and zinc.

Plant foods, however, are sometimes suboptimal mineral sources. For example, whole grains and beans have the antioxidant phytic acid, which combines with iron, zinc, manganese, and calcium, reducing their absorption. Calcium and oxalate anions $(C_2O_4)^{2-}$, prominent in leafy green vegetables and grains, compound this problem by worsening iron absorption. In contrast, vitamin C improves iron absorption.[75] The body absorbs iron better from meat, poultry, and seafood than from plants. Animal iron is designated heme because it is in blood's hemoglobin. Animals also harbor iron in muscles' myoglobin. Plant iron is nonheme.

2.7 VITAMINS

2.7.1 Inadequacy of Carbohydrates, Fat, Protein, and Minerals Alone

The enervation of rats fed pure carbohydrates, fat, protein, and minerals in the early twentieth century implied that such diets lacked an unknown nutrient or nutrients. The search for this substance or substances—what British biochemist Frederick Gowland Hopkins (1861–1947) in 1912 termed "unsuspected dietetic factors"—involved scientists and physicians in Asia, Europe, and North America.[76] That year Polish biochemist Casimir Funk (1884–1967) invented the term "vitamine," now spelled without the "e," for Hopkins' factors.[77] Its root is the Latin *vita*, meaning "life." The original spelling conveyed the initial but incorrect belief that all vitamins had an amine group characteristic of amino acids and proteins. During the twentieth century, researchers named thirteen to sixteen vitamins—depending on which are counted as such—classifying them by whether they dissolved in water or fat.[78] Unlike carbohydrates, fats, and proteins and like minerals, the body needs vitamins in only small quantities. Fractions of a gram suffice and superabundance may harm the body. Vitamins resemble the macronutrients in being organic and often benefit specific metabolic pathways. In cases where effects are additive, shortage or absence of one vitamin disables or diminishes another.

2.7.2 Fat-Soluble Vitamins

Scientists ordered vitamins by letter, with the first discovery receiving "A". The fat-soluble vitamins—A, D, E, and K—are in the fatty parts of plants, animals, and animal products. Fat-free foods cannot contain them. The body cannot absorb them unless it consumes some fat and can store them only in adipose and fatty structures within other cells. Because these vitamins do not dissolve in water, the body cannot excrete them in urine. Storage poses risk of superabundance, which, although uncommon, can harm the body. Vitamins A and D display greatest potential for injury in excess.

Taking the fat-soluble vitamins in order, A aids vision, cell growth, and the immune system. Animal products contain this vitamin in complete form, though the body can manufacture it from plant compounds known as carotenoids, which are vitamin A precursors. A later section examines these molecules, beta carotene prominent among them. Vitamin A is in eggs, dairy, the liver of various animals, and fish. Red and yellow vegetables and fruits contain carotenoids. This category includes carrots, red peppers (*Capsicum annuum*), tomatoes, apricots (*Prunus armeniaca*), peaches (*Prunus persica*), and mangoes (*Mangifera indica*). Additionally, dark green leafy vegetables and broccoli have carotenoids. The National Research Council of the National Academies of Sciences, Engineering, and Medicine in Washington, DC, having established the recommended dietary allowances (RDA) for nutrients, urges men to consume 900 micrograms (mcg) of vitamin A and women 700.[79]

Discussed in Chapter 1 and a previous section, vitamin D is atypical because the body can manufacture it independent of food. For this reason, Canadian biochemist Glenville Jones disputed its designation as a vitamin, instead terming it a "nutritional entity."[80] Curiosity about the relationships among sunlight, skin, and pigmentation and between sunlight and bone health contributed to understanding vitamin D's synthesis and functions. Sunlight's benefits were apparent before the 1910s, when nutritionists and dieticians began recommending consumption of cod liver oil to combat rickets and osteomalacia.[81] Considered from nutrition's vantage point, vitamin D is in egg yolks, liver, fish oils, veal, beef, and fortified foods like dairy products. The RDA is 10–20 micrograms, or 400–800 international units (IU), depending on age and on pregnancy and lactation for women.[82]

Vitamin E (tocopherol) is an antioxidant, a class of compounds whose benefits a later section describes. Tocopherol stabilizes LDL, whose function was noted. Vitamin E aids red-blood-cell formation and helps the body store vitamins A and K and minerals iron and selenium. Tocopherol is in vegetable oils, peanuts, nuts, spinach, broccoli, and fortified products like breakfast cereals and margarine. The RDA is 4–15 milligrams (mg) or 6–22.4 IU depending on age and on pregnancy and lactation for women.[83] Because natural sources are best, people who consume vitamin E in fortified products should aim for 33 IU per day. Superabundance does not appear to harm the body.

Vitamin K activates the protein cascade necessary to clot blood in a wound and strengthens bones by binding calcium to proteins in them. Vitamin K is a broad designation for the compounds phylloquinone (K_1), menaquinone (K_2), and menadione (K_3), which share properties and tend to occur in leaves. Good options are dark green leafy vegetables, broccoli, cauliflower, soybeans and their products, green tea, and wheat bran. Animal sources include liver and fermented dairy products. Laboratories synthesize menadione, whose potential harm diminishes its suitability in nutritional supplements. Vitamin K's RDA is 90 micrograms for women and 120 for men.[84] Diets are seldom deficient.

2.7.3 Water-Soluble Vitamins

Unlike their fat-soluble counterparts, the B vitamins and C, dissolving in water, tend to store poorly in the body due to excretion in urine and must be consumed regularly. Rather than storage in the manner of fat-soluble vitamins, the B complex and C congregate with enzymes whose function they enhance. Care must be taken in preparing foods with these vitamins, which may be lost through cooking and exposure to air and light.

Nutritionists and dieticians concentrate on eight B vitamins: B_1 (thiamine or thiamin), B_2 (riboflavin), B_3 (niacin or nicotinic acid), B_5 (pantothenic acid), B_6 (pyridoxine), B_7 (biotin), B_9 (folate, folic acid, or pteroylmonoglutamic acid), and B_{12} (cobalamin). The omitted four are B_4 (adenine), B_8 (inositol), B_{10} (para amino benzoic acid or PABA), and B_{11} (salicylic acid). This book concentrates on the standard eight. B vitamins help the body derive energy from food and manufacture red blood cells. As coenzymes, B vitamins enhance enzymes, a noteworthy function given that vitamins are not proteins and so cannot be enzymes. An example of a coenzyme, vitamin B_3 is part of nicotinamide adenine dinucleotide (NAD) and nicotinamide adenine dinucleotide phosphate (NADP), both necessary for deriving energy from foods. B vitamins are in beef, fish, poultry, eggs, dairy products, dark green leafy vegetables, and legumes. B-vitamin deficiencies cause diseases examined below.

The remaining water-soluble vitamin, C, receives attention elsewhere. Chapter 3 treats it from an evolutionary perspective. This paragraph restricts commentary to the publicity that American chemist and two-time Nobel laureate Linus Carl Pauling (1901–1994) garnered the vitamin by promoting it against the common cold. This belief generated controversy and the questionable practice of consuming large amounts (megadoses) of vitamin C in hopes of averting illness.

2.7.4 Vitamin Deficiency Diseases

The histories of scurvy, rickets, and osteomalacia, referenced earlier, indicate that attempts to fight deficiency diseases brought vitamins to the fore. Some ailments, known for thousands of years, defied solution until scientists isolated vitamins in the twentieth century. For example, the Chinese, Egyptians, and Greeks documented the failure of vision in poor light, a condition known as night blindness or nyctalopia.[85] Greek physician Hippocrates (c. 460–c. 375 BCE)—medicine's putative founder, though several authors wrote his texts—is thought to have recommended liver's consumption. In contrast to his recommendation, Egyptians, Indians (not American Indians), and Chinese put liquid from liver into the eyes. Japanese urged ingestion of fish oils and bird livers. As with scurvy, scientists sought the compound effective against nyctalopia common to these treatments. Vitamin A's 1912 discovery provided the answer.

B-vitamin shortages cause at least three diseases. Beriberi, which may weaken the heart, circulation, muscles, and nerves, persisted among people whose staple was white rice. (All cultivated rice is in the genus *Oryza* and receives treatment in Chapter 12.) Restoration of rice bran, present in whole-grain rice, cured the disease. Success was due to vitamin B_1, discovered in 1910 and named a vitamin in 1926. Pellagra resisted cure, Chapter 1 noted, until it was conceived not as a skin affliction but as nutritional shortfall. Suspicion fell on corn (*Zea mays*), which fed several peoples including blacks and poor whites in the southern United States. Attempts to blame the disease on corn's deterioration in storage led nowhere. Only vitamin B_3's discovery in 1937 and fortification of cornmeal and other foods cured pellagra. Anemia may result from deficiencies in B_9 or B_{12}. Anemia may also stem from inadequate iron or dearth of both iron and B_9 or B_{12}. When both iron and a B vitamin are culprits, neither deficit need be large to cause anemia. Chapter 1 detailed these factors and anemia's nondietary causes.

The battle against deficiency diseases spurred governments to mandate foods' fortification. These efforts have produced milk with vitamin D; breakfast cereals, pasta, and breads with several vitamins and minerals; juices with vitamin C; rice and some vegetable oils with vitamin A; iodized salt; eggs with omega-3 fatty acids; soybean foods with calcium and vitamins A and D; and snacks with calcium. Those who want more nutrients may take supplements as pills, beverages, or powders. Some products contain a single nutrient whereas others supply several. Supplements may target men, women, children, or seniors. The consensus holds that supplements are less nourishing than whole foods.

2.8 PHYTOCHEMICALS

The observation that plant eaters tend to be healthier than those who favor animal products implies that plants must contain compounds, known as phytochemicals or phytonutrients, that confer benefits beyond those available in carbohydrates, fat, protein, minerals, and vitamins and beyond what meat and kindred items supply.[86] This book eschews the term "phytonutrient" absent consensus about nutritional status. Phytochemicals' novelty as research subjects cautions against generalizations, particularly because findings have been ambivalent and occasionally contradictory and counterintuitive. More scrutiny is necessary to untangle their effects.

Yet pessimism and circumspection are unnecessary in all cases. The subject of ongoing research, beneficial phytochemicals appear to be numerous in vegetables, fruits, legumes, and whole grains. Phytochemicals may be conspicuous, giving carrots, tomatoes, and other vegetables and fruits their distinctive appearance and enhancing aroma and flavor in onions, leeks (*Allium ampeloprasum*), garlic (*A. sativum*), chives (*A. schoenoprasum*), kurrat or wild leek (*A. ampeloprasum*), and shallots (*A. cepa*). Chemical structure shapes attributes and functions.

Structure divides phytochemicals into five classes. The largest polyphenols includes flavonoids, which impart color to plant parts as mentioned, likely an adaptation for attracting insects to pollinate flowers. Flavonoids in legume roots attract nitrifying bacteria. More generally, flavonoids may protect plants against pathogens and help transmit intracellular and extracellular messages. In the body, flavonoids are antioxidants, which appear to protect cells against free radicals. Free radicals are electrically neutral, reactive atoms or molecules.

Consider hydrogen, the simplest atom. It has a single positively charged proton in the nucleus. To retain electrical neutrality, hydrogen has one negatively charged electron to counterbalance the proton's positive charge. This single electron occupies what chemists and physicists term the lowest orbital or shell, which is stable with two electrons rather than one. Consequently, hydrogen reacts with other atoms or ions to achieve a full lowest orbital of two electrons. Free radicals may damage cells by bonding with proteins, membranes, and DNA in a type of electron theft known as oxidation. Such damage may make cells cancerous. Antioxidants protect cells by donating electrons to free radicals, thereby preventing them from scavenging electrons. Antioxidants may protect the body against pathogens, inflammation, and heart disease.

A second category, phytoestrogens, includes isoflavones, which appear to protect the body against heart disease, osteoporosis, and some cancers. Soybeans have the isoflavones genistein and daidzein, which may partly explain lower chronic-disease rates among East Asian than among Americans and Europeans. Another type of phytoestrogen, lignan, may offer comparable benefits and is numerous in flaxseeds (*Linum usitatissimum*). A third class of phytochemicals, phytosterols, resembles cholesterol and appears to lower it in blood. Soybean oil contains phytosterols, another factor that may help explain East Asians' health. Fourth, glucosinolates may reduce damage from carcinogens and toxins by speeding their excretion, though clinical trials have yet to confirm this effect. Research focuses on glucosinolates sinigrin and progoitrin in hopes of evaluating their promise. These compounds are abundant in crucifers (also known as cole crops): broccoli, cauliflower, turnip (*Brassica rapa ssp. rapa*), kale, Brussels sprouts, garden cress (*Lepidium sativum*), bok choy (*Brassica rapa ssp. chinensis*), cabbage, and related plants. Fifth, the carotenoids include some 600 chemicals, notably vitamin A precursor beta carotene.[87]

Other carotenoids are less valuable in this regard. Beta carotene is thought to protect the body against heart disease, though clinical results are disappointing. A 1996 study yielded higher rates of lung cancer and heart disease among smokers who ingested beta carotene than among smokers who did not.[88] Beta carotene's potential harm may stem from its antioxidant properties. Because they donate electrons, beta carotene and other antioxidants may become free radicals capable of the damage outlined above. Resembling beta carotene, lycopene, plentiful in tomatoes, may protect against heart disease, stroke, and prostate cancer. Other sources are watermelon, pink grapefruit, guava (*Psidium guajava*), and apricots.

2.9 WATER

Although this book focuses on foods, water's importance mandates mention. The Egyptians thought it the universe's original building block, a belief that Greek philosopher Thales of Miletus (c. 625–c. 547 BCE) reiterated, though its formula was unknown until 1813, when Swedish physician and chemist Jons Jacob Berzelius (1779–1848) published its 2:1 ratio of hydrogen to oxygen.[89] Water appears to be a precondition for life, which probably arose in the ocean roughly 3.8 billion years ago. Water supports life's chemical reactions and is a solvent for polar as well as organic molecules. The body's proportion of water varies with age, sex, leanness, activity, and diseases and ranges between 45 and 75 percent of body mass, with American anthropologist Clark Spencer Larsen (b. 1952) estimating the amount at roughly two-thirds.[90] Most foods, especially those with few calories, contain it. Fruits and vegetables tend to be over four-fifths water. For example, lettuce, cucumbers, celery, peppers, spinach, tomatoes, carrots, watermelon, strawberries, and cantaloupe (*Cucumis melo*) are at least 90 percent water.[91] Such items hydrate the body besides supplying other nutrients. Caloric foods like peanuts have little water.

The body stores around two-thirds of its water inside cells, though adipose has none, a circumstance that explains why such tissue stores so much energy.[92] The remaining one-third, outside cells, is in blood plasma, body cavities, organs, and other tissues. The body uses minerals—chiefly sodium, potassium, calcium, chlorine, phosphorus, and magnesium—as electrolytes to achieve and perpetuate this balance inside and outside cells. Digestion requires water. Saliva, digestion's initiator, is 97–99.5 percent water.[93] At suitable temperatures, water cools an individual when consumed and so is an aid in hot weather. An overheated body cools itself through perspiration, a mechanism that requires rehydration to avoid heat stroke and related problems. Water moistens mucus membranes and helps eliminate wastes through urination. Water's importance is evident in the fact that dehydration can kill. Someone who neither drinks water nor eats foods with it will perish within a week, though an adequately hydrated person can survive "several weeks without food."[94]

Water intake replenishes loss through perspiration, urination, respiration, and other functions. By increasing metabolism, activity increases demand for water. Even without exertion, people lose 2.5–3 liters (0.7–0.8 gallons) of water daily, all of which must be replaced.[95] Water's ingestion replaces losses liter per liter. Other suitable beverages include tea (*Camellia sinensis*) and coffee (*Coffea* species) because they are primarily water. Their preparation by boiling water kills pathogens, benefitting people without access to safe water. Milk, discussed in Chapter 7, also has water and may be recommended as a source of other nutrients. Soft drinks supply water, but nutritionists and dieticians dislike their sucrose, HFCS, or similar sweeteners. Although they may contain vitamins and minerals, fruit juices may be little better than soft drinks as water substitutes because of their sweeteners and absence of fiber. By increasing urine production, alcohol subverts the attempt to quench thirst.

Illnesses can dehydrate the body. Crohn's disease, ulcerative colitis, irritable bowel syndrome, and celiac disease deplete water through diarrhea. Waterborne diseases like cholera and dysentery bring diarrhea, misery, and death to societies that lack potable water. Since 1817 cholera has assailed the world in seven pandemics.[96] During the fifth (1881–1896), Russian composer Peter Ilyich Tchaikovsky (1840–1893) perished after ignoring warnings not to drink water without first boiling it.[97] Other casualties included Prussian military theorist Carl Philipp Gottfried von Clausewitz (1780–1831), eleventh U.S. President James Knox Polk (1795–1849), and French engineer and contributor to the science of thermodynamics Nicolas Leonard Sadi Carnot (1796–1832).

Waterborne diseases still plague developing nations, with cholera entrenched in several African countries. Turning to southwestern Asia's Arabia, Yemen surpassed 1 million infections and tallied almost 2,500 deaths between 2016 and 2018.[98] Each year since 2010, cholera has infected some

4 million people worldwide, killing as many as 130,000 annually.[99] Poverty, disorder, and violence encourage such diseases to spread, imperiling humanity on a scale difficult to comprehend wherever sanitation yields clean water. These episodes highlight water's centrality to humankind as well as the chaos that results from contamination.

NOTES

1 T. Colin Campbell, *Whole: Rethinking the Science of Nutrition* (Dallas, TX: BenBella Books, 2013), 40.
2 Vishwanath Sardesai, *Introduction to Clinical Nutrition*, 3rd ed. (Boca Raton, FL: CRC Press, 2012), 249.
3 R. E. Hughes, "Scurvy," in *The Cambridge World History of Food*, vol. 1, ed. Kenneth F. Kiple and Kriemhild Conee Ornelas (Cambridge, UK: Cambridge University Press, 2000), 989.
4 Bill Laws, *Fifty Plants that Changed the Course of History* (Buffalo, NY and Richmond Hill, Ontario: Firefly Books, 2015), 50; Pierre Laszlo, *Citrus: A History* (Chicago, IL and London: University of Chicago Press, 2008), 84.
5 Kaori O'Connor, *Pineapple: A Global History* (London: Reaktion Books, 2013), 45.
6 Kenneth J. Carpenter, *The History of Scurvy and Vitamin C* (Cambridge, UK: Cambridge University Press, 1986), 76–77.
7 Hughes, "Scurvy," 991–992.
8 "The Nutrients—Deficiencies, Surfeits, and Food-Related Disorders," in *The Cambridge World History of Food*, vol. 1, ed. Kenneth F. Kiple and Kriemhild Conee Ornelas (Cambridge, UK: Cambridge University Press, 2000), 739.
9 Richard D. Semba, "The Discovery of the Vitamins," *International Journal of Vitamin and Nutrition Research* 82, no. 5 (October 2012): 312; R. E. Hughes, "Vitamin C," in *The Cambridge World History of Food*, vol. 1, ed. Kenneth F. Kiple and Kriemhild Conee Ornelas (Cambridge, UK: Cambridge University Press, 2000), 756.
10 Ernst Mayr, *The Growth of Biological Thought: Diversity, Evolution, and Inheritance* (Cambridge, MA and London: Belknap Press of Harvard University Press, 1982), 97–98.
11 J. D. L. Hansen, "Protein-Energy Malnutrition," in *The Cambridge World History of Food*, vol. 1, ed. Kenneth F. Kiple and Kriemhild Conee Ornelas (Cambridge, UK: Cambridge University Press, 2000), 977.
12 Mike Lean and Emilie Combet, *Barasi's Human Nutrition: A Health Perspective*, 3d ed (Boca Raton, FL: CRC Press, 2017), 314.
13 Allan Borushek, *The CalorieKing Calorie, Fat, and Carbohydrate Counter* (Huntington Beach, CA: Family Health Publications, 2019), 101, 158–160.
14 Ibid., 159.
15 Ibid., 99–100, 130; "Olives," *Sizes*, last modified July 29, 2011, accessed October 10, 2019, https://www.sizes.com/food/olives.htm; "Egg, Yolk, Raw, Fresh," *USDA FoodData Central*, April 1, 2019, accessed October 10, 2019, https://fdc.nal.usda.gov/fdc-app.html#/food-details/172184/nutrients.
16 Lean and Combet, 315; Julian E. Spallholz, L. Mallory Boylan, and Judy A. Driskell, *Nutrition Chemistry and Biology*, 2d ed. (Boca Raton, FL: CRC Press, 1999), 202.
17 Sharon Durham, "Nuts for Calories!" last modified March 22, 2018, accessed January 23, 2019, https://www.ars.usda.gov/news-events/news/research-news/2018/nuts-for-calories.
18 "Appendix E-3.1.A3. Energy Levels Used for Assignment of Individuals to USDA Food Patterns," *U.S. Department of Health and Human Services*, last modified November 1, 2019, accessed February 6, 2020, https://health.gov/our-work/food-nutrition/2015-2020-dietary-guidelines/advisory-report/appendix-e-3/appendix-e-31a3.
19 Anne Maczulak, *The Smart Guide to Nutrition*, 2nd ed. (Norman, OK: Smart Guide Publications, 2014), 59.
20 Louise Eaton and Kara Rogers, ed., *Examining Basic Chemical Molecules* (New York: Britannica, 2018), 246.
21 Willem M. Jongman, "The Early Roman Empire: Consumption," in *The Cambridge Economic History of the Greco-Roman World*, ed. Walter Scheidel, Ian Morris, and Richard P. Saller (Cambridge, UK: Cambridge University Press, 2007), 599.
22 Sarah Brewer, *Nutrition: A Beginner's Guide* (London: Oneworld, 2013), 42–43.
23 John M. Kim, "Nutrition and the Decline of Mortality," in *The Cambridge World History of Food*, vol. 2, ed. Kenneth F. Kiple and Kriemhild Conee Ornelas (Cambridge, UK: Cambridge University Press, 2000), 1385.
24 Leslie Sansone, "Calorie Burn per Mile?" *Walk at Home*, accessed October 8, 2019, https://walkathome.com/calorie-burn-per-mile.

25 Paul Clayton and Judith Rowbotham, "How the Mid-Victorians Worked, Ate and Died," *International Journal of Environmental Research and Public Health* 6, no. 3, March 2009, accessed January 23, 2019, https://www.ncbi.nlm.nih.gov/pmc/articles/PMC2672390.

26 John Reader, *Potato: A History of the Propitious Esculent* (New Haven, CT and London: Yale University Press, 2008), 156; Shelley Barber, ed. *The Prendergast Letters: Correspondence from Famine-Era Ireland, 1840–1850* (Amherst and Boston: University of Massachusetts Press, 2006), 193; John Percival, *The Great Famine: Ireland's Potato Famine, 1845–51* (New York: Viewer Books, 1995), 36.

27 "Potatoes, Flesh and Skin, Raw," *USDA FoodData Central*, April 1, 2019, accessed January 19, 2020, https://fdc.nal.usda.gov/fdc-app.html#/food-details/170026/nutrients.

28 Betty Fussell, *The Story of Corn* (New York: Knopf, 1992), 273–274; Gary Taubes, *The Case against Sugar* (New York: Knopf, 2016), 25.

29 Lean and Combet, 314.

30 William Rubel, *Bread: A Global History* (London: Reaktion Books, 2011), 11–12.

31 John R. Holum, *Organic and Biological Chemistry* (New York: Wiley, 1996), 216.

32 "Potatoes, Flesh and Skin, Raw."

33 David M. Peterson and J. Paul Murphy, "Oat," in *The Cambridge World History of Food*, vol. 1, ed. Kenneth F. Kiple and Kriemhild Conee Ornelas (Cambridge, UK: Cambridge University Press, 2000), 129; "Oats, Raw," *USDA FoodData Central*, April 1, 2019, accessed January 19, 2020, https://fdc.nal.usda.gov/fdc-app.html#/food-details/340734/nutrients.

34 "New CDC Report: More than 100 Million Americans Have Diabetes or Prediabetes," *CDC*, last modified July 18, 2017, accessed January 23, 2019, https://www.cdc.gov/media/releases/2017/p0718-diabetes-report.html.

35 "Pepperidge Farm Classic 100% Whole Wheat Hamburger Bun," *CalorieKing*, accessed October 9, 2019, https://www.calorieking.com/us/en/foods/f/calories-in-bread-rolls-buns-classic-100-whole-wheat-hamburger-bun/ONAUaxnlRoyb3sHP1TYtlA.

36 "Buns and Rolls: Hamburger Buns," *Ball Park Buns & Rolls*, accessed October 9, 2019, https://www.ballparkbuns.com/product/hamburger-buns.

37 "Mustard," *USDA FoodData Central*, April 1, 2019, accessed October 9, 2019, https://fdc.nal.usda.gov/fdc-app.html#/food-details/343665/nutrients; "Ketchup," *USDA FoodData Central*, April 1, 2019, accessed October 9, 2019, https://fdc.nal.usda.gov/fdc-app.html#/food-details/467734/nutrients; "Mayonnaise," *USDA FoodData Central*, April 1, 2019, accessed October 9, 2019, https://fdc.nal.usda.gov/fdc-app.html#/food-details/458881/nutrients.

38 "Nutrition Calculator," McDonald's, 2017–2018, accessed January 23, 2019, https://www.mcdonalds.com/us/en-us/about-our-food/nutrition-calculator.html.

39 "Hostess Twinkies," *Nutritionix Grocery Database*, last modified December 11, 2018, accessed October 9, 2019, https://www.nutritionix.com/i/hostess/twinkies/54e4e87590108d0f348f5117; "Hostess Ho Ho's," *Nutritionix Grocery Database*, last modified April 23, 2016; accessed October 9, 2019, https://www.nutritionix.com/i/hostess/ho-hos/54982f654112493933526356; "Hostess Cup Cakes," *Nutritionix Grocery Database*, last modified September 14, 2016, accessed October 9, 2019, https://www.nutritionix.com/i/hostess/cup-cakes/55408cf6f9fa949f499079bd; "Hostess Ding Dongs Chocolate Cake with Creamy Filling," *Nutritionix Grocery Database*, last modified November 24, 2014, accessed October 9, 2019, https://www.nutritionix.com/i/hostess/ding-dongs-chocolate-cake-with-creamy-filling/527aa053cc1bd44b08000372.

40 "Donuts," *Dunkin' Donut*, 2017, accessed January 23, 2019, https://www.dunkindonuts.com/en/food-drinks/donuts/donuts.

41 "Pop-Tarts Brown Sugar Cinnamon," *Pop-Tarts*, last modified January 22, 2019, accessed January 23, 2019, http://smartlabel.kelloggs.com/Product/Index/00038000311109.

42 Brewer, 22.

43 "About Glycemic Index," *Glycemic Index Foundation*, 2017, accessed January 23, 2019, https://www.gisymbol.com/about-glycemic-index.

44 Eaton and Rogers, 221.

45 Stephanie Green, *Optimum Nutrition* (New York: Alpha, 2016), 72; Holum, 444.

46 David Perlmutter, *Grain Brain: The Surprising Truth about Wheat, Carbs, and Sugar—Your Brain's Silent Killers*, rev. ed. (New York: Little, Brown Spark, 2018), 82–85.

47 Veronica Childs and Laura Childs, *The Complete Low Carb, High Fat, No Hunger Diet: A User Manual for Our KetoHybrid Diet Constructed from the Best Practices of Low Carb, Ketogenic, & Paleo-Inspired Diets* (Delhi: Hula Books, 2014), 17.

48 Sandra Woodruff, *Secrets of Good-Carb/Low-Carb Living* (New York: Avery, 2004), 27.

49 Steven R. Gundry, *The Plant Paradox: The Hidden Dangers in "Healthy" Foods that Cause Disease and Weight Gain* (New York: Harper Wave, 2017), 170–171.
50 William H. Brown, Christopher S. Foote, and Brent L. Iverson, *Organic Chemistry*, 4th ed. (Belmont, CA: Thomson Brooks/Cole, 2005), 1038.
51 Green, 97–99.
52 "Trans Fat," *U.S. Department of Health and Human Services*, last modified May 18, 2018, accessed January 23, 2019, https://www.fda.gov/food/ucm292278.htm.
53 Tom Mueller, *Extra Virginity: The Sublime and Scandalous World of Olive Oil* (New York and London: Norton, 2012), 137.
54 Eaton and Rogers, 221.
55 C. Murray Skeaff and Jim Mann, "Lipids," in *Essentials of Human Nutrition*, ed. Jim Mann and A. Stewart Truswell, 5th ed. (Oxford: Oxford University Press, 2017), 40.
56 Eaton and Rogers, 215–216.
57 "Hostess Original Twinkies," *MyFoodDiary*, 2019, accessed January 23, 2019, https://www.myfooddiary.com/foods/849238/hostess-original-twinkies.
58 "100 Grams—Salmon, Cooked," *Myfitnesspal*, accessed January 23, 2019, https://www.myfitnesspal.com/food/calories/165152846.
59 "Nutrition Calculator."
60 Elmer Verner McCollum, *A History of Nutrition: The Sequence of Ideas in Nutrition Investigations* (Boston: Houghton Mifflin, 1957), 93–94.
61 K. J. Carpenter, "The History of Enthusiasm for Protein," *Journal of Nutrition* 116, no. 7 (July 1986): 1364.
62 Alan A. Jackson and A. Stewart Truswell, "Protein," in *Essentials of Human Nutrition*, ed. Jim Mann and A. Stewart Truswell, 5th ed. (Oxford: Oxford University Press, 2017), 76–77.
63 Milicent L. Hathaway, "Trends in Heights and Weights," in *Yearbook of Agriculture, 1959*, ed. Alfred Stefferud (Washington, DC: GPO, 1959), 182, ps://naldc.nal.usda.gov/download/IND43861419/PDF.
64 Eaton and Rogers, 69; Green, 85.
65 Jackson and Truswell, 63; Lean and Combet, 32; Eaton and Rogers, 69; Green, 85; Holum, 444; Peter L. Pellett, "Energy and Protein Metabolism," in *The Cambridge World History of Food*, vol. 1, ed. Kenneth F. Kiple and Kriemhild Conee Ornelas (Cambridge, UK: Cambridge University Press, 2000), 899; Clark Spencer Larsen, "Dietary Reconstruction and Nutritional Assessment of Past Peoples: The Bioanthropological Record," in *The Cambridge World History of Food*, vol. 1, ed. Kenneth F. Kiple and Kriemhild Conee Ornelas (Cambridge, UK: Cambridge University Press, 2000), 13; Brewer, 13.
66 Pellett, 899.
67 Green, 89.
68 Jackson and Truswell, 61.
69 Brown, Foote, and Iverson, 1092.
70 J. Luke Pryor and Deanna M. Dempsey, "Should Sodium (Via Foods, Salt Tablets, or Pickle Juice) Be Consumed prior to or during Endurance Activities for the Prevention of Exertional Heat Illness?" in *Quick Questions in Heat-Related Illness and Hydration: Expert Advice in Sports Medicine*, ed. Rebecca M. Lopez and Eric L. Sauers (Thorofare, NJ: Slack, 2015), 173–174.
71 Linsay McCallum, Stefanie Lip, and Sandosh Padmanabhan, "The Hidden Hand of Chloride in Hypertension," *Pflugers Archiv* 467, no. 3 (January 27, 2015): 595–603.
72 Larsen, 26.
73 Glenville Jones, "Vitamin D," in *The Cambridge World History of Food*, vol. 1, ed. Kenneth F. Kiple and Kriemhild Conee Ornelas (Cambridge, UK: Cambridge University Press, 2000), 763.
74 Yella Hewings-Martin, "Does Magnesium Hold the Key to Vitamin D Benefits?" *MedicalNewsToday*, December 30, 2018, accessed October 11, 2019, https://www.medicalnewstoday.com/articles/324022.php.
75 J. G. Vaughan and C. A. Geissler, *The New Oxford Book of Food Plants: A Guide to the Fruit, Vegetables, Herbs and Spices of the World*, rev. ed. (Oxford: Oxford University Press, 1997), 206.
76 F. Gowland Hopkins, "Feeding Experiments Illustrating the Importance of Accessory Factors in Normal Dietaries," *Journal of Physiology* 44, no. 5–6 (July 15, 1912): 450.
77 Semba, 310.
78 A. Stewart Truswell and Jim Mann, "Introduction," in *Essentials of Human Nutrition*, ed. Jim Mann and A. Stewart Truswell, 5th ed. (Oxford: Oxford University Press, 2017), 4; Larsen, 13.
79 "News from the National Academies," *National Academies of Sciences, Engineering, and Medicine*, January 9, 2001, accessed January 23, 2019, http://www8.nationalacademies.org/onpinews/newsitem.aspx?RecordID=10026.

80 Jones, 763.
81 Ibid., 764; Walter Gratzer, *Terrors of the Table: The Curious History of Nutrition* (Oxford and New York: Oxford University Press, 2005), 9.
82 "Vitamin D Fact Sheet for Health Professionals," *NIH*, last modified November 9, 2018, accessed January 23, 2019, https://ods.od.nih.gov/factsheets/VitaminD-HealthProfessional.
83 "Vitamin E Fact Sheet for Health Professionals," *NIH*, last modified August 17, 2018, accessed January 23, 2019, https://ods.od.nih.gov/factsheets/VitaminE-HealthProfessional.
84 Megan Ware, "Health Benefits and Sources of Vitamin K," *MedicalNewsToday*, last modified January 22, 2018, accessed January 23, 2019, https://www.medicalnewstoday.com/articles/219867.php.
85 George Wolf, "Vitamin A," in *The Cambridge World History of Food*, vol. 1, ed. Kenneth F. Kiple and Kriemhild Conee Ornelas (Cambridge, UK: Cambridge University Press, 2000), 742; Spallholz, Boylan, and Driskell, 63; Karl Y. Guggenheim, *Nutrition and Nutritional Diseases: The Evolution of Concepts* (Lexington, MA and Toronto: D. C. Health, 1981), 265–266.
86 Green, 138–139.
87 Ibid., 139.
88 Lean and Combet, 78.
89 Helge S. Kragh, *Conceptions of Cosmos: From Myths to the Accelerating University: A History of Cosmology* (Oxford: Oxford University Press, 2007), 7; Robert S. Brumbaugh, *The Philosophers of Greece* (Albany: State University of New York Press, 1981), 11; William H. Brock, *The History of Chemistry: A Very Short Introduction* (Oxford: Oxford University Press, 2016), 64, 66.
90 Green, 55; Larsen, 13.
91 "Foods with the Highest Water Content," *The Blend*, 2019, accessed January 23, 2019, https://greenblender.com/smoothies/2683/foods-with-the-highest-water-content.
92 Brewer, 143; Andrew Bahn, "Water, Electrolytes, and Acid-Base Balance," in *Essentials of Human Nutrition*, ed. Jim Mann and A. Stewart Truswell, 5th ed. (Oxford: Oxford University Press, 2017), 113.
93 Patricia Daniels, Trisha Gura, Susan Tyler Hitchcock, Lisa Stein, and John Thompson, *The Body: A Complete User's Guide*, rev. ed. (Washington, DC: National Geographic, 2014), 184.
94 Green, 55.
95 Ibid., 57.
96 Myron Echenberg, *Africa in the Time of Cholera: A History of Pandemics from 1817 to the Present* (Cambridge, UK: Cambridge University Press, 2011), 1.
97 Joseph Machlis, *The Enjoyment of Music: An Introduction to Perceptive Listening* (New York: Norton, 1955), 163.
98 "Mystery of Yemen Cholera Epidemic Solved," *ScienceDaily*, January 2, 2019, accessed January 23, 2019, https://www.sciencedaily.com/releases/2019/01/190102140745.htm.
99 "People Who Died from Cholera," 2019, accessed January 23, 2019, https://www.geni.com/projects/People-who-died-from-Cholera/27963.

3 Changing Circumstances and Diets

3.1 AUTOTROPHS

Typifying Rome's enthusiasm for botany and books, lawyer and politician Marcus Tullius Cicero (106–143 BCE) remarked that "If you have a garden and a library, you have everything you need."[1] Despite this praise, few contrivances betray plants' vulnerability more than a garden. Cabbage (*Brassica oleracea var. capitata*) seedlings mature in neat rows, in time filling their heads with delectable leaves. But anticipation of the harvest is premature. Within striking distance of a meal, groundhogs (*Marmota monax*) probe the perimeter for weaknesses, burrowing under fences. In a single evening, they devour weeks of toil. Rooted in the soil, cabbage and other treats cannot flee the assault. This shortcoming is understandable because plants need not search for food. It comes to them as sunlight, carbon dioxide, water, and minerals. Plants' majesty stems from their status as autotrophs.

3.2 HETEROTROPHS

3.2.1 Disadvantages

In contrast, animals' heterotrophy condemns them to seek food. Genesis, the first book in the Hebrew scriptures, conveys something of the difficulties. According to it, God banished humans from Eden, mandating that they thereafter labor for sustenance.[2] Nothing comes easily to them. This book cannot match Genesis' poetry, but, like it, this chapter aims to trace part of humanity's prehistory and history. The task is too immense for a single volume, necessitating concentration on a single aspect of our past: diet and nutrition's effects on health. This chapter puts this objective in an evolutionary context in hopes of illuminating how our biology and development over many millennia shaped our diet. This chapter also endeavors to indicate how foods influenced our biology and evolution. Not only have foods affected humanity, but people have modified them through a variety of interactions culminating in the rise of farming and livestock raising and subsequent genetic manipulations through selective breeding and biotechnology.

3.2.2 Classification of Heterotrophs

Heterotrophs may be classified by what they eat, with the range of foods determining degree of specialization. Herbivores eat only plants. This category includes specialists like the panda (*Ailuropoda melanoleuca*), which derives almost all its nourishment from bamboo (species in subfamily Bambusoideae) leaves, stems, and shoots. Such narrowness poses risks because the staple's endangerment causes hunger and starvation. Eradication of that food triggers extinction. At the other end of the spectrum are herbivores that eat many species. Elephants (*Elephas maximus* and *Loxodonta africana*), for example, consume several plants' bark, branches, roots, leaves, and fruits. Herbivores feed carnivores. Lions (*Panthera leo*), for example, target the African savanna's herbivores. Not necessarily restricted to herbivores, carnivores may also eat other carnivores and omnivores. Carnivory is not unique to animals because the Venus flytrap (*Dionaea muscipula*) and allied plants consume insects. Such organisms are both autotroph and heterotroph.

Herbivores and carnivores' specialization does not characterize omnivores, including humans, which differ from the others by feeding at more than one trophic level. To be sure, people may narrow their diets to one level, as do vegans mentioned in Chapter 1. Such restriction may be voluntary, though this book emphasizes that throughout history, poverty prevented commoners from affording meat. Biology does not, however, require abstinence from meat. To be sure, diseases may limit diets. Celiac disease, for example, prohibits consumption of wheat (*Triticum monococcum*, *T. dicoccon*, *T. aestivum*, and *T. durum*), rye (*Secale cereale*), barley (*Hordeum vulgare*), and triticale (*Triticale hexaploide*). Some with the malady cannot eat oats (*Avena sativa*). Yet even these cases neither prevent omnivory nor typify humanity.

3.3 HUMAN ADAPTATIONS FOR OMNIVORY AND ECLECTICISM

Far from excluding options, biology equips humans for a range of foods. Evolution adapted the teeth for omnivory. Molars and premolars crush and grind tough materials like seeds. Such activities help process plants as a first step in digestion. Additionally, premolars are adept at tearing meat. Incisors and canines bite and slice plants and meat. Due to the absence of enzyme cellulase, humans cannot digest cellulose—$(C_6H_{10}O_5)_n$, where "n" is a positive integer—in plant cell walls and so are not adapted to eating just plants. At the same time, humans do not consume only meat because it cannot satisfy cravings for sweetness, which orient the taste buds toward fruits, honey, and the sucrose ($C_{12}H_{22}O_{11}$) conspicuous in sugarcane (*Saccharum officinarum*) stalks and sugar beet (*Beta vulgaris spp. vulgaris*) taproots. Moreover, consumption of only meat is fatal, a phenomenon known as rabbit starvation.[3] Marbled meats and oily fish, nuts, seeds, fruits, and legumes demonstrate that omnivory can satiate fat cravings. In addition, humans have neither the four-chambered stomach that equips cows (*Bos taurus*) for herbivory nor the fleetness that enables cheetahs (*Acinonyx jubatus*) to outrun prey.

Rather than specializing in either of these directions, humans are generalists who consume plants, fungi, fermented foods and beverages, animals, and animal products. To put the matter another way, humans specialize in eclecticism and flexibility, modifying behaviors to fit changing circumstances. Such plasticity is an evolutionary outcome and a reason why people have colonized every continent. Scientists maintain facilities even in Antarctica. Despite the norm of only one child per birth, humans number in the billions. The adaptability inherent in omnivory helps explain our success as a species.

3.4 DIETARY BREADTH

3.4.1 The Role of Choice in Dietary Breadth

Skill in manipulating crops has given people over 20,000 species of edible plants.[4] Addition of animals and their products enlarges this tally. Despite omnivory and eclecticism, humans eat only a fraction of this total, with only about twenty plant species supplying nine-tenths of food.[5] Detractors blame farming for reducing dietary breadth, a development examined later, though this criticism may be unfair. If Americans stopped eating hot dogs and demanded okra (*Abelmoschus esculentus*), Swiss chard (*Beta vulgaris ssp. vulgaris*), kale (*Brassica oleracea ssp. sabellica*), garden cress (*Lepidium sativum*), brussels sprouts (*Brassica oleracea ssp. gemmifera*), pinto beans (a variety of *Phaseolus vulgaris*), and Chinese cabbage (*Brassica rapa ssp. pekinensis*), farmland, restaurants, and supermarkets would change.

3.4.2 The Role of Preferences in Dietary Breadth

This example underscores the importance of choice in determining what people eat. Preferences shape decisions and develop early. Babies and children become unruly when forced to eat what displeases them. Earliness implies that preferences are inborn. Cravings for the salt sodium chloride (NaCl), fat, sweetness, and tanginess are widespread, again suggesting a hereditary component honed by evolution. Habits, which depend on culture, also influence choice and may cause indignation when parents raise children on processed foods.

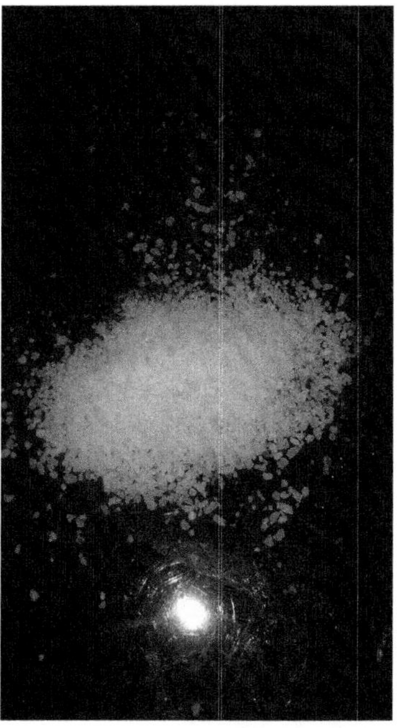

FIGURE 3.1 Sodium chloride. (Photo from author.)

3.4.3 The Role of Inequalities in Dietary Breadth

A factor that deserves scrutiny is the degree to which inequalities determine what people eat. For example, introduction of potatoes (*Solanum tuberosum*), treated in Chapter 13, into Europe in the sixteenth century met resistance. Europeans were accustomed to eating bread, peas (*Pisum sativum*), lentils (*Lens culinaris*), cabbage, and other foods that originated in seeds. Most of their food plants produced their edibles above ground. In contrast, *S. tuberosum* yielded food underground, the stems, leaves, flowers, fruits, and seeds being toxic. Moreover, it was not ideally propagated by seeds in contrast to grains, lettuce (*Lactuca sativa*), turnips (*Brassica rapa ssp. rapa*), cabbage, peas, lentils, chickpeas (*Cicer arietinum*), and other crops familiar to Europeans. Being misshapen, the tubers were thought to cause leprosy.

These traits slowed potatoes' integration into diets but could not vanquish necessity. Tubers thrived in the cool climate of northern Europe, where poverty drove the masses to it. Paying meager wages, industrialization left workers little alternative. In Ireland, absentee landlords extorted high rents, compelling tenants to plant almost all land to cash crops like wheat or to let livestock monopolize it as pasture. Either way, they had little land for their own needs and had to plant potatoes for maximum edible biomass per hectare. Chapter 1 and a later section emphasize that potatoes fed commoners on the eve of Ireland's famine and examine monoculture and destitution's consequences.

Inequality is no abstraction of distant times but remains prevalent. The affluent eat steak, duck, expensive cheeses, and other foods that have many nutrients and calories whereas developed nations' poor grow fat on empty calories and their developing world counterparts have too little to eat. Where meat is available, as in the United States, the underclass frequents hamburger joints and greasy diners. Vitamin C comes not from whole vegetables and fruits but from French fries and potato chips. Schools perpetuate an emphasis on junk by serving tater tots and deeming ketchup a vegetable.

Government aggravates these problems. Under fortieth U.S. President Ronald Wilson Reagan (1911–2004), the U.S. Department of Agriculture (USDA) in 1981 loosened restrictions on lunch programs, allowing schools to classify pickle relish and ketchup as vegetables, cake, cookies, and corn (*Zea mays*) chips as bread, and cake made with eggs as meat to perpetuate an illusion of wholesomeness.[6] More recently, following 2018 mandates that schools need not serve whole grains and reduce salt, the USDA in January 2020 announced its intention to allow more pizza, burgers, and fries in student lunches.[7] In these ways, inequalities and the delusion that unhealthiness can be reconceptualized as vitality worsen chronic diseases.

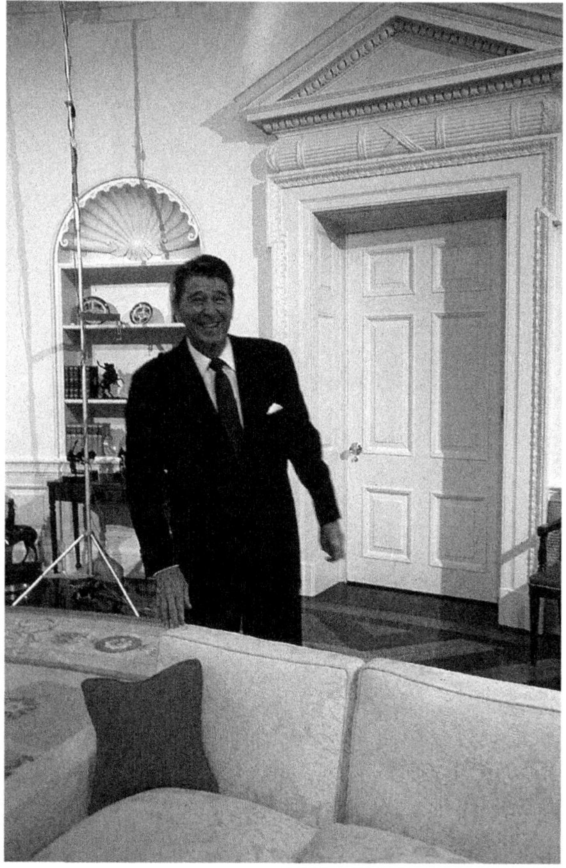

FIGURE 3.2 Ronald Reagan. (Photo courtesy of Library of Congress. https://www.loc.gov/pictures/item/2011632924/.)

3.4.4 The Role of Several Factors in Dietary Breadth

The foregoing indicates that many factors shape what people eat and their ability to acquire food in the first place. Although inequalities limit choices, modernity has made food almost effortless to obtain. A drive to the grocer or Burger King fills the stomach. But this ease is recent. For almost its entire tenure on Earth, humanity had to search for food. The quest for edible plants is known as foraging, gathering, or collecting. The term "hunting" ennobles the pursuit of game, though scavenging might have been more important throughout much of prehistory. The fact that the kidneys and liver detoxify the body implies that humans have long eaten rancid meat. Decomposition set in because humans were latecomers to a carcass. They scavenged before they hunted and continued to steal kills when opportunity arose, hunting yielded nothing, or edible plants dwindled. Chronicling this development, American anthropologist Clark Spencer Larsen (b. 1952) wrote that as scavengers, our ancestors accessed meat about 1.5 million years ago, becoming hunters about 800,000 years later.[8]

3.5 PRIMATE ORIGINS, EVOLUTION, AND DIETS

3.5.1 Primate Characteristics

Food-acquisition strategies may be studied from an evolutionary perspective. Although all life shares a common ancestry, evolution has produced too many species to permit global treatment. An apt starting point is our order, the primates, whose hallmarks include possession of nails rather than claws and flexible hands and feet capable of grasping objects like branches, an adaptation to arboreal life. Primates have large heads relative to the body. The skull houses a sizable brain, prompting the inference that primates are intelligent. Primate behaviors appear to corroborate this notion. Nevertheless, the study of intelligence is inexact because this trait is not easy to quantify even among humans. Primates tend to be helpless as newborns because their large brain is immature at birth, necessitating parental care. Intelligence and parent–child bonds facilitate sociability. Primate eyes are close together, permitting binocular vision. Relative to other animals, especially insects, primates live long lives. A person may surpass a century, though such longevity is uncommon. Being mammals, primates have fur (hair) rather than scales or feathers, though humans have less than other primates.

3.5.2 The Necessity of Comparing Kindred Primates

Primates number between roughly 230 and 270 species.[9] Precision is elusive because taxonomists cannot always agree whether similar individuals are alike enough to merit inclusion in a single species or possess differences warranting classification in separate species. This debate is part of a larger fissure between splitters and lumpers. Splitters magnify differences by partitioning alike individuals into different species whereas lumpers group small variations into a single species. The large number of primate species precludes discussion of all. Were such treatment possible, it would not enlighten readers because the less a species resembles humans, the less relevance it holds for understanding human diet, nutrition, and health. Regrettably, the primates most resembling us—archaic species like *Homo neanderthalensis* known as Neanderthals or Neandertals—are extinct. Their diets can sometimes be reconstructed but cannot be observed firsthand.

3.5.3 Degree of Relatedness and Definition of Species

This discussion mandates the definition of species. The most straightforward is a group of individuals that can mate to produce fertile offspring. Different dog breeds belong to one species (*Canis lupus familiaris*) because they yield fertile progeny. This fact justifies their designation as breeds rather than species. In contrast, crosses between a horse (*Equus caballus*) and donkey (*Equus asinus*) produce the mule, whose sterility confirms the parents as different species.

Returning to humankind, extinction limits but does not obliterate what can be known about Neanderthals. The name *H. neanderthalensis* differentiates them from us (*Homo sapiens*). The forgoing definition of species and designation of Neanderthals as separate require that they did not mate with us to produce children capable of having children of their own upon maturation. This rationale embeds assumptions about Neanderthals and us, including that they must have been sufficiently unlike modern humans to have deterred interbreeding. Putative and actual dissimilarities often convey the belief that Neanderthals were inferior to us and that inferiority doomed them to extinction. Couplings between the two must have been infrequent and seldom produced children. The few from such unions would have been oddities ostracized by their communities. Ostracism would have imperiled survival. Had they reached puberty, they could not have had children because these hybrids were sterile.

This thinking is incorrect. Studies reveal that we have Neanderthal genes. The amount varies by individual, but such variations do not negate Neanderthal ancestry, however remote those forbearers may be. This reality implies that wherever modern humans encountered other peoples, the two mated. Accordingly, prehistoric peoples' division into different species is likely inaccurate. Notions of separateness stem from belief that we are unique and exceptional, a comforting but inaccurate idea. This book uses conventional species names for different humans while rejecting radical notions of separateness.

3.5.4 The Value of Comparison between Humans and Extinct Peoples and between Humans and Apes

Returning to general considerations of relatedness, this chapter places human diets within a primate context. This context requires investigation of extinct peoples and their diets, topics of later sections. The study of human diets also benefits from examination of our closest extant relatives, the apes: chimpanzee (*Pan troglodytes*), bonobo (*Pan paniscus*), gorilla (*Gorilla gorilla* and *G. beringei*), orangutan (*Pongo pygmaeus*, *P. abelii*, and *P. tapanuliensis*), and gibbon (species in genera *Hoolock*, *Hylobates*, *Symphalangus*, and *Nomascus*).

3.5.5 Early Primates and Their Diets

Viewed from an evolutionary vantage point, primates are latecomers to the biota. Life originated roughly 3.8 billion years ago, but primates are no older than 65 million years, when the dinosaurs' demise at the end of the Cretaceous Period (145–165 million years ago) opened niches for mammals and promoted speciation. Even this date may be too early because the first species with primate characteristics may not have been primates and are probably best thought precursors rather than true to type.[10] Fossils suggest that these animals resembled squirrels (*Sciurus* species) and tree shrews (*Tupaia* species). Small, the proto primates radiated heat because of a large surface to volume ratio. But being warm-blooded like all mammals, these creatures had to sustain a high metabolism to offset heat loss and so needed many nutrients and calories.

They satisfied this requirement by eating insects, a diet that supplied protein, fat, minerals, and vitamins. The visual predation hypothesis holds that primates and their immediate forebears evolved their defining characteristics to hunt insects.[11] For example, visual acuity and dexterity enabled primates to see insects in dim light and grab them with their fingers. Insectivory (entomophagy) may explain the origins of humans' preference for meat and fat. Insect capture may be classified as hunting, suggesting another parallel to people, at least before agriculture and animal husbandry replaced hunting and gathering.

Insects feed several primates, including chimpanzees, numerous monkeys, *G. gorilla*, lemurs (species in the superfamily Lemuroidea), and humans. Although most Westerners abhor insects as filthy and repulsive, disgust is atypical. African, Asian, Australian, New Zealand, and American indigenes practiced entomophagy. As much as 80 percent of people eat one or more of the roughly

1,500 insect species on the global buffet.[12] The celebrated cave art in Altamira, Spain, suggests that its inhabitants ate insects roughly 30,000 years ago. Silkworms (*Bombyx mori*) fed ancient China. Colombians and Brazilians prize the leafcutter ant *Atta laevigata*. South Africans eat caterpillars of the moth *Gonimbrasia belina*. Indonesians consume grasshoppers (species in the superfamily Acridomorpha), crickets (species in the genera *Gryllus*, *Gryllodes*, *Teleogryllus*, and *Acheta*), termites (species in the infraorder Isoptera), honeybees (*Apis mellifera*), and sago palm weevils (*Rhynchophorus ferrugineus*). A 1525 account described Amerindian consumption of fleas, spiders, and worms.[13] Alaska's Nunamiut ingest maggots of the fly *Hypoderma tarandi*. The beetle *Udonga montana* is popular in India. Local markets in Thailand bulge with termites, ant eggs, honeybees, silkworms, grasshoppers, and crickets.

A type of carnivory, entomophagy, invites broader treatment of meat eating. Examining meat's dietary roles, the next chapter critiques the assumption that it and hunting were central to our ancestors. This chapter lays the groundwork for this criticism by noting plants' importance to many primates, including our lineage. In contrast to the visual predation hypothesis, the angiosperm radiation hypothesis notes that primates became numerous only with the spread of angiosperms (flowering plants).[14] These plants provided fruits for primates. This perspective argues that primates, rather than being primarily insectivores, favored fruits. Corroboration comes from the fact that humans are unusual among mammals in inability to manufacture vitamin C, necessitating its consumption in fruits, vegetables, and kindred items. Our ancestors must have regularly eaten these foods, a practice that conferred no selective advantage to people whose bodies made the nutrient. Absent selective pressure, our ancestors lost the ability to synthesize it perhaps 60 million years ago.[15] Over the next 30 million years, humanity's ancestors ate primarily fruits, becoming frugivores.

Frugivory honed the brain and senses. Frugivores developed color vision to identify changes in hue that signaled ripening. These animals needed an ability to map their surroundings in the brain in order to remember locations rich in fruit trees or allied resources. They also had to sequence areas, recalling and visiting those that yielded ripe fruits in spring, after which they migrated to spots that ripened fruits later. This process, repeated over seasons and years, helped protect frugivores from lulls in food availability and hunger. In requiring concrete applications of cognition, frugivory spurred brain enlargement, an aspect of human evolution.

American anthropologist Stephen Le, mentioned elsewhere, doubted the wisdom of this diet given the dangers of excessive fructose ($C_6H_{12}O_6$) consumption.[16] Chapter 2 defined fructose, noting its benefits and shortcomings. Chapter 11 treats it in the context of high fructose corn syrup (HFCS), whose derivation Chapter 2 mentioned. Criticisms against fruits, treated in Chapter 14, are part of a general wariness of plant foods. Chapters 1 and 2 mentioned that American cardiac surgeon Steven R. Gundry displayed this hostility in *The Plant Paradox* (2017), an approach that contradicts some nutritionists and dieticians' advice and thereby exacerbates confusion about what to eat.

Returning to the issue of size, massiveness, like smallness, influenced what our ancestors ate. The line leading to humans and its branches—best visualized as a bush—produced species larger than the first primates. Bigness reduced the ratio of surface area to volume, metabolism, and the need to eat insects and other energy and nutrient dense edibles. Only during the last century or so has food become plentiful—perhaps too abundant—for the masses. Before then, consumption of caloric foods like animal products was the best hedge against hunger. The fact that our taste buds detect salt, fat, sweetness, and tanginess, mentioned earlier, guides the body toward calories. These preferences must have evolved to sustain humans when and where food was scarce, at least seasonally. A later section discusses famine.

As the largest primate and probably a vegetarian, *Gigantopithecus*, originating some 8 million year ago and now extinct, proved that enormity need not require meat consumption.[17] About 3 meters (10 feet) tall and 300 kilograms (660 pounds), it likely consumed nuts and seeds given robust jaws and teeth for crushing these items. The biggest extant primate, *Gorilla beringei* likewise eats plants. Leaves, stems, and shoots predominate with fruits constituting a small portion. Seldom does it consume insects. The smaller species, *G. gorilla*, favors plants, though it derives about 3 percent of its diet from termites, snails, and slugs.[18] At least one study indicates that this species will eat monkeys.[19]

These creatures are branches on the primate bush, though *Gigantopithecus*' twig has withered. The base of this bush regresses roughly 55 million years, when the first true primates likely arose.[20] This time marked the beginning of the Eocene Epoch (55–34 million years ago). Temperatures rose, producing tropical climates worldwide, conditions that favored plants and insects, both mentioned as components of primate diets. Remote eras have not yielded abundant fossils from which to infer diet. Those from Egypt's Fayum desert suggest consumption of fruits and seeds about 34 million years ago, the boundary between the Eocene and Oligocene (34–23 million years ago) Epochs.[21] Temperature reductions around this time imply diminution in number of plants and insects. Primates dependent on them may have suffered deprivation. The Oligocene witnessed the emergence of anthropoids, primates that resembled us more closely than their forebearers did and that today include monkeys, the apes, and humans.

Following the Oligocene, the Miocene Epoch (25–23 million years ago) marked the evolution of apes that ate leaves, fruits, and nuts. Gaps in the fossil record complicate attempts to pinpoint modern apes' origins. Their diets need not be rehashed, though comparisons between chimpanzees and humans are instructive. Like humans, chimps use tools to extract food. For example, they insert twigs into logs to gather termites. Such technology resembles digging sticks, which prehistoric peoples employed to unearth roots and tubers. Chimpanzees also resemble humans in hunting game. They target some thirty-five species, red colobus monkeys (*Piliocolobus* species) being their favorite. Although chimpanzees may hunt alone, at other times they hunt collectively, increasing probability of success. The fact that chimps and humans share over 98 percent of deoxyribonucleic acid (DNA), discussed in Chapter 2, suggests that their common ancestor might have hunted because genes may canalize behavior and that chimpanzee hunting might prefigure early human hunting.[22]

3.5.6 Bipedalism and Food Acquisition

Historians and philosophers have emphasized discontinuities between scientific and biblical accounts of human origins. These contrasts yielded insights, but among intellectuals the real battle focused on cognition. An Aristotelian faith in rationality, mentioned in Chapter 1, undergirded the nineteenth-century conviction that brain enlargement directed our evolution. This belief persisted into the twentieth century, explaining why zoologists and anatomists were willing to accept big-brained hoaxes like Piltdown Man as genuine. Pre-human discoveries since the 1920s have discredited faith in cognition as our evolution's actuator.

Accumulation of fossils fingers bipedalism as the adaptation that distinguished our lineage from other primates. This innovation appears to have arisen roughly 6 million years ago, some 4 million years before the brain's enlargement.[23] Bipedalism must confer advantages; otherwise competition for resources should have exterminated its possessors. That extinction has claimed all but one biped—*H. sapiens*—warns against exaggerating its advantages. Nonetheless, since the nineteenth century, naturalists, anthropologists, and biologists have labored to detail how upright carriage benefitted our lineage.

As in much of evolutionary discourse, the starting point is British naturalist Charles Robert Darwin (1809–1882). He understood the obvious: erect posture freed the hands to do something besides support the body during locomotion. Ability to oppose the thumb to the other fingers permits hands to grasp objects. Darwin asserted in *The Descent of Man* (1871) that the hands made and used weapons to hunt.[24] Hunting and meat consumption must therefore be humanity's hallmarks. Since Darwin, anthropologists have debated hunting and meat's importance to our evolution. Examining meat, Chapter 4 considers hunting's social and economic dimensions from an evolutionary perspective.

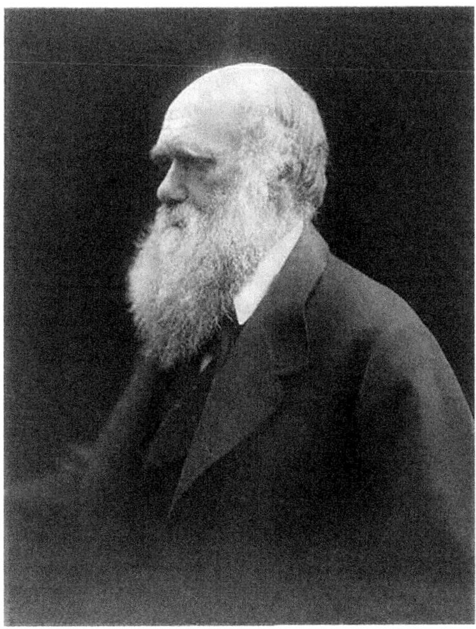

FIGURE 3.3 Charles Darwin. (Photo courtesy of Library of Congress. https://www.loc.gov/pictures/item/2004674431/.)

Debate over bipedalism has not produced unanimity. Twentieth and twenty-first century pre-human discoveries challenged Darwin's hunting thesis. Upright posture appears to have arisen some 5 million years before people began to hunt.[25] The earliest bipeds must have used their hands for another purpose. American anthropologist Claude Owen Lovejoy (b. 1943) hypothesized that our ancestors used their hands to gather food, which they carried back to camp.[26] Focusing on reproduction and child rearing, Lovejoy noted that many primate mothers raise offspring without the father. This burden reduces number of offspring because she must concentrate on acquiring food for one child until it is old enough to undertake this task. Lovejoy believed that our ancestors were different; the father used his hands to collect food, which he brought to mother and child, feeding both. Adequately nourished and spared from caring for children on her own, mothers could have more children without waiting for each to achieve autonomy. By feeding mother and child, fathers increased odds of survival for both. Lovejoy's ideas thus explained the origins and benefits of monogamy and the nuclear family.

In contrast to Darwin and Lovejoy, American anthropologists Peter S. Rodman (b. 1945) and Henry Malcolm McHenry (b. 1944) focused on feet rather than hands. They asserted that bipedalism is more efficient than quadrupedy, allowing our ancestors to cover long distances while foraging, scavenging, or hunting.[27] Efficiency implies that bipedalism reduced the need for calories. Rodman and McHenry's view supported Darwin and Lovejoy's contentions that bipedalism improved food acquisition, survival, and reproduction, explaining why bipedalism, once developed, persisted.

3.5.7 Australopithecine and *Paranthropus* Origins, Evolution, and Diets

Returning to the image of primate lineages as a bush, an analogy applicable to all life, the base represents primates' origins 55 million years ago. Movement up the bush is transition through time with the apex representing the present. This ascent is chronological progress but should not be construed as anatomical or behavioral improvement. Movement through time is not advancement from inferiority to superiority, primitiveness to perfection, or any language implying a trend. In mentioning *H. neaderthalensis*, an earlier section asserted that extinction does not evince inferiority any more than survival proves superiority. Geology and biology teach that extinction claims all species. None is immortal.

Movement up the bush produces many branches that spread from the base. Each twig represents a species. Many twigs are dead, signaling extinction, and are not immediately relevant to this discussion. Attention focuses on the twig that symbolizes humans and on its nearest live twigs, which represent chimpanzees, bonobos, gorillas, orangutans, and gibbons. Geography, anatomy, and genetics demonstrate that chimpanzees, bonobos, and gorillas are closer to humans than are orangutans and gibbons. Of the African apes—chimpanzees, gorillas, and bonobos—chimps are humans' nearest relatives, the two sharing their last common ancestor between 8 and 6 million years ago.[28] From this point of divergence, the path leading to us occupies the rest of this chapter.

This route is littered with extinct species more like us than extant apes. These extinct creatures plus humans constitute the hominins. Although only one trail among hominin paths leads to us, the others illuminate our lifeways. As context for the rest of this book, this chapter examines extinct hominins' diets and their relationship to our own. The previous section noted that bipedalism influenced how our ancestors obtained food. As an innovation, it thickened the primate bush, producing several genera and species.

Among the best known is the genus *Australopithecus*, which arose about 4 million years ago and whose fossils number in the hundreds.[29] Representing seven species, the australopithecines have received scrutiny since the 1920s. Naming the genus in 1924, South African anatomist Raymond Arthur Dart (1893–1988) thought it a carnivore.[30] Chapter 4 details his ideas.

British anthropologist Mary Douglas Leakey (1913–1996) complicated matters in 1959, discovering at Olduvai Gorge, Tanzania the first specimen of what is now classified *Paranthropus boisei*, a contemporary of *Australopithecus* and early *Homo*.[31] She found the remains among eggshells and bones of several animals, including mice (*Mus* species), rats (*Cricetomys* species), frogs (species in the order Anura), tortoises (species in the family Testudinidae), snakes (species in the suborder Serpentes), lizards (species in the order Squamata), birds (species in the class Aves), antelopes (species in the family Bovidae), and boars (*Sus scrofa*).[32] *P. boisei*'s large teeth capable of crushing nuts, seeds, and other hard materials led to the nickname "Nutcracker Man."[33] *Paranthropus*' dietary breadth, although the range is debated, focused attention on omnivory and eclecticism rather than carnivory.[34]

Australopithecus and *Paranthropus* appear to have eaten many items: nuts, seeds, tubers, roots, leaves, fruits, insects, eggs, and perhaps meat. They may have used twigs or slender bones to extract termites from logs in the manner of chimpanzees. Stone tools may have helped them unearth tubers and roots. Diverse strategies doubtless promoted survival, reproduction, and dispersal throughout Africa. They do not appear, however, to have mastered fire and so could not have cooked.

As noted, Australopithecines arose around 4 million years ago during the Pliocene Epoch (5–2.6 million years ago). Early in the Pliocene ocean temperatures were roughly 4 degrees Celsius (7.2 degrees Fahrenheit) above current averages.[35] Worldwide warmth supported plants, insects, and other animals that fed *Australopithecus*. Arising about 2.3 million years ago, *Paranthropus* benefited from grasslands' expansion in Africa by eating grass seeds.[36] Food supplies varied with temperature and rainfall during this time. Dearth stressed *Paranthropus*, probably causing its extinction. Species with the largest jaws and teeth likely ate leaves, nuts, seeds, roots, tubers, and other plant parts, though tooth wear suggests concentration on fruits. It may also have eaten meat. To the degree that they restricted diets to primarily plants, jaws and dentition may have hastened *Paranthropus*' demise.

3.5.8 *Homo habilis* and *Homo rudolfensis*: Origins, Evolution, and Diets

Although Leakey found *P. boisei* amid stone tools, her husband, Kenyan anthropologist Louis Seymour Bazett Leakey (1903–1972) deemed it too primitive to have made them.[37] This opinion, now out of favor, motivated the pair to seek the supposed first toolmaker. Others had unearthed but not classified its fossils in the late 1940s. The Leakeys added to these finds in 1959 and 1960.[38] In 1964 Louis Leakey, South African anthropologist Phillip Vallentine Tobias (1925–2012), and British physician and primatologist John Russell Napier (1917–1987) designated the creature *Homo habilis*, the earliest member of our genus.[39] The name means "handy man," emphasizing belief that it had been the first human to make tools.

The tag stirred controversy. Anatomy and geography usually determine classification of a species, but Leakey, Tobias, and Napier based the label *H. habilis* partly on tool making, which is a behavior rather than an anatomical trait. To be sure, anatomy shapes behavior. Without hands, for example, humans could not make the vast range of implements and other technologies that characterizes them. Nevertheless, such considerations complicate identification of species because behaviors must be inferred for extinct animals whereas anatomy permits measurement and description.

Moreover, emphasis on tool making may not be the watershed that the name *H. habilis* implies. *Australopithecus* and *Paranthropus* modified bones, twigs, and other objects for use as tools. As noted, chimpanzees use twigs to extract termites from logs. Sea otters (*Enhydra lutris*) use stones to break shells in order to eat shellfish, demonstrating that tool use is not exclusive to primates. Whether these animals make tools is debatable. Otters do not modify rocks in the way that human ancestors shaped them into blades, axes, scrapers, choppers, and points, though tool use reveals otters' ability to conceive an object not merely as static but as capable of manipulation to yield food. This thinking involves mental manipulation of objects even if the outcome is not their physical crafting into tools.

From this perspective, *H. habilis*' uniqueness is questionable. Moreover, it resembled *Australopithecus* in size and body proportions, suggesting membership in that genus rather than ours. For example, *H. habilis*' short legs may have made it walk like Australopithecines rather than us.[40] Yet *H. habilis* had smaller teeth and jaws and may have eaten an even greater diversity of foods than its predecessors and contemporaries. It may have used stone tools to unearth roots and tubers in a manner akin to *Australopithecus* and *Paranthropus*. Tools allowed *H. habilis* to process foods before eating them, lightening the load on teeth and jaws, which shrank over time. Although teeth were smaller, their enamel was thick, an adaptation to crushing and grinding tough materials like nuts, seeds, leaves, and even bark and wood. Like *Paranthropus*, *H. habilis* arose amid expansion of grasslands in Africa and ate grass seeds. Insects and other animals supplemented plants. Although *H. habilis* may not have hunted, it scavenged carcasses to increase protein intake. Beyond meat, *H. habilis* fractured animal bones to access marrow.

Like *Australopithecus* and *Paranthropus*, *H. habilis* never controlled fire and did not cook. Raw meat harbored pathogens, whose ingestion must have sped evolution of an immune system, kidneys, and liver. Energy and nutrient dense, meat accelerated enlargement of the brain, which has a voracious appetite. Our brain, though about 2 percent of body mass, devours some 20 percent of calories.[41] These considerations indicate that diet shaped *H. habilis*, yielding an animal with smaller face, jaws, and teeth and a bigger brain than *Australopithecus* and *Paranthropus*. *Australopithecus* averaged a brain between 380 and 550 milliliters.[42] Having larger bodies, *Paranthropus* had a brain, around 550 milliliters, at *Australopithecus*' upper bound.[43] *H. habilis* averaged about 600 milliliters.

Another early member of our genus, *H. rudolfensis*, had larger molars and premolars than those of *H. habilis*, intimating greater ability to crush and grind fibrous foods. Like robust Australopithecines and *Paranthropus*, *H. rudolfensis* housed teeth in powerful jaws. This dental anatomy equipped it to eat plants. On the other hand, it had a brain, at 775 milliliters, bigger than *Australopithecus*, *Paranthropus*, and *H. habilis*, implying that it ate meat for the energy and nutrients necessary to fuel cognition.[44] *H. rudolfensis* may therefore have been an omnivore like other hominins and primates in general. Despite its distinctiveness, *H. rudolfensis*' similarities to *H. habilis* convince some anthropologists that the two occupy one species.[45]

3.5.9 *Homo erectus*, Globalism, and Diets

Similarities to Australopithecines diminished with *H. erectus*, whose anatomy and behavior resembled ours. *H. erectus*' humanlike attributes make it is our genus' earliest unequivocal member.[46] Arising in Africa about 1.8 million years ago, *H. erectus* perished as late as 25,000 BCE.[47] During these millennia, its brain expanded from 650 milliliters to an average of 950 milliliters, with the largest being 1,200 milliliters.[48] Part of this increase stemmed from overall growth. *H. erectus* stood nearly 2 meters (2.2 yards or 6.6 feet), well within the range of modern peoples.[49] By contrast, *H. habilis* was between 1 meter (1.1 yards or 3.3 feet) and 1.3 meters (1.4 yards or 4.3 feet), roughly the stature of *Australopithecus* and *Paranthropus*.[50] *H. erectus'* fossils intimate a powerful physique with stout bones and large muscles.

The species resembled us not merely in size but also in behavior. *H. erectus* was the first to control fire about 1 million years ago, using it for warmth and cooking.[51] Anthropologists emphasized cooking's importance in making many items, including meat, more palatable and digestible. By tenderizing foods, cooking reduced chewing. Diminution of teeth, jaws, and face, observable in *H. habilis*, accelerated in *H. erectus*, giving it a more modern appearance. Aiding digestion, cooking shortened the large intestine (colon) and kept the stomach unspecialized. Chapter 4 notes that cooking let *H. erectus* eat more meat than its forebearers. Meat, acquired through hunting and scavenging, provided the nutrients and calories to enlarge brain and body.

Fire's control permitted colonization of temperate lands. Whereas no prior hominin left Africa, *H. erectus* displayed the modern penchant for migration, colonizing Asia and Europe in addition to its homeland. In Asia, migrants went as far east and south as Indonesia between 1 and 2 million years ago, staying within the tropics, though others moved north to Zhoukoudian (also spelled Choukoutien) near Beijing, China.[52] Other temperate Asian settlements included Majuangou, China, and Dmanisi, Georgia. In Europe, *H. erectus* penetrated north to Boxgrove, England, and Heidelberg, Germany. The Heidelberg specimen provokes disagreement over whether it is a unique species or *H. erectus*.

As is true of all animals, climate shaped *H. erectus*' diets. The tropics yielded edible plants year-round, though animals, including hominins, had to monitor them for signs of ripeness. This approach to food acquisition typified *H. erectus* in tropical Africa and Asia. But Zhoukoudian, Majuangou, Dmanisi, Boxgrove, and Heidelberg presented new challenges. Edible plants were available in warm weather but not in cold. Without plant foods during winter, *H. erectus* must have targeted game. Yet these animals faced the same stresses as people and were unusually lean. Winter fare in temperate regions must have featured protein but few carbohydrates and fat, threatening rabbit starvation, as mentioned earlier. Winter's paucity must have favored individuals who easily accumulated adipose during plentitude, the extra fat nursing them through winter. This chapter's final section explores the consequences of this adaptation.

3.5.10 Archaic *H. sapiens*: Origins, Evolution, and Diets

Anthropologists label early members of our species archaic. Connoting obsolescence or primitivism, the word risks disparagement. This book rejects any intimation that archaic peoples were inferior to their modern counterparts. Physical differences between them and us were small. Disparities stemmed from culture, of which technology is an element, more than biology. All organisms pass genes to the next generation, but humans bequeath much else: ideas, technologies, laws, mores, and other non-biological constructs and objects known collectively as culture.

Archaic peoples had a richer culture than their predecessors. Their tools included generic and specialist items and were more numerous than earlier versions. The best-known archaic group, Neanderthals buried their dead with grave goods, possibly including flowers, evidence that they pondered life's transience. Some burials oriented east and west, perhaps indicating sun worship.[53] Such beliefs evince complex minds and similarities to us. Their reputation as "cave men" ignores the reality that Neanderthals did not simply occupy their surroundings. They modified the environment by constructing dwellings. For example, roughly 45,000 years ago, *H. neanderthalensis* made abodes from mammoth bones and skins in what is today Ukraine.[54]

Like *H. erectus*, archaic species inhabited Africa, Asia, and Europe. In Africa, *H. erectus* appears to have evolved into anatomically modern peoples. *H. erectus* persisted in Asia until around 70,000 years ago, when moderns spread through the continent, replacing or mating with it. Europe remains a contentious space. Some anthropologists classify the earliest archaic peoples within *H. erectus*, whereas others move them into a new species, *Homo heidelbergensis*. These people, exposed to cold winters, evolved a compact, stocky frame in accord with Bergmann's rule, described in Chapter 1, and short, stout limbs to conserve heat in keeping with Allen's rule, formulated by American zoologist Joel Asaph Allen (1838–1921). From *H. heidelbergensis* arose Neanderthals, also adapted to cold.

Also like *H. erectus*, archaic peoples cooked. Absent laborious chewing, molars continued to shrink, though front teeth enlarged, a development unrelated to diet. As with *H. erectus*, attention has focused on meat. *H. heidelbergensis* and *H. neanderthalensis* sought large mammals, whose meat fed many mouths. Chapter 1 noted that the archaeological record preserves bones better than perishable plants. This bias buttresses perception of *H. neanderthalensis* as carnivores. One site in Hungary, for example, yielded bones from some 1,200 bison (*Bison bonasus*).[55] Neanderthals also ate mammoths (*Mammuthus* species), cattle (*Bos* species), boars, reindeer or caribou (*Rangifer tarandus*), rhinoceroses (*Rhinoceros* species), horses (*Equus ferus*), elk (*Cervus species*), wild donkeys (*Equus africanus*), deer (*Odocoileus* species), ibex (*Capra* species), chamois (*Rupicapra rupicapra*), and bears (*Ursus arctos*). *H. neanderthalensis* killed entire herds for meat. When large mammals were unavailable, Neanderthals targeted small game, including mice.

Israeli anthropologist and archaeologist Ofer Bar-Yosef (1937–2020) questioned preoccupation with meat, suggesting that its acquisition characterizes anatomically modern peoples better than their predecessors.[56] Like other animals and peoples, archaic *H. sapiens* ate what their surroundings supplied. Ecologists emphasize that plants are more numerous than animals in a biome, implying that archaic peoples consumed primarily plants. Evidence comes from Wadi Kebara, Israel's Kebara cave, which preserved seeds and nuts, including acorns (*Quercus* species). Bar-Yosef believed that the cave's inhabitants gathered these items primarily in March and April and again between October and December.[57] Scientists and scholars might oppose generalization of this cave's contents to all archaic diets, though extrapolation helps offset poor plant preservation in middens, noted in Chapter 1. Insects and meat supplemented this diet. Fish and shellfish's place in archaic diets is controversial and receives commentary in Chapter 5. Archeological evidence suggests that premodern peoples occasionally caught aquatic prey, which never constituted primary nutrients and calories. Referencing modern hunter-gatherers, Bar-Yosef estimated that plants gave archaic peoples in Africa and Asia's tropics and the Mediterranean basin over three-fifths of calories, with the rest coming from animals.[58] A previous section mentioned that meat was more important at high latitudes.

3.5.11 Modern *H. sapiens*: Origins, Evolution, and Diets

Previous sections intimated Africa's centrality to human origins. Darwin rooted humanity there.[59] Home to our closest relatives, the chimpanzee and gorilla, Africa must also have birthed humankind, he reasoned. Although he championed many of Darwin's ideas, German biologist Ernst Heinrich Philipp August Haeckel (1834–1919) rejected Africa as cradle, instead in the 1860s linking humans to Asia's orangutans.[60] In this scheme, he initially favored Indonesia, where in 1891 Dutch physician and anatomist Marie Eugene Francois Thomas Dubois (1858–1940) discovered the first *H. erectus* fragments.[61] Subsequent discoveries, beginning with Dart's 1924 identification of *Australopithecus africanus*, mentioned earlier, in Taung, South Africa, vindicated Darwin rather than Haeckel.

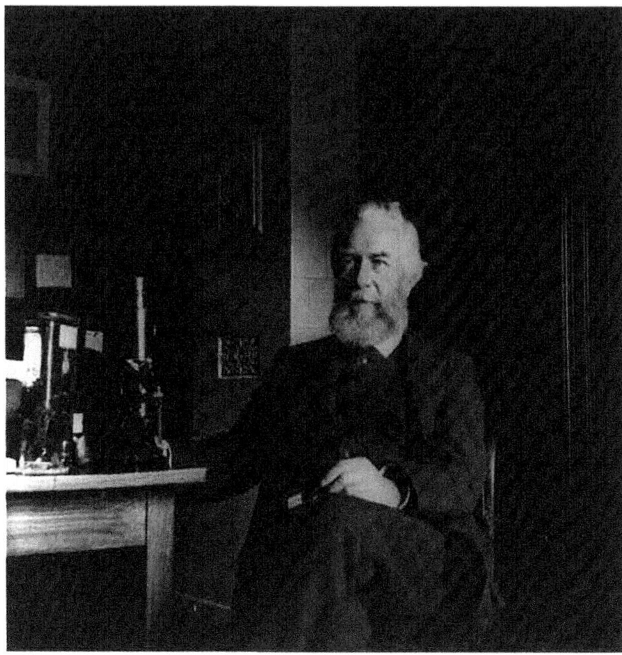

FIGURE 3.4 Ernst Haeckel. (Photo courtesy of Library of Congress. https://www.loc.gov/pictures/item/2016653104/.)

Modern humans arose in Africa within the last 200,000 years. In an evolutionary context, what constitutes modernity is open to interpretation. Anthropologists seek features like ours: gracile build, bulbous cranium with a brain as large as ours, flat face, small jaws and teeth, and a chin. The location and date of the oldest specimens with these traits are debatable, though Ethiopia in East Africa and Morocco in north-westernmost North Africa have yielded suitable fossils roughly 160,000 to 150,000 years old, approximating our origins.[62] From Ethiopia, humans could have reached Egypt and the Sinai Peninsula in southwestern Asia by following the Red Sea coast north. From Morocco, humans could have reached Egypt and the Sinai Peninsula by migrating east.

The Sinai permitted access to the Levant and Turkey in the north, Arabia in the southeast, and the rest of Asia to the east. Once in Turkey, the trek west approached modern Istanbul and the Bosporus Strait, across which was Europe. North of Morocco were the Strait of Gibraltar and Iberia (Spain and Portugal). Either path or both entered Europe.

These journeys were not instantaneous. Climate, topography, and food availability regulated the advance. Warmth enticed humans into the Levant—Chapter 14 describes southwestern Asia's geography—around 130,000 years ago, but cooling temperatures pushed them back into Egypt some 50,000 years later, when *H. neanderthalensis* recolonized the Levant.[63] These events occurred during the Pleistocene Epoch (2.6 million years ago–12,000 years ago), whose climate alternated between warm periods and ice sheets' spread across continents.

During cool periods, modern humans lived in Africa's tropics, but roughly 50,000 years ago they exited the continent even though temperatures were diminishing.[64] During the next 10,000 years, they colonized Europe to the northwest and penetrated Asia eastward. Moving southeast through Thailand, Cambodia, Vietnam, and Malaysia, humans reached Indonesia, New Guinea, and Australia. Other migrants moved north rather than south through Asia, settling Siberia before 20,000 years ago. Fire and warm clothes permitted life so far from the equator.

From Siberia, modern humans became the first peoples to colonize the Americas, though the time of this transition is debated. It was not a single event, but a series of migrations around 15,000 years ago made possible by the last ice age (115,000–11,700 years ago), during which more polar ocean water was ice than today.[65] With water locked in ice, the amount left as liquid diminished so that sea level dropped, exposing Beringia, a land bridge between northeastern Asia and northwestern North America. Asians, following grazing herds, crossed Beringia into North America. Because this land was exposed for millennia, people crossed it in many waves over many generations. Retreat of ice around 12,000 years ago and Beringia's disappearance beneath the ocean ended these migrations, separating the Americas from Asia. By 10,000 BCE humans, settling North and South America, had reached every habitable continent.

Such expanses of land, each with constellations of florae and faunae, gave humans diverse diets over time and space. Variety negates the idea of a paleo diet. Instead, people invented numerous paleolithic diets in adapting to their localities. Were it possible to pinpoint a single paleo diet, its resurrection today is unrealistic given that virtually everyone subsists on domesticates rather than wild plants and animals.

All dietary permutations cannot receive treatment, though a sampling of options in preagricultural North America underscores diversity. Chapter 9 documents that California indigenes harvested acorns millennia before Italian-Spanish mariner Christopher Columbus (1451–1506) reached the West Indies. They also ate fish, game, insects, berries, and roots. Pacific Northwest rivers yielded salmon (*Oncorhynchus* species) and other fish, whose plentitude permitted sedentism. In the American Southwest, people hunted mammoths, whose extinction about 6,000 years ago focused diets on wild turkeys (*Meleagris gallopavo*), pine or pinon nuts (*Pinus edulis*, *Pinus monophyla*, and *Pinus cembroides*), cacti (species in Cactaceae family), century plants (*Agave americana*), insects, berries, acorns, antelopes, deer, rabbits (species in Leporidae family), bears (*Ursus* species), snakes, owls (species in Strigidae and Tytonidae families), and coyotes (*Canis latrans*). Bison (*Bison bison*) sustained Great Plains Amerindians as salmon did those in the Pacific Northwest. Other game included elk, moose (*Alces alces*), deer, wolves (*Canis lupus*), coyotes, lynx (*Lynx* species), rabbits, gophers (*Thomomys* species), and North American prairie chickens (*Tympanuchus cupido*). Berries were eaten fresh in season and dried to last through winter. North toward the Arctic Circle, Inuit—discussed in Chapter 5—ate walrus (*Odobenus rosmarus*), seal (*Phoca vitulina*), whale (species in infraorder Cetacea), reindeer, polar bear (*Ursus maritimus*), muskox (*Ovibos moschatus*), trout (*Oncorhynchus mykiss*), cod (*Gadus* species), char (*Salvelinus alpinus*), capelin (*Mallotus villosus*), crowberry (*Empetrum* species), cloudberry (*Rubus chamaemorus*), fireweed (*Chamaenerion angustifolium*), seaweed (*Sargassum* species), and several grasses, roots, and tubers. Along the Missouri and Mississippi Rivers, diets featured fish, berries, and nuts. East of the Mississippi River, Native Americans ate bear, wild turkey, turtle (species in the order Testudines), grouse (species in the genera *Bonasa*, *Falcipennis*, *Tympanuchus*, and *Dendragapus*), palmetto berries (*Serenoa repens*) in Florida, numerous fish, pine nuts, wild sunflower (*Helianthus quinquelobus*) seeds, wild rice (*Zizania aquatica*), venison, pigeon (*Columba livia*), rabbit, acorns, and honey. This smorgasbord highlights our tendencies toward omnivory and opportunism. Past or present, variety supplies more nourishment than monotony.

3.5.12 From Food Acquisition to Food Production

Humans have long manipulated the environment to yield caloric foods, a trend that accelerated with agriculture and animal husbandry. Having starch, sugars, and fat, crops and livestock products are energy dense at the expense of nutrients and fiber.[66] From this observation follows the likelihood that foods were more nourishing before agriculture than afterward.[67] The wild animals that fed humans had to fend for themselves and were leaner than livestock, notes Chapter 10. What fat they had contained more omega 3 fatty acids—whose benefits Chapters 2 and 10 treat—than meat from livestock. Wild-caught fish retain this characteristic. Fat from game was less saturated than unsaturated, again differing from today's meat.

From these contrasts and from observations of today's hunter-gatherers, American radiologist Stanley Boyd Eaton (b. 1938) and coauthors asserted that preagricultural diets supplied over 30 percent of calories as protein, below one-quarter as fat, and about 100 grams daily of fiber, much of it soluble.[68] Fats were chiefly unsaturated and in a 1:1 ratio of omega 6 to omega 3. Diets contained abundant minerals, except sodium, and vitamins. Preagricultural peoples consumed many nutrients due to foods' quality and quantity. Being active, they ate plenty without becoming obese. Such fare contrasts with current preferences for little fiber and abundant sugars, saturated fat, and salt. Moreover, people now are inactive, a topic discussed later and throughout this book.

As had their predecessors, modern humans acquired foods by gathering, scavenging, hunting, and fishing before the advent of agriculture and livestock rearing. Writing about hunter-gatherers in 1965, American anthropologist Francis Clark Howell (1925–2007) gushed at the spectacle of fit men pursuing game over many kilometers of difficult terrain.[69] When necessary, they tracked a wounded animal for days of sustained walking and jogging, eating virtually nothing. Hunter-gatherers had abundant reserves of stamina and the vitality that come from occupying the pinnacle of health, a description that borders on romanticism.

Emphasis on hunter-gatherers' virtues transformed them into noble savages, a seventeenth-century literary creation. Uncorrupted by civilization, they represented humankind's original purity and goodness. This conviction underpinned Genesis' first chapters.[70] By implication, what they ate was wholesome. Aware of this attitude, food manufacturers celebrate a product's naturalness, true or not, because the public equates "natural" with "healthful." This conflation elevates the status and price of organic foods above agribusiness' produce. Preference for natural foods is reasonable in many cases, as noted. Their benefits are evident to gardeners, whose home-grown tomatoes (*Solanum esculentum*) have more flavor and nutrients than their commercial counterparts, picked green and exposed to ethylene gas (C_2H_4) to redden them.

Attention on hunting and gathering acknowledges their longevity as subsistence. Originating about 150,000 years ago, as mentioned, modern humans gathered, scavenged, hunted, and fished for all but the last 10,000 years. In some instances, these activities persisted into modernity. For example, Dutch sailors who landed on Australia in 1606 found no evidence of agriculture, though recent scholarship defines the aborigines as more than hunter-gatherers.[71] That hunting and gathering occupied over 90 percent of modern humans' tenure on Earth, and the entirety of our Australopithecine, *Paranthropus*, and *Homo* predecessors, allowed evolution to shape us and our diets for this mode of existence. From an evolutionary perspective, therefore, hunter-gatherers are the gold standard for evaluating us.[72]

Regrettably, the result is dualism between them and us. Stephen Le hammered home the contrast between hunter-gatherers' physical and mental vigor and our slothfulness. He estimated that hunter-gatherer men walked some 14.5 kilometers (9 miles) and women 9.5 kilometers (6 miles) daily compared to 4 kilometers (2.5 miles) for the average American adult.[73] He remarked that Americans spend lots of time in a car and in front of a television, computer, or both. Such inactivity causes and worsens chronic diseases.

As convincing as this example may seem, contrast between nomadism and sedentism risks overstating the divide. Where lifestyle is at issue, dissimilarity between activity and inertness does not appear to be rooted in the contrast between hunter-gatherers and us because modern humans lived strenuous existences long after they stopped searching for food. Although one example should not be pushed too far, in October 1705 German composer Johann Sebastian Bach (1685–1750) walked nearly 400 kilometers (250 miles) to visit a prominent organist, returning on foot the following February.[74] Beyond Bach, the bicycle's nineteenth-century debut occasioned gatherings of riders who devoted Sundays, often the only day free from work, to pedaling a century—a trek of one hundred miles (161 kilometers). These ventures were popular in the 1890s, the decade of the bicycle craze. Around then, men competed over one or many days to determine who could walk farthest per unit time. In 1808, British naval officer Robert Heriot Barclay (1786–1837) walked 1,000 miles in 1,000 hours.[75] In 1909, American pedestrian Edward Payson Weston (1839–1929), aged seventy, walked nearly 6,440 kilometers (4,000 miles) from New York City to San Francisco.[76] A year later he returned to the Big Apple from Los Angeles, covering 5,794 kilometers (3,600 miles). Both ways crowds greeted him as newspapers updated his progress daily. Those with money bet on pedestrian races, rejoicing or groaning their favorite's performance.

This vigor seems rare today in the United States and other developed countries. Walking and cycling have ceded ground to the automobile with results that should have been predictable a century ago. On average, the more time drivers spend on the road, the more obese they become.[77] Once at their destination, people do everything in their power not to exert themselves. Parking lots have become a battle zone where cars jostle for the closest spot. Tempers flare whenever someone believes an interloper has stolen a prized space that was about to be vacated. Stories proliferate about drivers, many young and able bodied, who park in handicapped zones to minimize walking. Others park on the wrong side of the road to be nearer their destination. Some drive rather than walk to get the mail even when the mailbox is no farther than driveway's end.

In this context, Weston, healthy to the end, suffered an ironic fate, dying not of natural causes but because a bus struck him. The automobile has killed countless people in accidents, though its corrosive effects are more insidious. It, along with other labor-saving machines, has idled too many people. As they retreated to their computers and televisions, heart disease, cancers, type 2 diabetes, and related maladies proliferated. The body no longer wears out from a lifetime of strenuous activities but instead deteriorates from disuse. In other words, the dichotomy is less between hunter-gatherers and us than between the eras before and after the automobile's invention.

Another problem with Le's characterization is its tenuousness. He omitted citations for distances that preagricultural women and men walked, though the numbers likely came from studies of modern hunter-gatherers. Chapter 1 advised caution when comparing peoples from radically different times. Such comparisons may be weak because modern hunter-gatherers occupy areas inadequate for farming or livestock raising. Their marginality implies that these people must work hard for food. In contrast, some preagricultural groups inhabited choice areas. Pacific Northwest Amerindians, mentioned earlier, had access to enough fish to permit sedentism. Yet the American Southwest's aridity likely generated conditions closer to those hunter-gatherers face today. Disparities between Pacific Northwest and American Southwest underscore the futility of trying to calculate an average number of kilometers walked daily.

Nonetheless, the generalization that hunter-gatherers led more arduous lives than we do must be correct, at least partly because, as mentioned, we have cars, airplanes, and other machines that they lacked. It must also be true because they had more robust physiques than we do.[78] Stouter bones require larger muscles to move them. All else being equal, large muscles are stronger than small ones. But large muscles require many calories to maintain, a potential liability whenever food is scarce. Evolution could have favored robusticity only if it provided a survival or reproductive advantage greater than its liabilities. That is, brawn's advantages must have outweighed high metabolism's disadvantages because life was sufficiently strenuous to favor strength over weakness even where countervailing forces operated.

Taking all factors into account, this chapter warns against wreathing our preagricultural past in a halo of sanctity. The temptation to venerate the remote past as a golden age, evident in Genesis' creation story, attempts to create a utopia that never existed. People mythologize the past because such thinking promotes optimism. If humans achieved perfection or something near it in the past, then they should be capable of elevating present and future to an exalted state.

Although these notions comfort us, they are untrue. English philosopher Thomas Hobbes (1588–1679) judged the state of nature, absent "culture of the earth," as "solitary, poor, nasty, brutish, and short."[79] Only about one-quarter of Neanderthals and contemporary modern humans lived to age forty, and few surpassed twenty during prehistory.[80] Early agriculturists fared no better. Although a small sample from Table 3.1, ten skeletons from Anatolia—Asia Minor or Asian Turkey—dating between roughly 550 and 333 BCE, evinced death before age forty in all but one case.[81]

Table 3.2, also concerning Anatolia, uses age ranges different from those in Table 3.1 and so defies close comparison with its predecessor. Nonetheless, it shows high mortality before age fourteen and after twenty-one. Only adolescence exhibited fewer deaths, a feature common to premodern populations.

TABLE 3.1
Age at Death (yr) in Anatolia from Senyurek

Period	Time	0–12	13–20	21–40	41–60	60+	Total Individuals
Chaleolithic-Copper	c. 5800–c. 3750 BCE	13 (20.9%)	8 (12.9%)	22 (35.4%)	15 (34.1%)	4 (6.4%)	62
Early Bronze	c. 3750–c. 1600 BCE	N/A	1 (33.1%)	1 (33.3%)	1 (33.3%)	N/A	3
Hittite Empires	c. 1600–c. 1200 BCE	2 (14.2%)	1 (7.1%)	9 (64.2%)	1 (7.1%)	1 (7.1%)	14
Post-Hittite–Phrygian	c. 1200–c. 550 BCE	2 (14.2%)	2 (14.2%)	7 (50%)	2 (14.2%)	1 (7.1%)	14
Medo-Persian–Hellenistic	c. 550–c. 333 BCE	3 (30%)	N/A	6 (60%)	1 (10%)	N/A	10
Roman–Byzantine	c. 332 BCE–c. 600 CE	1 (11.1%)	2 (22.2%)	3 (33.3%)	2 (22.2%)	1 (11.1%)	9
Total series		21(18.7%)	14(12.5%)	48(42.8%)	22(19.6%)	7(6.2%)	112

TABLE 3.2
Age at Death (yr) in Anatolia from Krogman

Time	Date	0–14	14–21	21+	Total
Chaleolithic	c. 5800–c. 4500 BCE	8 (66.7%)	1 (8.3%)	3 (25%)	12
Copper	c. 4500–c. 3750 BCE	9 (19.5%)	3 (6.5%)	34 (73.9%)	46
Early Bronze	c. 3750–c. 1600 BCE	N/A	1 (20%)	4 (80%)	5
Hittite Empire	c. 1600–c. 1200 BCE	29 (40.2%)	5 (6.9%)	38 (52.7%)	72
Post-Hittite–Phrygian	c. 1200–c. 550 BCE	3 (37.5%)	N/A	5 (62.5%)	8
Medo-Persian–Hellenistic	c. 550–c. 333 BCE	4 (36.3%)	N/A	7 (63.6%)	11
Roman–Byzantine	c. 332 BCE–c. 600 CE	7 (25.9%)	4 (14.8%)	16 (59.2%)	27
All periods		60 (33.1%)	14 (7.7%)	107 (59.1%)	181

High infant mortality kept life expectancy at birth (e^0) around twenty years. For example, estimates for ancient Egypt range between nineteen and twenty-five years.[82] Egyptian women who survived to age five, thereby escaping death in infancy, could expect another twenty-five years. Men averaged twenty-nine additional years. Into the Middle Ages, forty years marked life's end.[83]

French anthropologist and paleontologist Henri Victor Vallois (1889–1981) lamented that "few individuals passed forty years, and it is only quite exceptionally that any passed fifty."[84] Regressing some 750,000 years, he calculated in Table 3.3 that just 18.2 percent of Chinese *H. erectus* reached forty.[85] The percentage was 10.2 for Neanderthals between around 400,000 and 30,000 years ago, 12 for Eurasians between roughly 40,000 and 10,000 years ago—a period known as the Upper Paleolithic—3.7 for North Africans between about 25,000 and 11,000 years ago, and 4.2 percent for Eurasians from around 10,000 to 8000 BCE, a time known as the Mesolithic or Middle Stone Age. None of the 163 North Africans, only two of the seventy-six Upper Paleolithic individuals, and two of the seventy-one Mesolithic people lived beyond fifty years.

TABLE 3.3
Age at Death (yr) from Vallois

Place and Number of Persons	Age at Death (yr) from Vallois											
China, *Homo erectus* (c. 1.7 million–c. 300,000 yr ago) 22	0–14	%	15–30	%	31–40	%	41–50	%	51–60	%		
	15	68.2	3	13.6	N/A	N/A	3	13.6	1	4.6		
	Age group at death											
Indonesia, *H. erectus* (c. 1.65 million–c. 250,000 yr ago) 11	Young	%	Adolescent	%	Adult	%	Old Adults	%				
	1	9.1	4	36.1	2	18.2	4	36.4				
	Age range (yr) at death											
	Infants		Juveniles	Old Adults								
	0–11	%	12–20	%	21–30	%	31–40	%	41–50	%	51–60	%
Neanderthal, Eurasia (c.400,000–c. 30,000 yr ago) 39	15	38.5	4	10.3	6	15.4	10	25.6	3	7.7	1	2.5
Modern *H. sapiens*, Eurasia (c. 40,000–c. 10,000 yr ago) 76	29	38.2	12	16.0	15	20.0	11	14.7	7	9.2	2	2.8
Modern *H. sapiens*, North Africa (c. 25,000–c. 11,000 yr ago) 163		101	62%		31	19.0	25	15.3	6	3.7		
Modern *H. sapiens*, Eurasia (c. 10,000–c. 8000 BCE) 71	21	29.5	6	8.5	35	49.3	6	8.5	1	1.4	2	2.8

Summarizing humanity's frailty, Vallois wrote that prehistoric peoples survived little longer than apes.[86] Although some demographers and anthropologists disputed this conclusion—see American anthropologists Michael D. Gurven and Hillard Seth Kaplan's *Longevity among Hunter-Gatherers: A Cross-Cultural Examination* (2007)—research on Thai skeletons dating between roughly 2000 and 400 BCE reiterated Vallois' finding that few exceeded forty years.[87] Western hemisphere skeletons of Amerindians, Africans, and Europeans revealed that before roughly 1900 CE, few surpassed forty-five.[88]

The number forty's repetition is intriguing. Although some 40,000 years separated Neanderthals and early modern humans from their medieval counterparts, the same pattern prevailed: few people surpassed their fortieth year. Stasis implies that changes in diet and nutrition over these millennia—notably transition to agriculture and animal husbandry about 10,000 years ago—did not affect longevity. If farming harmed humanity, as critics charge, the injuries are not evident in attempts to gauge lifespan.

Admittedly, quantification poses problems. Data from Neanderthals and contemporary modern humans derive from partial and complete skeletons, which document these individuals. At issue is whether information about them can be extrapolated to countless early peoples whose skeletons have not been discovered or no longer exist. Turning to the Middle Ages, lifespan data come primarily from church records of births and deaths in Europe's cities and countryside. At issue is these statistics' applicability beyond Europe. Onlookers might wonder what they reveal about longevity in Africa, Asia, Australia, Oceania, and the Americas. Moreover, the problem of sample size is acute because the distant past lacked modern bureaucracies' comprehensive records.

These difficulties persist. Chapter 1 mentioned that Francis Clark Howell in 1965 reported lifespans over many millennia. Table 3.4 lists his figures for Europe between roughly 40,000 years ago and the fourteenth century CE, the period under review in previous paragraphs. Although he did not cite the source for these data, Howell put Neanderthal longevity at 29.4 years, the Cro-Magnons who settled France roughly 40,000 years ago at 32.4 years, and Bronze Age (c. 3700–c. 500 BCE) Austrians and fourteenth-century Britons at thirty-eight years.[89] Howell's silence about the origin of these numbers complicates their interpretation. Comparison of his figures to those already cited for antiquity indicates that he must have omitted newborns and infants. Chapter 1 and an earlier paragraph noted that high infant mortality, when counted, reduces e^0. Moreover, as noted, concentration on Europe may reveal little about the rest of the world.

Howell's numbers match those in a 1960 *Scientific American* article tabulated in Table 3.5, whose perusal suggests that he cherry picked data. Its author, American ecologist and limnologist Edward Smith Deevey Jr. (1914–1988), computed decreases in longevity from the Bronze Age to ancient Greece and Rome, figures that Howell ignored.[90] Deevey admitted that all estimates were too high because they omitted juvenile mortality given that immature skeletons, being delicate, preserved poorly.[91]

He surmised that between Neanderthal prehistory and 1900 CE, e^0 seldom departed over five years either way of age twenty-five and that half of all children perished before puberty. These numbers put e^0 between twenty and thirty years, a range that mirrors Austrian historian

TABLE 3.4
Longevity in Europe from Howell

Europe	Time	Lifespan (yr)
Neanderthal	c. 100,000 yr ago	29.4
Cro-Magnon	c. 40,000 yr ago	32.4
Bronze Age Austria	c. 3700–c. 500 BCE	38
England	14th century CE	38

TABLE 3.5
Longevity Absent Youth Mortality from Deevey

Place	Time	Lifespan (yr)
Eurasia	c. 100,000 yr ago	29.4
Eurasia	c. 40,000–c. 10,000 yr ago	32.4
Eurasia	c. 7000–c. 5000 BCE	31.5
Anatolia	c. 7000–c. 5800 BCE	38.2
Austria	c. 1750–c. 900 BCE	38
Greece	c. 2000–c. 30 BCE	35
Rome	c. 750 BCE–c. 500 CE	32
England	1276 CE	48
England	1376–1400	38
United States	1900–1902	61.5
United States	1950	70

TABLE 3.6
E^0 from Weiss

Place	Time	E^0 (yr)
Africa, Australopithecus	c. 3 million yr ago	c. 15
Eurasia	c. 100,000 yr ago	c. 18
World, preagriculture	<c. 8000 BCE	19–25
World, Neolithic	c. 7000–c. 5800 BCE	20–27
World, modern hunter-gatherers	c. 1900 CE	22–29
Eurasia	c. 3000 BCE–c. 1400 CE	22–29
Sweden	1780	38
United Kingdom	1861	43
Guatemala	1893	24
Sweden	1903	54
Sweden	1960	73

Walter Scheidel's (b. 1966) estimate for antiquity and American sociologist and demographer Karl Eschbach's for premodern times.[92] Corroboration of high juvenile mortality comes from twelve Anatolian skeletons listed in Table 3.2—admittedly a small sample—interred around 4500 BCE. Two-thirds died before age fifteen.[93] Over 6,300 years later, a Sangamon County, Illinois physician stated in 1840 that half of deaths occurred before age five, an estimate confirmed by county statistics a decade later.[94] As late as 1991, up to half the developing world's newborns died before age five.[95]

These harsh statistics have not eradicated notions of progress. American anthropologist and geneticist Kenneth M. Weiss (b. 1941) calculated, in Table 3.6, that e^0 nearly doubled from roughly fifteen years for Australopithecines to between twenty-two and twenty-nine years for ancient and medieval peoples.[96] Advancing the idea that chronological progress entails demographic improvement, Weiss reckoned that modern hunter-gatherers outlived their preagricultural predecessors even though, as noted, moderns likely have access to a narrower range of foods than their forebearers did. Despite difficulties in computation and interpretation, longevity is, this book emphasizes, a potentially important health index. Accordingly, later chapters compare lifespans, among other factors, over time and space to illuminate foods' effects on vitality.

3.5.13 The Debate over Agriculture and Animal Husbandry

The transition to farming and livestock raising, noted earlier, changed humanity in innumerable ways. Agriculture reinforced the trend toward sedentism and yielded a surplus, both of which were necessary for civilizations to flourish. By freeing a minority from the drudgery of tilling the land, farming permitted urbanites to specialize as craftspeople, artists, record keepers, priests, merchants, physicians, lawyers, inventors, architects, soldiers, bankers, and bureaucrats. A market economy—though not trade—appears to require the stability that farming provides. Government beyond the parameters of clan or tribe also seems improbable absent agriculture. Technology, although present to a degree among hunter-gatherers, progressed little before farming. These developments indicate that the modern world would not exist without agriculture and animal husbandry.

American internist and Rockefeller Foundation president John Hilton Knowles (1926–1979) summarized farming and livestock raising's benefits, asserting in 1977 that they provided a stable food supply and improved nutrition worldwide.[97] More and better crops, meat, poultry, eggs, and dairy products increased birthrates and diminished mortality. Although this book disputes the notion that agriculture and animal husbandry lengthened lifespan, Knowles is correct to attribute global population increases to their origin and development.

Agriculture's benefits have not silenced critics. Journalists have publicized modern farming's faults. Factory farms pollute air, land, and water. Pesticides, herbicides, and fertilizers taint the environment and food supply. Crops deplete soils of nutrients, erosion reduces organic matter, and salts from irrigation water diminish fertility. Cattle emit the greenhouse gas methane (CH_4). Poultry raisers immobilize chickens (*Gallus gallus domesticus*) in tiny cages. Pigs (*Sus scrofa domesticus*) and cattle wallow in their own excrement. Bacteria like *Salmonella enterica* and *Salmonella bongori* threaten us by multiplying in meat, vegetables, and fruits. Antibiotics and hormones pass from animal products to humans. Critics fault biotechnology for engineering foods whose consequences may be unknown.

Popular books accuse modern agriculture of undermining health. Chapters 1 and 12 mention that in *Wheat Belly* (2011), American cardiologist William R. Davis (b. 1957) blamed wheat for sickening and fattening consumers.[98] He wrote that modern cultivars have unnatural proteins (gliadin) due to scientific breeding since the 1960s.[99] Gliadin, he believed, affects the brain like opium, producing an addiction that causes overeating. (Readers might note that opium tends to suppress appetite.) In other words, wheat was an acceptable food until modern science perverted it. Chapter 12 evaluates these criticisms.

Modern farming is not alone in suffering condemnation. Anthropologists and economists critique farming at the other end of its chronology by focusing on origins, dismantling Knowles' opinion. For example, American anthropologist Robert Jurmain and coauthors remarked that "Although we might reasonably expect that nutrition and health would have improved with the development of agriculture, human health actually declined in most parts of the world beginning about 10,000 years ago."[100] American geographer Jared Mason Diamond (b. 1937) asserted that "the adoption of agriculture, supposedly our most decisive step toward a better life, was in many ways a catastrophe from which we have never recovered."[101] Clark Spencer Larsen wrote that "the shift from foraging to farming occasioned a reduction in nutrition."[102]

As noted, crops and livestock tend to have fewer nutrients than their wild counterparts. To be fair, scientists have bioengineered crops with extra nutrition. For example, in 1999, the International Rice Research Institute (IRRI) in Los Banos, Philippines developed "golden rice," which has beta carotene.[103] Chapter 2 introduced it and other carotenoids as vitamin A precursors, allowing golden rice to combat night blindness, a problem that Chapter 12 describes. Such benefits, however, were unavailable to early farmers.

Besides the claim that farming yields unnourishing foods, critics charge that agriculture reduced nutritional breadth by narrowing the range of foods. An earlier section noted this criticism's failure to acknowledge that farmers and stockmen raise what consumers want. As mentioned, farmers plant only about twenty of nature's over 20,000 edible plants on a large scale. Agriculture's emphasis, as noted, is on plants that yield many calories per hectare: sugarcane, potatoes, sweet potatoes (*Ipomoea batatas*), yams (*Dioscorea* species), cassava (*Manihot esculenta*), and similar items.

Overreliance on few plants undermines the omnivory and eclecticism typical of primates, including us, and can cause diseases. Chapters 2 and 12 implicate corn in pellagra and anemia, and polished rice in beriberi. Agriculture and animal husbandry appear to have worsened anemia, whose incidence rose upon their adoption.[104] This book indicates that diet was not always to blame because sedentism and crowding enabled parasites, pathogens, rodents, and insects to multiply, causing several maladies including anemia.

As this book does in detail, agriculture's detractors attempt to evaluate foods' effects on populations that consumed them. Larsen emphasized that when people became farmers and stockmen in Europe, southwestern Asia, Nubia—now southern Egypt and Sudan—Afghanistan, India, Pakistan, Bangladesh, Sri Lanka, Nepal, Bhutan, and Maldives in South Asia, and Illinois and lands along the Ohio River in North America they became shorter than their hunter-gatherer predecessors.[105] Echoing this view, Stanley Boyd Eaton and American anthropologist Melvin Joel Konner (b. 1946) wrote that the transition from hunting and gathering to agriculture and animal husbandry shortened Europeans 15.2 centimeters (6 inches) on average.[106] Because undernutrition stunts growth and because this phenomenon occurred in disparate areas, Larsen believed farming and livestock raising, the commonalities, must have been the culprits.[107]

But another explanation is possible. Height reductions were part of a trend toward smallness. Having slenderer bones and smaller muscles, agriculturalists were more lightly built (gracile) than their forebearers.[108] This development is difficult to interpret because it did not begin with farming. Modern humans have grown more gracile over time, not just since agriculture.[109] As mentioned, robusticity permitted strenuous exertions. Its decreases, therefore, may indicate that life became easier. Our ancestors may have become progressively better at using brain rather than brawn to survive. Whatever insights come from the trend toward gracility, it underscores this book's cautions against comparing radically dissimilar peoples. In other words, the fact that our hunter-gatherer predecessors were robust and lived physically taxing lives complicates comparison between them and us.

Returning to agriculture, dependence on few staples brought scarcity when they failed. Hunter-gatherers minimized risk by feeding on whatever the environment provided. If one tree was barren, they searched the next for berries, nuts, or another commodity. In this way, failure of a single resource did not threaten privation or starvation. Agriculture seldom permitted this luxury. Dependence on one crop was especially perilous because its failure could induce famine.

In this context, Chapter 2 mentioned the Irish potato famine. In 1845 and 1846, late blight of potato, caused by the mold *Phytophthora infestans*, destroyed Ireland's sustenance. Hunger drove people to eat bark, soil, weeds, leather, insects, rodents, and feces.[110] Too weak to leave their beds, families perished in their hovels, mothers clutching infants as all expired. [111] Dogs, cats (*Felis catus*), pigs, and rats (*Rattus* species) devoured corpses too numerous for burial. The dead awaiting this fate clogged gutters and streets. The disease recrudesced in subsequent years, causing over 1 million Irish to starve and 1.5 million to flee the island.[112]

British physician and botanist Redcliffe Nathan Salaman (1874–1955) judged the catastrophe Europe's worst since the Black Death (1347–1351), mentioned elsewhere.[113] The famine was unique only in magnitude. With dismal results, the Irish had subsisted on potatoes over a century before the cataclysm. Between 1724 and 1749 the harvest failed five times.[114] The fifteen years before the famine also produced misfortune, the yield being inadequate in 1830, 1832, 1835, 1837, 1839, 1840, and 1842. Such statistics underscored monoculture's dangers, particularly when uniformity exposed a crop to pathogens or pests, as in Ireland.

The island was not alone in suffering deprivation given famine's antiquity. It recurred often in southwestern Asia and Egypt between roughly 4000 and 500 BCE.[115] In this context, Genesis mentioned two in the Levant and a third in Egypt.[116] If these instances were real, then they must predate

Genesis' composition in the first millennium BCE. The Romans held an annual festival to seek god Robigus' protection against the grain diseases that presaged famine.[117] Between roughly 750 and 1100 CE Europe counted over fifty-five famines.[118] Diminishing crop yields hastened classical Mayan civilization's demise around 1000.[119] In 1065, Egyptians ate one another after exhausting the supply of dogs and cats.[120] Hunger and starvation afflicted Europe in 1312, 1315, 1316, 1317, 1339, and 1340, setting the stage for the Black Death.[121] The century or so afterward was no better, witnessing famines in 1352, 1362, 1397, 1416, 1426, and 1467.[122]

Crop failures in Germany between 1637 and 1639 induced consumption of cats, mice, and carrion. When these items ran short, Wittenberg instituted a lottery to decide who would be sacrificed to feed others. Poor harvests, low yields even in satisfactory years, and warfare multiplied famines before the eighteenth century.[123] Scarcity plagued the German states every fourth or fifth year until the nineteenth century.[124] Bread shortages sparked revolutions in France (1789–1799) and Russia (1917).

From 1891 to 1921, recurrent famines killed 834,000 Indians in Bombay Province.[125] Three million Bengalis starved in 1943.[126] Between 1968 and 1974, drought in West and Central Africa exacerbated the problems of overgrazing and deforestation, starving 1 million.[127] In 1974 warfare, floods, overpopulation, poverty, and the rice harvest's failure extirpated 1.5 million Bangladeshis.[128] With little arable land, North Korea suffered floods, droughts, and government corruption that starved 3 million between 1994 and 1998.[129] Malnutrition, starvation, and deficiency diseases killed over 3 million in the Democratic Republic of the Congo from 1998 to 2004.[130] Over 30,000 Somali children died from a famine that killed some 285,000 people in Somalia, Kenya, Ethiopia, and Djibouti in 2011 and 2012.[131] Since 2016 famines have penetrated Yemen, South Sudan, Somalia, and Nigeria. In 2018, the United Nations International Children's Emergency Fund (UNICEF) in New York City estimated that malnutrition kills 3 million children annually.[132] Summarizing famine's ubiquity, French historian Fernand Paul Braudel (1902–1985) wrote that it "recurred so insistently for centuries on end that it became incorporated into man's biological regime and built into his daily life."[133]

Food shortages unleashed the worst in humankind. Larsen believed that warfare became more savage with agriculture and animal husbandry's origins, as hungry rivals fought for land and livestock.[134] Conflicts sometimes pitted pastoralists against farmers, as the story of Cain and Abel implied.[135] In the American Southwest, aridity limited food production (see Chapter 6), exacerbating hunger and violence in pre-Columbian times. Skeletons displayed evidence of mutilation, including scalping. Droughts between roughly 950 and 1,250 caused brutality to devolve into cannibalism in what is today Cowboy Wash, Colorado, where the victors turned to human flesh to supplement inadequate nourishment.[136]

Cannibalism, mentioned here and in Egypt and Germany, traced its prehistory to Neanderthals, who must have been famished to have extracted marrow from human bones.[137] Such activity discredits any attempt to blame the practice on agriculture.

At issue is a phenomenon known as the Malthusian trap, named after English economist and cleric Thomas Robert Malthus (1766–1834). Born during the Enlightenment, he rejected the prevailing optimism that science and rationality could improve and perhaps perfect humanity. In *An Essay on the Principle of Population* (1798), he challenged the faith in progress, arguing that humans produce more children than the food supply can support.[138] Nature reduces excess through war, famine, and disease, as earlier examples indicated.[139]

Agriculture's detractors note that the third Malthusian check, contagion, spread among farmers, stockmen, and the urbanites who consumed their surpluses more easily than among nomads. Whereas gathering, scavenging, hunting, and fishing supported sparse populations, farming supplied the calories for large settlements. Free from the need to follow herds, agriculturists formed cities. Human and animal wastes aggregated in these places, allowing pathogens to multiply. These germs circulated among people who lived and worked together. Furthermore, livestock were likely the source of some infections. For example, humans probably contracted smallpox from cows and influenza from pigs, chickens, or possibly another bird. Measles may have arisen in cattle, passing to humans during domestication. Supplying carbohydrates, agriculture worsened oral diseases like caries. In contrast to farming's critics, however, this book emphasizes crowding and poor sanitation more than agriculture as contagion's abettor, a position consonant with research.[140]

Additionally, food supply impinges on economics because food sharpens inequalities.[141] Whenever it is scarce, prices rise absent subsidies. These increases do not trouble the rich but may prevent the masses from eating enough. Inequality's ultimate expression, slavery let owners deny their property sustenance. From the Caribbean islands to Sugar Land, Texas, sugar planters truncated lives by underfeeding slaves or convicts reduced to chattel.[142] Chapter 1 mentioned that in the Pacific Northwest—where inequalities were less stark—scarcity led Chinook elites to seize the poor's food.[143]

Dearth also affects biology. In several contexts, this chapter emphasized the precariousness of seeking food or growing it. Nature may produce less than expected. Alternatively, the environment may remain fecund, but population may exceed supply in Malthusian fashion, producing hunger at best and starvation at worst. As noted, scarcity favored the wealthy, who afforded high prices. Commoners lacked resources and had to economize. In this vein and from a biological perspective, paucity favored a low metabolism, which conserved calories and nutrients.[144] Nature rewarded individuals who easily accumulated adipose during plentitude and husbanded it during shortages. These children and adults tended to have better immune systems, fewer intestinal ailments, and less anemia than gaunt individuals. Adipose enabled girls to begin menarche earlier than their lean counterparts. With a longer reproductive life, all else equal, plump women had more children than slender ones, populating the next generation with their genes. That is, the race to leave offspring crowned plodders who retained fat and had what is known as a thrifty genome, not speedsters whose engines devoured fuel.

In 1962, American geneticist James Van Gundia Neel (1915–2000) articulated the notion of such a genome, proposing existence of what might be termed 'fat genes' that aid fat storage.[145] They guard their possessor against famine but cause obesity and other chronic maladies when food is bountiful. Neel's ideas remain controversial, though obesity must have a hereditary component; otherwise identical twins reared apart would not display similar masses and adipose distributions.[146] A corollary of humanity's evolution amid food insecurity is that attempts to lose mass distress countless people. Under such torment, few succeed over the long term. This situation may prompt Americans to question the wisdom of spending over $60 billion annually on mass reduction programs and products, according to a 2019 calculation.[147]

3.5.14 Agriculture and Animal Husbandry in Perspective

Deprivation, hunger, famine, violence, and warfare have destabilized societies for millennia, threatening quality of life and longevity. Despite imperfections, agriculture and animal husbandry have potential to diminish these threats. Despite flaws, this system remains operable absent an alternative to feed the world's billions. Organic farming has virtues, but its lower yields would exacerbate hunger, starvation, and related problems. Reversion to hunting and gathering would plummet populations and wreck the global economy. Even the core criticism that farming and livestock raising produce unhealthy foods is open to debate amid efforts to breed or bioengineer better crops and livestock. This book joins the discourse, scrutinizing such captiousness by evaluating several domesticates.

NOTES

1 "Marcus Tullius Cicero Quotes," *BrainyMedia Inc*, 2019, accessed January 4, 2019, https://www.brainyquote.com/quotes/marcus_tullius_cicero_104340.
2 Gen. 3:16–24 (New American Bible).
3 Stanley Ulijaszek, Neil Mann, and Sarah Elton, *Evolving Human Nutrition: Implications for Public Health* (New York: Cambridge University Press, 2012), 50.

4 "Plants for a Future," 1996–2012, accessed January 16, 2019, https://pfaf.org/user/edibleuses.aspx.
5 Ibid.
6 Susan Levine, *School Lunch Politics: The Surprising History of America's Favorite Welfare Program* (Princeton, NJ and Oxford, UK: Princeton University Press, 2008), 176–177.
7 Allison Aubrey, "More Salt, Fewer Whole Grains: USDA Eases School Lunch Nutrition Rules," *National Public Radio*, December 7, 2018, accessed January 18, 2020, https://www.npr.org/sections/thesalt/2018/12/07/674533555/more-salt-in-school-lunch-fewer-whole-grains-usda-eases-school-lunch-rules; Liz Crampton, "USDA Changes Obama-Era School Lunch Rules, Citing 'Flexibility,'" *Politico*, January 17, 2020, accessed January 18, 2020, https://www.politico.com/news/2020/01/17/school-lunch-rule-changes-100578.
8 Clark Spencer Larsen, "Dietary Reconstruction and Nutritional Assessment of Past Peoples: The Bioanthropological Record," in *The Cambridge World History of Food*, vol. 1, ed. Kenneth F. Kiple and Kriemhild Conee Ornelas (Cambridge, UK: Cambridge University Press, 2000), 13–14.
9 Robert Jurmain, Lynn Kilgore, Wenda Trevathan, and Russell L. Ciochon. *Introduction to Physical Anthropology*, 2013–2014 ed. (Belmont, CA: Wadsworth Cengage Learning, 2014), 135.
10 Clark Spencer Larsen, *Our Origins: Discovering Physical Anthropology*. (New York and London: Norton, 2017), 238–239.
11 Ibid., 236, 238.
12 Damian Carrington, "Insects Could Be the Key to Meeting Food Needs of Growing Global Population," *The Guardian*, July 31, 2010, accessed January 16, 2019, https://www.theguardian.com/environment/2010/aug/01/insects-food-emissions.
13 Waverly Root and Richard de Rochemont, *Eating in America: A History* (Hopewell, NJ: Ecco Press, 1995), 15.
14 Larsen, *Our Origins*, 238.
15 Stephen Le, *100 Million Years of Food: What Our Ancestors Ate and Why It Matters Today* (New York: Picador, 2016), 18.
16 Ibid., 17–18.
17 Larsen, Our Origins, 259–260.
18 Grahame Turner, "The Silverback Gorilla's Diet," *Sciencing*, last updated April 5, 2018, accessed January 16, 2019, https://sciencing.com/silverback-gorillas-diet-6548298.html; "Diet and Eating Habits," *Sea World Parks and Entertainment*, 2019, accessed January 16, 2019, https://seaworld.org/animals/all-about/gorilla/diet.
19 Ker Than, "First Proof Gorillas Eat Monkeys? Mammal DNA in Gorilla Feces Hints the Big Apes Might Eat Meat After All," *National Geographic*, March 7, 2010, accessed January 16, 2019, https://news.nationalgeographic.com/news/2010/03/100305-first-proof-gorillas-eat-monkeys-mammals-feces-dna.
20 Larsen, *Our Origins*, 239.
21 Ibid., 244.
22 Craig Stanford, "The Predatory Behavior and Ecology of Wild Chimpanzees," accessed January 17, 2019, https://www-bcf.usc.edu/~stanford/chimphunt.html.
23 Larsen, *Our Origins*, 12; Jurmain, Kilgore, Trevathan, and Ciochon, 300.
24 Charles Darwin, *The Descent of Man, and Selection in Relation to Sex* (London: Penguin Books, 2004), 68; Larsen, *Our Origins*, 278.
25 Larsen, *Our Origins*, 12; Larsen, "Dietary Reconstruction and Nutritional Assessment of Past Peoples," 14.
26 Larsen, *Our Origins*, 280.
27 Ibid.
28 Ibid., 226; Jurmain, Kilgore, Trevathan, and Ciochon, 25.
29 Larsen, *Our Origins*, 286.
30 F. Clark Howell, *Early Man* (New York: Tim-Life Books, 1965), 48; Raymond A. Dart, "The Predatory Transition from Ape to Man," *International Anthropological and Linguistic Review* 1, no. 4 (1953), http://www.users.miamioh.edu/erlichrd/350website/classrel/dart.html.
31 Glenn C. Conroy, *Reconstructing Human Origins: A Modern Synthesis* (New York and London: Norton, 1997), 167; "*Paranthropus boisei*," Smithsonian National Museum of Natural History, last modified August 24, 2018, accessed October 16, 2019, http://humanorigins.si.edu/evidence/human-fossils/species/paranthropus-boisei; Jurmain, Kilgore, Trevathan, and Ciochon, 298.
32 Ulijaszek, Mann, and Elton, 77; Ruth Moore, *Evolution*, rev. ed. (New York: Time-Life Books, 1968), 151.
33 Conroy, 167.

34 Jurmain, Kilgore, Trevathan, and Ciochon, 294.
35 David Biello, "Climate Change Future Suggested by Looking Back 4 Million Years," *Scientific American*, April 3, 2013, accessed January 17, 2019, https://blogs.scientificamerican.com/observations/climate-change-future-suggested-by-looking-back-4-million-years.
36 Alice Roberts, *Evolution: The Human Story*, 2nd ed. (New York: DK Publishing, 2018), 94–95; Ulijaszek, Mann, and Elton, 79.
37 Moore, 152.
38 Conroy, 258–259.
39 Ibid., 257.
40 Larsen, *Our Origins*, 308.
41 Cecil Adams, "Does Thinking Hard Burn More Calories?" *Washington City Paper*, December 7, 2012, accessed January 17, 2019, https://www.washingtoncitypaper.com/columns/straight-dope/article/13043347/straight-dope-does-thinking-hard-burn-more-calories.
42 "Hominid Species," *Talk Origins*, last modified April 30, 2010, accessed January 17, 2019, http://www.talkorigins.org/faqs/homs/species.html.
43 "Brain Size and Cultural Evolution," accessed January 17, 2019, http://www.bradshawfoundation.com/origins/australopithecus_afarensis.php.
44 "*Homo rudolfensis*," *Smithsonian National Museum of Natural History*, last modified August 24, 2018, accessed January 17, 2019. http://humanorigins.si.edu/evidence/human-fossils/species/homo-rudolfensis.
45 Larsen, *Our Origins*, 306–307.
46 Howell, 77.
47 Jurmain, Kilgore, Trevathan, and Ciochon, 301; Carl Zimmer, *Smithsonian Intimate Guide to Human Origins* (Washington, DC: Smithsonian Books, 2005), 138.
48 Larsen, *Our Origins*, 325–326.
49 Ibid., 321.
50 Ibid., 307–308; "*Homo habilis*," *Smithsonian National Museum of Natural History*, last modified August 24, 2018, accessed January 17, 2019. http://humanorigins.si.edu/evidence/human-fossils/species/homo-habilis; "*Paranthropus boisei*."
51 Jurmain, Kilgore, Trevathan, and Ciochon, 321.
52 Peter Bellwood, "Archaeology of Southeast Asian Hunters and Gatherers," in *The Cambridge Encyclopedia of Hunters and Gatherers*, ed. Richard B. Lee and Richard Daly (Cambridge, UK: Cambridge University Press, 1999), 284; Larsen, *Our Origins*, 316–317.
53 Howell, 130.
54 Bob Yirka, "Neanderthal Home Made of Mammoth Bones Discovered in Ukraine," *Phys.org*, December 19, 2011, accessed January 17, 2019, https://phys.org/news/2011-12-neanderthal-home-mammoth-bones-ukraine.html.
55 Thom Holmes, *Early Humans: The Pleistocene and Holocene Epochs* (New York: Chelsea House, 2009), 85.
56 Ofer Bar-Yosef, "Eat What Is There: Hunting and Gathering in the World of the Neanderthals and Their Neighbors," *International Journal of Osteoarchaeology* 14, nos. 3–4 (May 2004): 333.
57 Ibid., 336.
58 Ibid., 337.
59 Darwin, 182.
60 Geoffrey G. Pope, "Asian Paleoanthropology," in *History of Physical Anthropology: An Encyclopedia*, vol. 1: A-L, ed. Frank Spencer (New York and London: Garland Publishing, 1997), 127.
61 Larsen, *Our Origins*, 303–304.
62 Zimmer, 101; Chris Stringer and Peter Andrews, *The Complete World of Human Evolution* (London: Thames and Hudson, 2005), 160–161.
63 Zimmer, 121, 123, 129.
64 Ibid., 136–137.
65 Stringer and Andrews, 142.
66 Mark R. Jenike, "Nutritional Ecology: Diet, Physical Activity and Body Size," in *Hunter-Gatherers: An Interdisciplinary Perspective*, ed. Catherine Panter-Brick, Robert H. Layton, and Peter Rowley-Conwy (Cambridge, UK: Cambridge University Press, 2001), 208–211.
67 "Part I: Determining What Our Ancestors Ate," in *The Cambridge World History of Food*, vol. 1, ed. Kenneth F. Kiple and Kriemhild Conee Ornelas (Cambridge, UK: Cambridge University Press, 2000), 11.

68 Jenike, 208–209.
69 Howell, 173.
70 Gen. 1:26–2:25.
71 Cameron Wilson, "Rethinking Indigenous Australia's Agricultural Past," *Bush Telegraph*, May 15, 2014, accessed January 23, 2019, https://www.abc.net.au/radionational/programs/archived/bushtelegraph/rethinking-indigenous-australias-agricultural-past/5452454.
72 Kenneth F. Kiple, "The Question of Paleolithic Nutrition and Modern Health: From the End to the Beginning," in *The Cambridge World History of Food*, vol. 2, ed. Kenneth F. Kiple and Kriemhild Conee Ornelas (Cambridge, UK: Cambridge University Press, 2000), 1704.
73 Le, 4–5.
74 Danny Riley, "Walk on the Wild Side: Bach and Buxtehude," *Bachtrack*, April 23, 2017, accessed March 9, 2019, https://bachtrack.com/feature-at-home-guide-bach-buxtehude-lubeck-arnstadt-august-2017.
75 Tom Osler, *Serious Runner's Handbook: Answers to Hundreds of Your Running Questions* (Mountain View, CA: World Publications, 1978) 147.
76 Ibid., 154.
77 Phil Ciciora, "Study: Surge in Obesity Correlates with Increased Automobile Usage," *Illinois News Bureau*, May 11, 2011, accessed April 2, 2019, https://news.illinois.edu/view/6367/205328.
78 Jurmain, Kilgore, Trevathan, and Ciochon, 311.
79 Thomas Hobbes, *Leviathan* (Oxford: Oxford University Press, 1996), 84.
80 Sindya N. Bhanoo, "Life Span of Early Man Same as Neanderthals'," *New York Times*, January 10, 2011, accessed January 18, 2019, https://www.nytimes.com/2011/01/11/science/11obneanderthal.html; Walter Gratzer, *Terrors of the Table: The Curious History of Nutrition* (Oxford: Oxford University Press, 2005), 44.
81 Muzaffer Suleyman Senyurek, "A Note on the Duration of Life of the Ancient Inhabitants of Anatolia," *American Journal of Physical Anthropology* 5, no. 1 (March 1947): 59.
82 Ann E. M. Liljas, "Old Age in Ancient Egypt," March 2, 2015, accessed January 18, 2019, https://blogs.ucl.ac.uk/researchers-in-museums/2015/03/02/old-age-in-ancient-egypt; Roger S. Bagnall and Bruce W. Frier, *The Demography of Roman Egypt* (Cambridge, UK and New York: Cambridge University Press, 2006), 109.
83 John P. McKay, Bennett D. Hill, John Buckler, Clare Haru Crowston, Merry E. Wiesner-Hanks, and Joe Perry, *Understanding Western Society: A Brief History* (Boston and New York: Bedford/St. Martin's, 2012), 212; Edward S. Deevey Jr., "The Human Population," *Scientific American* (September 1, 1960), 200.
84 Henri V. Vallois, "The Social Life of Early Man: The Evidence of Skeletons," in *Social Life of Early Man*, ed. Sherwood L. Washburn (Chicago: Aldine, 1961), 222.
85 Ibid., 223.
86 Ibid., 224.
87 Michael Gurven and Hillard Kaplan, "Longevity among Hunter-Gatherers: A Cross-Cultural Examination," *Population and Development Review* 33, no. 2 (June 2007): 4–6, 40, https://www.academia.edu/17979487/Longevity_Among_Hunter-_Gatherers_A_Cross-Cultural_Examination?auto=download; Kathryn M. Domett, *Health in Late Prehistoric Thailand* (Oxford, UK: Archaeopress, 2001), 139.
88 Richard H. Steckel and Jerome C. Rose, "Introduction," in *The Backbone of History: Health and Nutrition in the Western Hemisphere*, ed. Richard H. Steckel and Jerome C. Rose (Cambridge, UK: Cambridge University Press, 2002), 6; Richard H. Steckel, Paul W. Sciulli, and Jerome C. Rose, "A Health Index from Skeletal Remains," in *The Backbone of History: Health and Nutrition in the Western Hemisphere*, ed. Richard H. Steckel and Jerome C. Rose (Cambridge, UK: Cambridge University Press, 2002), 72.
89 Howell, 174.
90 Deevey, 200.
91 Ibid., 202.
92 Walter Scheidel, "Demography," in *The Cambridge Economic History of the Greco-Roman World*, ed. Walter Scheidel, Ian Morris, and Richard Saller (Cambridge, UK: Cambridge University Press, 2007), 38; Karl Eschbach, "Longevity," in *Encyclopedia of Health & Aging*, ed. Kyriakos S. Markides (Los Angeles: SAGE Reference, 2007), 330.
93 Senyurek, 61.
94 Clark Spencer Larsen, *Skeletons in Our Closet: Revealing Our Past through Bioarchaeology* (Princeton, NJ and Oxford, UK: Princeton University Press, 2000), 208.

95 Peter G. Lunn, "Nutrition, Immunity and Infection," in *The Decline of Mortality in Europe*, ed. R. Schofield, D. Reher, and A. Bideau (Oxford: Clarendon Press, 1991), 131.
96 Kenneth M. Weiss, "Demographic Models for Anthropology." *American Antiquity* 38, no. 2 (April 1973): 50.
97 John H. Knowles, "The Responsibility of the Individual," *Daedalus* 106, no. 1 (Winter 1977): 57.
98 William Davis, *Wheat Belly: Lose the Wheat, Lose the Weight, and Find Your Path Back to Health* (New York: Rodale, 2011), x.
99 Ibid., 14.
100 Jurmain, Kilgore, Trevathan, and Ciochon, 447.
101 Jared Diamond, "The Worst Mistake in the History of the Human Race," *Discover*, May 1, 1999, accessed July 21, 2019, http://discovermagazine.com/1987/may/02-the-worst-mistake-in-the-history-of-the-human-race.
102 Larsen, *Skeletons in Our Closet*, 229.
103 Jorge Mayer, "The *Golden Rice* Project," 2005–2018, accessed January 18, 2019, http://www.goldenrice.org/Content4-Info/info.php.
104 Jurmain, Kilgore, Trevathan, and Ciochon, 447.
105 Larsen, *Our Origins*, 410–411.
106 S. Boyd Eaton and Melvin Konner, "Paleolithic Nutrition: A Consideration of Its Nature and Current Implications," in *Nutritional Anthropology: Biocultural Perspectives on Food and Nutrition*, 2d ed., ed. Darna L. Dufour, Alan H. Goodman, and Gretel H. Pelto (New York and Oxford: Oxford University Press, 2013), 52–53.
107 Larsen, *Our Origins*, 410–411.
108 *The Illustrated Encyclopedia of Fruits, Vegetables, and Herbs* (New York: Chartwell Books, 2017), 19.
109 Jurmain, Kilgore, Trevathan, and Ciochon, 311.
110 Cecil Woodham-Smith, *The Great Hunger: Ireland, 1845–1849* (New York: Harper and Row, 1962), 136, 141.
111 Cecil Woodham-Smith, "The Great Hunger: Ireland, 1845–1849," in *European Diet from Pre-Industrial to Modern Times*, ed. Elborg Forster and Robert Forster (New York: Harper Torchbooks, 1975), 16–17.
112 Gail L. Schumann and Cleora J. D'Arcy, *Hungry Planet: Stories of Plant Diseases* (St. Paul, MN: American Phytopathological Society, 2012), 12; Jessie I. Wood, "Three Billion Dollars a Year," in *Plant Diseases: The Yearbook of Agriculture, 1953*, ed. Alfred Stefferud (Washington, DC: GPO, 1953), 6; "White Potato," in *The Cambridge World History of Food*, vol. 2, ed. Kenneth F. Kiple and Kriemhild Conee Ornelas (Cambridge, UK: Cambridge University Press, 2000), 1879; Helen Sanderson, "Roots and Tubers," in *The Cultural History of Plants*, ed. Ghillean Prance and Mark Nesbitt (New York and London: Routledge, 2005), 64.
113 Redcliffe N. Salaman, *The History and Social Influence of the Potato*, rev. ed. (Cambridge, UK: Cambridge University Press, 1985), 305.
114 Henry Hobhouse, *Seeds of Change: Six Plants that Transformed Mankind* (New York: Shoemaker and Hoard, 2005), 257.
115 Donald J. Ortner and Gretchen Theobald, "Paleopathological Evidence of Malnutrition," in *The Cambridge World History of Food*, vol. 1, ed. Kenneth F. Kiple and Kriemhild Conee Ornelas (Cambridge, UK: Cambridge University Press, 2000), 41.
116 Gen. 12:10; Gen. 26:1; Gen. 41:53–54.
117 Wood, 5.
118 Linda Civitello, *Cuisine and Culture: A History of Food and People*, 3rd ed. (Hoboken, NJ: Wiley, 2011), 86.
119 Rebecca Storey, Lourdes Marquez Morfin, and Vernon Smith, "Social Disruption and the Maya Civilization of Mesoamerica: A Study of Health and Economy of the Last Thousand Years," in *The Backbone of History: Health and Nutrition in the Western Hemisphere*, ed. Richard H. Steckel and Jerome C. Rose (Cambridge, UK: Cambridge University Press, 2002), 286.
120 Peter Garnsey, *Food and Society in Classical Antiquity* (Cambridge, UK: Cambridge University Press, 1999), 37.
121 Mortimer Chambers, Raymond Grew, David Herlihy, Theodore K. Rabb, and Isser Woloch, *The Western Experience*, vol. 2, 4th ed. (New York: Knopf, 1987), 395; H. J. Teutenberg, "The General Relationship between Diet and Industrialization," in *European Diet from Pre-Industrial to Modern Times*, ed. Elborg Forster and Robert Forster (New York: Harper Torchbooks, 1975), 74.
122 Teutenberg, 74.
123 McKay, Hill, Buckler, Crowston, Wiesner-Hanks, and Perry, 526–527.
124 Teutenberg, 75.

125 Michelle B. McAlpin, "Famines, Epidemics, and Population Growth: The Case of India," *Journal of Interdisciplinary History* 14, no. 2 (Autumn 1983): 356.
126 Soutik Biswas, "How Churchill 'Starved' India," *BBC*, October 28, 2010, accessed March 6, 2019, http://www.bbc.co.uk/blogs/thereporters/soutikbiswas/2010/10/how_churchill_starved_india.html.
127 "State and Famine in the Sahel Region in the 20th Century," accessed January 19, 2019, http://www.msu.ac.zw/elearning/material/1180596897state%20and%20famine%20in%20the%20sahel%20region.doc.
128 Howard LaFranchi, "From Famine to Food Basket: How Bangladesh Became a Model for Reducing Hunger," *Christian Science Monitor*, June 17, 2015, accessed January 19, 2019, https://www.csmonitor.com/USA/Foreign-Policy/2015/0617/From-famine-to-food-basket-how-Bangladesh-became-a-model-for-reducing-hunger.
129 Jordan Weissmann, "How Kim Jong Il Starved North Korea," *The Atlantic*, December 20, 2011, accessed January 19, 2019, https://www.theatlantic.com/business/archive/2011/12/how-kim-jong-il-starved-north-korea/250244.
130 World Vision Staff, "East Africa Hunger, Famine: Facts, FAQs, and How to Help," World Vision, last modified July 10 2018, accessed January 19, 2019, https://www.worldvision.org/hunger-news-stories/east-africa-hunger-famine-facts.
131 Ibid.; Larry Short, "Disaster Response in 5 Hot Spots around the World," World Vision, last modified August 17, 2011, accessed January 19, 2019, https://www.worldvision.org/blog/disaster-response-hot-spots.
132 "Malnutrition in Children—UNICEF Data," *UNICEF*, May 2018, accessed January 19, 2019, https://data.unicef.org/topic/nutrition/malnutrition/#.
133 Fernand Braudel, *Capitalism and Material Life, 1400–1800*, trans. Miriam Kochan (New York: Harper Colophon Books, 1973), 38.
134 Larsen, *Our Origins*, 396.
135 Gen. 4:3–8.
136 Larsen, *Our Origins*, 396.
137 Helene Rougier, Isabelle Crevecoeur, Cedric Beauval, Cosimo Posth, Damien Flas, Christoph WiBing, Anja Furtwangler, Mietje Germonpre, Asier Gomez-Olivencia, Patrick Semal, Johannes van der Plicht, Herve Bocherens, and Johannes Krause, "Neandertal Cannibalism and Neandertal Bones Used as Tools in Northern Europe," *Scientific Reports* 6 (July 6, 2016), https://www.nature.com/articles/srep29005.
138 Thomas Malthus, *An Essay on the Principle of Population* (Amherst, New York: Prometheus Books, 1998), 13–14.
139 Ibid., 100, 139–140; John P. McKay, Bennett D. Hill, John Buckler, Clare Haru Crowston, Merry E. Wiesner-Hanks, and Joe Perry, *Understanding Western Society: A Brief History* (Boston and New York: Bedford/St. Martin's, 2012), 622.
140 George J. Armelagos, "Paleopathology," in *History of Physical Anthropology*, ed. Frank Spencer, vol. 2: M-Z (New York and London: Garland Publishing, 1997), 794.
141 Garnsey, 113.
142 Jessica Campisi and Brandon Griggs, "Nearly 100 Bodies Found at a Texas Construction Site Were Probably Black People Forced into Labor—after Slavery Ended," July 19, 2018, accessed January 18, 2019, https://www.cnn.com/2018/07/18/us/bodies-found-construction-site-slavery-trnd/index.html; Richard S. Dunn, *Sugar and Slaves: The Rise of the Planter Class in the English West Indies, 1624–1713* (Chapel Hill: Institute of Early American History and Culture, 1972) 302.
143 Wayne Suttles, "Coping with Abundance: Subsistence on the Northwest Coast," in *Man the Hunter*, ed. Richard B. Lee and Irven DeVore (Chicago: Aldine, 1968), 59.
144 Leslie Sue Lieberman, "Obesity," in *The Cambridge World History of Food*, vol. 1, ed. Kenneth F. Kiple and Kriemhild Conee Ornelas (Cambridge, UK: Cambridge University Press, 2000), 1067–1068; Kiple, 1707.
145 James V. Neel, "Diabetes Mellitus: A 'Thrifty' Genotype Rendered Detrimental by Progress?" *American Journal of Human Genetics* 14, no. 4 (December 1962): 353–358; Vishwanath Sardesai, *Introduction to Clinical Nutrition*, 3d ed. (Boca Raton, FL: CRC Press, 2012), 18; Kiple, 1707.
146 Adam Drewnowski and Victoria Warren-Mears, "Role of Taste and Appetite in Body Weight Regulation," in *Nutrition in the Prevention and Treatment of Disease*, ed. Ann M. Coulston, Cheryl L. Rock, and Elaine R. Monsen (San Diego: Academic Press, 2001), 539.
147 Geoff Williams, "The Heavy Price of Losing Weight," *U.S. News and World Report*, January 2, 2013, accessed January 28, 2019, https://money.usnews.com/money/personal-finance/articles/2013/01/02/the-heavy-price-of-losing-weight.

4 Meat

4.1 UBIQUITY OF MEAT

Graduate school introduced me to a group of agricultural scientists, among them a senior microbiologist. Our difference in ages created a natural mentoring relationship. Decades of experience convinced him that he had accumulated vast knowledge about the sciences, academe, and life's sundry affairs. He imparted this wisdom during lunch and dinner, where the entrees commanded his attention. Unfolding a menu, questioning a waitress about the specials, and ignoring the salad bar, he ordered a burger, steak, roast beef, corned beef, pastrami, beef stew, beef stroganoff, shish kebab, chili, lasagna, meatballs, bacon, ham, pork chops, shepherd's pie, barbequed ribs, sausage, meatloaf, salami, or some combination of these items. Delighted with these selections, he often remarked that a meal was incomplete without a dead animal as the main course. This sentiment affirmed belief that meat is humanity's chief sustenance and expressed the preferences of innumerable Americans on their way to a restaurant, picnic, party, banquet, buffet, deli, hot dog stand, cookout, game, sandwich shop, butcher, or supermarket.

Not only is it ubiquitous in the American diet, but meat has become a catchall. The U.S. Conference of Catholic Bishops defines it as flesh from terrestrial animals like cattle (*Bos taurus*), pigs (*Sus scrofa domesticus*), sheep (*Ovis aries*), chickens (*Gallus gallus domesticus*), turkeys (*Meleagris gallopavo f. domestica* and *M. ocellata*), ducks (*Anas platyrhynchos domesticus*), geese (*Anser* and *Branta* species), horses (*Equus caballus*), and goats (*Capra aegagrus hircus*).[1] This scheme makes warm bloodedness a criterion of meat. In this arrangement, beef, veal, pork, mutton, lamb, chevon, and capretto or kid are designated red meats because they have more iron than poultry, which constitutes white meats. As a religious matter, the distinction between these creatures and aquatic life, Chapter 1 noted, is rooted in the canonical gospels. Rather than this bifurcation, the U.S. Department of Agriculture's (USDA) Agricultural Marketing Service quarters flesh into meat, poultry, fish, and shellfish.[2] This partitioning seems haphazard, guided neither by warm or cold bloodedness nor habitat nor status as vertebrate or invertebrate. The broadest definition comes from the American Meat Science Association, which labels flesh from any animal meat.[3] In contrast to this breadth, *Meat Science*, a journal from Dutch health and science publisher Elsevier, excludes articles about seafood.[4] It publishes papers on poultry, though mammalian flesh is the focus. An emphasis on mammals aligns with this investigation. Restricting meat to beef, veal, pork, mutton, lamb, chevon, capretto, and game like bison and venison, this book favors a tripartite structure, with this chapter devoted to flesh from mammals, Chapter 5 to fish and shellfish, and Chapter 6 to poultry.

4.2 TYPES OF MEAT

Today's meats tend to be muscle, though definition of a cut varies by country. In the United States, pigs' belly and back furnish bacon. Flesh between the shoulder and hips supplies the tenderest cuts, namely loin and rib chops. The upper shoulder yields the inaptly termed pork butt, also known as Boston butt. Above the pork butt is fatty flesh made into sausage. Ham comes from the rear legs. American butchers derive T-bone, strip, and porterhouse steaks from the backs of beef cattle. In this area is beef loin, which supplies the choicest cuts, and from which are made filet mignon, tenderloin, and beef Wellington. The back also yields sirloin. As their names imply, ribeye and prime rib come from rib muscles. The breast, known as brisket, is made into pastrami and corned beef.

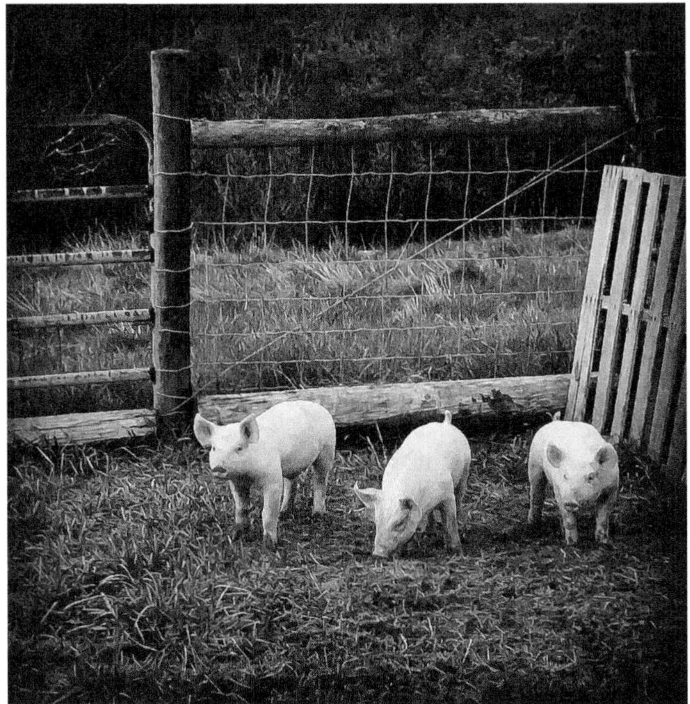

FIGURE 4.1 Pigs. (Photo courtesy of Jessica Vierling-West.)

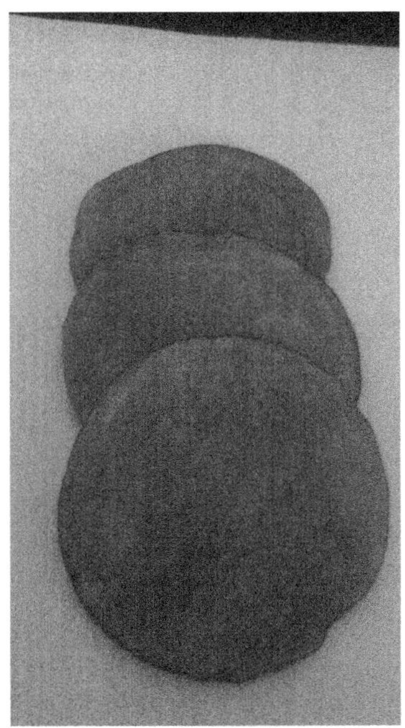

FIGURE 4.2 Canadian bacon. (Photo from author.)

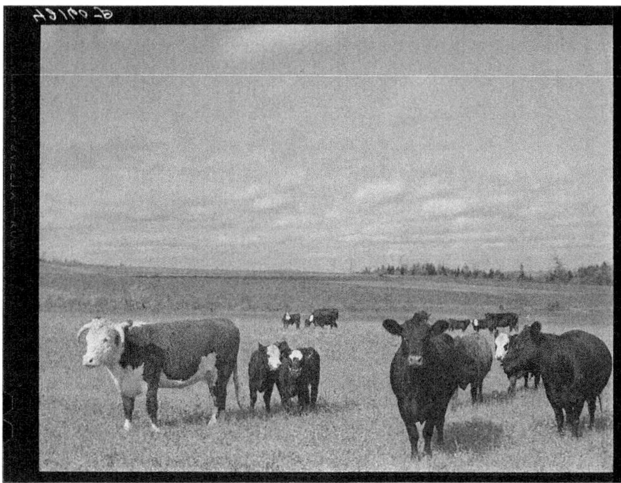

FIGURE 4.3 Beef cattle. (Photo courtesy of Library of Congress. https://www.loc.gov/pictures/item/2017792505/.)

Preoccupation with muscles as meat deviates from the past. Nineteenth-century English ate the joints, brain, heart, liver, pancreas, kidneys, and thymus gland of adult and juvenile cows, pigs, and sheep.[5] Sheep also furnished lungs and intestines. In the Americas, slaveowners consigned the least desirable animal parts to slaves. Pig intestines made chitterlings. Chicken gizzards and necks and pig chins, tails, snouts, and feet supplemented corn, garden vegetables, and legumes. Oxen buttocks furnished what were called ox tails. These items undergirded African American soul foods.

4.3 ECONOMICS, BIOLOGY, PSYCHOLOGY, AND HISTORY

At a minimum, economics, biology, psychology, and history explain meat's popularity. Chapter 1's observation that food sharpens inequalities applied to meat, whose price excluded the poor during most of history, leaving only the affluent as consumers.[6] Under such circumstances, it symbolized prestige, supplying visual confirmation that its possessor afforded the best in life. In this capacity, economics paired with psychology to validate meat eaters' status. Onlookers who could not afford meat aspired to have it when their fortunes improved. This hope gave the future promise and possibilities. This thinking created gradations of affordability. Someone too poor to purchase meat today may afford the cheapest cuts tomorrow. The fact that a commoner might secure inexpensive meats made them undesirable to his superior. The wealthy consume only the best as a way of preserving their status. The imperative of keeping abreast of elites helps explain why the developing world's middle class prizes meat.

Generalizing these dynamics, British classicist Peter David Arthur Garnsey (b. 1938) wrote that

> In strongly hierarchical and status-conscious societies, rich men use food as one of a number of ways of signaling their wealth and winning or maintaining prestige in the sight of the world. Food in pre-industrial society was the more effective as a marker of economic and social distinction for the fact that it consumed the greater proportion (perhaps 66–75%) of family income.[7]

Biology includes several factors inseparable from our evolution. Chapter 3 discussed the anatomical and dental traits that make humans omnivores and generalists. Ability to eat a variety of foods extends to meat. Modern humans have smaller jaws and teeth than their predecessors who specialized in nuts, seeds, leaves, and related tough or hard materials. Once cooked, meat became tender, lightening the load on jaws and teeth and permitting them to shrink. In this context, dental anatomy cannot be separated from cultural evolution, in this instance fire's mastery. Because meat has many nutrients and calories, humans did not develop the four-chambered stomach of herbivores like cattle. Meat kept the stomach small and unspecialized and shortened the colon. Our senses favor a combination of aromas and flavors—umami, saltiness, and the smell and taste of charred flesh and adipose—that is difficult to replicate apart from meat.[8] Modern hunter-gatherers accustomed to meat hesitate to sample grains and vegetables, though this phenomenon might be cultural as much as biological. The extent to which biology canalizes this behavior implies that humans have long eaten meat.

With humans, traits that elaborate over time tend to be both evolutionary and historical, complicating their treatment. The term "historical" or "history" includes investigation of the distant past given humankind's antiquity. This past is the domain of prehistory—defined in Chapter 1—though this chapter does not belabor the distinction between it and history. The remote past is difficult to interpret because it furnishes few clues about behavior. Too few fossils and technologies have survived to permit comprehensive understanding of early humans. Consequently, anthropologists do not know when humanity's ancestors began eating meat. Absence of certitude engenders debate and disagreement. Such exchanges reveal less about intellectual shortcomings than about scientists and scholars' commitment to testing ideas and evidence.

4.4 ORIGINS OF MEAT CONSUMPTION

North American mythology held that humans ate only meat during their formative period.[9] Shifting from stories to science, South African anatomist Raymond Arthur Dart (1893–1988)—who Chapter 3 mentioned as an advocate of the early origin of meat eating—provoked controversy by uniting meat consumption, hunting, and violence as prime movers in our evolution.[10] Discoverer of the first specimen of *Australopithecus africanus* in 1924, then the oldest known humanlike creature, Dart believed that a hazardous environment honed its survival instincts, leading it to destroy and devour without pity. Australopithecines, he wrote, smashed bones to extract marrow and "tore the battered bodies of their quarries apart limb from limbs and slaked their thirst with blood, consuming the flesh raw like every other carnivorous beast."[11]

This language is easier to dismiss as hyperbole than to acknowledge as insight into humanity's capacity for savagery. Rhetoric aside, Dart's position aligns with the realism of political philosophers Niccolò Machiavelli (1469–1527) and Thomas Hobbes (1588–1679). Without civilization's veneer, descent toward depravity is rapid. American dramatist and science writer Robert Ardrey (1908–1980) met Dart in 1955, coming under his influence. Ardrey reinforced the notion of "killer apes," pinpointing aggression as evolution's legacy to humanity.[12] Although disagreeable, these ideas concentrated attention on the quest for meat as a hallmark of humanity.

In 1967, South African paleontologist Charles Kimberlin Brain (b. 1931) undercut Dart's thesis by demonstrating the likelihood that animals larger than *Australopithecus* gnawed on bones in the caves it visited.[13] Rather than predator, it was likely prey to leopards (*Panthera pardus*), cheetahs (*Acinonyx jubatus*), and lions (*Panthera leo*). With Australopithecines relegated to gathering plants, attention focused on early *Homo*. In 1971, South African archeologist Glynn Llywelyn Isaac (1937–1985) asserted that from its inception our genus hunted.[14] Hunting parties enlarged into proto societies, whose division of labor dispatched men to hunt and women to collect plants and rear children. Men returned to camp with the kill, which nourished them, women, and children. Hunting thereby shaped sociability, hierarchy, and gender roles. Isaac's reconstruction of subsistence behaviors resembles American anthropologist Claude Owen Lovejoy's (b. 1943) provisioning hypothesis, discussed in Chapter 3, though Lovejoy did not focus on hunting.

Emphasis on hunting downplays the likelihood that *Australopithecus* and *Homo* scavenged carcasses when opportunities arose. Our evolution in Africa's tropics accelerated carrion's decay. By the time our ancestors secured such flesh, it was putrid, goading the liver, kidneys, and immune system's development. Cooking's invention was useful when heat was intense enough to kill pathogens.

By reducing early peoples to trash collectors, this scenario did not ennoble our lineage. American anthropologist Henry Bunn attempted to rehabilitate the behavior by characterizing it as aggressive patrolling of territory, what he called "power scavenging."[15] Such language cannot rival the gusto of humans and their forebears, who harnessed initiative, strength, stamina, and courage to pursue game. Desire to make humanity nature's conquerors conflicts with its relegation to the biota's margins as scavengers, which may have been our role until about 700,000 years ago.[16]

Irrespective of how and when the appetite for it developed, meat has powered the narrative of human evolution. As noted, fire's mastery led to cooking. By increasing digestibility, cooking meat and other items unlocked more nutrients for absorption. Nutrients and calories hastened brain expansion, accounting for the last 2 million years of enlargement. The tendency to regard cognition as our sine qua non prioritizes meat as human evolution's engine.

Last chapter mentioned American anthropologist Francis Clark Howell's (1925–2007) enthusiasm for the hunt, evoking it as way teen *Homo erectus* boys displayed courage and courted girls.[17] Meat's quest energized their European descendants, Neanderthals (*Homo neanderthalensis*), who lived "the hardy life of a roving band of hunters," he stated.[18] Skillful writers Dart, Ardrey, and Howell popularized belief that meat's pursuit was innately human. Seizing this idea, American cardiologist Robert Coleman Atkins (1930–2003) in 1972 minimized omnivory, discussed last chapter, remarking that "man was a hunter and our eating habits were largely carnivorous."[19]

This belief implies that prehistoric peoples wanted lots of meat. Plentitude meant access to numerous small animals or few large ones. Either approach should have been plausible in principle, though anthropologists emphasize that pursuit of large prey was time and labor efficient.[20] *Homo heildelbergensis* and *H. neanderthalensis* hunted mammoths (*Mammuthus* species) and similar behemoths. Early North Americans targeted the largest prey, whose extinction some 13,000 years ago fuels speculation that humans sped its demise.[21] From the tenet that sizable prey trumped all else follows belief that humans settled for fish, aquatic invertebrates, birds, rodents, insects, and plants only when big game failed to feed everyone.[22] These lesser items' consumption indicated a population under stress. According to this logic, difficulties procuring enough food for burgeoning populations forced people to invent agriculture and animal husbandry, a strategy that yielded the lowest-quality foods, as critics charged and as Chapter 3 mentioned.

4.5 DEBATE ABOUT MEAT'S HEALTHFULNESS

4.5.1 Context

Among agriculture's critics in Chapter 3, American anthropologist Clark Spencer Larsen (b. 1952) stated that "relative to plant foods, meat is a highly nutritional food resource."[23] This book affirms his accent on context and argues that meat is not healthful in an absolute sense. Chapter 3 emphasized that context determines a food's value or desirability, a caveat that applies to meat. Whenever food was scarce, meat benefited the hungry by supplying nutrients and calories, but it alone could not sustain humans. Europeans who settled in North America's hinterlands and who found nothing but rabbits (*Oryctolagus cuniculus*) and other small mammals to eat during winters died, a phenomenon discussed in Chapter 3 known as rabbit starvation or protein poisoning.[24]

Such foods provided too few carbohydrates and fat. Rabbits were lean, a problem winter compounded by reducing availability of plants they ate. Some Arctic populations survived on marine mammals, but these animals had enough fat to prevent protein poisoning. Additionally, meat has many calories, increasing obesity's risk whenever too abundant. Underscoring this effect, the 2004 documentary *Super Size Me* reported an American filmmaker's 11-kilogram (24-pound) increase during one month of nothing but McDonald's fare. Burgers were not the lone culprit given that fast foods furnish too many calories, saturated fat, sugars, and salt.

4.5.2 Meat in the Western Diet

McDonald's has succeeded because, returning to the senior microbiologist, a meal must feature a dead animal. This belief pervades developed nations and is central to the American experience of plentitude. West of Ohio stretches the Corn Belt, whose grains fatten hogs and cattle. In the nineteenth century, migrants west of the Mississippi River encountered vast grasslands ideal for grazing livestock. From their base in Texas, sheep and cattle consumed grasses while migrating north. By 1850, over 50 million cows populated the Great Plains.[25] By Civil War's end in 1865, Texas alone counted some 5 million longhorns.[26] By January 1919, the United States had over 74 million pigs and 68 million cattle.[27] That year U.S. slaughterhouses processed some 10.3 billion kilograms (22.6 billion pounds) of beef, pork, and mutton.[28] Amid this abundance, German economist Werner Sombart (1863–1941) in 1906 blamed "roast beef and apple pie" for pacifying American workers, blunting enthusiasm for socialism.[29] Americans devoured 50 billion burgers in 2017.[30] "Beef. It's What's for Dinner," announced the Cattlemen's Beef Board and National Cattlemen's Beef Association.[31]

Washington, DC's Worldwatch Institute ranked pork, beef, and mutton the planet's principal red meats.[32] One hundred grams of pork contain 212 calories, no carbohydrates, 27.8 grams of protein, and 15.3 grams of fat, over two-thirds being unsaturated.[33] Pork has more vitamin B_1 (thiamine) than beef or lamb.[34] Other nutrients include vitamins B_3 (niacin), B_6 (pyridoxine), and B_{12} (cobalamin) and minerals iron, phosphorus, selenium, and zinc. One hundred grams of ground beef have 305 calories, no carbohydrates, 36.1 grams of protein, and 5.8 grams of fat divided almost equally between saturated and unsaturated lipids.[35] Beef has abundant B_3, B_6, B_{12}, iron, selenium, zinc, and phosphorus. One hundred grams of mutton supply 234 calories, no carbohydrates, 33.43 grams of protein, and 11.09 grams of fat, slightly more being unsaturated.[36] Mutton is a rich source of B_3, B_{12}, iron, phosphorus, selenium, and zinc. It has vitamins E (tocopherol), B_1, B_2 (riboflavin), B_5 (pantothenic acid), and B_6 and minerals calcium, copper, magnesium, manganese, and potassium in lesser amounts. Methods of preparing meats vary, though many add too much sodium. Chapter 2 discussed these nutrients.

Summarizing and expanding the above, Table 4.1 compares calories and nutrients among beef, pork, mutton, goat, bison, and venison.[37]

4.5.3 Meat and Longevity

Meat consumption is highest in Luxembourg, the United States, and Australia.[38] In each, intake nearly triples the world's annual average of 46 kilograms (102 pounds) of meat per capita. Consumption is lowest in the Democratic Republic of the Congo, Bangladesh, and India at about one-tenth the global mean. In 2018, Luxembourg, the United States, and Australia had higher life expectancies at birth (e^0) than the bottom tier of meat eaters, though this circumstance alone reveals little about meat's healthfulness because the developing world trails its developed neighbors in economic and social indicators.[39] Interestingly, in 2018 the United States ranked fifty-third among nations in e^0. Fifty-one countries above it ate less meat per person. Only Luxembourg, ranking thirty-seventh in e^0, consumed more meat per capita than the United States. The thirty-six countries above Luxembourg ate less meat per person.

Interpretation of these numbers warrants caution because numerous factors affect lifespan, noted Chapter 1. Yet circumspection does not characterize all dietary discussions. Intentional or not, American cardiologist William R. Davis's (b. 1957) denigration of bread wheat (*Triticum aestivum*) and U.S. neurologist David Perlmutter's (b. 1954) broadside against all grains retain steak and potatoes (*Solanum tuberosum*) as favorites.[40] Although American cardiac surgeon Steven R. Gundry

TABLE 4.1
Nutrients in Meat 100 g

Nutrient	Beef	%DV	Pork	%DV	Mutton	%DV	Goat	%DV	Bison	%DV	Venison	%DV
Calories	305	N/A	212	N/A	234	N/A	143	N/A	146	N/A	190	N/A
Protein (g)	36.1	N/A	27.8	N/A	33.43	N/A	27.1	N/A	20.23	N/A	36.08	N/A
Fat (g)	5.8	N/A	15.3	N/A	11.09	N/A	3.03	N/A	7.21	N/A	3.93	N/A
Carb (g)	0	N/A	0	N/A	0.08	N/A	0	N/A	0.05	N/A	0	N/A
Fiber (g)	0	N/A	0	N/A	0	N/A	0	N/A	0	N/A	0	N/A
Minerals												
Ca (mg)	10	1	21	2.1	10	1	17	1.7	11	1.1	6	0.6
Fe (mg)	3.32	19	0.93	5	4.76	26.4	3.73	20.7	2.78	15.4	4.98	27.6
Mg (mg)	22	5.5	26	6.5	31	7.8	0	0	21	5.3	28	7
P (mg)	226	22.6	279	27.9	272	27.2	201	20.1	194	19.4	260	26
K (mg)	313	8.9	375	10.7	409	11.7	405	11.6	328	9.4	311	8.9
Na (mg)	62	2.6	59	2.5	135	5.6	86	3.6	70	2.9	268	11.2
Zn (mg)	4.56	26	2.92	17	5.93	39.5	5.27	35.1	4.59	30.6	8.59	57.3
Cu (mg)	0.12	7	0.1	6	0.06	3	0.3	15	0.14	7	0.28	14
Mn (mg)	0.05	2	0.01	0.5	0.03	1.5	0.04	2	0.01	0.5	0.03	1.5
Se (mcg)	36	51.4	45	64.3	38	54.3	11.79	16.8	20	28.6	17.6	25.1
Vitamins												
A (IU)	0	0	7	0.1	N/A	N/A	0	0	0	0	0	0
B_1 (mg)	0.07	4	0.97	55	0.06	4	0.09	6	0.14	9.3	0.15	10
B_2 (mg)	0.25	13	0.42	21	0.3	17.6	0.61	35.9	0.25	14.7	0.65	38.2
B_3 (mg)	3.81	19.1	5.95	29.8	6.52	32.6	3.95	19.8	5.3	26.5	7.39	37
B_5 (mg)	0.35	3.5	0.68	6.8	0.9	9	N/A	N/A	0.64	6.4	0.69	6.9
B_6 (mg)	0.33	16.5	0.43	21.5	0.38	19	0	0	0.38	19	0.48	24
B_9 (mcg)	7	1.8	6	1.5	0	0	5	1.3	12	3	11	2.8
B_{12} (mcg)	2.44	40.7	0.75	12.5	4.44	74	1.19	19.8	1.94	32.3	3.04	50.7
C (mg)	0	0	0.3	0.5	N/A	N/A	0	0	0	0	0	0
D (IU)	28	7	21	5.3	N/A	N/A	N/A	N/A	0	0	0	0
E (mg)	0.2	1.3	0.26	1.7	0.8	5.3	0.05	0.3	0.19	1.3	0.75	5
K (mcg)	0.1	0.01	0	0	N/A	N/A	2	2.5	1.2	1.5	1.5	1.9

criticized beef, pork, and lamb, his assault against plants leaves few foods safe for consumption.[41] If plants are suspect, then animals must fill the void. Israeli nutritionist Kadya Araki, echoing a familiar refrain, asserted that evolution shaped humans to eat primarily meat.[42] American anthropologist Stephen Le referenced his nephew as evidence that preference for meat over vegetables and legumes is inborn.[43]

4.5.4 Meat and Lifestyle

Preference for meat implies its healthfulness if natural selection shaped humans to crave what benefits them and to shun the rest. Such thinking, even if true, requires that modern lifestyles conform to the conditions that shaped our evolution. This book argues that reliance on machines rather than muscles and that food abundance rather than dearth deviate from these conditions, nullifying the value of craving caloric foods like meat. No less important in evaluating meat is evidence that meat may cause breast, colon, lung, and prostate cancers.[44] The association is strongest with red meat, though cooking methods may modify risks. All physicians—Davis, Perlmutter, and Gundry must know of these studies; yet they assail plants rather than meat.

Such behavior is familiar to students of American physicist and philosopher Thomas Samuel Kuhn's (1922–1996) *The Structure of Scientific Revolutions* (1962), which demonstrated that scientists invest themselves and their careers in a paradigm such that they explain away, ignore, or denounce contrary evidence.[45] All Americans, Davis, Perlmutter, Gundry, and Le crafted messages for readers in the country that consumes the second most meat per capita. For her part, Araki was born in the United States and educated at the University of Maryland.[46]

These opinions resemble attempts to preserve a paradigm that exalts meat as healthful irrespective of circumstances. Attention on diet deemphasizes lifestyle, maintaining the illusion that inactivity does not undermine health. This stance aligns with enthusiasm for machines and antipathy toward exertion. Crafting messages for a machine age, Davis, Perlmutter, and Gundry omitted idleness' hazards in contrast to ancient Greek medicine. The texts attributed to Greek physician Hippocrates (c. 460–c. 375 BCE), mentioned elsewhere, advocated exercise in addition to wholesome foods.[47] Also mentioned in other chapters, Greek anatomist and physician Galen (130–210 CE) thought exercise as indispensable as food, air (oxygen was then unknown), sleep, and cognition.[48] Returning to meat, the rest of this chapter tests the hypothesis that it invigorates the body by examining meat eaters' vitality.

4.6 MEAT IN ANCIENT EGYPT

4.6.1 Egypt as Case Study

Scrutinizing meat, this chapter turns to ancient Egypt as the first case study. Its civilization endured millennia and was largely stable and homogeneous. These characteristics recommend its examination as among the best-known early civilizations, one that has generated extensive scholarship. Readers may be familiar with the outlines of Egypt's civilization, making it a convenient point of departure.

4.6.2 Egypt's Geography

As elsewhere, geography shaped Egypt in north-easternmost Africa. Describing Egypt as the "gift of the Nile," Greek historian Herodotus (c. 485–c. 425 BCE) specified its principal feature.[49] The world's longest river, the Nile originates in Burundi nearly 6,700 kilometers (4,200 miles) south of the Mediterranean Sea. From its source, the river flows north, emptying into the sea. Ancient Egypt did not occupy the river's entirety because cataracts—unnavigable waterfalls—segment the Nile. In antiquity, Egypt stretched from the Mediterranean coast in the north to the first cataract at Aswan in the south. West and east of the Nile were deserts that deterred invaders, allowing Egypt to develop without continual interference. East was the Sinai Peninsula, which extended Egypt into Asia. The Sinai linked Egypt to the Levant, Arabia, and the rest of southwestern Asia. This region's empires occasionally conquered Egypt, though at other times Egypt penetrated northeast to enlarge its domains. South of the first cataract was Nubia, a kingdom with which Egypt traded.

Because movement south through Egypt necessitates travel up the Nile, the southernmost part is Upper Egypt. From Upper Egypt, the Nile flows north to the delta near Giza and Cairo, where the river divides into several smaller streams that branch west and east on the journey north to the Mediterranean Sea. The delta demarcates Lower Egypt in the north from Upper Egypt in the south.

4.6.3 Egypt's Settlement by Hunter-Gatherers

Having water and edible aquatic creatures, the Nile attracted settlers. Stone tools indicate settlement around 300,000 years ago.[50] These inhabitants must have been archaic peoples, whose evolution Chapter 3 discussed. The oldest skeletons near the Nile displayed modern anatomies and dated about 70,000 years ago.[51] Given that modern humans arose around 150,000 years ago in Africa (see Chapter 3), eighty millennia appear to separate these origins from Egypt's colonization, though their presence in Morocco from the beginning raises the possibility of equally early residence in Egypt given that the 3,700 kilometers (2,300 miles) between the two would not have been insuperable. People have continuously occupied Egypt for at least the last 11,000 years, collecting plants, fishing, and hunting game whose thirst brought them to the Nile. Egypt's adoption of agriculture from southwestern Asia around 5000 BCE deepened dependence on the river.[52]

4.6.4 Transition to Agriculture and Animal Husbandry

Unlike ancient Mesopotamia's (modern Iraq and parts of Syria, Turkey, and Iran) Tigris and Euphrates Rivers, the Nile's predictability made Egypt more stable than its northeastern neighbors. In the Ethiopian Mountains south of Egypt, summer rainfall and melting snow swelled the Nile, causing it to flood Egypt annually between June and September. As it overflowed its banks west and east, the Nile deposited silt, enriching soils for farming. Consequently, Egyptians did not need to manure their land. But fertility extended only as far as the river stretched at maximum inundation. West and east of this area, deserts prohibited farming. Egypt's geography, hydrology, and climate thus confined civilization to lands adjacent the Nile.

4.6.5 Literary and Artistic Evidence of the Past

An advantage of studying ancient Egypt is the presence of literary and artistic evidence. Not only locals documented Egypt's past, but neighbors wrote about a civilization they often judged superior to their own. Egypt was ancient even by Greek and Roman standards, and its durability comforted onlookers who revered constancy and feared change as misfortune's harbinger.

4.6.6 Literary Evidence of Diets

Ancient literature bifurcated Egypt's diets between rich and poor, reserving meat for the wealthy—a phenomenon noted elsewhere—who ate beef, pork, mutton, lamb, chevon, capretto, rabbits, hares (*Lepus* species), gazelles (*Gazella* species), and hedgehogs (species in the subfamily Erinaceinae). According to one source, priests at a temple to the god Amon managed a ranch with over 400,000 cattle during the New Kingdom (1570–1070 BCE).[53] Another operation employed nearly 1,000 men to tend its numerous herds. Other evidence that priests feasted on beef comes from middens near their dwellings at South Abydos, Upper Egypt; trash was about 95 percent cattle bones, an unsurprising statistic given beef's eminence as the chief meat.[54] Summarizing its status, French historian Pierre Tallet (b. 1966) wrote that "Meat was a luxury dish in Egypt."[55] In addition, the wealthy consumed fish and poultry, which Chapters 5 and 6 treat, respectively. In contrast, the poor afforded none of these luxuries, except perhaps during an occasional religious festival, when custom led them to indulge beyond their means.

4.6.7 Mummies as Evidence of Diets

A 2014 paper in the *Journal of Archaeological Science* challenged this dietary division between haves and have nots. French geophysicist Alexandra Touzeau and coauthors cast a wide net by examining mummies of forty-five Egyptians who lived between roughly 3500 BCE and 500 CE.[56] These millennia spanned Egyptian history from roughly the predynastic period (c. 4000–3150 BCE) through the first five centuries of Roman rule (30 BCE–c. 600 CE). Although these 4,000 years witnessed changes in who governed Egypt, the succession of pharaohs and emperors did not affect daily life. Rulers were more interested in collecting taxes than micromanaging events. More generally, ancient bureaucracies lacked the technology to control societies to the degree possible today.

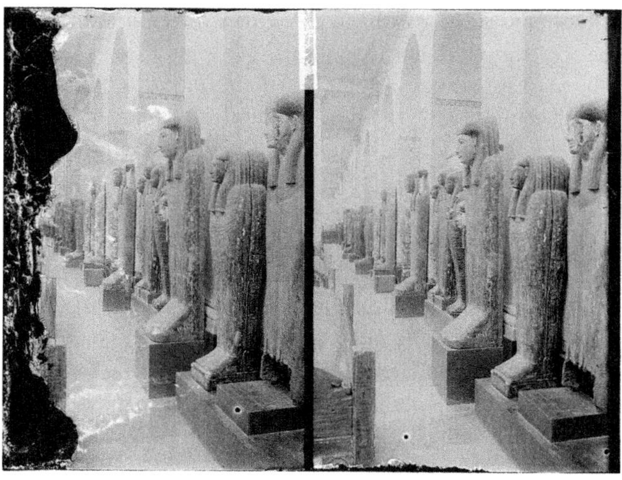

FIGURE 4.4 Egyptian coffins. (Photo courtesy of Library of Congress. https://www.loc.gov/pictures/item/2019700086/.)

Central to Touzeau and colleagues' argument is the link between mummification and affluence. Although Egyptian sources never quoted prices, United Kingdom (UK) microbiologist Tim Sandle must be right that mummification was the "preserve of royalty and the very wealthy."[57] Its use on pharaohs and their families, part of popular lore, corroborates his opinion. That the process, performed by special priests, took seventy days implies enormous expense.[58] Nothing less could have bought such time and effort. If nutrition may be inferred from mummies, this knowledge must illuminate what the wealthy ate. A corollary is that such information cannot indicate what the poor consumed unless everyone ate the same foods. As noted, Egypt's rigid stratification excluded this possibility.

Measuring carbon, nitrogen, and sulfur isotopes—Chapter 1 defined an isotope—in mummy hair, skin, bones, and teeth, Touzeau and colleagues confirmed Egypt's constancy, noting that elite diets changed little over 4,000 years.[59] They inferred from the ^{13}C to ^{12}C ratio in hair, skin, bones, and teeth that the wealthy consumed between one-tenth and half their protein from animals, an amount that resembles ovo-lacto-vegetarians' protein intake from animal sources.[60] (Chapter 1 defined vegetarianism's types.) In other words, dairy and eggs might have been wealthy Egyptians' only animal products.

But combinations of meat and plants can satisfy the restriction of not above 50 percent total protein from animals. For example, a holdover from U.S. slavery, Hoppin' John, discussed in Chapter 8, may contain cowpeas (*Vigna unguiculata*) or peas (*Pisum sativum*), pork, rice—*Oryza glaberrima* or *O. sativa* in the South—and vegetables. By mass, pork has roughly seven times more protein than cowpeas.[61] Considering just these ingredients, Hoppin' John met the criterion of not above 50 percent protein from animals whenever cowpeas totaled at least seven times the mass of pork. In this context, many combinations of meat and plants could have produced Touzeau and coauthors' ^{13}C to ^{12}C ratio. Ancient Egypt had pigs, and although critics might object that cowpeas, indigenous to southern Africa, were unknown in Egypt, it had other legumes like chickpeas (*Cicer arietinum*), broad beans (*Vicia faba*), lentils (*Lens culinaris*), and peas (*P. sativum*). The wealthy must have combined pork, beef, or other meats, legumes, nuts, and other plant protein in innumerable ways to consume not above 50 percent animal protein. None of these possibilities, however, denies that some elites ate meat in prodigious amounts, only that they were not among these dead. There is no reason, therefore, to infer from the ^{13}C to ^{12}C ratio that these mummified wealthy ate eggs and dairy but not meat.

Moreover, Touzeau and coauthors admitted that hair from these mummies had more ^{15}N, an isotope of nitrogen, than does that from today's Europeans and North Americans, who eat lots of meat.[62] Because meat contains nitrogen, whatever isotope, as a consequence of having protein (see Chapter 2), the most parsimonious explanation should be that Egyptian elites ate meat, possibly in larger amounts than modern Americans. The authors, however, attributed this finding to Egypt's aridity, which may have increased ^{15}N in plants to yield large amounts in hair even with little or no animal protein in diets. They pursued this rationale by ruling out sources of animal protein like Nile perch (*Lates niloticus*), whose ratio of nitrogen and sulfur isotopes in its tissues does not match these ratios in mummy hair.[63] If elites eschewed perch, then they probably did not eat other fish given the improbability that they all discriminated against just perch. This argument, however, depends on consumption of plants with lots of ^{15}N and minimal meat, fish, and poultry and so requires more assumptions than the hypothesis that Egypt's wealthy had ^{15}N in their hair because they ate meat and other animal protein.

Although Touzeau and colleagues' paper is provocative, a 2013 *Lancet* article countered it. Computed tomography (CT) scans of 137 mummies from Egypt, Peru, the American Southwest, and the Aleutian Islands allowed examination of arteries for plaque, whose presence indicated atherosclerosis (sometimes rendered arteriosclerosis).[64] The American Southwest and Aleutian Islands supplied only five mummies each and are omitted because the samples are small. Twenty-nine of the seventy-six (38.2 percent) Egyptian mummies displayed atherosclerosis compared to thirteen of the fifty-one (25.5 percent) Peruvian remains. Because consumption of red meat causes the condition, as the Cleveland Clinic affirmed, the *Lancet* study justifies the conclusion that wealthy Egyptians ate meat.[65] This chapter offers no hypothesis about whether Egyptians or Peruvians ate more meat because the samples are incomparable: the Egyptian sample necessarily preserved only elites whereas Peru's mummies, being natural, likely represented the more numerous commoners.

Comparisons aside, this chapter affirms that a chasm separated ancient Egypt's rich, who consumed meat, from the poor, who could not afford it. As noted, the wealthy maintained enormous herds of cattle.[66] A single cow, however, was worth a smallholder's harvest, or a laborer's wages, for a full year. Like any luxury, meat was too dear for the masses.

Absent meat, the poor ate bread or porridge made from wheat (*Triticum monococcum* or *T. dicoccon*) or barley (*Hordeum vulgare*), lettuce (*Lactuca sativa*), turnips (*Brassica rapa ssp. rapa*), cabbage (*Brassica oleracea var. capitata*), beets (*Beta vulgaris*), radishes (*Raphanus raphanistrum ssp. sativus*), broad beans, peas, lentils, chickpeas, garlic (*Allium sativum*), onions (*Allium cepa*), leeks (*Allium ampeloprasum*), cucumbers (*Cucumis sativus*), papyrus (*Cyperus papyrus*) roots, watermelons (*Citrullus lanatus*), figs (*Ficus carica*), dates (*Phoenix dactylifera*), grapes (*Vitis vinifera*) and raisins, and plums (*Prunus domestica*). Egyptians grew coconuts (*Cocos nucifera*), which fed the affluent rather than the poor. Touzeau and colleagues argued that few Egyptians ate native African grains like sorghum (*Sorghum bicolor*) and various millets (*Pennisetum glaucum* and *Eleusine coracana* being most important).[67] Roman conquest in 30 BCE introduced oleiculture into Egypt, though sesame (*Sesamum indicum*) competed with olives as a source of oil.[68] Chapter 10 discusses olive oil in the context of other fats. Although Egyptians ate local foods, around 400 CE the Romans began importing oranges (*Citrus sinensis* and *Citrus aurantium*), lemons (*Citrus limon*), peaches (*Prunus persica*), and bananas (*Musa x paradisiaca*) into Egypt from Asia. Being imports, these fruits were too expensive for the poor.

In addition to rich and poor, Egypt had *hemw*, a status difficult to define. These people were not free to work as they pleased but had to follow the master's dictates. Economic restrictions were not unique to *hemw* because commoners, though free in a narrow sense, could not choose their occupation. *Hemw* were bought and sold, and their children were unfree, other characteristics of slavery. Yet they sometimes earned wages, and could marry anyone irrespective of status, own property, and bequeath it to heirs, all attributes of freedom. Given that Egyptians were mindful of status and class and that social mobility was uncommon, these rights expressed aspiration more than actuality. Whatever this system's benefits, *hemw* disliked their status.

For example, the Hebrews described themselves as slaves while in Egypt, possibly in the mid second millennium BCE.[69] Some scholars doubt that they were ever in Egypt, let alone as slaves. But if the Pentateuch (Torah) is correct, it recounted that as *hemw*, the Hebrews ate no meat. Instead they had cucumbers, watermelons, leeks, garlic, onions, and fish.[70] Interesting is the intimation that they consumed abundant fish. Such reminiscences, written around a millennium after the events they purported to narrate, are likely exaggerations. Numbers list these foods in the context of the Hebrews' dissatisfaction with being homeless in the way that people in a new neighborhood might wish for their old acquaintances and familiar surroundings even when their former lives were unpleasant. Nonetheless, if the Hebrew account is reliable, it reinforces the likelihood that only affluent Egyptians ate meat.

This treatment of diet, as noted, depends on Egypt's division into two tiers: a tiny elite who monopolized almost everything and countless paupers. Absence of a middle class may seem strange given economists and historians' concern with it, though this preoccupation does not characterize antiquity. Although Roman naturalist Pliny the Elder (23–79 CE) likely exaggerated in claiming that just six men owned "half of North Africa," he understood that agrarian societies bifurcate into landowners and landless.[71] To flourish, a middle class appears to need numerous cities, infrastructure, banking, and vigorous commerce, all of which required food surpluses larger and more regular than were possible in antiquity. Frequent famines and shortages, discussed in Chapter 3, demonstrated agriculture's precariousness.

Examination of diet necessitates an attempt to gauge Egypt's food supply. Egyptologist and museum curator James Romano's claim that people "had as much food to eat as they desired" conflicts with Genesis' assertion that the region alternated between abundance and famine.[72] This book confirms that food was more scarce than plentiful before modernity. Whether harvests were adequate or meager, government took a portion through taxation. This policy persisted under Rome. First emperor Augustus (63 BCE–14 CE) and his successors declared Egypt their property, a policy that legalized grains' diversion to Rome, which imported roughly 493,347.4 cubic meters (14 million bushels) annually to feed the capital in the first century BCE.[73]

This situation harmed Egypt's masses, who suffered deprivation throughout antiquity. A 2013 paper documented undernutrition among inhabitants of Tell el-Amarna, the capital under Pharaoh Akhenaten (c. 1380–1336 BCE).[74] About 350 kilometers south of Cairo, Amarna is in Upper Egypt, where aridity preserved human remains better than the marshy delta. For this reason, researchers have focused on Upper Egypt. Amarna has attracted Egyptologists and anthropologists because people inhabited it only during Akhenaten's seventeen-year kingship (1353–1336), narrowing the time when someone buried there might have died.[75] Such precision is useful when the deceased was anonymous and undated, as was true for commoners.

Amarna's South Tombs Cemetery yielded 274 partial and complete skeletons.[76] Remains of ninety-five adults and sixty-four youths were at least half complete, allowing scrutiny.[77] Grave goods' paucity or absence identified the deceased as commoners. The sixty-four preadults displayed stunting as early as 7.5 months, near the start of weaning.[78] Transition to solids brought undernutrition that never abated. Adults remained stunted, with women on average shorter than their counterparts elsewhere in Egypt. Men were shorter than other Egyptian men except for those from roughly 4200 BCE. Cribra orbitalia, defined in Chapter 1, in Amarna skeletons indicated anemia. Although pathogens or parasites may cause the condition, the authors implicated diets deficient in iron or, less often, vitamin B_9 (folate, folic acid, or pteroylmonoglutamic acid) or B_{12} (cobalamin) deprivation, all discussed in Chapter 1. Meat's paucity was likely the culprit because, as Chapter 2 mentioned, the body absorbs iron better from animals than plants. Evidence of anemia indicated that a meatless diet harmed ordinary Egyptians.

Roughly 5 percent of juvenile remains exhibited porousness in the cranium's sphenoid, temporal, and occipital bones, evincing scurvy from inadequate vitamin C.[79] Because many vegetables and fruits have this vitamin (see Chapter 2), Egypt's masses must have lacked a varied diet from childhood, though they might have eaten figs and dates, neither of which has much vitamin C. With scant meat, vegetables, and fruits, they must have subsisted on grains, chickpeas, broad beans, and lentils. Barley and wheat lack vitamin C. Lentils, chickpeas, and broad beans have negligible amounts. Commoners must have eaten few peas, another legume known to them. Roughly 115 grams—under 1 cup in English units—supply over the daily 46 grams of vitamin C necessary to avert scurvy.[80]

A paltry diet did not fortify Amarna's residents for toil. Over three-quarters of adult skeletons exhibited osteoarthritis in the ankles, knees, hip, spine, elbows, shoulders, wrists, or their combination.[81] Adult bones had remodeled where tendons attached.[82] The condition—worse than for other Egyptians but less severe than for peoples in the Levant and North and South America—indicated strenuous exertions, which the authors attributed to the labor of carrying heavy stone blocks while building the city. Such toil was so hazardous that over two-thirds of adult skeletons displayed at least one fracture in various stages of healing. Amarna's opulence did not trickle down to the masses, who languished with little meat, vegetables, and fruits and whose lives overflowed with travails.

The poor of Tell Ibrahim Awad, Lower Egypt appear superficially to have been healthier than their Amarna compatriots. Of seventy-seven partial skeletons from the Old Kingdom (2600–2160 BCE), First Intermediate Period (2160–2040 BCE), and Middle Kingdom (2040–1700 BCE), only one (1.3 percent) displayed cribra orbitalia.[83] This number was not the percentage of anemic Tell Ibrahim Awad residents because it represented only anemia severe enough to have marked bones. Bones were silent about lesser deficiencies. Nonetheless, comparison of this condition across populations and times is valid because the same metric is applied.

In contrast to Tell Ibrahim Awad, human remains indicate that cribra orbitalia afflicted over one-quarter of those in Tell el-Daba, Lower Egypt and nearly two-fifth in Elephantine, an island in Upper Egypt.[84] Investigators asserted that Tell el-Daba and Elephantine better approximated ancient Egypt's nutrition and health and that Tell Ibrahim Awad would have aligned with their higher cribra orbitalia rates had centuries of irrigation not degraded so many skeletons.

Being better preserved than bones, teeth revealed undernutrition in Tell Ibrahim Awad; 38 percent of crania had teeth exhibiting enamel hypoplasia, defined in Chapter 1.[85] This thinning of enamel betrays the body's attempt, especially when young, to conserve energy and nutrients during privation. Percentages in predynastic Egypt and Nubia were 40 and in Tell el-Daba 46.[86] That is, between roughly two-fifths and half of ordinary Egyptians and Nubians may have been so undernourished that the ordeal stunted development. Amid food scarcity, meat—had the masses afforded it—might have provided the desperately needed calories and nutrients like iron, other minerals, and B vitamins to reduce instances of cribra orbitalia and enamel hypoplasia.

If meat might have benefitted commoners, excess harmed elites. Defined as intake above need, excess depended on life's rigors. Too much meat or another item for an inert person might have undernourished a laborer. Atherosclerosis in the Egyptian mummies mentioned earlier was no anomaly. Forty-four of fifty-two (84.6 percent) mummies in the Egyptian Museum in Cairo evinced it or other forms of cardiovascular disease.[87] A smaller sample revealed atherosclerosis in nine of sixteen (56.3 percent) mummies.[88]

Pharaoh Ramses II (c. 1303–c. 1213 BCE) had the disease, which may have killed son Merenptah (c. 1273–1203 BCE).[89] Priest Inemakhet (early second millennium BCE) had atherosclerosis and diabetes. Plaque clogged five arteries in Princess Ahmose Meryet Amon (c. 1580–c. 1550 BCE). Calcium salts in her heart imply that she suffered a heart attack.[90] Queen Hatshepsut (c. 1508–c. 1458 BCE) was obese and likely diabetic from eating "well and abundantly."[91] American cardiologist Michael Miyamoto blamed caloric foods, especially meat, and inactivity for cardiovascular disease among Egypt's royalty and wealthy.[92] Ancient Egypt's problems remain relevant today, when overconsumption, inactivity, and chronic diseases afflict many people in developed nations.

Longevity did not bless Egypt's masses. American anthropologist Delisa Phillips and colleagues fixed lifespan at 32.1 years for Tell Ibrahim Awad's poor, but this number omits youth mortality because the cemetery lacked juvenile remains.[93] British epidemiologist Ann E. M. Liljas computed ancient Egyptian e^0 at nineteen years, a number referenced in Chapter 3.[94] About half Roman Egypt's population died before age ten.[95] Of these deaths, around half occurred during the first year.[96] Human remains from Kulubnarti, Nubia indicate that between roughly 500 and 1500 CE, the death rate was high in infancy, early childhood, and after age twenty.[97] Adolescence alone provided sanctuary from high mortality. Almost no one survived beyond fifty years. In other words, and on average, commoners died young, an unsurprising reality given undernutrition and hardships. These realities indicate that Phillips and coauthors' calculation, absent juvenile mortality, was too high.

As noted, mummies illuminated elites' lives and deaths, indicating that most perished between ages thirty and forty.[98] Of thirty whose lifespans could be estimated from a collection in Lyon, France's Museum of Natural History, twenty-four died before age forty.[99] Of them, seven expired before age twenty. Six survived to or beyond their fortieth birthday. Although this sample is small, it reveals that one-fifth reached forty. Chapter 3 noted that into the Middle Ages few achieved such longevity.[100]

This contrast raises the issue of whether and to what extent meat advantaged Egypt's wealthy in a world where most people ate too little. At a time when contagion and parasites killed indiscriminately, elites do not appear to have suffered fewer infections.[101] Yet meat was not their only trump card because, as mentioned, they did not suffer the overwork and injuries that debilitated commoners. The reality that overwork truncated Caribbean slaves' lives, as noted in Chapter 1, implies that it prematurely killed Egypt's poor. Exhaustion and undernourishment impaired every aspect of their lives. On the other hand, indulgence and idleness gave elites heart disease.

4.7 MEAT IN NORTH AMERICA

4.7.1 North America's Settlement

Describing the evolution of humans and diets, Chapter 3 identified Africa as their homeland. As noted, modern peoples arose there about 150,000 years ago. From African Egypt, migrants moved east into the Sinai Peninsula some 50,000 years ago, beginning their colonization of every continent. Entrance into North America came comparatively late at roughly 13,000 BCE.[102] Northern latitudes supplied big game for hunters, whose proficiency may have hastened extinction of the largest, though the warming climate likely dealt the fatal blow by shrinking habitats. Eradication of the biggest prey left bison as North America's largest herbivore.

4.7.2 North American Bison

This chapter rejects conflation of the terms "bison" and "buffalo"—evident in American food writer Waverly Lewis Root (1903–1982) and American filmmaker Richard de Rochemont's (1903–1982)

Eating in America: A History (1995)—because bison are more closely related to cattle than buffaloes.[103] Although both have shaggy fur and horns and belong to the Bovidae family, they occupy different continents and have unique features. Buffaloes lack humps and have short fur at the chin and long horns. In this class are Asia's water buffalo (*Bubalus bubalis*) and Africa's cape buffalo (*Syncerus caffer caffer*). In contrast, the two bison species have a hump at the shoulders, long fur at the chin that resembles a beard, and short horns. The wisent (*Bison bonasus*) roamed northern Europe before hunters slaughtered it. Reintroduced into Belarus and Poland in 1929, the wisent is now a vulnerable species. The American bison (*Bison bison*) was also overhunted. Its meat nourished North American Indians into the nineteenth century.

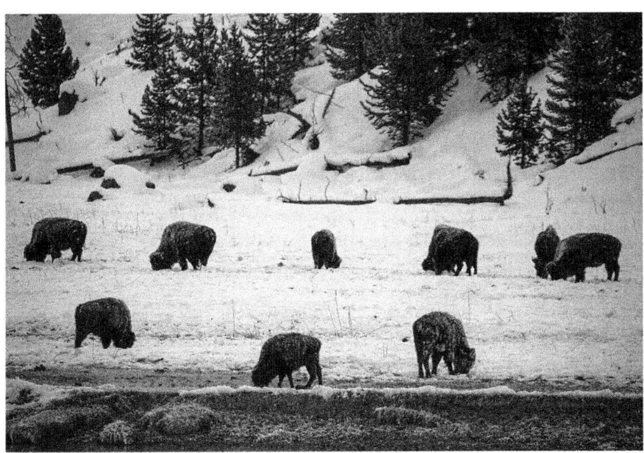

FIGURE 4.5 Bison. (Photo courtesy of Library of Congress. https://www.loc.gov/pictures/item/2017686037/.)

Pre-Columbian bison populations are unknown, with estimates between 60 million and 100 million.[104] At their apex, bison ranged south into Monterrey, Mexico and north into Alberta and Saskatchewan provinces, Canada. To the west they inhabited grasslands near the Rocky Mountains. Eastward they reached New York. In the sixteenth century, bison may have occupied roughly 70 percent of what are now the forty-eight contiguous U.S. states.[105]

Their presence on the Great Plains is central to the lore of the American West. Since the Lewis and Clark expedition (1804–1806), Americans have offered several definitions of the Great Plains. In 2017 American geologist Robert Francis Diffendal Jr. characterized the region as flatlands west of the Mississippi River with rainfall sufficient for grasses but not trees.[106] In keeping with these criteria, he fixed the western boundary at the Rocky Mountains.[107]

Northern and southern termini are less easy to pinpoint because the grasslands do not end abruptly. American anthropologist Joseph M. Prince and American economist Richard Hall Steckel (b. 1944) set these boundaries in the Canadian provinces of Manitoba, Saskatchewan, and Alberta to the north and in Texas to the south. Prince and Steckel, however, moved the eastern boundary west of the Mississippi River, fixing it with an imaginary vertical line from central Oklahoma to Manitoba.[108] Consequently, their geography of the Great Plains was smaller than Diffendal's. Most U.S. lands between the Mississippi River and Rocky Mountains receive under 51 centimeters (20 inches) of rain annually.[109]

4.7.3 Humans on the Great Plains

Burials in and near the plains suggest settlement between roughly 11,000 and 11,500 years ago.[110] These dates align with the Clovis culture's emergence between about 11,300 and 10,900 years ago.[111] In this fluid region, populations shifted over time as people collected plants and pursued bison, antelopes (species in Bovidae family), elk (*Cervus species*), deer (*Odocoileus* species), wolves (*Canis lupus*), foxes (*Vulpes vulpes*), bears (*Ursus americanus* and *Ursus arctos*), beavers (*Castor canadensis*), muskrats (*Ondatra zibethicus*), mink (*Mustela vison*), weasels (*Mustela nivalis*), and raccoons (*Procyon lotor*). Introduction of Old-World livestock led Native Americans to expand the hunt to sheep and cattle. Trade with Europeans gave indigenes horses and metal weapons: guns, knives, and arrowheads.

By increasing mobility, the horse prompted Plains Indians to concentrate on bison, which they had hunted since roughly 8000 BCE.[112] During much of the nineteenth century, firearms could not be reloaded quickly enough for the hunt, a problem that breechloading rifles solved around 1870. In addition to meat, Plains Indians ate prairie turnips (*Psoralea esculenta*), wild artichokes (*Cynara cardunculus*), wild onions (*Allium canadense*), chokecherries (*Prunus virginiana*), gooseberries (*Ribes uva-crispa*), buffaloberries (*Shepherdia* species), elderberries (*Sambucus nigra*), wild plums (*Prunus americana*), sand cherries (*Prunus pumila*), ground beans (*Falcata comosa*), sunflower seeds (*Helianthus annuus*), prickly pears (*Opuntia* species), and nuts from several tree species. Trade expanded diets to include corn, beans (*Phaseolus vulgaris, P. lunatus, P. acutifolius,* and *P. coccineus*), and squashes (*Cucurbita* species).

By mid-nineteenth century, several Plains indigenes competed for territory and, with it, access to water, game, edible plants, and trade. Some gathered plants, hunted, farmed, and traded, achieving varied diets. Among them were the Arikara in what are now North and South Dakota, the Omaha in South Dakota and Nebraska, and the Pawnee and Ponca in Nebraska. Plains nomads did not farm but instead hunted, collected plants, and traded. Among them, the Comanche roamed Texas, Oklahoma, and Kansas, the Arapaho and Cheyenne Kansas and Wyoming, the Crow Wyoming and Montana, the Kiowa Colorado, the Sioux the Dakotas, and the Assiniboine and Blackfeet the border between the United States and Canada.

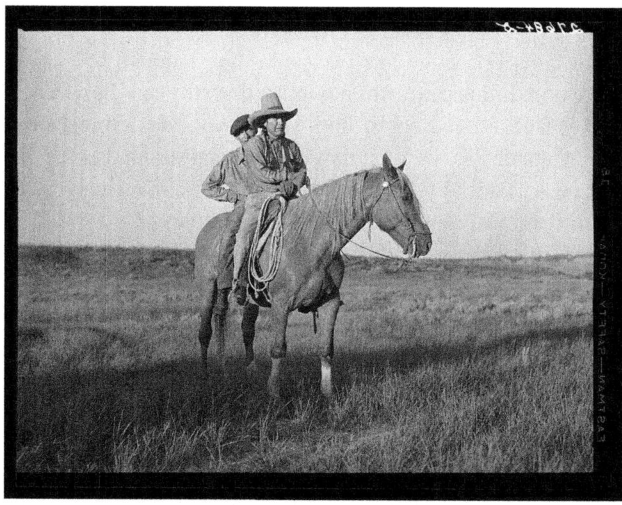

FIGURE 4.6 Cheyenne Indians. (Photo courtesy of Library of Congress. https://www.loc.gov/pictures/item/2017777944/.)

The nomads appear to have had the most bison and other meat. The Ponca may have eaten the least, their last bison kill occurring in 1855.[113] The Omaha stopped hunting bison in 1876.[114] Of the sedentary peoples, the Arikara and Pawnee probably ate the most bison. American demographer S. Ryan Johansson and American anthropologist Douglas Owsley praised the Arikara's "exceptionally diverse and healthy diet," which included bison, deer, corn, beans, squashes, sunflower seeds, prairie turnips, and several species of berries.[115]

4.7.4 Health on the Great Plains

Dietary diversity's benefits were evident on examination of 273 Arikara skeletons interred between the sixteenth and nineteenth centuries, most between 1680 and 1750.[116] Femur robustness evinced excellent nutrition, and iron, vitamin B_9, and B_{12} deficiencies were uncommon.[117] Bone density benefited from the fact that Arikara and other Plains Indians were active outdoors. Exertion and exposure to sunlight correlate with bone density, partly explaining Arikara's stout femurs. Of skeletons classified men, only 2 percent had porotic hyperostosis, defined in Chapter 1, and 8.3 percent had cribra orbitalia. Women exhibited no porotic hyperostosis and just 2 percent had cribra orbitalia. These data suggest adequate iron and vitamins B_9 and B_{12}. Because vitamin C aids iron absorption, it too was likely satisfactory in diets.

Other evidence indicated healthfulness. As noted, most Arikara skeletons dated between 1680 and 1750, prosperous decades when number of villages and size of storage pits and middens increased. These people must have been well nourished to have stored more food and generated more garbage. Population increase is harder to interpret. Vitamins B_9 and B_{12}, omega 3 fatty acids, olive oil, vegetables, fruits, fish, and nuts may increase fertility.[118] Soy foods, dairy, vitamin D, antioxidants, caffeine, and alcohol may contribute little or nothing to it. Junk foods and beverages, red meat, and potatoes are thought to depress fertility. Such thinking provides no insight into the fact that prehistory and history supply countless examples of population increase amid penury and dietary distress. Additionally, the premise that some foods enhance fertility whereas others diminish it is questionable. Against the opinion that potatoes reduce fertility, for example, Chapter 13 demonstrates that birthrate rose throughout northern Europe upon their widespread adoption in the eighteenth century.

Nonetheless, the Arikara inhabited no utopia. Food was scarce during winter. Every five to ten years, shortages were severe enough to kill weaklings, infants, and the old.[119] As noted, population increased amid abundance, crowding Arikara villages and polluting the nearby Missouri River. Pathogens, parasites, rodents, and insects multiplied in this environment. After roughly 1740, conflicts escalated with the Sioux. These problems offset good nutrition, dragging e^0 below twenty years.[120]

Where it occurred, anemia probably did not result from dietary deficiency. As mentioned and as Tables 4.2 and 4.3 indicate, porotic hyperostosis and cribra orbitalia were infrequent among the Arikara, and the ninety-seven Pawnee skeletons exhibited no instances of either among men.[121] Only two women suffered from porotic hyperostosis and none had cribra orbitalia. All seventy-six Omaha skeletons, both men and women, displayed no anemia.

TABLE 4.2
Porotic Hyperostosis in Great Plains Indians Adults

Group	% Men w/PH	% Women w/PH
Nomad	1.9	1.8
Arikara	2	0
Pawnee	0	3.6
Omaha	0	0

TABLE 4.3
Cribra Orbitalia in Great Plains Indians Adults

Group	% Men w/CO	% Women w/CO
Nomad	6	8.6
Arikara	8.3	2
Pawnee	0	0
Omaha	0	0

Arikara, Pawnee, and Omaha skeletons of children who died before age eleven had higher rates of porotic hyperostosis and cribra orbitalia, in Tables 4.4 and 4.5, than adults. Anemia must have stunted these youths during years normally devoted to growth and contributed to their demise.

Surprisingly, the 217 Cheyenne, Crow, and Sioux skeletons had the most adult and childhood porotic hyperostosis and cribra orbitalia.[122] These horsemen should have been least vulnerable to anemia because, as noted, they had access to the most bison and other game. Meat constituted two-thirds to 85 percent of their diet whereas sedentary Plains Indians got under half their calories from it.[123] Additionally, being more than transportation and status symbols, horses supplied meat when food was scarce. The wealthiest, owning as many as forty horses, had plenty of extra food during shortages.[124] The Plains staple was pemmican, a combination of dried bison, lard, and wild berries, cherries, or plums that stored years in an era before refrigeration.

Although these horsemen compared poorly to their sedentary neighbors in skeletal pathologies, Table 4.6 demonstrates that they lived longest. Omitting youth mortality, Table 4.6 shows that the Cheyenne, Crow, and Sioux as a group outlived the Omaha by 16.3 years, the Arikara by 13.7 years, and the Pawnee by 11.1 years.[125] Unlike skeletal pathology data, differences in lifespan are unsurprising given nomad mobility and greater bison consumption.

TABLE 4.4
Porotic Hyperostosis in Great Plains Indians Children

Group	% Children, Ages 1–10 yr, with PH
Nomad	0
Arikara	2.9
Pawnee	2.8
Omaha	2.2

TABLE 4.5
Cribra Orbitalia in Great Plains Indians Children

Group	% Children, Ages 1–10 yr, w/ CO
Nomad	25
Arikara	14.3
Pawnee	2.9
Omaha	2.3

TABLE 4.6
Age at Death of Great Plains Indians

Group	Age at Death (yr)
Nomad	32.5
Arikara	18.8
Pawnee	21.4
Omaha	16.2

Unlike beef, bison does not raise low-density lipoproteins (LDL), whose role in transporting cholesterol to cells Chapter 2 discussed.[126] When allowed to eat grasses, as is their preference, bison store unsaturated fat as omega 6 and omega 3 fatty acids in a 4:1 ratio.[127] Grain-fed cattle yield beef with a ratio around 13.6:1, and modern diets approach 30:1.[128] In contrast, studies of modern hunter-gatherers indicate a ratio near 1:1.[129] Chapter 2 examined the structure, naming, and function of fatty acids, including omega 3 and omega 6.

Returning to anemia, an earlier section mentioned iron and vitamins B_9 and B_{12} as crucial nutrients. Table 4.1 indicates that 100 grams of bison supply 15.4 percent of the U.S. Food and Drug Administration's (FDA) daily value (DV) for iron, 3 percent for B_9 and 32.3 percent for B_{12}. Focusing on iron, Table 4.1 shows that by mass bison trails beef, mutton, goat, and venison but surpasses pork. Nevertheless, Prince and Steckel judged bison intake adequate in iron to enable Plains Indians, even the poorest, to attain maximum heights.[130] Under this circumstance, iron cannot have been deficient.

That is, bison eaters should have been unlikely anemics. The contradiction between bison consumption and anemia amplified the larger incongruity that Plains Indians who ate a varied diet exhibited signs of dietary distress. Movement beyond this problem requires examination of the mythology of the hunt. Always on the move, Cheyenne, Crow, and Sioux seldom resided anywhere long enough to accumulate the wastes that nourished germs, parasites, rodents, and insects. These peoples lived in small bands, not in cramped cities that incubated contagion. Getting plenty of sunshine and feasting on bison, other game, and a variety of plants, these nomads must have been hale.

Yet this image of Plains peoples as paragons of vitality was an anachronism by the late nineteenth century, when anthropologists began to study them. By then, reservations warehoused the remnants of tribes that had once relished their independence, giving them too much white flour and alcohol, too many canned goods, too little fresh meat, and too few fresh vegetables and fruits.[131] Among students of native peoples, German-American anthropologist Franz Uri Boas (1858–1942) measured Plains Indians in the 1880s, presenting these data at the 1892 Columbian Exposition in Chicago, Illinois.[132] Marking the quatercentenary of Italian-Spanish mariner Christopher Columbus' (1451–1506) first encounter with Amerindians, the event heightened scholarly and popular interest in them.

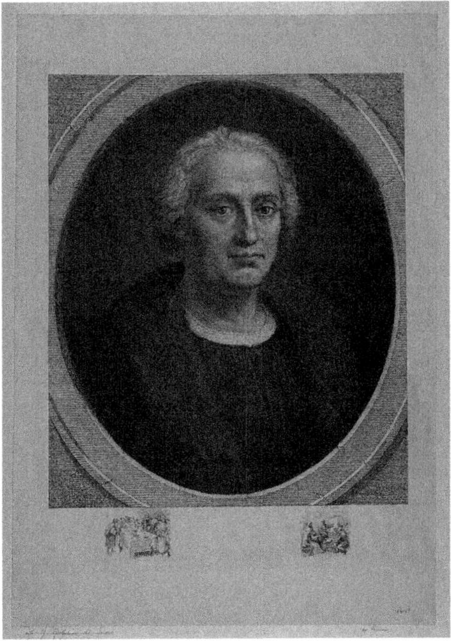

FIGURE 4.7 Christopher Columbus. (Photo courtesy of Library of Congress. https://www.loc.gov/pictures/item/96513605/.)

These measurements came at a crucial moment. As mentioned, the Plains Indians then occupied unhealthy reservations. The bison that had nourished them faced extermination as whites slaughtered them to clear land for cattle, sheep, railroads, and towns. Yet the 1880s were not distant from good times. Older adults had eaten bison and other game as children. Their heights therefore recorded nutrition during youth's growth spurt. Boas and his assistants measured men and women from eight Plains tribes: the Arapaho, Assiniboine, Blackfoot, Cheyenne, Comanche, Crow, Kiowa, and Sioux. Table 4.7 shows that men averaged 172.2 centimeters (67.8 inches) and women 159.7 centimeters (62.9 inches).[133] The tallest were the Cheyenne, whose men were 176.7 centimeters (69.6 inches) and women 161.5 centimeters (63.6 inches). The shortest were the Comanche, whose men stood 168 centimeters (66.1 inches) on average. The mean for women was 156.7 centimeters (61.7 inches).

The Comanche occupying the southernmost Plains, temptation exists to apply Bergmann's rule, introduced in Chapter 1, to them. German biologist Carl Georg Lucas Christian Bergmann (1814–1865) described size as an adaptation to climate. Near the equator, people tend to be small because smallness dissipates heat, an advantage in hot climates. Away from the equator, largeness conserves heat, a benefit in cold climates.

Height is an aspect of size, though largeness may be achieved through bulk irrespective of stature. For example, the Romans described Mediterranean peoples as shorter than northern Europeans, evidence that shortness might be an adaptation to warmth.[134] Yet skeletal measurements do not entirely confirm this impression because remains interred in Greece between roughly 3000 and 146 BCE indicated that women were 2 centimeters (0.8 inches) shorter—but men 0.5 centimeters (0.2 inches) taller—than their counterparts in Roman Germania.[135] Even had heights differed north and south, dietary dissimilarities rather than climatic adaptation might have been the cause.

Returning to the Great Plains, the Comanche, occupying the southern Plains, confirmed the expectation of smallness if shortness were always an adaptation to warmth. Yet the two cannot be equated because the Assiniboine were the second shortest Plains people despite inhabiting the U.S.-Canada border. Not a consequence of Bergmann's Rule, Plains tallness—and possibly height across time and place—must illuminate nutrition, making it a metric for comparing nutrition among various peoples. This view aligns with Dutch historian Willem Marinus Jongman's judgment that "Stature is no doubt the best generalized indictor of nutritional status."[136]

In 2012, the U.S. Centers for Disease Control and Prevention (CDC) in Atlanta, Georgia reported a mean height of 176.5 centimeters (69.5 inches) for American men.[137] The average American woman stood 161.8 centimeters (63.7 inches).[138] These heights almost mirror 1880s Cheyenne stature, an achievement given that food is more plentiful in the United States today than at any time in the past. Equally impressive, global measurements indicate that in the 1880s the Cheyenne were the world's tallest people.[139] As a group, Plains nomads stood 1–2 centimeters (0.4–0.8 inches) above

TABLE 4.7
Plains Indians Heights

Group	Men (cm)	Women (cm)
Arapaho	174.3	161.8
Assiniboine	169.6	159.2
Blackfeet	172.0	160.5
Cheyenne	176.7	161.5
Comanche	168.0	156.7
Crow	173.6	159.1
Kiowa	170.4	158.5
Sioux	172.8	160.6
Mean	172.2	159.7

whites in nineteenth century United States and Australia and 6–12 centimeters (2.4–4.7 inches) over Europeans.[140] These data do not guarantee that abundance produces health. People are tall today despite prevalence of junk foods, cigarettes, and inactivity.

4.7.5 Meat and Health in North America

Reaching North America some fifteen millennia after the first arrivals, Europeans and their descendants ate beef and pork rather than game like bison. Despite this difference, European Americans also benefitted from meat. Data from pensions certified between 1654 and 1830 in Middlesex County, Massachusetts demonstrated that widows' meat allowances increased over time.[141] Between 1675 and 1750 the annual allotment per widow rose from 36.3 to 76.2 kilograms (80 to 168 pounds). American historian, economist, and 1993 Nobel laureate in economics Robert William Fogel (1926–2013) extrapolated this trend, noting that by roughly 1750, Americans' meat intake reached an amount that Britons would not match until after 1900. By 1750 Americans were taller than Brits on average and had reached twentieth-century developed world heights, indicating nourishment equal to recent times.

Stature and lifespan grew until about 1790, when gains reversed as entrepreneurs created factories.[142] Management underpaid workers, inequalities widened, and nutrition, height, and longevity fell. Since the 1880s these measures rebounded. Over the long term, meat consumption increased and mortality fell 35 percent in the United States and 21 percent in the United Kingdom between 1700 and 1980.[143] This book emphasizes that diet alone did not determine longevity. Chapter 7 notes that pasteurization, clean water, sewage treatment and disposal, antisepsis in hospitals, and hygiene in the home reduced deaths.

4.8 MEAT IN TWENTIETH-CENTURY PARAGUAY

4.8.1 Settlement of South America

Chapter 3 and the previous section mentioned that migrants from northeastern Asia entered northwestern North America around 15,000 years ago. Population pressure and pursuit of game may have driven the first Americans south and east. Some hugged the Pacific coast as they moved south, crossing the isthmus of Panama—sometimes designated the isthmus of Darien—into what is today Colombia in north-westernmost South America.[144] Stone tools, animal bones, and plant debris in Peru are nearly 15,000 years old, implying rapid migration from arctic to South America.[145]

From Peru, Amerindians moved southeast through Bolivia and into Paraguay. South of the equator and mostly within the Tropic of Capricorn, Paraguay experiences less annual temperature variation than temperate countries. Rainfall supported dense forests with insects, amphibians, reptiles, birds, and mammals, all feeding humans. During the last 10,000 years, people settled near the Parana River, which flows south from Brazil through Paraguay and Argentina and into the Atlantic Ocean. Among them were eastern Paraguay's Ache, sometimes named the Guayaki. They may have combined hunting, collecting plants, and farming, but conflicts with the Guarani and other neighbors during the last millennium drove them into Paraguay's hills and away from agriculture.

4.8.2 The Ache in Paraguay

In the seventeenth century, Jesuit missionaries were the first Europeans to encounter the Ache. Spain's enslavement of the Guarani in the seventeenth and eighteenth centuries removed a threat, allowing Ache numbers to increase. Four groups, each with a unique language, persisted into the twentieth century, when anthropologists studied them. Interest stemmed from reports of cannibalism, infanticide, bellicosity, polyandry, and promiscuity. Some anthropologists depicted them as throwbacks to humanity's original primitivism. Such thinking defined their value as illuminating our earliest behaviors.

4.8.3 Ache Diets

Our concerns, however, are diet, nutrition, and health. American anthropologists Kim R. Hill (b. 1953) and Ana Magdalena Hurtado estimated that as hunter-gatherers, the Ache got 2,106 calories (78 percent) of the daily 2,700 from meat.[146] This percentage is within the range, cited earlier, of Plains hunters' two-thirds to 85 percent of calories from meat. Transition to reservations after 1963 did not drop Ache meat intake below about 55 percent of calories.[147] As hunters, they derived roughly nine-tenths of meat in order of importance from the nine-banded armadillo (*Dasypus novemcinctus*), capuchin monkey (*Cebus* species), white-lipped peccary (*Tayassu peccary*), paca (*Cuniculus paca*), coati (*Nasua nasua*), brocket deer (*Mazama* species), and collared peccary (*Pecari tajacu*).[148]

Another 8 percent of calories came from honey—a sweetener discussed in Chapters 2 and 11—and the rest from palm (*Acrocomia aculeata*) starch and hearts, insect larvae, and fruits. Hunters shared the kill with kin and nonrelatives. Honey was likewise shared widely, though the Ache tended to keep insect larvae within families. Hunting occupied men about seven hours per day.[149] Women gathered plants two hours daily, relocated camp another two hours, and cared for children. Ubiquitous insects, spiders, ticks, and snakes prevented mothers from leaving children alone. Ache hunter-gatherers seldom traded with sedentary neighbors for foods, notably cassava (*Manihot esculenta*), corn, and yams (*Dioscorea* species).

4.8.4 Ache Health

Ache suffered high mortality from violence, accidents, and pathogens and parasites from insects and arachnids.[150] Additionally, they had almost no possessions and lived in rudimentary circumstances by Western standards.[151] The rest of this section argues that they were vigorous despite hazards and penury. Because their healthiness cannot be ascribed to material conditions, diet must have played a large—and possibly primary—role. Being preponderant, meat must have been crucial.

Twenty-year-olds could expect another forty years if women and another thirty-four years if men.[152] The mean between these numbers, thirty-seven, was life expectancy at age twenty (e^{20}). Skeletons from nine locations in Ecuador indicate that native Ecuadorians did not match this longevity. Between roughly 3400 and 1500 BCE farmers in Real Alto did best, with an average e^{20} of twenty-one years.[153] The other sites lagged, with e^{20} in the low teens in two locations.

Critics might reject these comparisons because the Ecuadorians lived over 3,000 years before twentieth-century Ache. This criticism relies on the premise that longevity improved during these millennia. Even if an argument may be made to support this assumption—which Chapter 3 doubted—its application here would be inappropriate. Ache impoverishment and technological crudity imply that they enjoyed no material advantages over prehistoric Ecuadorians. Moreover, Real Alto's inhabitants farmed whereas the Ache hunted and gathered. The fact that demographers calculated greater longevity for farmers than hunter-gatherers implies that Real Alto's residents should have outlived the Ache, not the reverse.[154]

Enlarging this insight, hunter-gatherers died youngest compared with farmers and people who grew crops to supplement wild foods.[155] This trend should have condemned Ache to the earliest deaths. Longevity in defiance of this trend intimated a healthful diet, especially because they appear to have had no other advantages.

Moreover, in a study of five hunter-gatherers—Ache, Tanzania's Hadza, Colombia and Venezuela's Hiwi, Namibia, Angola, and Botswana's !Kung (sometimes designated Ju/'hoansi), and the Philippines' Agta—Ache had the least youth mortalities at about half the others' rates.[156]

Between ages fifteen and forty, Ache mortality was around 1 percent annually, roughly the rate of the others, hunter-gathers or sedentary, and only one-quarter !Kung mortality.[157] But meat, if the principal cause of Ache success, may not extend absolute lifespan. The largest number (mode) of Ache died at age seventy-one.[158] Both !Kung and Hadza lived longer as measured by mode whereas the Hiwi died sooner. Data were absent for the Agta.

Enlarging these comparisons, in 1993 about 12 percent of Ache newborns died in their first year, whereas first year mortality was around 10 percent in the United States in 1900.[159] This outcome is unsurprising because the average American was worth over $4,000 in 1900 in contrast to just $12 for an entire Ache family in 1993.[160] Despite the wealth chasm, just 2 percent separated Ache and Americans.

Interpretation of menarche (menses' onset) may be less straightforward than longevity. Age of first menstruation correlates with calories, protein, iron, zinc, calcium, and vitamin B_9.[161] Calories alone may be decisive such that junk, fatty, and sugary foods may hasten menarche. Although overweight and obesity may precipitate menarche, junk foods were unavailable to the Ache, leaving high-quality diet to initiate puberty. On average, Ache girls began menstruation at age thirteen.[162] By contrast, !Kung girls typically began at seventeen.

Diet, however, is not the lone variable because poverty correlates with early menarche.[163] Ache girls may have experienced their first period at thirteen because of penury, though this rationale does not explain late onset among !Kung. More generally, as a group, poor nations exhibited later onset than Ache. In 2001, Papua New Guinea, Haiti, Nepal, Algeria, Bangladesh, Cameroon, Kenya, Malaysia, Nicaragua, Nigeria, Senegal, Somalia, Tanzania, and Yemen averaged first menstruation at least a full year later than Ache girls.[164] If diseases delay menarche, then Ache, beset by pathogens and parasites, should have bloomed late.[165] Meat must have countered this effect.

Other signs of Ache health included rarity of heart disease, stroke, cancers, and obesity.[166] Blood pressure, cholesterol, and triglycerides—all discussed in Chapter 2—were low and dementia absent. These attributes are common among hunter-gatherers, who share lifestyle even when diets diverge. Lifestyle more than meat, therefore, may explain Ache freedom from Western maladies. Even so, meat must have enhanced vitality.

4.9 MEAT IN PERSPECTIVE

That Egyptian elites, Plains Indians, and Ache ate much meat invites comparison with Americans, who trailed only Luxembourgers as meat consumers, as noted. Ancient Egypt best approximated the United States given inactivity and derivation of meat from livestock rather than game. Both suffered heart disease, to which meat contributes, as mentioned. Yet Ache, who consumed 78 percent of calories from meat, exhibited neither coronary conditions nor other chronic maladies common in the United States and the developed world in general. Ache health implies that meat is far from being the chief impetus for these problems.

Instead, bad habits—for example sloth and smoking—may do more harm than inordinate meat intake. This conclusion undermines belief that "nutrition is the master key to human health."[167] In addition to diet and lifestyle, genes influence health, but because they are fixed at conception, contemplation of inadequacies benefits no one. Until gene therapy is possible, those who want vitality should emulate twenty-sixth U.S. President Theodore Roosevelt's (1858–1919) "strenuous life," referenced in Chapter 1.[168] To the extent that diet is the problem, meat appears to deserve little blame. Fault lies at least partly with developed countries' dietary superabundance. Unlike past peoples, we experience no seasonal shortages. Famines are now so unusual in Europe, Australia, and North America that historians—perhaps no longer mindful of food insecurity—omit them from textbooks. Supermarkets always have plenty, especially the dead animals that constitute our meals.

NOTES

1 Heather Brown, "Good Question: Why Isn't Seafood Considered Meat?" *CBS Minnesota*, March 13, 2014, accessed January 24, 2019, https://minnesota.cbslocal.com/2014/03/13/good-question-why-isnt-seafood-considered-meat.
2 "Meat, Poultry, Fish, and Shellfish CIDs," *USDA*, accessed January 24, 2019, https://www.ams.usda.gov/grades-standards/cid/meat.
3 Xue Zhang, Casey M. Owens, and M. Wes Schilling, "Meat: The Edible Flesh from Mammals Only or Does It Include Poultry, Fish, and Seafood?" *Animal Frontiers* 7, no. 4 (October 1, 2017): 12.
4 "Meat Science," *Elsevier*, 2019, accessed January 24, 2019, https://www.journals.elsevier.com/meat-science.
5 Paul Clayton and Judith Rowbotham, "How the Mid-Victorians Worked, Ate and Died," *International Journal of Environmental Research and Public Health* 6, no. 3 (March 2009): 1235–1253, https://www.ncbi.nlm.nih.gov/pmc/articles/PMC2672390.
6 Stanley Ulijaszek, Neil Mann, and Sarah Elton, *Evolving Human Nutrition: Implications for Public Health* (Cambridge, UK and New York: Cambridge University Press, 2012), 219–222.
7 Peter Garnsey, *Food and Society in Classical Antiquity* (Cambridge, UK: Cambridge University Press, 1999), 113.
8 Nigel Barber, "Do Humans Need Meat?" *Psychology Today*, October 12, 2016, accessed January 24, 2019, https://www.psychologytoday.com/us/blog/the-human-beast/201610/do-humans-need-meat.
9 Alvin Silverstein and Virginia Silverstein, *Beans: All about Them* (Englewood Cliffs, NJ: Prentice-Hall, 1975), 5–6.
10 Raymond A. Dart, "The Predatory Transition from Ape to Man," *International Anthropological and Linguistic Review* 1, no. 4 (1953), http://www.users.miamioh.edu/erlichrd/350website/classrel/dart.html.
11 Ibid.
12 Robert Ardrey, *African Genesis: A Personal Investigation into the Animal Origins and Nature of Man* (New York: Atheneum, 1970), 1.
13 Henry T. Bunn, "Meat Made Us Human," in *Evolution of the Human Diet: The Known, the Unknown, and the Unknowable*, ed. Peter S. Ungar (Oxford and New York: Oxford University Press, 2007), 191.
14 Ibid., 191–192.
15 Ibid., 198.
16 Clark Spencer Larsen, "Dietary Reconstruction and Nutritional Assessment of Past Peoples: The Bioanthropological Record," in *The Cambridge World History of Food*, vol. 1, ed. Kenneth F. Kiple and Kriemhild Conee Ornelas (Cambridge, UK: Cambridge University Press, 2000), 14.
17 F. Clark Howell, *Early Man* (New York: Tim-Life Books, 1965), 98–99.
18 Ibid., 132.
19 Robert C. Atkins, *Dr. Atkins' Diet Revolution: The High Calorie Way to Stay Thin Forever* (New York: David McKay, 1972), 55.
20 Steven L. Kuhn and Mary C. Stiner, "The Antiquity of Hunter-Gatherers," in *Hunter-Gatherers: An Interdisciplinary Perspective*, ed. Catherine Panter-Brick, Robert H. Layton, and Peter Rowley-Conwy (Cambridge, UK and New York: Cambridge University Press, 2001), 101–103.
21 John S. Compton, *Human Origins: How Diet, Climate and Landscape Shaped Us* (Cape Town, South Africa: Earthspun Books, 2016), 269.
22 Mark Nathan Cohen, *The Food Crisis in Prehistory: Overpopulation and the Origins of Agriculture* (New Haven, CT: Yale University Press, 1977), 90–97.
23 Larsen, 15.
24 Ulijaszek, Mann, and Elton, 129.
25 J. Allen Barksdale, "American Bison," in *The Cambridge World History of Food*, vol. 1, ed. Kenneth F. Kiple and Kriemhild Conee Ornelas (Cambridge, UK: Cambridge University Press, 2000), 452.
26 Alan Brinkley, *American History: A Survey*, vol. 2, *Since 1865*, 9th ed. (New York: McGraw-Hill, 1995), 462.
27 "Live Stock, 1920," in *Yearbook of Agriculture, 1920* (Washington, DC: GPO, 1921), 701.
28 "Miscellaneous Agricultural Statistics," in *Yearbook of Agriculture, 1920* (Washington, DC: GPO, 1921), 826.
29 Miguel Requena, "Socialism, Roast Beef, and Apple Pie: Werner Sombart on Socialism a Hundred Years Later," *Sociologica* 2–3 (May–December 2009): 7, http://citeseerx.ist.psu.edu/viewdoc/download?doi=10.1.1.882.2203&rep=rep1&type=pdf.

30 Nick Hines, "Americans Eat Enough Burgers to Circle the Earth 32 Times Every Year," Vinepair, April 12, 2017, accessed January 25, 2019, https://vinepair.com/cocktail-chatter/how-many-burgers-americans-eat-per-year.

31 "Beef. It's What's for Dinner," Cattlemen's Beef Board and National Cattlemen's Beef Association, 2019, accessed January 25, 2019, https://www.beefitswhatsfordinner.com.

32 "Global Meat Production and Consumption Continue to Rise," *Worldwatch Institute*, last modified January 26, 2019, accessed January 26, 2019, http://www.worldwatch.org/global-meat-production-and-consumption-continue-rise.

33 J. Samuel Godber, "Nutritional Value of Muscle Foods," in *Muscle Foods: Meat, Poultry, and Seafood Technology*, ed. Donald M. Kinsman, Anthony W. Kotula, and Burdette C. Breidenstein (New York and London: Chapman and Hall, 1994), 438, 441, 445–446.

34 Atli Arnarson, "Pork 101: Nutrition Facts and Health Effects," Healthline, April 1, 2015, accessed January 26, 2019, https://www.healthline.com/nutrition/foods/pork.

35 Atli Arnarson, "Beef 101: Nutrition Facts and Health Effects," *Healthline*, March 30, 2015, accessed January 26, 2019, https://www.healthline.com/nutrition/foods/beef; Godber, 438, 441, 445–446.

36 "Mutton, Roasted (Navajo), Cooked," NutritonValue.org, 2019, accessed January 26, 2019, https://www.nutritionvalue.org/Mutton%2C_roasted_%28Navajo%29%2C_cooked_nutritional_value.html.

37 Godber, 438, 441, 445–446; W. Stephen Damron, *Introduction to Animal Science: Global Biological, Social, and Industry Perspectives*, 3d ed. (Upper Saddle River, NJ and Columbus, OH: Pearson/Prentice Hall, 2006), 335, 458, 501; "Bison, Ground, Grass-Fed, Raw," *USDA FoodData Central*, April 1, 2019, accessed January 21, 2020, https://fdc.nal.usda.gov/fdc-app.html#/food-details/175293/nutrients; "Venison/Deer, NFS," *USDA FoodData Central*, April 1, 2019, accessed January 21, 2020, https://fdc.nal.usda.gov/fdc-app.html#/food-details/337054/nutrients; "Amount of Vitamin D in Beef," *Diet and Fitness Today*, 2005–2020, accessed January 21, 2020, http://www.dietandfitnesstoday.com/vitamin-d-in-beef.php; "Amount of Vitamin D in Ground Pork," *Diet and Fitness Today*, 2005–2020, accessed January 21, 2020, http://www.dietandfitnesstoday.com/vitamin-d-in-ground-pork.php; "Amount of Manganese in Bison," *Diet and Fitness Today*, 2005–2020, accessed January 21, 2020, http://www.dietandfitnesstoday.com/manganese-in-bison.php; "Manganese in Deer Calculator," *Diet and Fitness Today*, 2005–2020, accessed January 21, 2020, http://www.dietandfitnesstoday.com/manganese-in-deer.php; Daisy Whitbread, "Top 10 Foods Highest in Selenium," *My Food Data*, last modified November 10, 2019, accessed January 21, 2020, https://www.myfooddata.com/articles/foods-high-in-selenium.php; "Game Meat, Goat, Cooked, Roasted," *Self Nutrition Data*, 2018, accessed January 21, 2020, https://nutritiondata.self.com/facts/lamb-veal-and-game-products/4638/2; "Game Meat, Raw, Ground, Bison," *Nutrition Value*, 2020, accessed January 21, 2020, https://www.nutritionvalue.org/Game_meat_%2C_raw%2C_ground%2C_bison_nutritional_value.html; "Game Meat, Raw, Ground, Deer," *Nutrition Value*, 2020, accessed January 21, 2020, https://www.nutritionvalue.org/Game_meat%2C_raw%2C_ground%2C_deer_nutritional_value.html; "Beef, Raw, 97% Lean Meat/3% Fat, Ground," *Nutrition Value*, 2020, accessed January 21, 2020, https://www.nutritionvalue.org/Beef%2C_raw%2C_97%25_lean_meat_%252F_3%25_fat%2C_ground_nutritional_value.html; "Goat Meat," *Calorie Slism*, accessed January 21, 2020, https://slism.com/calorie/111204; "Mutton, Cooked, Roasted (Navajo)," *USDA FoodData Central*, April 1, 2019, accessed January 21, 2020, https://fdc.nal.usda.gov/fdc-app.html#/food-details/167634/nutrients.

38 Eliza Barclay, "A Nation of Meat Eaters: See How It All Adds Up," *NPR*, June 27, 2012, accessed January 26, 2019, https://www.npr.org/sections/thesalt/2012/06/27/155527365/visualizing-a-nation-of-meat-eaters.

39 "The World: Life Expectancy (2018)," *geoba.se*, 2019, accessed January 26, 2019, http://www.geoba.se/population.php?pc=world&type=015&year=2018&st=country&asde=&page=1.

40 William Davis, *Wheat Belly: Lose the Wheat, Lose the Weight, and Find Your Path Back to Health* (Emmaus, PA: Rodale, 2011), x; David Perlmutter, *Grain Brain: The Surprising Truth about Wheat, Carbs, and Sugar—Your Brain's Silent Killers*, rev. ed. (New York: Little, Brown Spark, 2018), 12.

41 Steven R. Gundry, *The Plant Paradox: The Hidden Dangers in "Healthy" Foods that Cause Disease and Weight Gain* (New York: Harper Wave, 2017), 157–158; T. Colin Campbell and Thomas Campbell, "'The Plant Paradox' by Steven Gundry MD—A Commentary," *Center for Nutrition Studies*, August 23, 2017, accessed January 26, 2019, https://nutritionstudies.org/the-plant-paradox-by-steven-grundy-md-commentary.

42 Kadya Araki, "Why All Humans Need to Eat Meat for Health," accessed January 26, 2019, https://breakingmuscle.com/healthy-eating/why-all-humans-need-to-eat-meat-for-health.

43 Stephen Le, *100 Million Years of Food: What Our Ancestors Ate and Why It Matters Today* (New York: Picador, 2016), 43.

44 Cheryl L. Rock and Wendy Demark-Wahnefried, "Nutrition and Breast Cancer," in *Nutrition in the Prevention and Treatment of Disease*, ed. Ann M. Coulston, Cheryl L. Rock, and Elaine R. Monsen (San Diego: Academic Press, 2001), 343; Martha L. Slattery and Bette J. Caan, "Nutrition and Colon Cancer," in *Nutrition in the Prevention and Treatment of Disease*, ed. Ann M. Coulston, Cheryl L. Rock, and Elaine R. Monsen (San Diego: Academic Press, 2001), 359–360, 365; Susan T. Mayne, "Nutrition and Lung Cancer," in *Nutrition in the Prevention and Treatment of Disease*, ed. Ann M. Coulston, Cheryl L. Rock, and Elaine R. Monsen (San Diego: Academic Press, 2001), 392–393; Laurence N. Kolonel, "Nutrition and Prostate Cancer," in *Nutrition in the Prevention and Treatment of Disease*, ed. Ann M. Coulston, Cheryl L. Rock, and Elaine R. Monsen (San Diego: Academic Press, 2001), 375.

45 Thomas S. Kuhn, *The Structure of Scientific Revolutions*, 4th ed. (Chicago and London: University of Chicago Press, 2012), 149–151.

46 "Kadya Araki," accessed January 26, 2019, https://breakingmuscle.com/coaches/kadya-araki.

47 John Wilkins, "Medical Literature, Diet, and Health," in *A Companion to Food in the Ancient World*, ed. John Wilkins and Robin Nadeau (Malden, MA: Wiley Blackwell, 2015), 61.

48 Ibid., 59.

49 J. Gwyn Griffiths, "Hecataeus and Herodotus on 'a Gift of the River'," *Journal of Near Eastern Studies* 25, no. 1 (January 1966): 57.

50 Beatrix Midant-Reynes, *The Prehistory of Egypt: From the First Egyptians to the First Pharaohs*, trans. Ian Shaw (Oxford, UK and Malden, MA: Blackwell, 2000), 25.

51 Chris Stringer and Peter Andrews, *The Complete World of Human Evolution* (London: Thames and Hudson, 2005), 161.

52 Naomi F. Miller and Wilma Wetterstrom, "The Beginnings of Agriculture," in *The Cambridge World History of Food*, vol. 2, ed. Kenneth F. Kiple and Kriemhild Conee Ornelas (Cambridge, UK: Cambridge University Press, 2000), 1129–1130.

53 Lionel Casson, *Everyday Life in Ancient Egypt*, rev. ed. (Baltimore, MD and London: Johns Hopkins University Press, 2001), 39.

54 Lisa Sabbahy, "A Decade of Advances in the Paleopathology of the Ancient Egyptians," in *Egyptian Bioarchaeology: Humans, Animals, and the Environment*, ed. Salima Ikram, Jessica Kaiser, and Roxie Walker (Leiden: Sidestone Press, 2015), 116; Pierre Tallet, "Food in Ancient Egypt," in *A Companion to Food in the Ancient World*, ed. John Wilkins and Robin Nadeau (Chichester, UK: Wiley Blackwell, 2015), 321.

55 Tallet, 321.

56 Alexandra Touzeau, Romain Amiot, Janne Blichert-Toft, Jean-Pierre Flandrois, Francois Fourel, Vincent Grossi, Francois Martineau, Pascale Richardin, and Christoph Lecuyer, "Diet of Ancient Egyptians Inferred from Stable Isotope Systematics," *Journal of Archaeological Science* 46 (June 2014): 117; Alexander Hellemans, "What Did Ancient Egyptians Really Eat?" *Inside Science*, May 8, 2014, accessed January 31, 2019, https://www.insidescience.org/news/what-did-ancient-egyptians-really-eat.

57 Tim Sandle, "Pharaohs and Mummies: Diseases of Ancient Egypt and Modern Approaches," *Journal of Infectious Diseases and Preventive Medicine* 1, no. 4 (2013), https://www.omicsonline.org/open-access/pharaohs-and-mummies-diseases-of-ancient-egypt-and-modern-approaches-2329-8731.1000e110.php?aid=20477.

58 "Egyptian Mummies," *Smithsonian Institution*, accessed January 31, 2019, www.si.edu/spotlight/ancient-egypt/mummies.

59 Touzeau, et al., 117.

60 Ibid., 121.

61 "Pork," USDA FoodData Central, April 1, 2019, accessed October 24, 2019, https://fdc.nal.usda.gov/fdc-app.html#/food-details/410519/nutrients; "Cowpeas (Blackeyes), Immature Seeds, Raw," *USDA FoodData Central*, April 1, 2019, accessed October 24, 2019, https://fdc.nal.usda.gov/fdc-app.html#/food-details/169220/nutrients.

62 Touzeau, et al., 121.

63 Ibid., 122.

64 R. C. Thompson, A. H. Allam, G. P. Lombardi, L. S. Wann, M. L. Sutherland, J. D. Sutherland, M. A. Soliman, B. Frohlich, D. T. Mininberg, J. M. Monge, C. M. Vallodolid, S. L. Cox, G. Abd el-Maksoud, I. Badr, M. I. Miyamoto, A. el-Halim Nur el-Din, J. Narula, C. E. Finch, and G. S. Thomas, "Atherosclerosis across 4000 Years of Human History: The Horus Study of Four Ancient Populations," *Lancet* 381 (April 6, 2013), https://www.ncbi.nlm.nih.gov/pubmed/23489753.

65 "New Link between Heart Disease and Red Meat: New Understanding of Cardiovascular Health Benefits of Vegan, Vegetarian Diets," *Science Daily*, April 7, 2013, accessed January 31, 2019, https://www.sciencedaily.com/releases/2013/04/130407133320.htm.
66 Bob Brier and Hoyt Hobbs, *Ancient Egypt: Everyday Life in the Land of the Nile* (New York: Sterling, 2009), 119.
67 Touzeau, et al., 120.
68 Garnsey, 14.
69 Gen. 47:19–21 (New American Bible).
70 Num. 11:5 (New American Bible).
71 Pliny, *Natural History*, trans. H. Rackman, vol. 5 (Cambridge, MA: Harvard University Press, 1949), 213.
72 James F. Romano, *Daily Life of the Ancient Egyptians* (Pittsburgh: Carnegie Museum of Natural History, 1990), 35; Gen. 41:1–7.
73 The Editors, "Introduction," in *The Cambridge World History of Food*, vol. 1, ed. Kenneth F. Kiple and Kriemhild Conee Ornelas (Cambridge, UK: Cambridge University Press, 2000), 2.
74 Barry Kemp, Anna Stevens, Gretchen R. Dobbs, Melissa Zabecki, and Jerome C. Rose, "Life, Death and beyond in Akhenaten's Egypt: Excavating the South Tombs Cemetery at Amarna," *Antiquity* 87, no. 335 (March 1, 2013): 67.
75 Jerome C. Rose and Melissa Zabecki, "The Commoners of Tell el-Amarna," in *Beyond the Horizon: Studies in Egyptian Art, Archaeology and History in Honour of Barry J. Kemp*, ed. Salima Ikram and Aidan Dodson, vol. 2 (Cairo: Supreme Council of Antiquities, 2009), 408.
76 Kemp, Stevens, Dobbs, Zabecki, and Rose, 67.
77 Ibid., 68.
78 Ibid., 71–72.
79 Ibid., 72.
80 "Peas, Green, Raw," *USDA FoodData Central*, April 1, 2019, accessed February 8, 2020, https://fdc.nal.usda.gov/fdc-app.html#/food-details/170419/nutrients; Anitra C. Carr and Balz Frei, "Toward a New Recommended Dietary Allowance for Vitamin C Based on Antioxidant and Health Effects in Humans," *The American Journal of Clinical Nutrition* 69, no. 6 (June 1, 1999): 1086.
81 Kemp, Stevens, Dobbs, Zabecki, and Rose, 73.
82 Ibid., 74.
83 Delisa L. Phillips, Jerome C. Rose, and Willem M. van Haarlem, "Bioarchaeology of Tell Ibrahim Awad," *Egypt and the Levant* 19 (December 2009): 157, 166.
84 Ibid., 166.
85 Ibid., 164.
86 Ibid., 164–165.
87 Sabbahy, 116.
88 Colleen Story, Kristeen Cherney, and Rachel Nall, "The History of Heart Disease," *Healthline*, July 9, 2018, accessed February 5, 2019, https://www.healthline.com/health/heart-disease/history.
89 Ibid.; Renate Germer, *Mummies: Life after Death in Ancient Egypt* (Munich and New York: Prestel, 1997), 127.
90 Sabbahy, 117.
91 Meredith F. Small, "Mummy Reveals Egyptian Queen Was Fat, Balding and Bearded," *Live Science*, July 6, 2007, accessed February 5, 2019, https://www.livescience.com/7336-mummy-reveals-egyptian-queen-fat-balding-bearded.html.
92 James Owen, "Egyptian Princess Mummy Had Oldest Known Heart Disease," *National Geographic News*, April15,2011,accessedFebruary5,2019,https://news.nationalgeographic.com/news/2011/04/110415-ancient-egypt-mummies-princess-heart-disease-health-science.
93 Phillips, Rose, and Haarlem, 161, 163.
94 Ann E. M. Liljas, "Old Age in Ancient Egypt," March 2, 2015, accessed January 18, 2019, https://blogs.ucl.ac.uk/researchers-in-museums/2015/03/02/old-age-in-ancient-egypt.
95 Walter Scheidel, *Death on the Nile: Disease and the Demography of Roman Egypt* (Leiden: Brill, 2001), 30.
96 Ibid., 31.
97 Ibid., 139.
98 Germer, 128.
99 Guillaume Herzberg and Raoul Perrot, "Paleopathologie de 31 Cranes Egyptiens Momifies du Museum d' Histoire Naturelle de Lyon," *Paleobios* 1, no. 1–2 (1983): 105.

100 John P. McKay, Bennett D. Hill, John Buckler, Clare Haru Crowston, Merry E. Wiesner-Hanks, and Joe Perry, *Understanding Western Society: A Brief History* (Boston, MA and New York: Bedford/St. Martin's, 2012), 212; Edward S. Deevey Jr., "The Human Population," *Scientific American* (September 1, 1960): 200.
101 Scheidel, 59–95; Germer, 127–128.
102 Stringer and Andrews, 142.
103 Barksdale, 450; Waverley Root and Richard de Rochemont, *Eating in America: A History* (Hopewell, NJ: Ecco Press, 1995), 72.
104 Peter Farb, *Ecology* (New York: Time, 1963), 159; Root and Rochemont, 201.
105 Barksdale, 450.
106 R. F. Diffendal Jr., *Great Plains Geology* (Lincoln and London: University of Nebraska Press, 2017), xix-xx.
107 Ibid., 1.
108 Joseph M. Prince and Richard H. Steckel, *Tallest in the World: Native Americans of the Great Plains in the Nineteenth Century* (Cambridge, MA: National Bureau of Economic Research, 1998), 5.
109 Ibid.
110 Joseph F. Powell, *The First Americans: Race, Evolution, and the Origin of Native Americans* (Cambridge, UK: Cambridge University Press, 2005), 137, 139, 148.
111 Jack L. Hofman and Russell W. Graham, "The Paleo-Indian Cultures of the Great Plains," in *Archaeology on the Great Plains*, ed. W. Raymond Wood (Lawrence: University Press of Kansas, 1998), 93.
112 Barksdale, 450–451.
113 "Ponca History," *Ponca Tribe of Indians of Oklahoma*, 2018, accessed February 7, 2019, http://ponca.com/ponca-history.
114 David J. Wishart, *An Unspeakable Sadness: The Dispossession of the Nebraska Indians* (Lincoln: University of Nebraska Press, 1994), 230.
115 S. Ryan Johansson and Douglas Owsley, "Welfare History on the Great Plains: Mortality and Skeletal Health, 1650 to 1900," in *The Backbone of History: Health and Nutrition in the Western Hemisphere* (Cambridge, UK: Cambridge University Press, 2002), 537.
116 Ibid., 535–536, 540.
117 Ibid., 539, 550.
118 Robert H. Shmerling, "Fertility and Diet: Is There a Connection?" *Harvard Health Publishing*, May 31, 2018, accessed February 7, 2019, https://www.health.harvard.edu/blog/fertility-and-diet-is-there-a-connection-2018053113949.
119 Johansson and Owsley, 537.
120 Ibid., 535.
121 Ibid., 550.
122 Ibid.
123 Prince and Steckel, 7.
124 Ibid., 8–9.
125 Johansson and Owsley, 543.
126 "Bison vs. Beef—Which Red Meat Reigns Supreme?" *Onnit Labs*, August 24, 2016, accessed February 7, 2019, www.onnit.com/academy/bison-vs-beef.
127 Ted Slanker, "Omega-3 Fatty Acids," *Slanker Grass-Fed Meat*, 2000–2019, accessed February 7, 2019, https://www.texasgrassfedbeef.com/grass-fed-meat-education/omega-3-fatty-acids.
128 Cynthia A. Daley, Amber Abbott, Patrick S. Doyle, Glenn A. Nader, and Stephanie Larson, "A Review of Fatty Acid Profiles and Antioxidant Content in Grass-Fed and Grain-Fed Beef," *Nutrition Journal* 9 (March 10, 2010), https://www.ncbi.nlm.nih.gov/pmc/articles/PMC2846864.
129 Artemis P. Simopoulos, "An Increase in the Omega-6/Omega-3 Fatty Acid Ratio Increases the Risk for Obesity," *Nutrients* 8, no. 3 (March 2016): 128, https://www.ncbi.nlm.nih.gov/pmc/articles/PMC4808858.
130 Prince and Steckel, 12.
131 Johansson and Owsley, 547.
132 Prince and Steckel, 2–3.
133 Ibid., 29.
134 Tacitus, *The Germania*, in *The Agricola and The Germania*, trans. H. Mattingly and S. A. Handford (London: Penguin Books, 1970), 118; Nikola C. G. Kopke, "Regional Differences and Temporal Development of Nutritional Status in Europe from the 8th Century B.C. until the 18th Century A.D." (PhD diss., Universitat Tubingen, 2008), 139.

135 Sitta von Reden, "Classical Greece: Consumption," in *The Cambridge Economic History of the Greco-Roman World*, ed. Walter Scheidel, Ian Morris, and Richard P. Saller (Cambridge, UK: Cambridge University Press, 2007), 388; Willem M. Jongman, "The Early Roman Empire: Consumption," in *The Cambridge Economic History of the Greco-Roman World*, ed. Walter Scheidel, Ian Morris, and Richard P. Saller (Cambridge, UK: Cambridge University Press, 2007), 607.
136 Jongman, 607.
137 "Anthropometric Reference Data for Children and Adults: United States, 2007–2012," *Vital and Health Statistics*, October 2012, accessed February 8, 2019, https://www.cdc.gov/nchs/data/series/sr_11/sr11_252.pdf; Dani Arbuckle, "What Is the Average Adult Male Height and Weight?" *Livestrong*, 2019, accessed February 8, 2019, https://www.livestrong.com/article/289265-what-is-the-average-adult-male-height.
138 Vincent Iannelli, "What Is the Average Height for an Adult Woman?" *Verywellfit.com*, last modified October 25, 2018, accessed February 8, 2019, https://www.verywellfit.com/average-height-for-a-woman-statistics-2632136.
139 Prince and Steckel, 10.
140 Ibid., 9.
141 Robert William Fogel, "Nutrition and the Decline in Mortality Since 1700: Some Preliminary Findings," in *Long-Term Factors in American Economic Growth*, ed. Stanley L. Engerman and Robert E. Gallman (Chicago and London: University of Chicago Press, 1986), 466.
142 Robert William Fogel, *The Escape from Hunger and Premature Death, 1700–2100: Europe, America, and the Third World* (Cambridge, UK: Cambridge University Press, 2004), 17–19.
143 Ibid., 439.
144 "Ancient Humans Arrived in South America in Multiple Waves," *Science Daily*, February 24, 2017, accessed February 9, 2019, https://www.sciencedaily.com/releases/2017/02/170224121748.htm.
145 Lizzie Wade, "Traces of Some of South America's Earliest People Found under Ancient Dirt Pyramid," *ScienceMag*, American Association for the Advancement of Science, May 24, 2017, accessed February 9, 2019, https://www.sciencemag.org/news/2017/05/traces-some-south-america-s-earliest-people-found-under-ancient-dirt-pyramid?r3f_986=https://www.google.com.
146 Kim Hill and A. Magdalena Hurtado, "The Ache of Paraguay," in *The Cambridge Encyclopedia of Hunters and Gatherers*, ed. Richard B. Lee and Richard Daly (Cambridge, UK: Cambridge University Press, 2002), 93.
147 "Ache," *Cengage*, last modified January 13, 2020, accessed February 10, 2020, https://www.encyclopedia.com/places/latin-america-and-caribbean/south-american-political-geography/ache.
148 Hill and Hurtado, "Ache of Paraguay," 93.
149 Ibid.
150 Kim Hill and A. Magdalena Hurtado, *Ache Life History: The Ecology and Demography of a Foraging People* (New York: Aldine, 1996), 152–154.
151 Hill and Hurtado, "Ache of Paraguay," 95.
152 Hill and Hurtado, *Ache Life History*, 194.
153 Douglas H. Ubelaker and Linda A. Newson, "Patterns of Health and Nutrition in Prehistoric and Historic Ecuador," in *The Backbone of History: Health and Nutrition in the Western Hemisphere*, ed. Richard H. Steckel and Jerome C. Rose (Cambridge, UK: Cambridge University Press, 2002), 353, 355.
154 Michael Gurven and Hillard Kaplan, "Longevity among Hunter-Gatherers: A Cross Cultural Examination," *Population and Development Review* 33, no. 2 (June 2007): 326.
155 Ibid.
156 Ibid.
157 Gurven and Kaplan, 332–333, 348.
158 Ibid., 335.
159 Hill and Hurtado, *Ache Life History*, 186; "Achievements in Public Health, 1900–1999: Healthier Mothers and Babies," *CDC*, October 1, 1999, accessed February 10, 2019, https://www.cdc.gov/mmwr/preview/mmwrhtml/mm4838a2.htm.
160 "Economy > GDP Per Capita in 1900: Countries Compared," *Nation Master*, 2003–2019, accessed February 10, 2019, https://www.nationmaster.com/country-info/stats/Economy/GDP-per-capita-in-1900; Hill and Hurtado, "Ache of Paraguay," 95.
161 Ashraf Soliman, Vincenzo De Sanctis, and Rania Elalaily, "Nutrition and Pubertal Development," *Indian Journal of Endocrinology and Metabolism* 18 (November 2014), https://www.ncbi.nlm.nih.gov/pmc/articles/PMC4266867.

162 Hill and Hurtado, *Ache Life History*, 362.
163 "Poorer Girls over Twice as Likely to Start Period by 11," *Economic and Social Research Council*, October 12, 2016, accessed February 10, 2019, https://esrc.ukri.org/news-events-and-publications/news/news-items/poorer-girls-over-twice-as-likely-to-start-period-by-11.
164 Frederic Thomas, Francois Renaud, Eric Benefice, Thierry de Meeus, and Jean-Francois Guegan, "International Variability of Ages at Menarche and Menopause: Patterns and Main Determinants," *Human Biology* 73, no. 2 (April 2001): 274–276.
165 Kathleen O'Grady, "Early Puberty for Girls. The New 'Normal' and Why We Need to Be Concerned," *Canadian Women's Health Network*, Fall-Winter 2008–2009, accessed February 10, 2019, www.cwhn.ca/en/node/39365.
166 Hill and Hurtado, *Ache Life History*, 161.
167 T. Colin Cadvmpbell, *Whole: Rethinking the Science of Nutrition* (Dallas, TX: BenBella Books, 2013), xii.
168 Theodore Roosevelt, "The Strenuous Life," Speech before the Hamilton Club, April 10, 1899, accessed February 10, 2019, https://en.wikisource.org/wiki/The_Strenuous_Life.

5 Fish and Shellfish

5.1 ANTIQUITY OF FISH

Of the animals that humans eat, fish are among the oldest. The waters they inhabit formed on Earth perhaps 4 billion years ago.[1] Life originated during the next 700 million years in the ocean, the first creatures being microbes.[2] The first vertebrates, fish arose roughly 520 million years ago during the Cambrian Period (540–485 million years ago).[3] The ocean harbored early species, which thereafter colonized freshwater lakes and rivers. These pioneers resembled worms more than fish, though scales and fins were early adaptations to aquatic environments. During the Devonian Period (405–345 million years ago), known as the age of fishes, species began to diversify.[4] Their numbers increased during the Jurassic (180–135 million years ago) and Cretaceous (135–165 million years ago) Periods and today constitute over 31,000 species.[5]

Water covers roughly two-thirds of Earth, most of the unpolluted portions being suitable for fish.[6] Although scientists once thought the deepest ocean inhospitable, telegraph cables' deposition and retraction on the ocean floor in the nineteenth century revealed fish at the bottom. Even the deepest part—in the Pacific Ocean's Mariana Trench—which plummets to 11,030 meters (12,062.6 yards or 36,187.7 feet), has fish.[7] Most occupy continental shelves, the portions of continents covered by ocean. They are comparatively shallow at under 200 meters (218.7 yards or 656.2 feet). Beyond them, depths plunge.

Apart from the ocean, fish inhabit lakes and rivers. For example, Lake Erie has about half the fish despite holding just 2 percent of their waters.[8] Dubbed Florida's inland sea, Lake Okeechobee bills itself "the crappie capital of the world" and "the best panfish lake in the world."[9] Tanzania's Lake Malawi has chambo (*Oreochromis* species), sardine (*Engraulicypris sardella*), and kampango catfish (*Bagrus meridionalis*). Siberia's Lake Baikal supports sculpins (species in the superfamily Cottoidea), golomyankas (*Comephorus baicalensis* and *Comephorus dybowskii*), omul (*Coregonus migratorius*), Baikal whitefish (*Coregonus baicalensis*), white grayling (*Thymallus brevipinnis*),

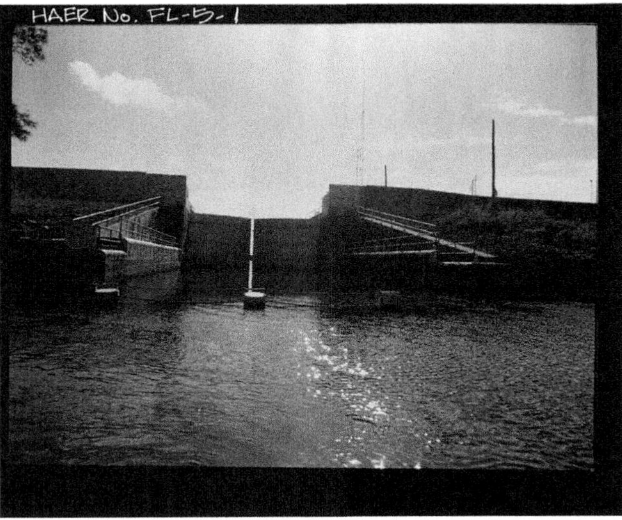

FIGURE 5.1 Lake Okeechobee. (Photo courtesy of Library of Congress. https://www.loc.gov/pictures/item/fl0306.photos.184074p/.)

black grayling (*Thymallus baicalensis*), and sturgeon (*Acipenser baerii baicalensis*). Nile perch (*Lates niloticus*), mentioned last chapter, inhabit northeastern Africa's Nile River. The Nile also has bolti (*Oreochromis niloticus*), barbel (Schilbe mystus), elephant-snout fish (*Gnathonemus petersii*), African lungfish and mudfish (*Protopterus* species), catfish (species in the suborder Siluroidea), and tigerfish (*Hydrocynus* species).

5.2 FISH CONSUMPTION AMONG PRIMATES AND EARLY HUMANS

5.2.1 Pre-Human Fish Consumption

Many primates, including macaques (*Macaca* species), baboons (*Papio* species), chimpanzees (*Pan troglodytes*), bonobos (*Pan paniscus*), and orangutans (*Pongo pygmaeus*, *P. abelii*, and *P. tapanuliensis*), infrequently eat fish. Canadian psychologist Anne E. Russon suspected that humanity's ancestors resembled orangutans in using sticks to catch fish.[10] Our predecessors—for example, *Australopithecus* and *Paranthropus* (see Chapter 3)—were probably omnivores and might have eaten fish. The earliest fish bones—from catfish—in middens are nearly 2 million years old.[11]

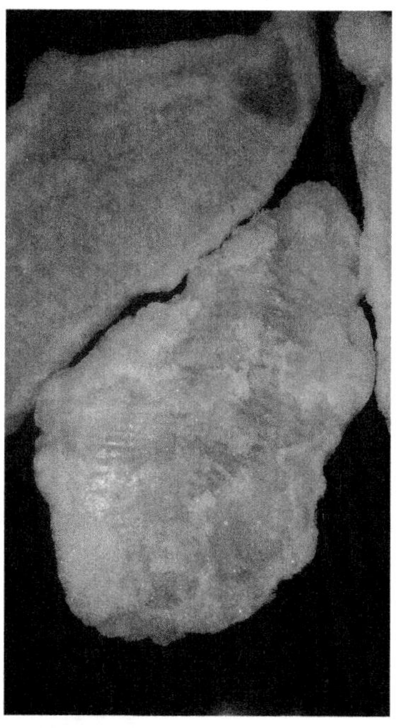

FIGURE 5.2 Catfish. (Photo from author.)

5.2.2 Role of Fish in Human Evolution

Anthropologists associate them with our genus, *Homo*, whose evolution Chapter 3 recounted. If these bones marked fishing's origin, they indicate that our ancestors ate fish as the brain expanded.[12] Fish must therefore have provided nutrients and calories for enlargement, an argument Chapter 4 summarized in favor of meat. Fish fatty acids may have spurred brain and central nervous system (CNS) development. Chapter 2 mentioned fatty acids' role in forming neural membranes. This rationale accentuates fish's significance to human evolution.

Emphasizing fish's dietary antiquity, British zoologist Francis Downes Ommanney (1903–1980) stated that fishing and hunting originated together, occupying humanity "a good long time."[13]

This opinion neglects fishing's primacy if British-American anthropologist Brian Murray Fagan (b. 1936) is correct that the activity began around 2 million years ago and if American anthropologist Clark Spencer Larsen (b. 1952)—mentioned throughout this book—is right that hunting is about 700,000 years old.[14] People depended on fish and shellfish as especially concentrated protein, a nutrient indispensable to growing global populations, Ommanney believed.[15]

A variant of the Paleo diet favors fish. American nutritionist and exercise physiologist Loren Cordain (b. 1950) asserted that for some 2.5 million years lean animals fed hunter-gatherers.[16] During this duration, evolution shaped humans to eat animals with little saturated fat. What fats they had were omega 3, a type of fatty acid that Chapter 2 defined. In other words, evolution fashioned us to consume seafood and game. Rather than being substandard, fish provided fatty acids, protein, vitamins, and minerals suited to our biology and lifeways. People suffered obesity, type 2 diabetes, and heart disease only upon eschewing fish and other sources of lean protein. This reasoning makes sense, though these maladies also stem from inactivity, this book argues. Chapters 1 and 3 discussed the use of hunter-gatherers as models for us.

Another thesis, however, deemphasizes fish. Chapter 4 reprised the argument that our ancestors prioritized meat. They turned to fish and other items only when the hunt did not feed everyone.[17] Far from being desirable, fish indicated privation. Anthropologists in this camp, rejecting the idea that fishing and hunting are equally old or that fishing predated hunting, believe that inclusion of fish and shellfish in diets came late in human evolution. Even if humankind sampled them early, they were uncommon as food until modern peoples arose roughly 150,000 years ago.

Even if it occupied the second tier, as some anthropologists believe, seafood might have given modern peoples an advantage over *Homo neanderthalensis* (Neanderthals or Neandertals), whose evolution Chapter 3 discussed. A 2009 study of carbon and nitrogen isotopes—Chapter 1 defined an isotope—suggested that Neanderthals in what are today France, Germany, Belgium, and Croatia ate large mammals rather than fish but that modern humans had a broader diet that included fish and shellfish.[18] Such breadth may have helped us survive scarcity better than Neanderthals.

American anthropologist Bruce Hardy and French anthropologist Marie-Helene Moncel disagreed. Their 2011 examination of Payre in France's Rhone Valley yielded stone tools whose wear indicated processing of fish and shellfish.[19] Because Neanderthals occupied Payre, they must have eaten a diet as varied as ours. Neanderthals may have consumed sea bream (*Pagrus major* and *Pagellus bogaraveo*) and mussels (*Mytilus galloprovincialis*) along the Mediterranean coast and salmon (*Oncorhynchus* species) near the Black Sea. Such diversity supports Israeli anthropologist Ofer Bar-Yosef's (1937–2020) argument in Chapter 3 that Neanderthals ate what their surroundings provided.

German bio-geologists Herve Bocherens and Dorothee Drucker rejected fish, however, tracing high nitrogen isotope ^{15}N concentrations in fossils from Crimea to the mammoths (*Mammuthus* species), rather than seafood, that modern humans ate.[20] Chapters 1 and 4 discussed use of isotopes to determine what people ate. Belief that moderns and Neanderthals consumed similar foods implies that Neanderthals also seldom ate fish and shellfish, an idea that affirms the above opinion about them.

5.3 FISHING AND HUMANITY

Despite this attempt to demote fish, humans pursued it avidly enough to invent the fishhook before 21,000 BCE and the fishing net around 6800 BCE.[21] Because nets degrade and so escape discovery, an earlier date is possible. Egyptian, Greek, and Roman texts describe how ancients fished in the Mediterranean Sea, rivers, and lakes. Naturalist Pliny the Elder (23–79 CE) wrote that Greeks and Romans fermented fish intestines to make a sauce known as garum, which remained popular in the eastern Mediterranean basin throughout the Middle Ages.[22] Around 1000 CE the English began eating more ocean fish, evidence of overfishing in lakes and rivers.[23]

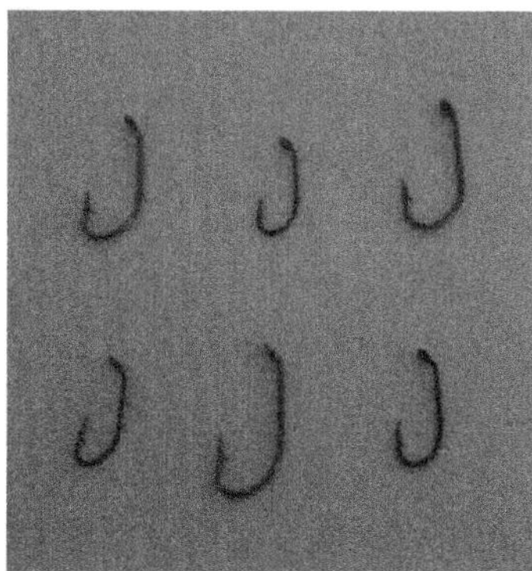

FIGURE 5.3 Fishhooks. (Photo from author.)

Besides these developments, Amerindians on California's Channel Islands, treated in Chapter 9, harvested abundant shellfish around 9500 BCE.[24] South of the equator Peruvians on the Pacific coast used spears to impale fish 500 years later.[25] In the second millennium BCE, they began fishing in reed boats, catching Peruvian anchovies (*Engraulis ringens*) with cotton nets.[26] New Guineans made nets from spider webs.[27] In other cases, people fashioned human hair, wool, or leather into nets. About 500 BCE, occupants of Vancouver Island, Canada, harvested mollusks (species in the phylum Mollusca) some 20 meters (21.9 yards or 65.6 feet) below the surface.[28] In shallow water, women and children gathered shellfish. In addition, women made nets. Men fished at depth with lines, nets, and spears. New Zealand's Maori collected shellfish from lakes and rivers when large prey failed to feed everyone.

In the fourteenth century CE, sailboats trawled the Baltic and North Seas.[29] Along nineteenth-century British, Belgian, and Californian coasts, horses (*Equus caballus*) pulled nets ashore.[30] California and the Pacific Northwest supplied salmon. Nineteenth-century France and Britain began trawling with steamboats.[31] In the twentieth century, gasoline and diesel engines powered fishing boats.[32] In 2018, the United Nations Food and Agriculture Organization (FAO) in Rome, Italy, listed China, Indonesia, the United States, Russia, Peru, India, and Japan as catchers of most fish.[33]

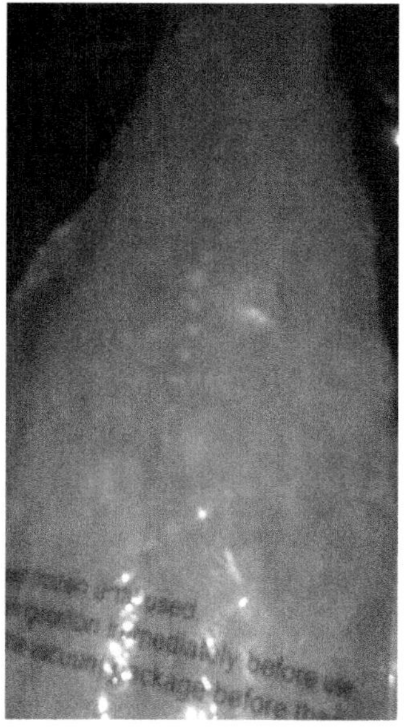

FIGURE 5.4 Salmon. (Photo from author.)

5.4 FISH AND SHELLFISH CONSUMPTION IN MODERNITY

5.4.1 Geography and Economics of Consumption

Before globalism and as implied above, fish and shellfish fed people near coasts, lakes, and rivers and at high latitudes during winters, when plants are unavailable. Communities in such environs and outside the global economy eat the local catch. East, South, and Southeast Asia consume fish and shellfish as a staple. Outside these areas, they feed Mexico, Cote d'Ivoire, and Mozambique. Europeans also tend to eat much fish, though Africa and the Levant consume the least. The poor get animal protein, if any, from fish and shellfish.

5.4.2 Nutrients in Fish

Beyond economic and geographic considerations, fish has the most vitamin D of any food and ample selenium, iodine, calcium, phosphorus, iron, zinc, vitamins A, B_3 (niacin or nicotinic acid), B_6 (pyridoxine), and B_{12} (cobalamin), protein, and omega 3 fatty acids.[34] "Indeed, with their unsaturated fats, vitamins, minerals, and trace elements, fish and shellfish constitute a near-perfect food for the human body," wrote American aquaculture researcher Colin E. Nash in 2000.[35] With less fat and fewer calories than many meats, fish and shellfish attract dieters.

Cod (*Gadus morhua* and *G. macrocephalus*) supplies abundant protein, phosphorus, and vitamins B_3 and B_{12}. Sardines (*Sardina pilchardus*) are rich in vitamins B_3, B_{12}, and D, selenium, phosphorus, calcium, iron, protein, and omega 3 fatty acids. One hundred grams of mackerel (species in genera *Rastrelliger* and *Scomber*) have above the U.S. Food and Drug Administration's (FDA) daily value (DV) of vitamins B_{12} and D and plentiful protein, magnesium, potassium, and vitamin B_6. Fish tends to provide more protein, vitamins, and minerals per calorie than livestock. Like meat, fish lacks vitamin C, fiber, and phytochemicals. Chapter 2 discussed these nutrients and others. Table 5.1 lists calories and nutrients in tuna, tilapia, pollock, cod, and mackerel.[36]

TABLE 5.1
Nutrients in Fishes 100 g

Nutrient	Tuna	%DV	Tilapia	%DV	Pollock	%DV	Cod	%DV	Mackerel	%DV
Calories	86	N/A	96	N/A	56	N/A	82	N/A	189	N/A
Protein (g)	25.5	N/A	20.08	N/A	12.19	N/A	17.81	N/A	19.08	N/A
Fat (g)	0.96	N/A	1.70	N/A	0.41	N/A	0.67	N/A	11.91	N/A
Carbs (g)	0	N/A	0	N/A	0	N/A	0	N/A	0	N/A
Fiber (g)	0	N/A	0	N/A	0	N/A	0	N/A	0	N/A
					Minerals					
Ca (mg)	17	1.7	10	1	15	1.5	16	1.6	16	1.6
Fe (mg)	1.53	9	0.56	3.1	0.22	1.2	0.38	2.1	1.48	8.2
Mg (mg)	23	5.8	27	6.8	16	4	32	8	60	15
P (mg)	163	16.3	170	17	284	28.4	203	20.3	187	18.7
K (mg)	179	5.1	302	8.6	160	4.6	413	11.8	344	9.8
Na (mg)	247	10.3	52	2.2	333	13.9	54	2.3	89	3.7
Zn (mg)	0.77	5.1	0.33	2.2	0.31	2.1	0.45	3	0.64	4.3
Cu (mg)	0.05	3	0.08	4	0.04	2	0.03	1.5	0.08	4
Mn (mg)	0.01	0.5	0.04	2	0.01	0.5	0.02	1	0.02	1
Se (mcg)	70.6	101	41.8	59.7	15.9	22.7	33.1	47.3	41.6	59.4

(Continued)

TABLE 5.1 (*Continued*)
Nutrients in Fishes 100 g

Nutrient	Tuna	%DV	Tilapia	%DV	Pollock	%DV	Cod	%DV	Mackerel	%DV
					Vitamins					
A (IU)	20	0.4	0	0	46	0.9	40	0.8	167	3.3
B_1 (mg)	0.03	2	0.04	2.4	0.03	2	0.08	4.7	0.16	10.7
B_2 (mg)	0.07	4.1	0.06	3.5	0.08	4.7	0.07	4.1	0.35	20.6
B_3 (mg)	13.28	66.4	3.9	19.5	0.65	3.3	2.06	10.3	8.83	44.2
B_5 (mg)	0.12	1.2	0.49	4.9	0.36	3.6	0.15	1.5	0.86	8.6
B_6 (mg)	0.32	16	0.16	8	0.07	3.5	0.25	12.5	0.38	19
B_9 (mcg)	4	1	24	6	3	0.8	7	1.8	1	0.3
B_{12} (mcg)	2.55	42.5	1.58	26.3	1.63	27.2	0.91	15.2	7.29	121.5
C (mg)	0	0	0	0	0	0	1	1.7	0.9	1.5
D (IU)	80	20	124	31	42	10.5	36	9	643	160.8
E (mg)	0.33	2.2	0.40	2.7	0.49	3.3	0.64	4.3	1.35	9
K (mcg)	0.2	0.3	1.4	1.8	0.1	0.1	0.1	0.1	3.4	4.3

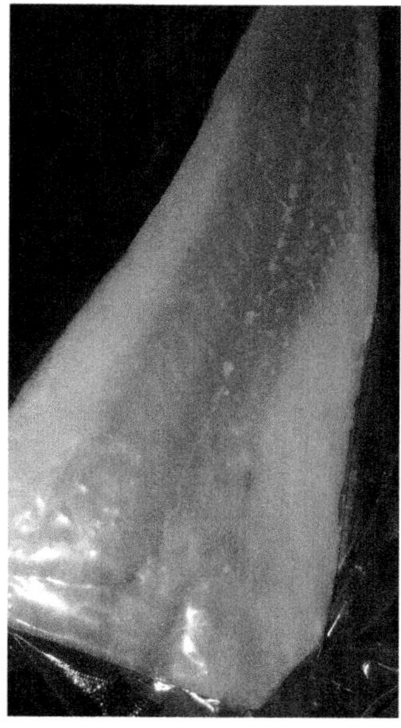

FIGURE 5.5 Cod. (Photo from author.)

5.4.3 Nutrients in Shellfish

In addition to fish, aquatic environments supply shellfish. Although nutritionists and dieticians group both as seafood, shellfish resembles insects more than fish in lacking bones, making both invertebrates. Shellfish includes mollusks, which may encompass 100,000 species.[37] Unlike insects, mollusks lack legs. Their calcium carbonate ($CaCO_3$) shell may be a single unit as is true of snails (species in the class Gastropoda) or two as with clams (species in the class Bivalvia). Mollusks also include oysters (species in the genera *Ostrea*, *Crassostrea*, *Ostreola*, *Magallana*, and *Saccostrea*), mussels, scallops (species in the family Pectinoidea), limpets (*Patella vulgata*), and cockles (*Cerastoderma edule*).

The second class of shellfish, the subphylum Crustacea, matches insects in having exoskeletons of the tough organic compound chitin and calcium. Crustaceans have four antennae, a head, mouth, body, and ten appendages. Examples include crabs (species in the infraorder Brachyura), shrimp (species in the infraorder Caridea), lobster (species in the family Nephropidae), crayfish (species in the families Astacidae, Parastacidae, and Austraostracidae), krill (species in the order Euphausiacae), and barnacles (*Cirripedia* species).

Nutrients depend on type, though shellfish often have protein, iodine, selenium, and vitamin A. Mostly water, they have little fat and few calories. When cooked to remove much water, shrimp, crab, clams, and mussels are over half protein by mass.[38] One hundred grams of shrimp have 71 calories, 20.9 grams of protein, 1.1 grams of fat, no carbohydrates, 54 milligrams of calcium, 22 milligrams of magnesium, and 3.09 milligrams of iron.[39] One hundred grams of lobster contain 77 calories, 0.75 grams of fat, no carbohydrates, 16.52 grams of protein, 200 milligrams of potassium, and small quantities of iron and vitamin C. One hundred grams of mussels supply 115 calories, 2.6 grams each of fat and carbohydrates, 21.2 grams of protein, 50 milligrams of calcium, 2.1 milligrams of iron, and 36 micrograms of vitamin A.[40] Some nutritionists recommend mussels for vitamin B_{12} and crab, shrimp, lobster, prawn, and crayfish for selenium.[41] As noted, shells supply calcium. Despite these benefits, shellfish may contain abundant cholesterol and sodium.

Table 5.2 shows calories and nutrients in shrimp, oysters, lobster, clams, and crab.[42]

TABLE 5.2
Nutrients in Shellfish 100 g

Nutrient	Shrimp	%DV	Oysters	%DV	Lobster	%DV	Clams	%DV	Crab	%DV
Calories	71	N/A	51	N/A	77	N/A	86	N/A	87	N/A
Protein (g)	20.9	N/A	14.1	N/A	16.52	N/A	14.67	N/A	18.06	N/A
Fat (g)	1.1	N/A	1.71	N/A	0.75	N/A	0.96	N/A	1.08	N/A
Carbs (g)	0	N/A	2.72	N/A	0	N/A	3.57	N/A	0.04	N/A
Fiber (g)	0	N/A	0	N/A	0	N/A	0	N/A	0	N/A
Minerals										
Ca (mg)	54	5.4	59	5.9	84	8.4	39	3.9	89	8.9
Fe (mg)	3.09	18	13.4	76	0.26	1.4	1.62	9	0.74	4.1
Mg (mg)	22	5.5	18	4.5	38	9.5	19	4.8	34	8.5
P (mg)	137	13.7	278	27.8	161	16.1	198	19.8	229	22.9
K (mg)	113	3.2	156	4.5	200	5.7	46	1.3	329	9.4
Na (mg)	566	23.6	85	3.5	423	17.6	56	2.3	293	12.2
Zn (mg)	1.56	9	181.9	1,213	3.53	23.5	0.51	3.4	3.54	23.6
Cu (mg)	0.19	11	8.9	506	1.35	67.5	0.05	2.5	0.67	33.5
Mn (mg)	0.03	2	0.36	18	0.06	3	0.09	4.5	0.15	7.5
Se (mcg)	29.6	42.3	19.7	28.1	63.6	90.9	30.6	43.7	37.4	53.4
Vitamins										
A (IU)	180	3.6	100	2	4	0.08	300	6	5	0.1
B_1 (mg)	0.03	2	0.02	1.3	0.02	1.3	0.02	1.3	0.08	5.3
B_2 (mg)	0.03	2	0.33	17	0.01	0.6	0.04	2.4	0.04	2.4
B_3 (mg)	2.59	15	2.49	14	1.59	8	0.35	1.8	2.7	13.5
B_5 (mg)	N/A	N/A	0.2	2	1.45	14.5	0.15	1.5	0.35	3.5
B_6 (mg)	0.16	8	0.03	1.5	0.1	5	0.01	0.5	0.15	7.5
B_9 (mcg)	19	4.8	7	1.8	10	2.5	5	1.3	44	11
B_{12} (mcg)	1.11	18.5	8.75	145.8	1.25	20.8	11.28	188	9	150
C (mg)	2	3.3	0	0	0	0	0	0	3	5
D (IU)	152	38	0	0	1	0.3	1	0.3	0	0
E (mg)	1.32	8.8	0.85	5.7	0.87	5.8	0.68	4.5	1.84	12.3
K (mcg)	N/A	N/A	1	1.3	0	0	0.2	0.3	0.3	0.4

5.4.4 Aquaculture and Nutrients

Aquaculture tends to yield less-nourishing fish than nature because farm fish eat rapeseed (*Brassica napus*), wheat (*Triticum aestivum*), corn (*Zea mays*), rice (*Oryza sativa*), soybeans (*Glycine max*), pulverized feathers, yeast (*Saccharomyces cerevisiae*), chicken fat, or their combination, the accent being on plant foods rather than multiple trophic levels.[43] Farm fish tend to have more fat and thus more calories than wild because fish swim less and eat more in captivity.[44] For example, Table 5.3 shows that by mass wild catfish in the same species has more protein, calcium, iron, magnesium, phosphorus, potassium, zinc, manganese, selenium, and vitamins A, B_1 (thiamine or thiamin), B_5 (pantothenic acid), C, and D, less fat, and fewer calories than its farm counterpart.[45] This table also compares calories and nutrients in wild and farm salmon.

On the other hand, because aquaculture permits growers to control ponds, the metal mercury and other contaminants should be absent. These pollutants, coming from factories and utilities, caution against eating predators like swordfish (*Xiphias gladius*), king mackerel (*Scomberomorus cavalla*), shark (species in the superorder Selachimorpha), orange roughy (*Hoplostethus atlanticus*), tilefish

TABLE 5.3
Nutrients in Salmon and Catfish Wild versus Farm 100 g

Nutrient	Wild Salmon	%DV	Farm Salmon	%DV	Wild Catfish	%DV	Farm Catfish	%DV
Calories	42	N/A	208	N/A	95	N/A	119	N/A
Protein (g)	19.84	N/A	29.42	N/A	16.38	N/A	15.23	N/A
Fat (g)	6.34	N/A	13.42	N/A	2.82	N/A	5.94	N/A
Carbs (g)	0	N/A	0	N/A	0	N/A	0	N/A
Fiber (g)	0	N/A	0	N/A	0	N/A	0	N/A
Minerals								
Ca (mg)	12	1.2	9	0.9	14	1.4	8	0.8
Fe (mg)	0.80	4.4	0.34	1.9	0.3	1.7	0.23	1.3
Mg (mg)	29	7.3	27	6.8	23	5.8	19	4.8
P (mg)	200	20	240	24	209	20.9	204	20.4
K (mg)	490	14	363	10.4	358	10.2	302	8.6
Na (mg)	44	1.8	59	2.5	43	1.8	98	4.1
Zn (mg)	0.64	4.3	0.36	2.4	0.51	3.4	0.48	3.2
Cu (mg)	0.25	12.5	0.05	2.5	0.03	1.5	0.03	1.5
Mn (mg)	0.02	1	0.01	0.5	0.03	1.5	0.02	1
Se (mcg)	36.5	52.1	24.0	34.3	12.6	18	8.2	11.7
Vitamins								
A (IU)	40	0.8	193	3.9	50	1	1	0.02
B_1 (mg)	0.23	15.3	0.21	14	0.21	14	0.02	1.3
B_2 (mg)	0.38	22.4	0.16	9.4	0.07	4.1	0.08	4.7
B_3 (mg)	7.86	39.3	8.67	43.4	1.91	9.6	2.11	10.6
B_5 (mg)	1.66	16.6	1.55	15.5	0.77	7.7	0.67	6.7
B_6 (mg)	0.82	41	0.64	32	0.12	6	0.15	7.5
B_9 (mcg)	25	6.3	26	6.5	10	2.5	10	2.5
B_{12} (mcg)	3.18	53	3.23	53.8	2.23	37.2	2.88	48
C (mg)	0	0	3.69	6.5	0.7	1.2	0	0
D (IU)	361	90.3	441	110.3	500	125	9	2.3
E (mg)	0.73	4.9	3.55	23.7	NA	NA	0.81	5.4
K (mcg)	0.1	0.1	0.5	0.6	NA	NA	2.1	2.6

(*Lopholatilus* species), and bigeye tuna (*Thunnus obesus*).[46] Carp (*Cyprinus carpio*), catfish, trout (species in genera *Oncorhynchus*, *Salmo*, and *Salvelinus*), and perch (*Perca fluviatilis*, *P. schrenkii*, and *P. flavescens*) from ponds and streams also tend to have toxins. The attempt to balance seafood's benefits and perils leaves consumers unsure what to eat, how much, and how often.[47]

5.4.5 History and Opinions about Aquaculture

The Egyptians invented aquaculture about 2500 BCE, from where it spread west through North Africa.[48] Before 1000 BCE, China was farming fish to feed its people.[49] Around 600 BCE, Celts in Gaul (today France, Belgium, and Luxembourg) began raising mollusks.[50] Aquaculture persisted in Europe, which in the 1960s farmed trout and salmon. Farm fish increased from under 4 percent of the total harvest by mass in 1970 to nearly 52 percent in 2005.[51] No livestock sector grew as much during these years.

Critics deem farm fish unnourishing, insipid, and sometimes full of antibiotics, hormones, and pesticides. Hazards are greatest where governments do not regulate production. In a global economy, consumers cannot always determine whether fish comes from farm or the wild. In the case of farm fish, labels do not always disclose country of origin. Proponents like FAO and the World Health Organization (WHO) in Geneva, Switzerland hope that aquaculture will make fish abundant enough to afford the poor animal protein, an urgent need in Africa and Asia.[52] Unlike many plants, animals supply protein with all essential amino acids, noted Chapter 2.

5.4.6 Fish Consumption and Longevity

Chapter 4 compared longevity among countries with the greatest per capita meat consumption. Applying this procedure here, China has the highest per person fish consumption but in 2018 ranked 111th in life expectancy at birth (e^0) at 75.7 years.[53] Myanmar and Vietnam, ranking second and third in fish consumption, trailed China's e^0. The fourth largest per person consumer, Japan, ranked second in e^0 at 85.5 years. Tokyo's National Centre for Global Health and Medicine credits Japanese longevity to consumption of fish, rice and other whole grains, soy foods, vegetables, and fruits.[54] Monaco's residents had the highest e^0 at 89.4 years and eat seafood, cod being popular.[55] Singapore ranked third, trailing Japan by under two months.[56] Singaporeans eat lobster, oysters, swordfish, cod, salmon, scallops, mussels, and clams.[57]

China, Myanmar, and Vietnam prove that seafood cannot be longevity's sole determinant. Chapter 1 indicated that many factors influence lifespan. Seeking clarity unavailable in the above e^0s, the remainder of this chapter examines seafood's healthfulness throughout history.

5.5 ALASKA, CANADA, GREENLAND, AND THE PACIFIC NORTHWEST

5.5.1 Distribution of Fish in Alaska, Canada, Greenland, and the Pacific Northwest

North American waters have many fish species. Canada totals some 1,200 indigenous species, roughly 990 marine, 180 freshwater, and the rest diadromous in splitting their time among brine, brackish water, and freshwater.[58] In this last category, anadromous fishes live in the ocean and mate in freshwater whereas catadromous species do the reverse. American species are most numerous in the Great Lakes and Ontario, with little diversity in Nunavut, the Northwest Territories, the Yukon, Alberta, and Saskatchewan. The Arctic Ocean has some 240 species, most anadromous.[59] Able to tolerate brine, brackish water, and freshwater, these species are known as euryhaline.

Around 55 percent of Arctic species are in the suborders Cottoidei and Zoarcoidei.[60] The first contains sculpines, snailfishes, and alligator fishes. Eelpouts and pricklebacks belong to Zoarcoidei. Although it supplies fewer Arctic species than Cottoidei or Zoarcoidei, the Salmonids include commercial fish like salmon, trout, char (*Salvelinus* species), whitefish (*Coregonus* species), and cisco (*Coregonus artedi*). British Columbia's Pacific waters have over 400 species.[61] At the other end of the continent, the North Atlantic Ocean has attracted fishers since prehistory. The catch included cod (*G. morhua*), herring (*Clupea herengus*), mackerel (*Scomber scombrus*), horse mackerel (*Trachurus*

trachurus), capelin (*Mallotus villosus*), blue whiting (*Micromesistius poutassou*), tuna (*Thunnus alalonga* and *T. thynnus*), swordfish, and blue marlin (*Makaira nigricans*).

5.5.2 Human Migrations into North America

As elsewhere in the western hemisphere, Canada's original inhabitants were Asians who entered what is now Alaska about 13,000 BCE. Chapters 3 and 4 detailed migrations from an evolutionary vantagepoint. Where apparent, mongoloid features identified Asian origins, though such characteristics typified neither all Asians nor all Amerindians. Entrance into North America was not one event but a series of forays over millennia. The last ice age abetted these migrations by holding large amounts of water as ice. With less water as liquid, sea levels fell, exposing land—known as Beringia—between eastern Siberia and western Alaska. Humans may have followed the herbivores they hunted across Beringia. The ocean reclaimed this land about 9700 BCE as the climate warmed. Beringia's disappearance largely isolated Amerindians from the eastern hemisphere until the late fifteenth century CE, though Vikings settled Greenland between the tenth and fourteenth centuries.

These Norse were the first Europeans to encounter the Inuit. Early literature coined the word "Eskimo" for Greenland and Canada's Inuit, Alaska's Inupiat, and Alaska and Siberia's Yupik. Now branded derogatory, the term has fallen from favor. Greenlander and Canadian scholars likewise reject the word "Indian," which properly applies only to India's people. The label, however, is still permissible in the United States, where scholars refer to American Indians to differentiate them from Indians, though a movement to remove names like Indians and Redskins from U.S. sports teams demonstrates that such language provokes discomfort. In casual and even scholarly usage, language sometimes confuses rather than clarifies. Anthropologists have termed Athapaskan speakers in Canada's Northwest Territories Dogrib Indians, Tlicho (dog's rib), or Thlingchadinne, though these indigenes eschew these labels, calling themselves Done, meaning "people."[62]

Precise and consistent terminology guards against confusing or conflating large numbers of peoples. In 2016, Canada alone totaled over 1.6 million indigenes.[63] Since 1910 linguists and anthropologists have attempted to differentiate them by language. Canada's government prefers a tripartite division. The Inuit inhabit northern Canada, mostly within the Arctic Circle. South of them, the First Nations consider themselves Canada's original occupants. The third category, Metis, have aboriginal and European lineages. Canada's largest groups of indigenes identify as Inupiat, Yupik, Aleut, Eyak, Tlingit, Haida, or Tsimshian. Outside Canada, indigenes inhabit Alaska and Greenland. Athapaskan speakers occupy northernmost Alaska. Roughly nine-tenths of Greenlanders are Inuit and the rest Danish.[64]

5.5.3 Role of Geography and Climate in Fishing in Alaska, Canada, Greenland, and the Pacific Northwest

Geography and climate shaped diets. Alaska, Greenland, and Canada's provinces of British Columbia, Alberta, Saskatchewan, and Manitoba are north of the forty-ninth parallel, a line roughly 5,440 kilometers (3,380 miles) above the equator. Movement away from the equator and toward the poles reduces sunlight, which contacts Earth at an angle rather than directly as latitude increases. Because the sun is the ultimate source of energy, high latitudes receive less energy to sustain life than low latitudes, diminishing biomass of plants and animals. Away from the equator, temperature fluctuations produce seasons. Winters are long and harsh, eliminating plant foods when florae are dormant, and frozen soils trap roots and tubers.

5.5.4 Fishing Supplied Much More Food than Gathering

Alaska, Canada, and Greenland's indigenes adapted to their geography and climate by hunting and fishing. Plants, whose collection was possible during warm weather, were scant in diets. For example, between October 1953 and April 1954, a group of Cree in Canada's province of Newfoundland and Labrador collected five pails of blueberries (*Vaccinium angustifolium*) in contrast to nearly 5,500 kilograms (12,100 pounds) of fish and game.[65] The mass of these blueberries is unstated but cannot have been large. In nontechnical settings, the terms "pail" and "bucket" are interchangeable. Neither is precise, though Amazon.com sells buckets that hold 15 liters (4 gallons).[66] One cup of blueberries being about 150 grams (5.3 ounces) and 1 liter holding around 4 cups yield roughly 9 kilograms (19.8 pounds) of blueberries per bucket, bringing the total to 45 kilograms (99.2 pounds) or under 1 percent of food collected.

Almost all Cree food in this sample was meat or fish. Fish totaled 1,436 kilograms (3,165 pounds).[67] Among game, only moose (*Alces alces*), at 1,814 kilograms (4,000 pounds), represented a larger amount. The next most consequential mammals were beaver (*Castor canadensis*) at 962 kilograms (2,120 pounds) and caribou (*Rangifer tarandus groenlandicus* and *Rangifer tarandus caribou*) at 680 kilograms (1,500 pounds). Several mammals were unimportant. For example, squirrel totaled just 3.6 kilograms (8 pounds). Birds were still less significant, grouse (*Bonasa umbellus*) and owl (species in genera *Bubo*, *Surnia*, *Strix*, *Asio*, and *Aegolius*) at 0.5 kilograms (1 pound) each. Moreover, fish increased in diets as Cree overhunted caribou.[68]

5.5.5 Overhunting Increased Reliance on Fish

Nineteenth-century Inuit in the Northwest Territories and Nunavut overhunted bowhead whales (*Balaena mysticetus*), causing them to concentrate increasingly on fish and caribou in the twentieth century.[69] They ate nothing but fish, observed Icelandic-Canadian explorer Vilhjalmur Stefansson (1879–1962) in 1906.[70] The Northwest Territories' caribou hunt peaked about 1890, after which populations declined.[71] The Done filled the void with fish. Trade with whites yielded fishing nets, which increased catches. By 1910 Alaska's Inupiat, who overhunted bowhead whales, walruses (*Odobenus rosmarus*), and caribou, shifted diets toward fish.[72]

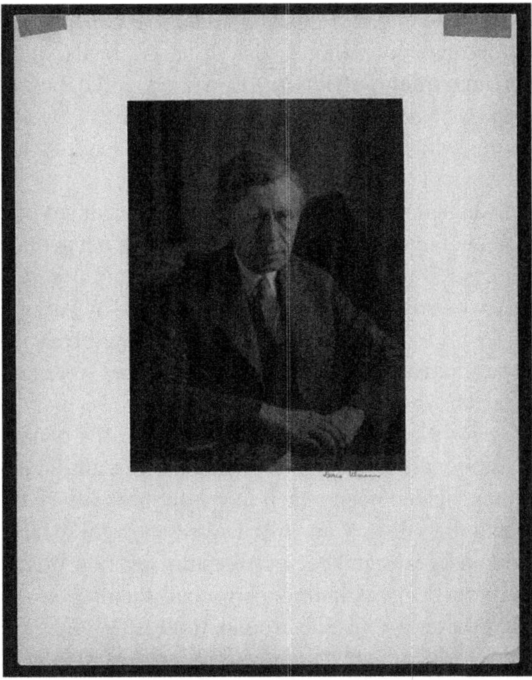

FIGURE 5.6 Vilhjalmur Stefansson. (Photo courtesy of Library of Congress. https://www.loc.gov/pictures/item/2009633849/.)

5.5.6 Fish Species Central to Amerindian Diets

Fish has been a northern staple since at least 5000 BCE, when pits along British Columbia's Pacific coast grew to store large aggregates of frozen salmon, implying fishing's intensification.[73] Europeans judged salmon so plentiful in the northwest at spawning that an onlooker could "walk across" a river "on their backs."[74] In recent times, British Columbia and Yukon's Witsuwit'en and Gitxsau caught sea trout (*Salmo trutta*) and salmon, both staples.[75] Among *Oncorhynchus* species, they targeted sockeye (*Oncorhynchus nerka*), steelhead trout (*Oncorhynchus mykiss*), and cutthroat trout (*Oncorhynchus clarkia*). Eulachon (*Thaleichthys pacificus*), known as candlefish, rounded out the menu. Plentiful fish, especially salmon, permitted sedentism. Surplus was preserved by smoking.

5.5.7 Fish Targeted throughout the Year

Cree ate brook or speckled trout (*Salvelinus fontinalis*), related char species, whitefish, pike (*Esox lucius*), walleye (*Sander vitreus*), sucker (*Catostomus catostomus*), burbot (*Lota lota*), ling or lingcod (*Ophiodon elongatus*), and sturgeon.[76] Walleye and sturgeon were less abundant because geography restricted their range. Whereas Cree hunted in spurts to match seasonal availability, they fished year-round.[77] Fishing intensified in September and October, though between June and August catches tended to be small. Fish were less bountiful during winter because they inhabited depths difficult to reach with nets. Cree settlements in eastern Canada's Quebec depended on fish and caribou.[78] Even those with traditional jobs fished when off duty.

Related to Cree are Innu—a name meaning "humans"—who have inhabited Quebec and Newfoundland and Labrador for at least 2000 years and possibly since 6000 BCE.[79] Rivers in these provinces, the Gulf of St. Lawrence, and the Atlantic Ocean long supplied fish. About 1500 CE, these waters attracted Basque, Portuguese, and French fishers, who competed with Innu. The gulf and ocean furnished cod, herring, and lobster, whereas rivers had salmon and trout. Fish, game, and wild berries sustained Innu, though shortages caused famine.

Emphasizing the Northwest Territories' diverse habitats, American anthropologist June Helm (1924–2004) noted the "thousands upon thousands" of lakes, ponds, and rivers with fish.[80] Done in this region ate whitefish, lake trout (*Salvelinus namaycush*), pike, burbot, sucker, pickerel (*Esox americanus*), inconnu (*Stenodus leucichthys*), and Arctic grayling (*Thymallus arcticus*). Most calories and nutrients came from whitefish, trout, pike, pickerel, suckers, hare (*Lepus americanus*), moose, and barren-ground caribou (*R. tarandus groenlandicus*).

The catch was meager in January and February when fish occupied deep waters.[81] Their return to the shallows in March meant larger hauls. By March 15, each net averaged fifteen to twenty-five fish daily, compared to the desired thirty.[82] During May and again in late June, fish were plentiful. The harvest declined in July when fish again sought deep waters. By August 1, hungry Done begged kin and neighbors for fish. By mid-month, better prospects allowed Done to report that "In August, we eat mostly fish."[83] Catches increased thereafter such that fishes were numerous between roughly September 10 and Christmas, the excess smoked.

Fish sustained Done lifeways. Needing dogs for hunting, a family owned five or six, each requiring at least 0.9 kilograms (2 pounds) of fish daily.[84] Rations increased during winter when hunting intensified. Trade with whites yielded nets, which Done put beneath ice during winter in hopes of catching enough for them and their dogs. Canoes patrolled lakes for fish in summer.

Related to the Done are indigenes in the southwestern portion of the Northwest Territories, northern Alberta, and northern British Columbia who call themselves "Dene," another word for "people."[85] Having occupied these lands since around 1000 BCE, they ate trout, burbot, grayling, whitefish, pike, and inconnu. Fish and game supplied most calories and nutrients, though they collected blueberries, rosehips (*Rosa* species), saskatoons (*Amelanchier alnifolia*), raspberries (*Rubus idaeus*), and strawberries (*Fragaria vesca*) and traded for flour, sucrose, tea (*Camellia sinensis*), lard, chocolate, alcohol, and tobacco (*Nicotiana tabacum*).

The Northwest Territories and Nunavut's Inuit fished lakes, rivers, the Arctic Ocean, Baffin Bay, Pelly Bay, Hudson Bay, and Labrador Sea for char, whitefish, trout, grayling, Arctic staghorn sculpin (*Gymnocanthus tricuspis*), tomcod (*Microgadus tomcod*) and cod, the first three ubiquitous in diets.[86] Inuit valued lakes for char and the ocean for cod. Pelly Bay supplied abundant fish, especially trout and tomcod. Trout were most numerous between mid-May and mid-July and again in November.[87] From mid-July to October, Inuit caught trout and char. Char peaked in August and September, the surfeit dried and frozen for consumption in November and December.[88] Near Pelly Bay, trout were most plentiful in August, though numbers were also large in July and October. Whereas game fluctuated, fish was the staple, especially between May and August, even though species' availability varied throughout the year. Since about 1910, trade with whites yielded fishing nets.[89] Decline in caribou populations after the mid-1950s strengthened fish's dietary role. Inuit consumed all trout they caught and some char, selling the rest. Inuit children and the old collected shellfish; what youths gathered supplied most of their diet. Men fished from canoes.

Among the world's richest fisheries into the twentieth century, Pacific Northwest rivers bulged with salmon in "tens and hundreds of thousands" and sturgeon as massive as 450 kilograms (0.5 U.S. tons).[90] Abundance permitted one of the densest hunter-gatherer populations worldwide, with only parts of California and the Arctic as rivals.[91] British Columbia's Nass River had halibut (*Hippoglossus stenolepis*) and eulachon. Vancouver Island's Nootka caught halibut, cod, herring, and chum salmon (*Oncorhynchus keta*). In the nineteenth century, a few hours' fishing near Washington State's Cape Flattery produced halibut for a week.[92] At Astoria, Oregon, where the Columbia River enters the Pacific Ocean, Chinook ate eulachon and salmon eggs. A confederation of Pacific Amerindians, Salish consumed sturgeon, halibut, lingcod, sockeye, chum salmon, pink salmon (*Oncorhynchus gorbuscha*), coho salmon (*Oncorhynchus kisutch*), and capelin. Being fattest, sockeye and chum salmon were preferred. Women dried the excess and gathered shellfish. Mussels preserved poorly and were eaten immediately. The Oohl—Yurok in early literature—fished northwestern California's Klamath-Trinity River for sturgeon, salmon, and eulachon and gathered mussels from the ocean. In 1968, American anthropologist and linguist Wayne Prescott Suttles (1918–2005) estimated fish at half Oohl diets and roughly 40 percent of Taa-laa-wa Dee-ni—Tolowa in anthropological studies—calories in northwestern California and southern Oregon.[93]

5.5.8 Health in Alaska, Canada, Greenland, and the Pacific Northwest

Interest in fish and shellfish quickened in the 1970s upon reports that Greenland Inuit had only one-tenth the rate of fatal heart attacks as whites in Denmark and the United States.[94] American nutritionist Ken Babal wrote that an unnamed Greenland hospital did not record a single Inuit heart attack death over an unspecified decade, citing *The Omega Diet* by American endocrinologist Artemis P. Simopoulos (b. 1933).[95] *The Omega Diet* stated this claim without a citation.[96] The closest endnote referenced an article in the medical journal *The Lancet*, but the article omitted Inuit.[97] Cordain asserted that the decade in question occurred between 1968 and 1978.[98]

These issues aside, American epidemiologists Faina Linkov and Barbara Stadterman and American surgeon and epidemiologist Emanuela Taioli contrasted European and American red meat intake with Inuit consumption of fish, whose omega 3 fatty acids reduced plaque in arteries and triglycerides in blood.[99] Chapter 2 defined fatty acids and triglycerides and illustrated their structures. Even small amounts of fish lowered risk of developing cancers in the mouth, pharynx, esophagus, stomach, colon, rectum, and pancreas. Fish consumption likely diminishes risk of breast cancer.[100] Moreover, fish and shellfish appear to reduce risks of prostate and lung cancers.[101] Conversely, meat and dairy products correlated with increases in prostate cancers in the United States between 1930 and 1992. These results led Linkov, Stadterman, and Taioli to recommend a diet of fish, poultry, low-fat dairy, vegetables, fruits, legumes, and whole grains.[102] Everyone should limit calories, sucrose, alcohol, and dairy, eschew smoking, and exercise regularly.[103]

Despite these findings, fish, especially salted, may cause nasopharyngeal and stomach cancers, the first of which Danish oncologist Jeppe T. Friborg and Danish epidemiologist Mads Melbye documented in Inuit.[104] Yet cancers were "almost non-existent" in them around 1900.[105] Their dearth might have resulted from Inuit's short lifespan by Western standards given that cancers tend to afflict the elderly. Friborg and Melbye, however, noted that cancers rose during the twentieth century as fish and sea mammal intake diminished and smoking surged. Examining diet, they noted that fish, seals (species in the clade Pinnipedia), and similar animals furnished calories as unsaturated fat and protein rather than carbohydrates. Although vegetables and fruits were lacking and vitamin C was probably inadequate, fish and marine mammals furnished vitamin A and omega 3 fatty acids, both thought to reduce cancer risks. But during the twentieth century, Inuit imported meat, flour, sucrose, and processed foods from Canada, Europe, and the United States, shifting consumption toward saturated fat and refined carbohydrates. By the 1980s, fish trailed coffee (*Coffea* species), sucrose, and bread in Inuit diets.[106] In 2009, Inuit under age thirty-nine derived a plurality of calories from sugary beverages.

Like Chapter 4's Plains Indians, this transition undermined health. As Inuit ate more calories and processed foods and became less active, they became obese and type 2 diabetes rates increased sixty times.[107] After roughly 1950, lung, colon, and breast cancers afflicted the population. Since the 1970s, lung cancer has totaled 20 percent of Inuit malignancies.[108] Inuit women have the world's highest rate, and men do not lag far. Friborg and Melbye faulted smoking, though the above dietary transition, idleness, obesity, and type 2 diabetes likely increased breast and colon cancers.[109] Since about 1980, Alaskan Inuit have had colon cancer in greater proportion than white Americans. Friborg and Melbye blamed these problems on the shift from lean fish to a fatty Western diet.

The authors' judgment that Inuit lives were brief is difficult to evaluate absent quantification. Being Danes, Friborg and Melbye might have idealized Denmark, where e^0 ranked forty-ninth in 2018 at 79.7 years.[110] Inuit data are sparse and contradictory. For example, the Sadlermiut Inuit languished on the Hudson Bay's Southampton, Coats, and Walrus Islands. Examination of 187 skeletons yielded none over age fifty-five.[111] Forty percent perished before age four. These numbers may not typify all Inuit because European diseases eradicated the Sadlermiut in 1903.[112]

Even were Sadlermiut mortality the norm, this book argues that life was short during prehistory and most of history. Few people surpassed age forty, global e^0 hovered around twenty-five years until about 1900 CE, and half of all lives ended before puberty.[113] Life's brevity across millennia and the world suggests that the Sadlermiut's experience was no aberration.

At the other end of the spectrum is information about the Aleutian Islands' Aleuts, who are related to the Inuit. In the nineteenth century, Russian Orthodox missionary Ivan Popov (1797–1879) recorded "quite a few" Aleuts on the eastern Aleutian Islands (Fox Islands) over age fifty-five and "a number of people between ages 90–100."[114] These numbers, coming from a theologian rather than a scientist, must be exaggerated.

A better health gauge was enamel hypoplasia—defined in Chapter 1—in Aleut and Inuit teeth.[115] The condition betrays undernutrition, especially during childhood when growth is normally rapid. An earlier section noted that Inuit children ate much shellfish. Providing few calories and almost no fat, shellfish might not have given them, active and inhabiting a harsh environment, enough energy.

This impression strengthens given Canadian anthropologist David John Damas' (1926–2010) 1972 remark that Nunavut Inuit girls began menarche late, though he did not quantify onset.[116] To this observation, June Helm added that Done men stood about 165.1 centimeters (65 inches).[117] This height is nearly 3 centimeters (1.2 inches) shorter than the average for Comanche men, Chapter 4 reported, the shortest Plains Indians in the late nineteenth century.[118] Because childhood nutrition influences adult height (see Chapter 1), shellfish might have given children inadequate calories if Inuit and Done children are comparable. This evidence is used cautiously because Done are not identical to Inuit, the groups likely having entered North America in separate waves. Done men were also over 8 centimeters (3.1 inches) shorter on average than northern Europe's men between roughly 800 and 1300 CE, suggesting that Done diets might have been inferior to medieval fare.[119]

During the past millennium, the shortest northern European men still averaged 7 millimeters (0.3 inches) above Done men.[120]

Nutrition alone does not explain these differences. Done are darker than northern Europeans because their skin has more melanin, a pigment that absorbs the sun's ultraviolet light. Done must therefore have originally lived near the equator, where darkness evolved as protection against the sun's intensity. Given this intensity, darkness did not prevent absorption of enough ultraviolet light to manufacture vitamin D. Chapters 1 and 2 discussed the connections among sunlight, vitamin D, minerals, the immune system, rickets, and osteomalacia. Northern Europeans, being lighter, evolved farther from the equator, where paleness admitted enough ultraviolet rays for vitamin-D synthesis at latitudes with less sunshine. Originally farther from the equator, they inhabited a colder climate and evolved large bodies that conserved heat according to Bergman's rule, discussed in Chapter 1. Near the equator, however, Done evolved small frames to dissipate heat. In other words, evolution, independent of nutrition, explains why northern Europeans are larger than Done. This section treats size as a proxy for stature while acknowledging that the two correlate imperfectly.

Also affecting health, food scarcity led roughly 10 percent of Northwest Territories' Inuit to starve in 1921 and 1922, stated Danish explorer Knud Johan Victor Rasmussen (1879–1933).[121] Trying to keep their numbers from outstripping food supply, these Inuit, like Chapter 4's Ache, practiced infanticide. In 1931, Rasmussen reported that parents killed thirty-eight of ninety-six female newborns.[122] Like the Ache, Inuit abandoned the old and ill who trailed the group.[123]

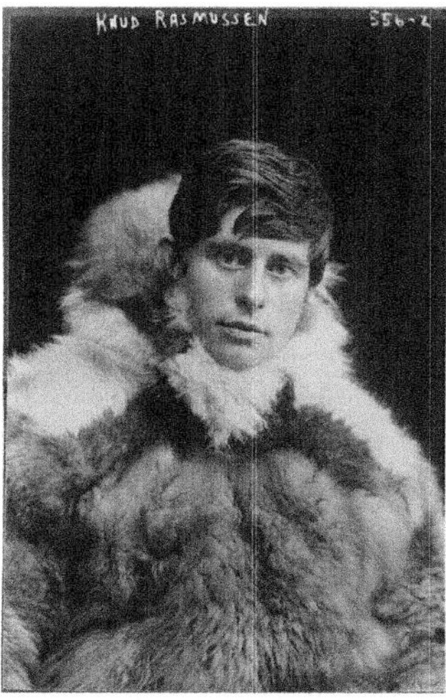

FIGURE 5.7 Knud Rasmussen. (Photo courtesy of Library of Congress. https://www.loc.gov/pictures/item/2014682626/.)

These circumstances presumably do not characterize affluent regions, where low-calorie options such as shellfish and fish may offset availability of too many fatty foods. Moreover, whatever seafood's drawbacks, Nunavut's Inuit remained spry into their seventh decade.[124] Americans, even those who do nothing more strenuous than sit in front of a computer, are ready to retire by then. In this context, research suggests that fish and fish fats preserve the elderly's strength and cognition.[125]

Fertility may be another seafood gauge. Chapter 4 cited research that fish consumption may increase fruitfulness.[126] Fertility, that chapter noted, may not measure vitality given that misery, deprivation, and squalor do not seem to limit reproduction. Instead, this book emphasizes that birthrate appears to correlate with infant mortality. Infanticide among Inuit, Ache, and other hunter-gatherers demonstrates that birthrate surpasses food supply in pitiless environments. Nonetheless, undernourishment may reduce fertility because women store sex hormones in fat. Below about

15 percent body fat, reproductivity diminishes.[127] Into the 1960s, the average Nunavut Inuit woman ate enough food and maintained enough body fat to deliver six to eight newborns.[128]

Another nutritional parameter was absence of osteoporosis, osteomalacia, and rickets—all discussed in Chapters 1 and 2—in early anthropological literature about Alaskan, Canadian, Greenland, and Pacific Northwest indigenes. Silence does not guarantee freedom from these conditions. Osteoporosis and osteomalacia are not evident upon inspection, though rickets' bow leggedness tends to be conspicuous. Before roughly the mid-twentieth century, reliance on fish, noted as the richest dietary source of vitamin D, appears to have prevented bone deformations severe enough to prompt detection.[129] In 2016, the Government of Northwest Territories recommended char for both vitamin D and calcium.[130] Other traditional vitamin D sources are seal liver, egg yolk, and blubber. Fish and comparable items must have been essential to bone health so far north, where, as mentioned, sunshine is inadequate much of the year. Although a 2005 study attributed differences in bone density between Greenland Inuit and whites to unequal body size rather than nutrition, reduction in fish intake has made rickets twelve times more prevalent among Nunavut Inuit than white Canadians.[131]

Besides research is the example of Vilhjalmur Stefansson. He arrived in the Northwest Territories in 1906 unenthusiastic about fish.[132] Displeasure abated after months living on fish and water. He grew more energetic and alert and came to appreciate the absence of overweight and obesity among Inuit despite fatty diets. Beyond fish and marine mammals, strenuous lives as hunter-gatherers contributed to their trimness. The experience led him to advocate fat over carbohydrates. Consequently, fat's proponents, treated in Chapter 10, gravitate to Stefansson's books.

5.6 GREAT BRITAIN

5.6.1 Geography and Settlement

Great Britain—Britain for our purposes—is an island north of France. England, Scotland, and Wales constitute the island, which humans occupied about 30,000 years ago.[133] During the last ice age (c. 115,000–c. 11,700 years ago), the poles held enough water as ice to diminish sea levels, connecting Britain with the rest of Europe and facilitating movement between both. A rising ocean made Britain an island in the fifth or fourth millennium BCE but did not end migrations, which continued during Europe's Neolithic Period (c. 4000–c. 2500 BCE), Bronze Age (c. 2500–c. 800 BCE), Iron Age (c. 800 BCE–42 CE), Roman antiquity (43–410), Anglo-Saxon rule (c. 500–1066), Viking raids (793–850), and Norman conquest (1066).[134]

5.6.2 Centrality of Fishing in Earliest Times and Antiquity

The North Sea, North Atlantic Ocean, rivers, lakes, and ponds supplied fish and shellfish. Spears for catching salmon in Northern Ireland's Bann River dated from the Mesolithic Period (9600–4000 BCE) and provided the earliest evidence for fishing near Britain.[135] During these millennia, Scots on Oronsay Island ate crab, limpet, mussel, whelk (*Busycon carica*), oyster, European conger (*Conger conger*), haddock (*Melanogrammus aeglefinus*), sea bream, ballan wrasse (*Labrus bergylta*), thornback ray (*Raja clavata*), skate (*Dipturus batis*), and shark. Throughout prehistory and history, shellfish fed the poor. The rich sometimes disdained it for that reason, eating it only occasionally. In modernity, however, all classes consumed shellfish. Seafood was most plentiful during summer. Transition to agriculture let farmers fish in early summer, when chores were not onerous.[136] During the Iron Age, cod fishing intensified. Around 600 BCE, Celts in Britain began salting fish and meats. Fishers salted the catch on the coast, selling it at inland markets.[137]

Conquering Britain in 43 CE, the Romans targeted cod, lingcod, haddock, crab, lobster, oyster, whelk, cockle, mussel, and limpet, shipping oysters to Rome.[138] The Romans taught Brits to prefer marine over freshwater species, partiality that persisted centuries. Although the Romans practiced aquaculture, evidence is absent from Britain.[139] Also unclear is the extent to which it adopted Rome's enthusiasm for garum, a fermented sauce of red mullet (*Mullus barbatus* and *Mullus surmuletus*), sprat (*Sprattus sprattus*), European anchovy (*Engraulis encrasicolus*), mackerel, and salt (sodium chloride).[140]

5.6.3 Fishing in the Middle Ages

Rome left the island in the early fifth century, leaving Germanic Anglo-Saxons and the Christian Church in charge. A unifying force, the church permitted fish but not meat on Fridays. Chapter 1 noted the biblical connection between fish and Jesus, unsurprising given that the canonical gospels were written in Greek and that the Greek *ichthys* means "fish" and is an acrostic for "Jesus Christ, Son of God, Savior."[141]

During the Middle Ages, abstinence from meat came to encompass all Lent, the forty weekdays between Ash Wednesday and Easter. This requirement made sense in temperate regions. Lent comes late in winter, after the slaughter of all livestock but what could be kept for reproduction given inability to graze when grasses were dormant. Moreover, until 1216 British monks obeyed the *Rule of St. Benedict* (c. 530), a set of guidelines by Italian abbot Benedict of Nursia (c. 480–c. 543), which forbade meat but not fish or poultry to all but the ill.[142] In addition to Fridays and Lent, the church banished meat from Wednesdays, Saturdays, and all fasting days, a total that eliminated it half the year. Readers, accustomed to the reality that few honor traffic laws when police are absent, might wonder whether people obeyed these strictures. Malcontents must have ignored regulations, but faith was strong in medieval Britain, and communities expected conformity.

Whatever the magnitude of compliance, consumption was large enough that Britain imported dried fish, chiefly cod, from Norway beginning in the ninth century.[143] The Anglo-Saxon practice of cooking fish in iron cauldrons must have been ubiquitous, inspiring the expression "kettle of fish." In the ninth and tenth centuries, Vikings settled Britain, targeting herring and whitefish. In 1066, French Normans conquered Britain. Enthusiasm for fish is evident in their promotion each year between September 29 and November 11 of a herring festival in Great Yarmouth, England.[144] Normans accepted rent as salted herring, mackerel, salmon, and eel (species in the order Anguilliformes). Church leaders like abbots and bishops took two or three courses of fish at meals, and Duchess of York Cecily Neville (1415–1495), mother of King Edward IV (1442–1483), served fish thrice daily—one salted and two fresh—during fasts.[145] Royalty employed fishers to supply this bounty. Laws gave lords half the fish and all unusual specimens caught on their property.[146] Royalty claimed all sturgeon. Twelfth-century texts listed consumption of plaice (*Pleuronectes platessa*), cod, European flounder (*Platichthys flesus*), gudgeon (*Gobio gobio*), loach (species in the superfamily Cobitoidea), roach (*Rutilus rutilus*), tench (*Tinca tinca*), Dover sole (*Solea solea*), mudfish (*Neochanna burrowsius*), and lamprey (*Lampetra fluviatilis*).

During the Middle Ages, salted herring became the Lenten staple.[147] In addition to herring, British food historian Constance Anne Wilson (b. 1934) asserted that during Lent, medieval Brits combined Atlantic salmon (*Salmo salar*), codling, or haddock with figs (*Ficus carica*), raisins (*Vitis vinifera*), apples (*Malus domestica*), pears (*Pyrus* species), and sucrose.[148] The last, however, was uncommon before the sixteenth-century establishment of plantations in tropical America. Before 1500, Brits and other Europeans seldom had sucrose, though fructose and glucose—both ($C_6H_{12}O_6$)—were available in honey. In the sixteenth century, the average European consumed just 4 grams (1 teaspoon) of sucrose annually.[149] The only commercial source then was sugarcane (*Saccharum officinarum*) because sugar beet (*Beta vulgaris ssp. vulgaris*) was unknown until the mid-eighteenth century. Chapters 2 and 11 discuss sweeteners.

5.6.4 Consumption of Salted Fish

By the thirteenth century, Britain's appetite for salt necessitated imports from France.[150] The prevalence of salting for preservation implies that everyone who ate salted fish consumed too much. Whereas preagricultural peoples ingested under 1 gram of salt daily, by roughly 1400 the average European ate 20 grams per day.[151] This peak doubled today's intake, which remains inordinate.

Chapter 2 implicated sodium in high blood pressure, heart disease, and kidney disease. Although bones contain sodium, too much in the diet depletes their calcium, causing osteoporosis.[152] Sodium raises the risk of stomach cancer, asthma, liver disease, and obesity. Children who overindulge undermine health into adulthood. Superfluity appears to weaken cognition in the old. Sodium especially harms sub-Saharan Africans, Indians, Pakistanis, and Bengalis.[153]

Despite hazards, Chapter 2 identified sodium and chloride as electrolytes. As noted above and in Chapter 2, sodium is in bones. With hydrogen, chloride forms hydrochloric acid (HCl) to aid digestion. From early times, salt was essential to replace electrolytes lost from perspiration in warm climates. Nomads did not cross deserts without it. Like several other nutrients and as indicated, however, surfeit damages rather than benefits the body. The generalization that if small amounts are good, then more must be better is untrue.

Wilson wrote that the poor ate more salted fish than the affluent, implying that poverty correlated with illnesses from excess sodium.[154] Fresh fish's expensiveness dissuaded the poor rather than the rich from buying it. Contradicting her, American economist, historian, and 1993 Nobel laureate in economics Robert William Fogel (1926–2013) asserted that British elites weakened their health by eating too much salted fish and meat before roughly 1725.[155] Britain's poor lived as long as members of the House of Lords (peers) because they ate healthier diets. The next section details these circumstances.

5.6.5 Increasing Demand for Fish and Shellfish

Whether salted or fresh, demand for fish drove the British, benefitting from improvements in navigation and shipbuilding, to seek cod near Iceland in the fifteenth century.[156] Leaving port in February or March, sailors salted cod aboard ship, returning in autumn to sell their catch. The masses purchased cod, pollock (*Pollachius virens*), sculpin, lingcod, and shellfish. After declining in late antiquity, shellfish sales rose after roughly 700, a trend that continued into modernity.[157] Large families bought hundreds on a single trip to market. London's poor ate oysters, which were much cheaper than fish. Wilson noted consumption of lobster, crayfish, or crab with sucrose, almond milk, cloves (*Syzygium aromaticum*), and mace (*Myristica fragrans*).[158] Her narrative must have omitted the masses because sucrose, cloves, and mace were expensive tropical imports in the fifteenth century. Beyond shellfish, perch, carp, bream, salmon, trout, grayling, barbel, chub (*Squalius cephalus*), tench, roach, Eurasian dace (*Leuciscus leuciscus*), bleak (*Alburnus alburnus*), ruff (*Arripis georgianus*), flounder, eel, pike, and minnow (*Phoxinus phoxinus*) were popular.[159] Commoners bought eel because it was the least expensive fish, making stew with it or other seafood, barley (*Hordeum vulgare*), oats (*Avena sativa*), herbs like parsley (*Petroselinum crispum*), or their combination.

Fish stoked the appetite. A sixteenth-century menu indicated that one wealthy couple shared two loaves of white bread (probably *Triticum aestivum*) known as manchet, ten herrings or sprats, and 0.9 liters (1 quart) each of beer and wine for breakfast.[160] Affluent Brits ate up to 1.4 kilograms (3 pounds) of fish or meat daily.[161] Even children consumed fish and beer.

This paragraph attempts to detail fish intake. Taking herring as an example, FAO graphed a range of masses, though a typical herring is between roughly 70 and 200 grams, whose average is 135 grams.[162] Ten herrings for a couple at breakfast allot five per person or 675 grams. But Neville served fish at every meal, a practice that triples our 675 grams to just over 2 kilograms. The mean between it and the above 1.4 kilograms is 1.7 kilograms of fish daily for a wealthy Briton.

Retaining herring as the example, Table 5.4 lists calories and nutrients in 1.7 kilograms.[163]

TABLE 5.4
Nutrients in Herring 1.7 kg

Nutrient	Herring	%DV
Calories	2,686	N/A
Protein (g)	305.3	N/A
Fat (g)	153.7	N/A
Carbs (g)	0	N/A
Fiber (g)	0	N/A
	Minerals	
Ca (mg)	969	96.9
Fe (mg)	18.7	103.9
Mg (mg)	544	136
P (mg)	4,012	401.2
K (mg)	5,559	158.8
Na (mg)	1,530	63.8
Zn (mg)	16.8	112
Cu (mg)	1.6	80
Mn (mg)	0.6	30
Se (mcg)	620.5	886.4
	Vitamins	
A (IU)	1,581	31.6
B_1 (mg)	1.6	106.7
B_2 (mg)	4	235.3
B_3 (mg)	54.7	273.5
B_5 (mg)	11	110
B_6 (mg)	5.1	255
B_9 (mcg)	170	42.5
B_{12} (mcg)	232.4	3,873.3
C (mg)	11.9	19.8
D (IU)	2,839	709.8
E (mg)	18.2	121.3
K (mcg)	1.7	2.1

Even at this mass, sodium is under DV. But one-third of Neville's fish was salted. Applying this proportion to our example, one-third of 1.7 kilograms equals 566.7 grams of salted herring. I know no way to pinpoint the amount of sodium in this quantity in the sixteenth century, but an estimate is possible using U.S. Department of Agriculture's (USDA) measurement of 1,181 milligrams of sodium per 100 grams of salted herring.[164] This value is 49.2 percent of sodium's DV, though 566.7 grams of salted herring exceed DV almost 2.8 times.[165]

Returning to the narrative, Parliament encouraged fish eating by reinstituting Wednesday and Saturday bans against meat that had lapsed in the late Middle Ages.[166] Overfishing resulted in the next century, increasing fish prices. Parliament further heightened prices by taxing salt.[167] Britain depleted, fishers in the sixteenth and seventeenth centuries entered waters near New England, Newfoundland and Labrador, and Nova Scotia.[168] At the same time, nobility relinquished sturgeon, allowing it to sell in markets. In the eighteenth century, Britain met the demand for fish partly by importing mullet and anchovies from the Mediterranean Sea.[169] That century, consumption of freshwater species, long overexploited as mentioned, declined in favor of ocean fish. Toward century's end, processors began packing fish in ice, obviating the need for salt.[170] This transition occurred first with salmon in Scotland, where fresh and frozen supplanted salted.

5.6.6 Dietary Trends

Besides this development, two trends affected nutrition. First, sixteenth- and seventeenth-century British cooks began garnishing fish with sour oranges (*Citrus aurantium*). Lemons (*Citrus limon*) followed in the eighteenth century. Depending on the amount, such additions supplied vitamin C, which fish lacks. Designated a serving, 85 grams of sour oranges have 120 percent of vitamin C's DV.[171] The same quantity of lemons furnishes roughly half as much vitamin C.[172] Second, by the 1870s, fried fish and potatoes (*Solanum tuberosum*), known as fish and chips and supplying fat and calories, were popular among laborers.[173] Advertised online, for example, Joey's Seafood fish and chips yield 56 percent of calories as fat.[174] By contrast, tuna canned in water supplies 10 percent of calories as fat.[175] Despite excess fat and calories, this combination increased the consumption of potatoes, which Chapter 13 judges the healthiest food.

5.6.7 Health in Britain

Fogel tabulated e^0 for British peers and commoners from 1551 to 1925. Peerage as an institution traced its lineage to the twelfth century when England's monarchs invited the largest, richest landowners to form Parliament. An onlooker might expect peers to have outlived commoners because, Chapter 1 noted, longevity correlates with wealth. For example, the richest 1 percent of U.S. men outlive the poorest 1 percent by almost fifteen years.[176] Because access to healthcare does not appear to be decisive, wealth may provide an advantage beyond other factors. If it alone lengthens life, then peers should have outlasted the commoner.

Yet Table 5.5 demonstrates that before 1725 they did not. Between 1601 and 1675, peers as a group died younger than the masses, and in other decades neither had an advantage of over a year or two.[177] Fogel faulted nobles for consuming too much salted fish and meat, bread, and alcohol and too few vegetables and fruits.[178] The last section supported this assessment, recalling one couple's breakfast menu as evidence that the wealthy likely ate more calories at one meal than they

TABLE 5.5
E^0 in England and Wales

Time	Peers (Yrs)	Commoners (Yrs)
1551–1575	38	35.6
1576–1600	37.2	38
1601–1625	34.7	37.3
1626–1650	33	35.5
1651–1675	31.9	34.2
1676–1700	34.2	33.5
1701–1725	36.2	35.1
1726–1750	38.1	33.8
1751–1775	40.2	36.3
1776–1800	48.1	37
1801–1825	50.6	41.5
1826–1850	55.3	44.6
1851–1875	58.6	N/A
1876–1900	60.2	N/A
1901–1925	65	N/A

needed all day. They compounded gluttony with idleness, having the money to hire servants for arduous jobs. They did not work their large hectarages but instead rented land to tenants. Those who owned plantations in the Caribbean bought slaves. In this context, Britain functioned like ancient Egypt, discussed in Chapter 4, with a chasm between indolent, flabby elites and overworked, underfed commoners and *hemw*.

Before 1725, Britain's masses ate more varied diets than aristocrats. The poor ate less meat but more vegetables and dairy and probably consumed more vitamins, minerals, and phytochemicals than elites, who were likely deficient in vitamins A, C, and D.[179] Like Done, however, British children's shortness indicated undernourishment. Between 1750 and 1800, London's poorest were shorter than slaves from the Caribbean island Trinidad.[180] These slaves, in turn, stood below 99 percent of all English laborers.[181] Oysters and other inexpensive seafood, noted as the poor's staples, must have nourished Britain's destitute children worse than Caribbean slaves, who themselves were underfed. A previous section and earlier chapters emphasized that children, who normally grow rapidly, are especially vulnerable to undernutrition. London's overcrowding and contagion joined inadequate diets in afflicting the poor. Moreover, poor children left school young to work long hours in factories. Deprived of sunshine, they suffered rickets, discussed in Chapters 1 and 2. Overwork exacerbated undernutrition and diseases.

Although spared poverty, British nobles as a group did not reach age forty before 1750.[182] Eliminating mortality before age ten should have increased longevity, but gains were elusive before 1925.[183] Awash in sodium, peers likely suffered kidney and heart disease. Too much alcohol throughout life worsened health. After 1725, however, a gap opened between aristocrats and the masses. By 1850, nobles lived on average eleven years longer than commoners.[184] Fogel could not explain this increase, but the answer may lie in Wilson's earlier remark that in the late eighteenth century fish began to be preserved with ice rather than salt. Diminution in sodium consumption must have lessened the burden on heart and kidneys. Readers might evaluate their salt intake against these data.

United Kingdom pharmacologist Paul Clayton and historian Judith D. Rowbotham (b. 1952), both introduced in Chapter 1, argued that Britain's masses lived long, vigorous lives between roughly 1850 and 1870. Subtracting mortality before age five, commoners lived as long as today's developed populations despite medical care that current physicians would deem substandard.[185] Fresh herring was a staple in autumn, winter, and spring. Other seafood included sprat, eel, cod, haddock, John Dory (*Zeus faber*), oyster, whelk, mussel, and cockle. Brits ate the whole fish rather than just muscles as is common today. In addition to fish and some meat, the masses consumed onions (*Allium cepa*), watercress (*Nasturtium officinale*), Jerusalem artichoke (*Helianthus tuberosus*), carrot (*Daucus carota ssp. sativus*), turnip (*Brassica rapa ssp. rapa*), cabbage (*Brassica oleracea var. capitata*), broccoli (*Brassica oleracea var. italica*), peas (*Pisum sativum*), beans, chestnuts (*Castanea sativa*), walnuts (*Jaglans regia*), hazelnuts (*Corylus avellana*), Brazil nuts (*Bertholletia excelsa*), almonds (*Prunus dulcis*), apples, plums (*Prunus domestica*), gooseberries (*Ribes uva-crispa*), chicken (*Gallus domesticus*), eggs, and cheese. Clayton and Rowbotham did not specify the beans, but they were likely *Phaseolus vulgaris*, which since the sixteenth century (see Chapter 8) had become global staples.

Fish and other wholesome foods did not alone confer vitality. Mid-nineteenth century Brits lived before machines like automobiles reduced exertion. Automation, explored throughout this book, is central to modernity's disconnect with the past. The automobile fosters inactivity and causes chronic diseases. These British and others who predated it walked wherever they went. Servants performed the drudgery that their employers evaded. Women hauled coal to heat homes, and men who built roads and railways metabolized as many as 5,000 calories daily.[186] Farm and factory labor was arduous. On average, commoners ate twice what we do because they worked harder and longer.

Chapter 3 contrasted this vigor with modern inertness and, with the rest of this book, argued that vitality requires exertion. Diet alone cannot scale the summit of health. Chapter 4 noted that Egypt's wealthy, Plains Indians, and Ache all ate much meat, but only Plains Indians and Ache were vigorous, at least before confinement on reservations. Their activity contrasted with Egyptian elites' indolence that combined with fatty meats to cause heart disease. This chapter emphasized the rarity of heart disease and cancers among Inuit who were active besides eating fish. Clayton and Rowbotham documented this phenomenon in Britain about 1850, quoting a physician who in 1869 showed medical students a cancerous lung, knowing it might be their only opportunity to study the malignancy.[187] The authors labeled cancers, heart disease, and stroke as "uncommon" in the mid-nineteenth century, blaming their current ubiquity on "chronic malnutrition" and "low energy lifestyles."[188]

NOTES

1 Christopher Lloyd, *Absolutely Everything!: A History of Earth, Dinosaurs, Rulers, Robots and Other Things too Numerous to Mention* (Tonbridge, UK: What on Earth Books, 2018), 18.
2 Kathryn Hennessy, ed., *Smithsonian Natural History: The Ultimate Visual Guide to Everything on Earth* (New York: DK, 2010), 22.
3 Carol Hand, *The Evolution of Fish* (Minneapolis, MN: ABDO Publishing, 2019), 5–6.
4 F. D. Ommanney, *The Fishes* (New York: Time, 1964), 68–69; Jacques Cousteau, *The Ocean World* (New York: Bradale Press/Harry N. Abrams, 1985.
5 Ommanney, 68–69; Hennessy, 320.
6 Hennessy, 13.
7 Doreen Gonzales, *The Huge Pacific Ocean* (Berkeley Heights, NJ: Enslow, 2013), 17; Michael Allaby, *Oceans: A Scientific History of Oceans and Marine Life* (New York: Facts on File, 2009), 120.
8 Mark Brush, "Lake Erie Has 2% of the Water in the Great Lakes, but 50% of the Fish," *Michigan Radio*, November 5, 2013, accessed February 14, 2019, http://www.michiganradio.org/post/lake-erie-has-2-water-great-lakes-50-fish.
9 "Lake Okeechobee Fishing Records Catch," accessed February 14, 2019, https://lakeokeechobee-bassfishing.com/fish-records.
10 Bruce Bower, "Orangutans Use Simple Tools to Catch Fish," *Wired*, April 18, 2011, accessed February 14, 2019, https://www.wired.com/2011/04/orangutan-tools-fishing.
11 Stephanie Pappas, "Ancient 'Brain Food' Helped Humans Get Smart," *Live Science*, June 3, 2010, accessed February 14, 2019, https://www.livescience.com/10664-ancient-brain-food-helped-humans-smart.html.
12 Ibid.
13 Ommanney, 169.
14 Brian Fagan, *Fishing: How the Sea Fed Civilization* (New Haven, CT and London: Yale University Press, 2017), 6; Clark Spencer Larsen, "Dietary Reconstruction and Nutritional Assessment of Past Peoples: The Bioanthropological Record," in *The Cambridge World History of Food*, vol. 1, ed. Kenneth F. Kiple and Kriemhild Conee Ornelas (Cambridge, UK: Cambridge University Press, 2000), 14.
15 Ommanney, 169.
16 Loren Cordain, *The Paleo Diet: Lose Weight and Get Healthy by Eating the Foods You Were Designed to Eat*, rev. ed. (Hoboken, NJ: Wiley, 2011), 5, 25–26.
17 Mark Nathan Cohen, *Health and the Rise of Civilization* (New Haven, CT and London: Yale University Press, 1989), 55–56; Mark Nathan Cohen, "History, Diet, and Hunter-Gatherers," in *The Cambridge World History of Food*, vol 1, ed. Kenneth F. Kiple and Kriemhild Conee Ornelas (Cambridge, UK: Cambridge University Press, 2000), 66.
18 Ewen Callaway, "Seafood Gave Us the Edge on the Neanderthals," New Scientist, August 12, 2009, accessed February 14, 2019, https://www.newscientist.com/article/dn17595-seafood-gave-us-the-edge-on-the-neanderthals.
19 Bruce L. Hardy and Marie-Helene Moncel, "Neanderthal Use of Fish, Mammals, Birds, Starchy Plants and Wood 125–250,000 Years Ago," *Plos One* 6, no. 8 (August 24, 2011), accessed February 14, 2019, https://journals.plos.org/plosone/article?id=10.1371/journal.pone.0023768.
20 "Early Modern Humans Consumed More Plants than Neanderthals But Ate Very Little Fish," *Phys. org*, August 8, 2017, accessed February 14, 2019, https://phys.org/news/2017-08-early-modern-humans-consumed-neanderthals.html.
21 Fagan, 38; Dietrich Sahrhage and Johannes Lundbeck, *A History of Fishing* (Berlin: Springer-Verlag, 1992), 22.
22 Andrew F. Smith, "From Garum to Ketchup. A Spicy Tale of Two Fish Sauces," in *Food in the Arts: Proceedings of the Oxford Symposium on Food and Cookery, 1997*, ed. Harlan Walker (Devon, UK: Prospect Books, 1998), 300.

23 James H. Barrett, Alison M. Locker, and Callum M. Roberts, "The Origins of Intensive Marine Fishing in Medieval Europe: the English Evidence," *Proceedings of the Royal Society* 271, no. 1556 (December 7, 2004): 2417–2421, https://royalsocietypublishing.org/doi/abs/10.1098/rspb.2004.2885.

24 Fagan, 100–101.

25 Anna. C. Roosevelt, "Archaeology of South American Hunters and Gatherers," in *The Cambridge Encyclopedia of Hunters and Gatherers*, ed. Richard B. Lee and Richard Daly (Cambridge, UK and New York: Cambridge University Press, 2004), 88.

26 Fagan, 230; D. F. Gartside and I. R. Kirkegaard, "A History of Fishing," UNESCO, accessed December 7, 2019, https://www.eolss.net/sample-chapters/C10/E5-01A-03-00.pdf.

27 E. W. Gudger, "Fishing with Spider's Webs," *Scientific American Supplement* 87, no. 2253 (March 8, 1919): 149.

28 Gartside and Kirkegaard.

29 Sahrhage, 104–106.

30 Gartside and Kirkegaard.

31 Sahrhage, 109.

32 Ibid., 117.

33 Food and Agriculture Organization, *The State of World Fisheries and Aquaculture* (Rome: Food and Agriculture Organization of the United Nations, 2018), 9.

34 Christos Pitsavos, Christina-Maria Kastorini, and Christodoulos Stefanadis, "Fish Consumption and Health," in *Fish Consumption and Health*, ed. George P. Gagne and Richard H. Medrano (New York: Nova Science Publishers, 2009), 2.

35 Colin E. Nash, "Aquatic Animals," in *The Cambridge World History of Food*, vol 1, ed. Kenneth F. Kiple and Kriemhild Conee Ornelas (Cambridge, UK: Cambridge University Press, 2000), 465.

36 J. Samuel Godber, "Nutritional Value of Muscle Foods," in *Muscle Foods: Meat, Poultry, and Seafood Technology*, ed. Donald M. Kinsman, Anthony W. Kotula, and Burdette C. Breidenstein (New York and London: Chapman and Hall, 1994), 438, 441, 445–446; L. Jahns, "Fish Intake in the United States," in *Fish and Fish Oil in Health and Disease Prevention*, ed. Susan K. Raatz and Douglas M. Bibus (Amsterdam: Academic Press, 2016), 4; "Tuna, Canned, Water Pack," USDA FoodData Central, April 1, 2019, accessed January 21, 2020, https://fdc.nal.usda.gov/fdc-app.html#/food-details/337833/nutrients; "Fish, Tuna, White, Canned in Water, Drained Solids," *USDA FoodData Central*, April 1, 2019, accessed January 21, 2020, https://fdc.nal.usda.gov/fdc-app.html#/food-details/175158/nutrients; "Fish, Tilapia, Raw," *USDA FoodData Central*, April 1, 2019, accessed January 21, 2020, https://fdc.nal.usda.gov/fdc-app.html#/food-details/175176/nutrients; "Fish, Pollock, Alaska, Raw," *USDA FoodData Central*, April 1, 2019, accessed January 21, 2020, https://fdc.nal.usda.gov/fdc-app.html#/food-details/173725/nutrients; "Mackerel, Raw," *USDA FoodData Central*, April 1, 2019, accessed January 21, 2020, https://fdc.nal.usda.gov/fdc-app.html#/food-details/337677/nutrients; "Fish, Mackerel, Atlantic, Raw," *USDA FoodData Central*, April 1, 2019, accessed January 21, 2020, https://fdc.nal.usda.gov/fdc-app.html#/food-details/175119/nutrients; "Fish, Cod, Atlantic, Raw," *USDA FoodData Central*, April 1, 2019, accessed January 21, 2020, https://fdc.nal.usda.gov/fdc-app.html#/food-details/171955/nutrients.

37 "Snails, Clams, Squids and Octopodes," *Biokids*, 2002–2019, accessed February 23, 2019, http://www.biokids.umich.edu/critters/Mollusca.

38 Ken Babal, *Seafood Sense: The Truth about Seafood Nutrition and Safety* (Laguna Beach, CA: Basic Health Publications, 2005), 18.

39 Godber, 438, 441, 445–446, Jahns, 4.

40 "Mussels," *Eat This Much*, 2019, accessed February 23, 2019, https://www.eatthismuch.com/food/nutrition/mussels,127416.

41 P. K. Newby, *Food and Nutrition: What Everyone Needs to Know* (New York: Oxford University Press, 2018), 186.

42 Godber, 438, 441, 445–446; Jahns, 4; "Crustaceans, Shrimp, Raw," *USDA FoodData Central*, April 1, 2019, accessed January 21, 2020, https://fdc.nal.usda.gov/fdc-app.html#/food-details/175179/nutrients; "100 G, Shrimp," *Fat Secret*, 2020, accessed January 21, 2020, https://www.fatsecret.com/calories-nutrition/usda/shrimp?portionid=60841&portionamount=100.000; "Oysters, Raw," *USDA FoodData Central*, April 1, 2019, accessed January 21, 2020, https://fdc.nal.usda.gov/fdc-app.html#/food-details/337923/nutrients; "Mollusks, Oysters, Eastern, Wild, Raw," *Self Nutrition Data*, 2018, accessed January 21, 2020, https://nutritiondata.self.com/facts/finfish-and-shellfish-products/4189/2; "Crustaceans, Lobster, Northern, Raw," *USDA FoodData Central*, April 1, 2019, accessed January 21, 2020, https://fdc.nal.usda.gov/fdc-app.html#/food-details/174208/nutrients; "Clams, Raw," *USDA FoodData Central*, April 1, 2019, accessed January 21, 2020, https://fdc.nal.usda.gov/fdc-app.html#/food-details/337892/nutrients; "Mollusks, Clam,

Mixed Species, Raw," *USDA FoodData Central*, April 1, 2019, accessed January 21, 2020, https://fdc.nal.usda.gov/fdc-app.html#/food-details/174214/nutrients; "Crustaceans, Crab, Blue, Raw," *USDA FoodData Central*, April 1, 2019, accessed January 21, 2020, https://fdc.nal.usda.gov/fdc-app.html#/food-details/174204/nutrients; "Amount of Vitamin D in Crab," *Diet and Fitness Today*, 2005–2020, accessed January 21, 2020, http://www.dietandfitnesstoday.com/vitamin-d-in-crab.php; "Amount of Vitamin K in Crab," *Diet and Fitness Today*, 2005–2020, accessed January 21, 2020, http://www.dietandfitnesstoday.com/vitamin-k-in-crab.php; "Amount of Vitamin E in Crab," *Diet and Fitness Today*, 2005–2020, accessed January 21, 2020, http://www.dietandfitnesstoday.com/vitamin-e-in-crab.php.

43 Newby, 75.

44 Nash, 465.

45 Jahns, 4; "Fish, Salmon, Atlantic, Wild, Raw," *USDA FoodData Central*, April 1, 2019, accessed January 21, 2020, https://fdc.nal.usda.gov/fdc-app.html#/food-details/173686/nutrients; "Fish, Salmon, Coho, Wild, Raw," *USDA FoodData Central*, April 1, 2019, accessed January 21, 2020, https://fdc.nal.usda.gov/fdc-app.html#/food-details/175136/nutrients; "Fish, Salmon, Atlantic, Farmed, Raw," *USDA FoodData Central*, April 1, 2019, accessed January 21, 2020, https://fdc.nal.usda.gov/fdc-app.html#/food-details/175167/nutrients; "Fish, Catfish, Channel, Wild, Raw," *USDA FoodData Central*, April 1, 2019, accessed January 21, 2020, https://fdc.nal.usda.gov/fdc-app.html#/food-details/174186/nutrients; "Fish, Catfish, Channel, Farmed, Raw," *USDA FoodData Central*, April 1, 2019, accessed January 21, 2020, https://fdc.nal.usda.gov/fdc-app.html#/food-details/175165/nutrients.

46 Newby, 191.

47 Jahns, 11.

48 Newby, 192.

49 Nash, 456.

50 Newby, 192.

51 Johnny O. Ogunji, "Fish Consumption: A Paradox of Good Health," in *Fish Consumption and Health*, ed. George P. Gagne and Richard H. Medrano (New York: Nova Science Publishers, 2009), 86.

52 Ibid.

53 "The World: Life Expectancy (2018)," *geoba.se*, 2019, accessed February 16, 2019, http://www.geoba.se/population.php?pc=world&type=015&year=2018&st=country&asde=&page=1.

54 Kashmira Gander, "Japan's High Life Expectancy Linked to Diet, Study Finds," *Independent*, March 28, 2016, accessed February 16, 2019, https://www.independent.co.uk/life-style/health-and-families/health-news/high-life-expectancy-in-japan-partly-down-to-diet-carbohydrates-vegetables-fruit-fish-meat-a6956011.html.

55 "The World: Life Expectancy (2018);" Chaya Shepard, "Food in Monaco," *Vagabond Journey*, November 6, 2011, accessed February 16, 2019, https://www.vagabondjourney.com/food-in-monaco.

56 "The World: Life Expectancy (2018)."

57 "Singapore: Seafood Report 2017," *USDA*, November 10, 2017, accessed February 16, 2019, https://www.fas.usda.gov/data/singapore-seafood-report-2017.

58 Joseph S. Nelson, "Fish," *The Canadian Encyclopedia*, October 25, 2010, last modified March 4, 2015, accessed February 23, 2019, https://www.thecanadianencyclopedia.ca/en/article/fishes.

59 "Arctic Ocean Diversity," *Census of Marine Life*, accessed February 23, 2019, http://www.arcodiv.org/Fish.html.

60 Ibid.

61 Alex Peden, "An Introduction to the Marine Fish of British Columbia," *Electronic Atlas of the Wildlife of British Columbia*, 2018, accessed February 23, 2019, http://ibis.geog.ubc.ca/biodiversity/efauna/IntroductiontotheMarineFishofBritishColumbia.html.

62 June Helm and Thomas D. Andrews, "Tlicho (Dogrib)," *The Canadian Encyclopedia*, August 6, 2009, last modified March 4, 2015, accessed February 21, 2019, https://www.thecanadianencyclopedia.ca/en/article/tlicho-dogrib.

63 Zach Parrott, "Indigenous Peoples in Canada," *The Canadian Encyclopedia*, March 13, 2007, last modified October 12, 2018, accessed February 21, 2019, https://www.thecanadianencyclopedia.ca/en/article/aboriginal-people.

64 "Indigenous Peoples in Greenland," *IWGIA*, accessed February 21, 2019, https://www.iwgia.org/en/greenland.

65 Edward S. Roger, "The Mistassini Cree," in *Hunters and Gatherers Today: A Socioeconomic Study of Eleven Such Cultures in the Twentieth Century*, ed. M. G. Bicchieri (Prospect Heights, IL: Waveland Press, 1972), 104.

66 "Black Builders Bucket. Holds 3 Gallons of Liquid." *Amazon.com*, 1996–2019, accessed February 21, 2019, https://www.amazon.co.uk/Black-Builders-Bucket-Gallons-Liquid/dp/B005COYVEA.
67 Roger, 104.
68 Ibid., 102.
69 Ernest S. Burch, Jr. and Yvon Csonka, "The Caribou Inuit," in *The Cambridge Encyclopedia of Hunters and Gatherers*, ed. Richard B. Lee and Richard Daly (Cambridge, UK and New York: Cambridge University Press, 2004), 57–58.
70 Andreas Eenfeldt, *Low Carb, High Fat Food Revolution: Advice and Recipes to Improve Your Health and Reduce Your Weight*, trans. Viktoria Lindback (New York: Skyhorse Publishing, 2014), 131.
71 June Helm, "The Dogrib Indians," in *Hunters and Gatherers Today: A Socioeconomic Study of Eleven Such Cultures in the Twentieth Century*, ed. M. G. Bicchieri (Prospect Heights, IL: Waveland Press, 1972), 61.
72 Rosita Worl, "Inupiat Arctic Whalers," in *The Cambridge Encyclopedia of Hunters and Gatherers*, ed. Richard B. Lee and Richard Daly (Cambridge, UK and New York: Cambridge University Press, 2004), 61.
73 Aubrey Cannon, "Archaeology of North American Hunters and Gatherers," in *The Cambridge Encyclopedia of Hunters and Gatherers*, ed. Richard B. Lee and Richard Daly (Cambridge, UK and New York: Cambridge University Press, 2004), 33.
74 Waverley Root and Richard de Rochemont, *Eating in America: A History* (Hopewell, NJ: Ecco Press, 1995), 21.
75 Richard Daly, "Witsuwit'en and Gitxsau of the Western Cordillera," in *The Cambridge Encyclopedia of Hunters and Gatherers*, ed. Richard B. Lee and Richard Daly (Cambridge, UK and New York: Cambridge University Press, 2004), 71–72.
76 Roger, 103, 112.
77 Ibid., 108–109.
78 Harvey A. Feit, "James Bay Cree," in *The Cambridge Encyclopedia of Hunters and Gatherers*, ed. Richard B. Lee and Richard Daly (Cambridge, UK and New York: Cambridge University Press, 2004), 43.
79 Ibid.
80 Helm, "Dogrib Indians," 55.
81 Ibid.
82 Ibid., 63, 71.
83 Ibid., 67.
84 Ibid.
85 Michael Asch and Shirleen Smith, "Slavey Dene," in *The Cambridge Encyclopedia of Hunters and Gatherers*, ed. Richard B. Lee and Richard Daly (Cambridge, UK and New York: Cambridge University Press, 2004), 46–47.
86 David Damas, "The Copper Eskimo," in *Hunters and Gatherers Today: A Socioeconomic Study of Eleven Such Cultures in the Twentieth Century*, ed. M. G. Bicchieri (Prospect Heights, IL: Waveland Press, 1972), 11–12.
87 Ibid., 15.
88 Ibid., 13.
89 Ibid., 18.
90 Wayne Suttles, "Coping with Abundance: Subsistence on the Northwest Coast," in *Man the Hunter*, ed. Richard B. Lee and Irven DeVore (Chicago: Aldine, 1968), 58.
91 Ibid., 56.
92 Ibid., 59.
93 Ibid., 61.
94 Faina Linkov, Barbara Stadterman, and Emanuela Taioli, "Fish Consumption and Cancer: Summary of Evidence," in *Fish Consumption and Health*, ed. George P. Gagne and Richard H. Medrano (New York: Nova Science Publishers, 2009), 118–119.
95 Babal, 14.
96 Artemis P. Simopoulos and Jo Robinson, *The Omega Diet: The Lifesaving Nutritional Program Based on the Diet of the Island of Crete* (New York: Harper, 1999), 56.
97 S. Renaud and A. Nordoy, "'Small is Beautiful': Alpha-Linolenic Acid and Eicosapentaenoic Acid in Man," *The Lancet* 321, no. 8334 (May 21, 1983): 1169.
98 Cordain, 6.
99 Linkov, Stadterman, and Taioli, 117.
100 Ibid., 124–125.

101 Ibid., 126–127.
102 Ibid., 126.
103 Ibid., 130.
104 Linkov, Stadterman, and Taioli, 117; Jeppe T. Friborg and Mads Melbye, "Cancer Patterns in Inuit Populations," *Lancet Oncology* 9, no. 9 (September 1, 2008): 892.
105 Friborg and Melbye, 892.
106 Jahns, 10.
107 Friborg and Melbye, 893; S. Boyd Eaton and Stanley B. Eaton III, "Hunter-Gatherers and Human Health," in *The Cambridge Encyclopedia of Hunters and Gatherers*, ed. Richard B. Lee and Richard Daly (Cambridge, UK: Cambridge University Press, 2004), 452.
108 Friborg and Melbye, 893.
109 Ibid., 897.
110 "The World: Life Expectancy (2018)."
111 "Discussion, Part 5," in *Man the Hunter*, ed. Richard B. Lee and Irven DeVore (Chicago: Aldine, 1968), 242.
112 Jean L. Briggs, "Sadlermiut Inuit," The Canadian Encyclopedia, March 1, 2012, last modified March 4, 2015, accessed February 24, 2019, https://www.thecanadianencyclopedia.ca/en/article/sadlermiut-inuit.
113 John P. McKay, Bennett D. Hill, John Buckler, Clare Haru Crowston, Merry E. Wiesner-Hanks, and Joe Perry, *Understanding Western Society: A Brief History* (Boston, MA and New York: Bedford/St. Martin's, 2012), 212; Edward S. Deevey Jr., "The Human Population," *Scientific American* 203, no. 9 (September 1, 1960), 202.
114 "Discussion, Part 5," 242.
115 Ibid., 243.
116 Damas, 42.
117 Helm, "Dogrib Indians," 54.
118 Joseph M. Prince and Richard H. Steckel, *Tallest in the World: Native Americans of the Great Plains in the Nineteenth Century* (Cambridge, MA: National Bureau of Economic Research, 1998), 29.
119 Richard H. Steckel, *Health and Nutrition in the Preindustrial Era: Insights from a Millennium of Average Heights in Northern Europe* (Cambridge, MA: National Bureau of Economic Research, 2001), i, 18.
120 Ibid., i.
121 Asen Balikci, "The Netsilik Eskimos: Adaptive Processes," in *Man the Hunter*, ed. Richard B. Lee and Irven DeVore (Chicago: Aldine, 1968), 82.
122 Knud Rasmussen, *The Netsilik Eskimos: Social Life and Spiritual Culture* (Copenhagen: Gyldendal, 1931), 141.
123 Balikci, 81.
124 Damas, 42.
125 L. C. Fernandes, "Fish Intake and Strength in the Elderly," in *Fish and Fish Oil in Health and Disease Prevention*, ed. Susan K. Raatz and Douglas M. Bibus (Amsterdam: Academic Press, 2016), 138; C. M. Butt and N. Salem Jr., "Fish and Fish Oil for the Aging Brain," in *Fish and Fish Oil in Health and Disease Prevention*, ed. Susan K. Raatz and Douglas M. Bibus (Amsterdam: Academic Press, 2016), 143.
126 Robert H. Shmerling, "Fertility and Diet: Is There a Connection?" *Harvard Health Publishing*, May 31, 2018, accessed February 7, 2019, https://www.health.harvard.edu/blog/fertility-and-diet-is-there-a-connection-2018053113949.
127 Gemma Askham, "There's a Reason Why Having a Low Body Fat Percentage Isn't Always Healthy," *Women's Health*, August 24, 2018, accessed February 25, 2019, https://www.womenshealthmag.com/uk/health/female-health/a708160/body-fat-percentage-women.
128 Damas, 42.
129 Sara Minogue, "Changes in Arctic Diet Put Inuit at Risk for Rickets," *The Globe and Mail*, June 8, 2007, last modified April 25, 2018, accessed March 4, 2019, https://www.theglobeandmail.com/life/changes-in-arctic-diet-put-inuit-at-risk-for-rickets/article20404517.
130 "Arctic Char," *Government of Northwest Territories*, October 2016, accessed March 4, 2019, https://www.hss.gov.nt.ca/sites/hss/files/resources/contaminants-fact-sheets-arctic-char.pdf.
131 S. Andersen, E. Boeskov, and P. Laurberg, "Ethnic Differences in Bone Mineral Density between Inuit and Caucasians in North Greenland Are Caused by Differences in Body Size," *Journal of Clinical Densitometry* 8, no. 4 (Winter 2005): 409; Sarah Rogers, "Rickets, Vitamin D Deficiency Still Plague Inuit Children," *Nunatsiaq News*, April 7, 2015, accessed March 4, 2019, https://nunatsiaq.com/stories/article/65674vitamin_d_deficiency_rickets_still_plagues_inuit_children.

132 Eenfeldt, 131–132.
133 Bernard Wood, *Human Evolution: A Very Short Introduction* (Oxford: Oxford University Press, 2005), 110.
134 C. Anne Wilson, *Food and Drink in Britain: From the Stone Age to the 19th Century* (Chicago: Academy Chicago Publishers, 1973), 13–14.
135 Ibid., 17.
136 Ibid., 18–19.
137 Ibid., 20.
138 Ibid., 21.
139 Ibid., 22.
140 Ibid., 23–24.
141 Elesha Coffman, "What Is the Origin of the Christian Fish Symbol?" *Christianity Today*, 2019, accessed February 26, 2019, https://www.christianitytoday.com/history/2008/august/what-is-origin-of-christian-fish-symbol.html.
142 *The Rule of St. Benedict*, trans. Anthony C. Meisel and M. L. del Mastro (New York: Doubleday, 1975). 80; Wilson, 26.
143 Wilson, 30.
144 Ibid., 27.
145 Ibid., 31.
146 Ibid., 29.
147 Ibid., 28.
148 Ibid., 41–42.
149 Henry Hobhouse, *Seeds of Change: Six Plants that Transformed Mankind* (New York: Shoemaker and Hoard, 2005), 54.
150 Wilson, 39.
151 Sarah Brewer, *Nutrition: A Beginner's Guide* (London: Oneworld, 2013), 159; Fernand Braudel, *Capitalism and Material Life, 1400 to 1800*, trans. Miriam Kochan (New York: Harper Colophon Books, 1973), 141.
152 Brewer, 161.
153 "Action on Salt," *Wolfson Institute of Preventive Medicine*, accessed February 27, 2019, http://www.actiononsalt.org.uk/salthealth/salt-and-ethnic-minorities.
154 Wilson, 31.
155 Robert William Fogel, "Nutrition and the Decline in Mortality Since 1700: Some Preliminary Findings," in *Long-Term Factors in American Economic Growth*, ed. Stanley L. Engerman and Robert E. Gallman (Chicago and London: University of Chicago Press, 1986), 445, 482
156 Wilson, 34.
157 Ibid., 28.
158 Ibid., 43.
159 Ibid., 36–37.
160 Ibid., 45.
161 J. C. Drummond and Anne Wilbraham, *The Englishman's Food: A History of Five Centuries of English Diet*, rev. ed. (London: Pimlico, 1991), 78–79.
162 G. D. Stroud, "FAO Ministry of Agriculture, Fisheries and Food," Torry Advisory Note No. 57, 2001, accessed November 3, 2019, http://www.fao.org/3/x5933e/x5933e01.htm#TopOfPage.
163 "Fish, Herring, Atlantic, Raw," *USDA FoodData Central*, April 1, 2019, accessed January 21, 2020, https://fdc.nal.usda.gov/fdc-app.html#/food-details/175116/nutrients.
164 "Herring, Dried, Salted," *USDA FoodData Central*, April 1, 2019, accessed November 3, 2019, https://fdc.nal.usda.gov/fdc-app.html#/food-details/337674/nutrients.
165 "FDA Vitamins and Minerals Chart," *FDA*, accessed April 24, 2019, https://www.accessdata.fda.gov/scripts/interactivenutritionfactslabel/factsheets/vitamin_and_mineral_chart.pdf.
166 Wilson, 46.
167 Ibid., 47.
168 Ibid., 48.
169 Ibid., 49.
170 Ibid., 50.
171 "Seville Oranges," *Eat This Much*, accessed February 27, 2019, https://www.eatthismuch.com/food/nutrition/seville-oranges,139834.
172 Jessie Szalay, "Lemons: Health Benefits and Nutrition Facts," *Live Science*, April 23, 2018, accessed February 27, 2019, https://www.livescience.com/54282-lemon-nutrition.html.

173 Wilson, 59.
174 "1 Piece Fish and Chips," *Nutritionnix*, accessed February 27, 2019, https://www.nutritionix.com/i/joeys-seafood/1-piece-fish-and-chips/c6404921a5eb068e82678a72.
175 Jahns, 4.
176 Peter Dizikes, "New Study Shows Rich, Poor Have Huge Mortality Gap in U.S." *MIT News*, April 11, 2016, http://news.mit.edu/2016/study-rich-poor-huge-mortality-gap-us-0411.
177 Fogel, 445.
178 Ibid., 482.
179 Ibid., 482; Drummond and Wilbraham, 79–80.
180 Fogel., 473–474.
181 Ibid., 471.
182 Ibid., 445.
183 Ibid., 445, 467.
184 Ibid., 445.
185 Paul Clayton and Judith Rowbotham, "How the Mid-Victorians Worked, Ate and Died," *International Journal of Environmental Research and Public Health* 6, no. 3 (March 2009), https://www.ncbi.nlm.nih.gov/pmc/articles/PMC2672390.
186 Ibid.
187 Ibid.
188 Ibid.

6 Poultry and Eggs

6.1 AVIAN EVOLUTION

This book seeks precision by specifying animals, plants, fungi, bacteria, and protists' scientific names. These names are part of the International Code of Phylogenic Nomenclature and are meant to standardize biology's language. The taxonomic rank class includes Aves, whose members are birds. These vertebrates lay eggs with hard shells, have wings and feathers, and are warm blooded.

Like all life, birds are evolutionary products with histories that recede ages into the past. Scientists and journalists have popularized birds' evolution from dinosaurs, tracing the avian lineage to species that behaved in ways reminiscent of modern birds. For example, these prehistoric creatures made nests for eggs, which mothers guarded, sitting on them to warm the embryos. These species, known as theropods, had hollow, light bones, a feature that would ease liftoff when their descendants evolved wings.

Theropods were carnivores that probably began to diverge from other dinosaurs between 227 and 174 million years ago.[1] This theropod class, known as coelurosaurs, included *Tyrannosaurus rex*, whose reputation for ferocity enthralled generations of children. In *Jurassic Park* (1993), American filmmaker Steven Allan Spielberg (b. 1946) popularized the genus *Velociraptor*, another coelurosaur. Bipedalism freed these animals' front arms, which their descendants would adapt for flight.

The chief adaptations appear to have evolved between roughly 200 and 150 million years ago and include feathers' origin and development, reduction in body size, forelimbs' elongation into wings, enlargement of shoulder bones and sternum to bear arm muscles' mass and strength, and increase in tail strength and stiffness to improve balance and maneuverability.[2] These changes are evident in fossils about 160–150 million years old. For example, a 160-million-year-old specimen of *Anchiornis huxleyi* in what is today Manchuria, China—Chapter 8 describes its geography—had claws for impaling prey and climbing and descending trees to pursue food or escape predators.[3] Feathers likely enabled flight and insulated the bird from cold, heat, and water. Since the 2009 find, scientists have unearthed over 200 kindred fossils. Rarer are the twelve of *Archaeopteryx lithographica*, which lived about 150 million years ago in what is now Germany.[4] The initial 1861 discovery came just two years after British naturalist Charles Robert Darwin (1809–1882) published *On the Origin of Species* and provided vivid evidence of transitional species by combining reptilian and avian traits.

Diminutive, these animals were not the behemoths whose fossils fill museums and excite children. They occupied faunal interstices and might have remained curiosities but for the mass extinction about 65 million years ago that extirpated around 90 percent of terrestrial species.[5] Their competitors gone, birds expanded to over 10,000 species and to every continent.[6] Even inhospitable Antarctica has forty-six species.[7]

6.2 BIRDS AND EGGS ENTERED DIETS

6.2.1 *Pre-Homo sapiens'* Consumption of Birds and Eggs

This radiation predated humanity's origins, which Chapter 3 recounted. That chapter and others emphasized humans' omnivory and eclecticism, characteristics consistent with early consumption of birds, eggs, and much else. This supposition gained credibility with the 1959 discovery of the first specimen of what is now classified *Paranthropus boisei* (see Chapter 3) amid bones from several animals and eggshells.[8] Besides *P. boisei*, anthropologists discovered ostrich (*Struthio camelus*) eggshells at Zhoukoudian, China, which *Homo erectus* occupied about 780,000 years ago.[9]

These finds do not prove pre-*H. sapiens*' egg eating because another predator might have been the consumer. Yet eggshells are intriguing because it is difficult to envision what else would have been careful enough to take an egg without prematurely breaking the shell. Moreover, the ostrich shells are charred, intimating cooking, a behavior that appears at be unique to *Homo*. The *P. boisei* fossils, roughly 1.8 million years old, may mark egg eating's origins, though doubts have arisen about the diversity of his diet. If eggs were consumed at the dawn of humanity, birds must likewise have entered diets early because it seems unreasonable to suppose that hungry hominids monitored birds closely enough to find the nest but were too obtuse to identify them as potential food.

6.2.2 *H. sapiens'* Early Consumption of Birds and Eggs

Like procurement of any plant or animal before agriculture and animal husbandry, birds had to be captured and eggs collected. The prospect of snaring an animal able to evade predators through flight may have been daunting, though American ornithologist Richard Fourness Johnston (1925–2014) stated that "Many kinds of birds can be caught readily."[10] Humans long ago appreciated them, especially young adults, as "superior fare" and "highly prized" eggs.[11]

By observing birds, prehistoric peoples tracked their habits and detected their vulnerability in spring during molting and nesting and in autumn when summer engorgement fattened them.[12] During the Mesolithic Period (9000–7000 BCE), humans reconnoitered wetlands for several species. For example, Danes hunted mallards (*Anas platyrhynchos*), swans (*Cygnus* species), grebes (species in the family Podicipedidae), Eurasian coots (*Fulica atra*), cormorants (species in the family Phalacrocoracidae), and gulls (*Larus* species). Near the North and Baltic Seas, hunters targeted Eurasian cranes (*Grus grus*), swans, cormorants, and sea eagles (*Haliaeetus* species). Mesolithic Germans consumed mallards. To the east, Baltic, Polish, and Russian wetlands yielded numerous bird bones as dietary evidence. Eighty-nine percent of bones from a Mesolithic site along Estonia's Narva River are waterfowl, chiefly mallards.[13] Likely wielding slings, Iron Age (800 BCE–42 CE) Britons near what is today Somerset, England, also hunted mallards.

6.3 OVERCONSUMPTION AND EXTINCTION

6.3.1 Dodo

The appetite for birds, eggs, or both eradicated the dodo (*Raphus cucullatus*). Although the bird was too large and heavy to fly, its smaller ancestors flew to the Indian Ocean island Mauritius during the last 8 million years, though the date of arrival has not been pinpointed.[14] Absent predators, dodos grew larger and lost or never developed a startle reflex. Enlargement is curious given that many species shrink on islands, a phenomenon known as island dwarfing. African, Arab, and Indian sailors identified but did not settle Mauritius in the tenth century CE.[15] The Portuguese arrived in 1507 but never mentioned a flightless bird.[16]

Dutch colonists, however, encountered it around 1598.[17] They must have sampled the bird, else they could not have lamented its toughness and unpalatability.[18] These defects may explain why a 2013 investigation found no dodo bones in island middens.[19] Even if humans disliked the flesh—excepting tasty breast, stomach, and intestines—they devoured the dodo to satiate hunger and enjoyed its eggs enough to imperil the species.[20] Moreover, their tagalongs—dogs, pigs, cats, and rats—also ate the eggs and outcompeted dodos for food.[21] Extinction came within eighty years of Dutch settlement.

6.3.2 Passenger Pigeon

Misfortune likewise befell passenger pigeons (*Ectopistes migratorius*). American journalist Barry Yeoman summarized their appeal, writing that they "were tasty...and their arrival guaranteed an abundance of free protein."[22] An onlooker might have thought their demise improbable given passenger pigeons' status as the most numerous bird in North America and perhaps the world. American ornithologist Alexander Wilson (1766–1813) estimated a single flock above 2 billion birds.[23] These creatures—"the most numerous bird ever to exist on earth"—may have totaled 9 billion at their zenith.[24] But their noisiness alerted hunters, and their habits were predictable. In the nineteenth century, American naturalist John James Audubon (1785–1851) warned that overhunting threatened them, though few heeded him.[25] In 1900, an Ohioan killed the last wild specimen, and fourteen years later the final captive died in Ohio's Cincinnati Zoo.

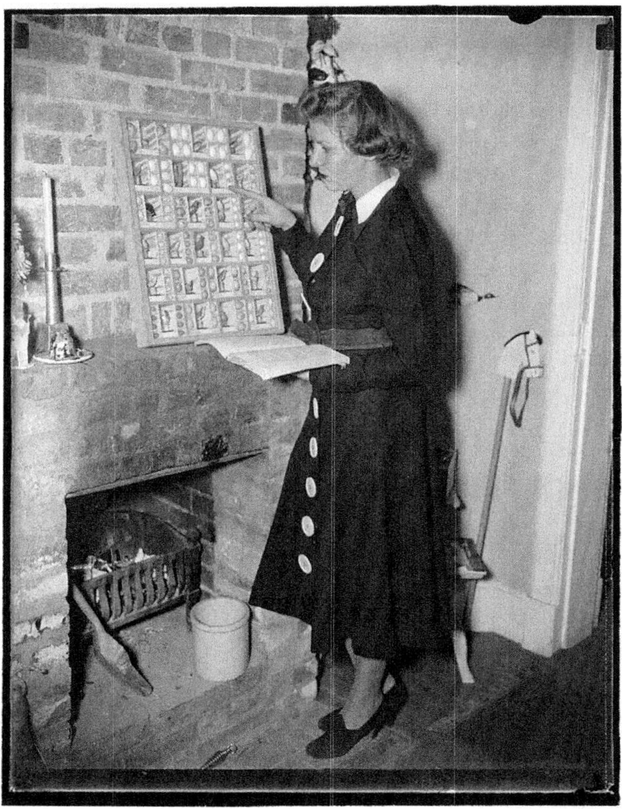

FIGURE 6.1 Passenger pigeon eggs. (Photo courtesy of Library of Congress. https://www.loc.gov/pictures/item/2016872686/.)

6.4 BIRD AND EGG CONSUMPTION IN THE AMERICAS

Earlier in North America, Mississippians ate these pigeons, wild turkeys (*Meleagris gallopavo*), mourning doves (*Zenaida macroura*), songbirds (species in the clade Passeri), herons (species in the family Ardeidae), ducks, and geese (*Branta canadensis* and *Anser* species).[26] Turkeys, ducks, and geese fed natives and Spaniards in Florida. Turkeys were eaten throughout Central America, Mexico, and the American Southwest. Later sections enlarge the discussion of turkeys and their eggs as food, evaluating their nutrition and healthfulness in pre-Columbian times.

Colonizing the Americas, Europeans intensified poultry husbandry and consumption. Into the mid-twentieth century, family farms raised birds, usually chickens, for meat, eggs, and income.[27] Farmers and consumers favored poultry because of inexpensiveness and efficient conversion of grains, notably corn (*Zea mays*), and soybeans (*Glycine max*) into protein as meat and eggs. The drive toward economy is evident in the fact that about 1940 the average chicken needed roughly 3 kilograms (6.5 pounds) of feed to produce 0.5 kilograms (1 pound) of flesh whereas around 2012 that chicken yielded the same mass on only 0.8 kilograms (1.8 pounds) of feed.[28] Moreover, poultry start-up costs have been, and are, low.[29] Feed and housing are cheap, and domestic birds tend to be hardy.

Pursuit of economy has made chicken cheaper than beef or pork. In 1960, 0.5 kilograms of chicken breast retailed for 42.7 cents in the United States.[30] That year the same mass of pork averaged 55.4 cents and beef fetched 82.1 cents. Chicken has held this advantage, retailing in the United States for $1.90 per 0.5 kilograms compared to $3.70 for the same quantity of pork and $5.95 for beef by a March 2019 estimate. Critics complain that agribusiness exploits chickens, though consumers want bargains at the grocer.[31]

6.5 WORLD CONSUMPTION OF BIRDS AND EGGS

Around 1995, chicken surpassed beef in global sales.[32] Since 1999, the world has produced more chicken than beef.[33] Only pork outstrips chicken in world sales and consumption.[34] Beyond chicken, turkeys rank fifth in global sales and consumption, ducks seventh, and geese ninth.[35] Outside the top ten, pigeons (*Columba livia domestica*) and unspecified birds are seventeenth. Among livestock, chicken production is growing fastest worldwide at roughly 5 percent annually, a rate that doubled metric tonnage between 1980 and 2003.[36] Between 1988 and 2003, countries with the largest income growth tripled chicken production and consumption. By comparison, global pork production is growing 3–4 percent yearly and beef 1–2 percent. World egg supply is increasing over 3 percent per year.[37] Turkeys, ducks, geese, and guineafowl (*Numididae meleagris*) furnish eggs, though most come from chickens.

6.6 POULTRY AS NOURISHMENT

6.6.1 Poultry as an Alternative to Beef and Pork

Interest in poultry stems at least partly from its reputation, crafted in the 1980s, as a low-fat, low-calorie alternative to beef and pork.[38] This thinking helped chicken infiltrate fast food without losing its appeal to dieters and health enthusiasts, though the generalization that poultry has little fat does not hold in all cases. Table 6.1 shows that 100 grams of duck and goose have 28.35 and 21.92 grams of fat, respectively.[39] By comparison, 100 grams of raw turkey with skin have 6.2 grams of fat, the amount being an average of samples from breast, wing, drumstick, thigh, and back.[40] One hundred grams of turkey breast without skin furnish just 2.1 grams of fat.[41] One hundred grams of chicken breast with skin have 13.6 grams of fat, and the same amount of chicken eggs supplies 10.6 grams of fat. Removal of skin reduces fat in 100 grams of chicken breast to just 1.2 grams.[42]

Because fat has more calories by mass than carbohydrates or protein, Chapter 2 noted, duck and goose have more calories than turkey, chicken, and chicken egg. Referencing Table 6.1, 100 grams of duck and goose have 337 and 305 calories, respectively, compared to 147 for the same quantity of turkey breast without skin, 239 for chicken, and 155 for egg.[43] Chapter 4's Table 4.1 listed 100 grams of bison at 146 calories and 7.21 grams of fat, of mutton at 234 calories and 11.09 grams of fat, of goat at 143 calories and 3.03 grams of fat, of beef at 305 calories and 5.8 grams of fat, of pork at 212 calories and 15.3 grams of fat, and of venison at 190 calories and 3.93 grams of fat.

6.6.2 Poultry's Nutrient Density

This book emphasizes neither calories nor fat alone, but nutrient density. American animal scientist W. Stephen Damron championed meat, fish, poultry, eggs, and dairy for this reason.[44] Confining this paragraph to equal masses of chicken, its eggs, turkey, duck, and goose and encouraging readers to survey the rest of this book for other foods, Table 6.1 indicates that these birds and eggs lack fiber or vitamin C, and that chicken ranks first in protein.[45] Turkey has the most magnesium, and vitamins B_3 (niacin or nicotinic acid) and B_6 (pyridoxine), duck has the most vitamin B_1 (thiamine or thiamin), goose has the most iron, phosphorus, potassium, zinc, copper, and vitamins B_5

TABLE 6.1
Nutrients in Poultry and Eggs 100g

Nutrient	Chicken	%DV	Egg	%DV	Turkey	%DV	Duck	%DV	Goose	%DV
Calories	239	N/A	155	N/A	114	N/A	337	N/A	305	N/A
Protein (g)	27.3	N/A	12.58	N/A	23.66	N/A	18.99	N/A	25.16	N/A
Fat (g)	13.6	N/A	10.61	N/A	1.48	N/A	28.35	N/A	21.92	N/A
Carbs (g)	0	N/A	1.12	N/A	0.14	N/A	0	N/A	0	N/A
Fiber (g)	0	N/A	0	N/A	0	N/A	0	N/A	0	N/A
Minerals										
Ca (mg)	15	1.5	50	5	11	1.1	11	1.1	13	1.3
Fe (mg)	1.26	7	1.19	6.6	0.71	5.7	2.7	15	2.83	15.7
Mg (mg)	23	5.8	10	2.5	28	7	16	4	22	5.5
P (mg)	182	18.2	172	17.2	201	20.1	156	15.6	270	27
K (mg)	223	6.4	126	3.6	242	6.9	204	5.8	329	9.4
Na (mg)	82	3.4	124	5.2	113	4.7	59	2.5	70	2.9
Zn (mg)	1.94	12.9	1.05	7	1.28	8.5	1.86	12.4	2.62	17.5
Cu (mg)	0.07	3.5	0.01	0.5	0.07	3.5	0.23	11.5	0.26	13
Mn (mg)	0.02	1	0.03	1.5	0.01	0.5	0.02	1	0.02	1
Se (mcg)	23.9	34.1	30.8	44	22.7	32.4	22.4	32	25.5	36.4
Vitamins										
A (IU)	161	3.2	560	11.2	20	0.04	210	4.2	70	1.4
B_1 (mg)	0.06	4	0.07	4.7	0.04	2.7	0.17	11.3	0.08	5.3
B_2 (mg)	0.17	10	0.51	30	0.15	8.8	0.27	15.9	0.32	18.8
B_3 (mg)	8.49	42.5	0.06	0.3	9.92	49.6	4.83	24.2	4.17	20.9
B_5 (mg)	1.03	10.3	1.4	14	0.78	7.8	1.1	11	1.53	15.3
B_6 (mg)	0.4	20	0.12	6	0.81	40.5	0.18	9	0.37	18.5
B_9 (mcg)	5	1.3	44	11	9	2.3	6	1.5	2	0.5
B_{12} (mcg)	0.3	5	1.11	18.5	0.39	6.5	0.3	5	0.41	6.8
C (mg)	0	0	0	0	0	0	0	0	0	0
D (IU)	5	1.3	82	20.5	5	1.3	3	0.8	3	0.8
E (mg)	0.27	1.8	1.05	7	0.06	0.4	0.7	4.7	1.74	11.6
K (mcg)	0.3	0.38	0.3	0.38	0	0	2.8	3.5	5.1	6.4

(pantothenic acid) and E, and eggs have the most calcium, manganese, selenium, and vitamins A, B_2 (riboflavin), B_9 (folate, folic acid, or pteroylmonoglutamic acid), B_{12} (cobalamin), and D.[46]

These numbers suggest that chicken egg and goose provide greater nutritional breadth than chicken or turkey. Goose has a minor place in American diets, though chicken eggs were a breakfast staple throughout much of U.S. history.[47] Consumption peaked in 1945 at 403 eggs per average American.[48] Thereafter, concern about cholesterol—Chapter 2 discussed its functions and regulation—caused eggs to decline to their 1991 nadir of 233 per average American. Since then, they rebounded to 279 annually per average American in March 2019.[49] The last figure equals roughly 0.8 eggs daily, or 40 grams given 50 grams per egg, the amount Damron specified.[50] Table 6.2 lists calories and nutrients in this mass.[51]

6.6.3 Poultry, Nutrients, and Anemia

Among these nutrients, attention focuses on iron and vitamins B_9 and B_{12} because deficits may cause or exacerbate anemia, which this book characterizes as an affliction of some premodern peoples and which later sections discuss. Chapter 1 remarked that when iron and a B vitamin are deficient,

TABLE 6.2
Nutrients in 0.8 Eggs 40 g

Nutrient	Eggs (40 g)	%DV
Calories	61.97	N/A
Protein (g)	5.07	N/A
Fat (g)	4.23	N/A
Carbs (g)	0.47	N/A
Fiber (g)	0	N/A
	Minerals	
Ca (mg)	20	2
Fe (mg)	0.48	2.7
Mg (mg)	4	1
P (mg)	68.8	6.9
K (mg)	50.4	1.4
Na (mg)	49.6	2.1
Zn (mg)	0.42	2.8
Cu (mg)	0.06	2.8
Mn (mg)	0.01	0.5
Se (mcg)	12.32	17.6
	Vitamins	
A (IU)	224	4.5
B_1 (mg)	0.03	1.9
B_2 (mg)	0.21	12.2
B_3 (mg)	0.03	0.1
B_5 (mg)	0.56	5.6
B_6 (mg)	0.05	2.3
B_9 (mcg)	17.6	4.4
B_{12} (mcg)	0.44	7.4
C (mg)	0	0
D (IU)	32.8	8.2
E (mg)	0.42	2.8
K (mcg)	0.12	0.2

neither shortage need be marked to produce anemia.[52] Table 6.3 lists these nutrients in chicken, chicken egg, turkey, duck, goose, beef, bison, pork, venison, and salmon.[53] These comparisons favor bison and venison over chickens, their eggs, turkeys, ducks, and geese for iron and vitamin B_{12}. Additionally, salmon surpasses poultry, though not eggs, in B_9, and salmon and beef have more B_{12} than poultry and eggs. Poultry and eggs do not best protect against anemia.

6.7 EASTERN HEMISPHERE

6.7.1 CHICKENS

The first section stated that birds evolved from theropods. Chickens appear to have descended from *T. rex* given that proteins from a 68-million-year-old femur best matched those in *Gallus gallus domesticus* among extant animals.[54] Another link between dinosaurs and chickens emerged from experimental combination of chick and mouse tissues, which prompted cells to manufacture teeth.[55] That is, mouse genes caused chick cells to express genes, latent millions of years, that directed formation of teeth, which dinosaurs and *Archaeopteryx lithographica* had. The genus

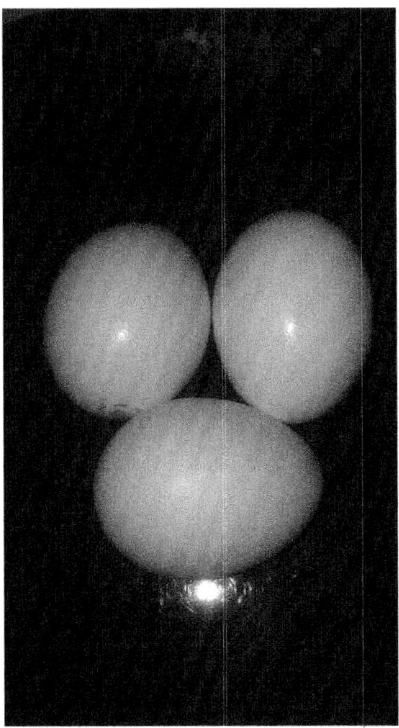

FIGURE 6.2 Chicken eggs. (Photo from author.)

TABLE 6.3
Iron Vitamins B_9 and B_{12} in Poultry Eggs Meat and Salmon 100g

Meat	Iron (mg)	%DV	B_9 (mcg)	%DV	B_{12} (mcg)	%DV
Chicken	1.26	7	5	1.3	0.3	5
Chicken egg	1.19	6.6	44	11	1.11	18.5
Turkey	0.71	5.7	9	2.3	0.39	6.51
Duck	2.7	15	6	1.5	0.3	5
Goose	2.83	15.7	2	0.5	0.41	6.8
Beef	3.32	19	7	1.8	2.44	40.7
Bison	2.78	15.4	12	3	1.94	32.3
Pork	10.93	5.0	6	1.5	0.75	12.5
Venison	4.98	27.6	11	2.8	3.04	50
Wild salmon	0.8	4.4	25	6.3	3.18	53

Gallus arose roughly 50 million years ago, with most early fossils in southern Europe.[56] When the climate warmed these birds dispersed from the equator, though during cool periods they retreated into the tropics and subtropics, behavior that suggests adaptation to warmth. By writing's invention around 3000 BCE, *Gallus* had settled Southeast Asia, no longer inhabited Europe, and was absent from early European texts.[57] Darwin wrote that chickens descended from the red junglefowl (*Gallus gallus*), whose presence in Thailand strengthened the case for chickens' Southeast Asian origins.[58] Genetic studies cemented the link between the two birds.

The need for food, whether flesh or eggs, may not have prompted domestication. American poultry scientist William J. Stadelman (1917–2007) and Annie Potts, English professor, codirector of the New Zealand Centre for Human-Animal studies, and author of *Chicken* (2012), asserted

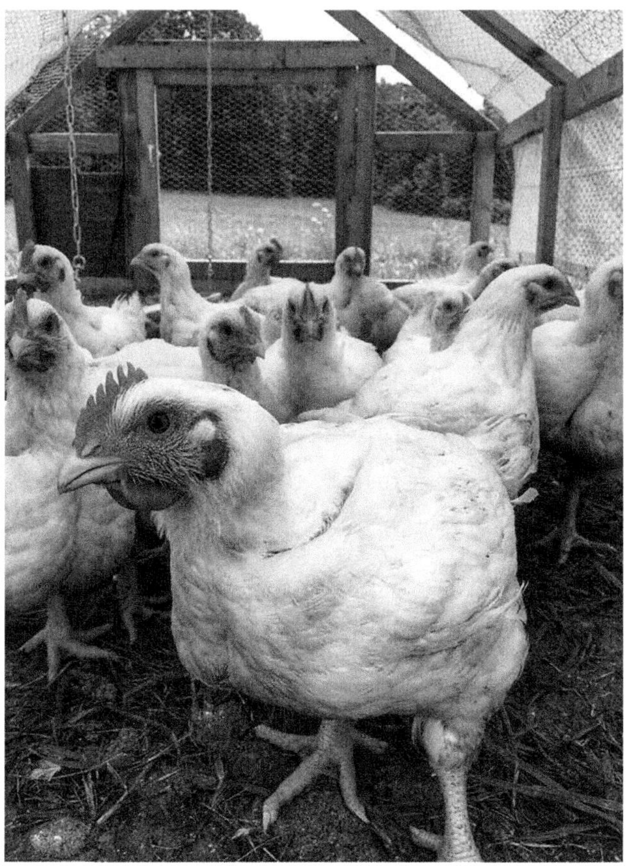

FIGURE 6.3 Meat chickens. (Photo courtesy of Jessica Vierling-West.)

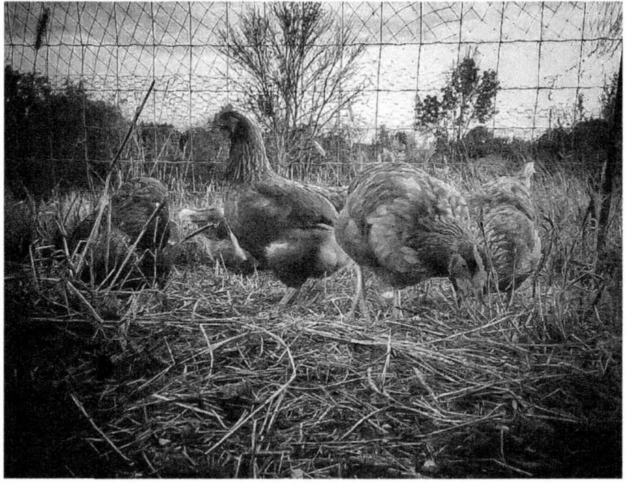

FIGURE 6.4 Laying hens. (Photo courtesy of Jessica Vierling-West.)

that humans tamed chickens first for religious purposes.[59] Damron wrote that the desire to raise cockfighters prompted domestication.[60] American journalist Andrew Lawler described domestication as an outcome of mutualism. Farmers appreciated chickens' appetite for insects that otherwise bedeviled crops and for weeds that competed for sunlight, water, and minerals.[61] Moreover, chickens vocalized the arrival of dawn or intruders. Reciprocating these benefits, people fed chickens, housed them, and protected them from predators. In contrast to these ideas, British sociologist Eric Chaline stated that hunger for meat and eggs spurred domestication.[62]

Focus on a single factor obscures the possibility that humans domesticated chickens to fill several needs. As was true of bison (*Bison bison*) and turkeys (discussed later), people used chickens as circumstances dictated. Raising these birds for sacrifice, divination, pest control, or biological proxies for alarm clocks does not preclude the likelihood that hungry people ate hens' eggs. Chickens that had outlived their original purpose might have been consumed. Ingestion is implicit in the notion of domestication, a status that relies on identification of bones bigger than those found in the wild.[63] Largeness was an asset for cockfighting or consumption but unnecessary for religious purposes.

Whatever combination of reasons prompted domestication, red junglefowls tended to stay near their home base.[64] This sedentism predisposed them to tolerate confinement, thereby facilitating taming. Moreover, Lawler asserted that these birds adapted to diverse foods, geographies, and climates, permitting an owner to take them wherever he migrated.[65] British anthropologist Roger Marsh Blench (b. 1953) and British archaeologist Kevin C. MacDonald, however, stated that red junglefowls tolerated tropical and subtropical climates better than the cold.[66] Consequently, their presence outside warm regions indicated human agency. Even if Blench and MacDonald are correct about climatic preferences, Lawler is right to emphasize that domestication made people and chickens travel companions.

Domestication appears to have occurred roughly when humans began raising crops, a development discussed in Chapter 3. Chaline suggested that Thais tamed chickens around 8000 BCE, however, a date that appears to predate farming in the region.[67] From Thailand, migrants, merchants, or both took chickens north to China by 6000 BCE.[68] Bones dated to 5500 BCE in Manchuria and Pakistan are larger than wild specimens. Over 3,400 years ago, red junglefowls were in India, where they hybridized with gray junglefowls (*Gallus sonneratii*), the second contributing a minority of genes to the modern chicken.[69] In 1474 BCE, Pharaoh Thutmose III brought chickens from Iraq to Egypt during military operations.[70] Domestic birds were no novelty because Egypt already raised geese for meat and eggs and to warn farmers of intruders. Yet Egyptians came to prefer chickens because they laid more eggs than geese, grew faster, and ate ticks and mosquitoes.[71] Egypt designed incubators able to hatch as many as 15,000 eggs at once.[72] Production on this scale fueled the inference that eggs sustained the pyramid builders. China may have done likewise to feed the Great Wall of China's laborers.

Egyptian merchants moved chickens south up the Nile River—Chapter 4 described Egypt's geography—into Nubia and elsewhere in East Africa by 500 CE.[73] Around then, chickens appeared in Mali southwest of what is today Algeria. Algeria's access to the Mediterranean Sea raises the possibility that seafarers introduced chickens into Algeria, from where they went inland to Mali. Alternatively, westward migration from Nubia was also possible.

The Persians, acquiring chickens from India about 400 BCE, may have taken them west to Greece.[74] Trading throughout the Mediterranean, Greeks likely introduced chickens to the Romans, who castrated roosters before gorging them to enlarge, fatten, and tenderize flesh. Rome bred some chickens for food and others for fighting. By crossbreeding different types, Romans witnessed the phenomenon of heterosis (hybrid vigor), whereby offspring displayed traits superior to those of parents.

Part of the Roman Empire, Spain bridged Old and New Worlds when Italian-Spanish mariner Christopher Columbus (1451–1506) in 1493 brought chickens to the Caribbean island Hispaniola, now Haiti and the Dominican Republic.[75] Sixteenth-century Dutch and Portuguese carried chickens from Africa to the Caribbean and Brazil. Genes from chicken bones that date from Spaniards' arrival in Florida most resemble those from today's Spanish chickens, evidence that American chickens originated in Spain.[76]

Some scholars argued, however, that chickens reached the western hemisphere before these events.[77] This perspective traces a route from Southeast Asia east through Polynesia to South America's Pacific coast. Fifty chicken bones from El Arenal, Chile, dated between 700 and 1390 CE, indicate that the bird was there at least a century before Columbus' voyages.[78] Moreover, some American hens lay blue eggs unknown elsewhere except in China, implying a Pacific migration to the New World.[79] Finally, Amerindians had names for chickens that did not derive from European languages, implying that Europe played no part in the first introduction of *G. gallus domesticus.*

6.7.2 Ducks

Most domestic ducks descended from the mallard, which colonized the world's wetlands. An earlier section stated that northern Europeans hunted waterfowl from an early date. Widespread enthusiasm for ducks spurred domestication in several areas. Asia, notably China, Vietnam, Indonesia, Thailand, Myanmar, the Philippines, and Bangladesh, has roughly three-quarters of domestic ducks.[80]

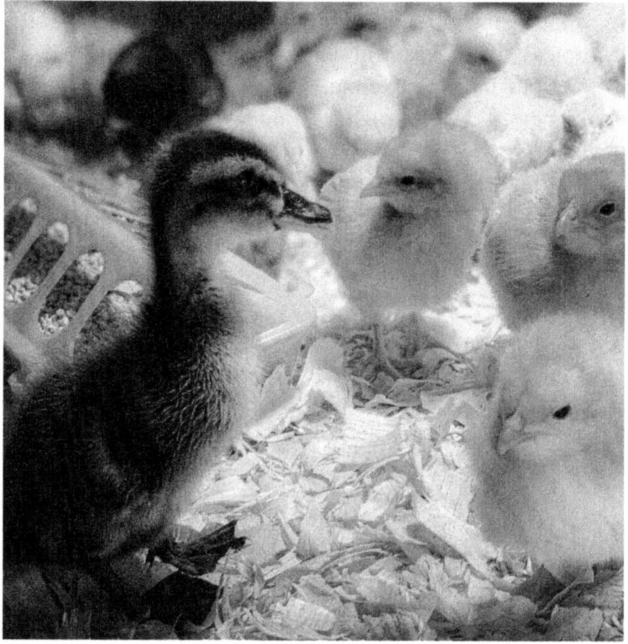

FIGURE 6.5 Ducklings and chicks. (Photo courtesy of Jessica Vierling-West.)

These birds benefited Asia's rice (*Oryza sativa*) growers. Whole grain rice (see Chapter 12) supplies starch, minerals, and vitamins but has little fat and lacks some essential amino acids. Ducks complemented the grass by furnishing abundant fat, as noted, and complete protein. Fat and calories made ducks valuable in premodern times when food was more often scarce than plentiful. A supply of complete protein was crucial to peoples who seldom afforded meat. Moreover, ducks thrived better than chickens in rice paddies, eating juvenile crabs (species in the infraorder Brachyura) and locusts (species in the order Orthoptera), both rice pests.[81] Suited to this environment, ducks laid more eggs than chickens, supplying more food. Rapid growth permitted slaughter and consumption at six or seven weeks.[82]

Chinese depictions of ducks dated about 2500 BCE.[83] Although possibly not that early, domestication occurred no later than the Warring States period (475–221 BCE) according to contemporary texts. Chinese south of the Yangtze River took the lead in taming various breeds. On the river, Jiangsu province along the Pacific coast was active in this endeavor. Regions near or in the tropics were best for duck keeping and taming because warmth favored hatchlings' survival. Among Chinese breeds, Peking duck is known worldwide.

Outside China, Egypt may have domesticated ducks, though interest lay with chickens, geese, and pigeons more than ducks. Greek botanist and philosopher Theophrastus (c. 371–c. 287 BCE) mentioned domestic ducks, though they may have been minor in Greek and Roman diets.[84] Like chickens, Romans force fed ducks, a practice that improved flavor and raised prices, reserving them for elites. Roman agriculturist Lucius Junius Moderatus Columella (4–70 CE) lamented that ducks were more expensive to raise than geese.

In the fourth century, Brits and Dutch ate wild ducks.[85] The Saxons who settled Britain between the fifth and seventh centuries may have kept ducks. Between the eighth and tenth centuries, the French kept fewer ducks than chickens and geese.[86] Germans likewise preferred chickens and geese over ducks. Medieval Europe appears to have tamed ducks in response to overhunting wild populations. After roughly 1500, duck bones became more numerous in middens, indicating increases in consumption. Enlargement of ducks in the eighteenth and nineteenth centuries evinced selective breeding. During these centuries, Europeans concentrated on breeds that laid many eggs, rapidly reached sizes suitable for slaughter, or both.

Turning to the western hemisphere, U.S. interest in ducks quickened in 1873 upon importation of the white pekin breed from China.[87] The most numerous duck in the United States, it matured to slaughter size fastest, laid numerous eggs, and tolerated confinement well. Small farmers tended to favor Rouen or Muscovy because it foraged better than white pekin. A Brazilian import, Muscovy was the only widespread commercial variety not descended from mallards. Hobbyists often kept bantam (small) breeds, including white or gray calls, black east indies, wood ducks, mandarins, and teals. In the United States, the leading duck producers are Indiana, California, New York, Wisconsin, and Pennsylvania.[88]

6.7.3 Poultry, Thailand, Vietnam, and Health

An earlier section named Thailand as chickens' probable cradle. Australian archaeologist and anthropologist Marc F. Oxenham, Vietnamese archaeologist Nguyen Lan Cuong, and Vietnamese biologist Nguyen Kim Thuy identified chicken bones—implying consumption and dating from roughly 2100 BCE to 200 CE—in Thai villages Ban Chiang, Nong Nor, Ban Lum Khao, Ban Na Di, and Noen U-Loke.[89] To chickens, American anthropologist Christopher A. King and American archaeologist Lynette Norr added wild birds, naming no species, in their study of Ban Chiang.[90] If Thailand's countryside today illuminates prehistory, villagers kept chickens more for eggs than flesh.[91] Other foods included fish, game, beef, rice, millet (species in Eragrostideae tribe), yams (*Dioscorea* species), and wild plants.[92] Between roughly 2100 BCE and 200 CE, these villagers likely increased consumption of carnivores. This class might have included birds that targeted only insects and other animals, though chickens and ducks tend toward omnivory rather than specialization.

Researchers—including Australian anthropologist Kathryn M. Domett in her 2001 study of four prehistoric Thai villages discussed later—mentioned no duck bones as biofacts. Readers might recall that bird bones, being light and hollow, preserve less than sturdy remains and posit this reason for duck bones' absence. Such thinking, however, should also apply to chicken bones, which are extant.

Lack of duck bones is puzzling given the probability that early Thais ate ducks. Chapter 12 remarks that Thailand acquired rice about 3500 BCE, and the previous section noted that paddies provided an environment better for ducks than chickens.[93] It would seem peculiar that, in an era of food insecurity, hungry Thais ate chickens but not ducks. Moreover, because rice cultivation characterized Thailand, Southeast Asia in general, southern China, and South Asia, duck consumption was widespread, as the previous section noted. This section therefore treats chickens and ducks as part of Thai diets such that examination of health illuminates both birds' contributions to it.

Oxenham, Cuong, and Thuy grouped skeletons, in Table 6.4, by age from the above Thai villages with those from Khok Phanom Di in Chachoengsao province, Thailand, and Non Nok Tha in Khon Kaen province, Thailand, and from three Vietnamese sites.[94] Absent from their discussion is information about deaths before age fifteen, a decision that excluded most if not all prepubescents. Childhood's rapid growth demands calories and nutrients such that juvenile skeletons and teeth tend to register deficiencies more than adult ones. Other chapters emphasize that pathologies may stem from dietary inadequacies, pathogens, parasites, or their combination. To be sure, skeletons and their provenance may supply little information or juvenile skeletons may be scarce. Nonetheless, youth skeletons' omission excludes data.

Obviously, juveniles' absence precludes calculation of infant and childhood mortality. Estimation, however, is possible given American ecologist and limnologist Edward Smith Deevey Jr.'s (1914–1988) generalization—see below and Chapters 1 and 3—that between Neanderthal prehistory and roughly 1900 CE half of all deaths occurred before puberty.[95] This magnitude agrees with Domett and New Zealand anthropologist Nancy Tayles' computation of 46 percent juvenile mortality in Ban Lum Khao and 44 percent in Noen U-Loke between roughly 500 BCE and 300 CE.[96] Beyond these figures, Domett computed, in Table 6.5, mortality before age fifteen at 55.8 percent, using 154 skeletons of villagers at Khok Phanom Di, occupied between roughly 2000 and 1500 BCE.[97] Of these deaths, 73.3 percent occurred during life's first year. Ban Na Di, whose seventy-eight skeletons dated between 600 and 400 BCE, totaled 35.9 percent mortality before age fifteen.[98] The lowest juvenile death rate came from Nong Nor, inhabited between 1100 and 700 BCE, at 21.3 percent, though 155 skeletons' poor preservation implies that youth bones deteriorated, reducing the appearance of childhood mortality below the true percentage.[99]

This mortality contextualizes and deepens Oxenham, Cuong, and Thuy's study. For example, they examined 142 skeletons from Ban Chiang, not specifying whether the total included juveniles and adults.[100] If both and if Deevey may be taken as a guide, seventy-one should have perished before age fifteen, the threshold year in the authors' tabulation, and the other seventy-one afterward.

TABLE 6.4
% Deaths by Age in Thailand and Vietnam from Oxenham Cuong and Thuy

Place	Date	15–19 yr	20–29 yr	30–39 yr	40+ yr
Da But, Vietnam	c. 4000–c. 3500 BCE	11.7	18.2	28.6	41.6
Khok Phanom Di, Thailand	c. 2000–c. 1500 BCE	11.8	33.8	36.8	17.6
Early Non Nok Tha, Thailand	c. 2800–c. 1400 BCE	5.1	17.9	25.6	51.3
Early Ban Chiang, Thailand	c. 2100–c. 900 BCE	6.9	20.7	20.7	51.7
Late Non Nok Tha, Thailand	c. 1400–c. 200 BCE	2.4	14.3	35.7	47.6
Nong Nor, Thailand	c. 1100–c. 700 BCE	2.4	30.6	50.6	16.5
Ban Lum Khao, Thailand	c. 1000–c. 500 BCE	8.5	42.4	28.8	20.3
Late Ban Chiang, Thailand	c. 900 BCE–c. 200 CE	15.2	18.2	33.3	33.3
Ban Na Di, Thailand	c. 600–c. 400 BCE	0.0	36.1	36.1	27.8
Ma, Ca, Vietnam	c. 500 BCE–c. 300 CE	11.9	38.1	23.8	26.2
Noen U-Loke, Thailand	c. 300 BCE–c. 300 CE	7.4	44.4	25.9	22.2
Red River, Vietnam	c. 200 BCE–c. 300 CE	13.6	36.4	27.3	22.7

TABLE 6.5
Age at Death in Thailand from Domett

SE Thailand	#	%	SE Thailand	#	%	NE Thailand	#	%	NE Thailand	#	%
Khok Phanom Di c. 2000–c. 1500 BCE			Nong Nor c. 1100–c. 700 BCE			Ban Lum Khao c. 1000–c. 500 BCE			Ban Na Di c. 600–c. 400 BCE		
<1 yr	63	40.9		17	10.9		21	19.1		15	19.2
1–4	11	7.1		6	3.9		14	12.8		8	10.3
5–9	7	4.5		4	2.6		11	10		2	2.6
10–14	5	3.3		6	3.9		5	4.5		3	3.8
Youths	86	55.8		33	21.3		51	46.4		28	35.9
15–19	8	5.2		2	1.3		5	4.5		0	0
20–29	23	14.9		26	16.8		25	22.7		13	16.7
30–39	27	17.5		43	27.7		17	15.5		13	16.7
≥40	10	6.5		14	9		12	10.9		10	12.8
Adults	68	44.2		85	72		59	53.6		36	64.1
Total	154	100		118	100		110	100		64	100
Unknown	0			37			0			14	

Referencing only adults, Oxenham, Cuong, and Thuy determined that before around 900 BCE, 51.7 percent of Ban Chiang's residents reached age forty, a figure that declined to one-third afterward.[101] But, assuming that the skeletons represented both youths and adults, and noting that these authors considered only adults, only roughly half (about seventy-one skeletons) should have been adults. Inclusion of juveniles doubles the population, halving the proportion that reached any age, Table 6.6 indicates. That is, before about 900 BCE, roughly one-quarter of Ban Chiang's occupants reached age forty. Afterward the percentage fell to only around 16.7. Domett and Tayles conceded as much, characterizing the fifth decade as "old age."[102]

In this light, Ban Chiang looks like medieval Europe (see Chapter 3), where age forty marked life's end.[103] The village confirms French anthropologist and paleontologist Henri Victor Vallois' (1889–1981) lament, quoted in Chapter 3, that "few individuals passed forty years, and it is only quite exceptionally that any passed fifty."[104] Domett repeated some of this language almost verbatim, noting that "Few individuals survived beyond 40 years in each of the samples."[105] Although some demographers and anthropologists, referenced in Chapter 3, dispute this conclusion, studies of skeletons from natives, Africans, and whites in the Americas reveal that before roughly 1900, few surpassed age forty-five.[106]

Of the other sites and employing the same method for calculating survival to forty, the approximate figures are one-quarter of inhabitants in Non Nok Tha, one-fifth in Da But in Vihn Loc district, Vietnam, 13 percent in Ban Na Di and a settlement along Vietnam's Ma River, one-tenth in Ban Lum Khao, Noen U-Loke, and a village along Vietnam's Red River, and 8 percent in Khok Phanom Di and Nong Nor.[107] My numbers may be compared with Domett's computation of survival to age forty at 12.8 percent for Ban Na Di, at 10.9 percent for Ban Lum Khao, 9 percent for Nong Nor, and 6.5 percent for Khok Phanom Di.[108] Overall, Domett's calculations of survivorship to forty are no bleaker than mine. That said, lifespan appears to have been greatest in early Ban Chiang and Non Nok Tha. Oxenham, Cuong, and Thuy's age distribution for adults reveals that mortality rose around age twenty and remained high thereafter.[109] This distribution and high prepubescent mortality imply that ages fifteen through nineteen were the only years comparatively free from death.

Yet these numbers reveal little about eggs, chickens, and ducks' contributions to health. Domett identified chicken bones at both southeastern villages, Khok Phanom Di and Nong Nor, but at neither in the northeast, Ban Lum Khao and Ban Na Di.[110] This division should have permitted contrasts

TABLE 6.6
Revised % Deaths by Age in Thailand and Vietnam

Place	<15 yr	15–19 yr	20–29 yr	30–39 yr	40+ yr
Da But	50	5.8	9.1	14.3	20.3
Khok Phanom Di	55.8	5.2	14.9	17.5	6.5
Early Non Nok Tha	50	2.55	9	12.8	25.65
Early Ban Chiang	50	3.45	10.4	10.4	25.85
Late Non Nok Tha	50	1.2	7.15	17.85	23.8
Nong Nor	28	1.3	16.8	27.7	9
Ban Lum Khao	46.4	4.5	22.7	15.5	10.9
Late Ban Chiang	50	c. 7.6	c. 9.1	c. 16.65	16.65
Ban Na Di	35.9	0	16.7	16.7	12.8
Ma, Ca	50	5.95	19.05	11.9	13.1
Noen U-Loke	50	3.7	22.2	13	11.1
Red River	50	6.8	18.2	13.65	11.35

between southeast and northeast, but the differences were temporal rather than geographic. That is, health—as measured by longevity, height, and enamel hypoplasia (all defined in Chapter 1)—improved over time not space.[111] The earliest village, Khok Phanom Di, displayed the worst health. Bronze Age Nong Nor and Ban Lum Khao (c. 1400 BCE) were intermediate, and Iron Age Ban Na Di (600–400 BCE) exhibited the best outcomes. Were diet a factor, the later sites may have been healthier because food supply was more dependable, or storage places held larger reserves to cover fluctuations in supply.

6.8 WESTERN HEMISPHERE

6.8.1 Turkeys in Pre-Columbian North America

The turkey's ancestors inhabited North America around 23 million years ago.[112] Unlike today's turkeys, these birds were light enough to fly, though their reproductive habits favored enlargement. Like many animals, including humans to a degree, the turkey's predecessors exhibited sexual dimorphism whereby males were larger than females.[113] This difference implies that females mated with large males, a preference that retained genes for size. Domestication would amplify this trend.

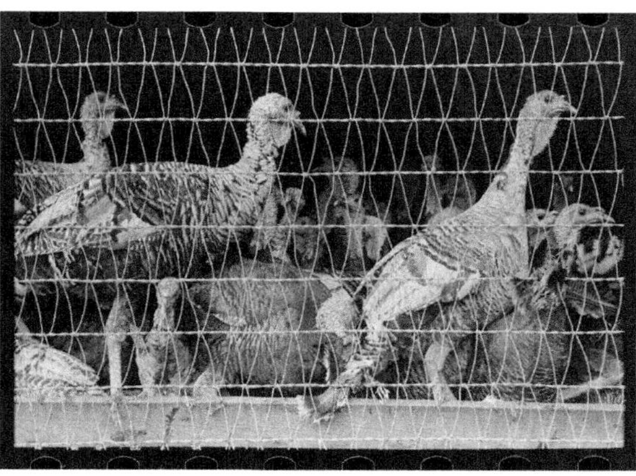

FIGURE 6.6 Turkeys. (Photo courtesy of Library of Congress. https://www.loc.gov/pictures/item/2017741384/.)

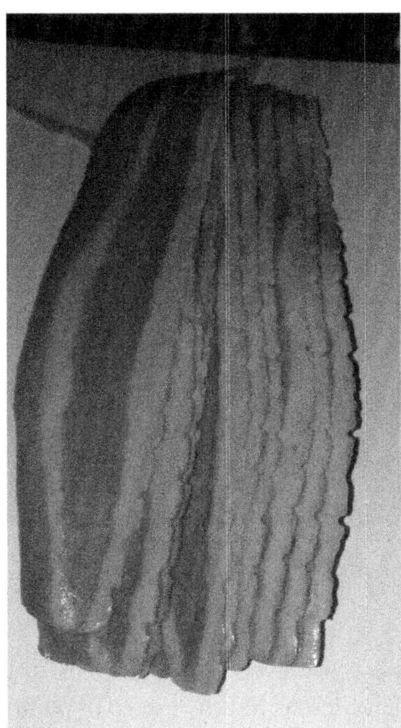

FIGURE 6.7 Turkey bacon. (Photo from author.)

Scientists have dated the genus *Meleagris* to the Pleistocene (2.6 million–12,000 years ago). Early finds may be *M. gallopavo*. The genus speciated repeatedly before humans entered the Americas, a development that Chapter 3 recounted. Amerindians domesticated two, *Meleagris ocellata* in Central America and southern Mexico and *M. gallopavo f. domestica* in the American Southwest. The first must have been plentiful enough for the Maya to characterize Central America and southern Mexico as lands of turkeys and deer.[114] Europeans who colonized what is today the United States encountered the second, making it a Thanksgiving staple. So complete was domestication that wild turkeys no longer exist. Aside from dogs, the turkey was prehistoric North America's only domestic animal.[115]

The taming of two species necessitated more than one episode of domestication. Mesoamericans may have tamed *M. ocellata* between 2500 and 200 BCE.[116] To the north, Ancestral Puebloans in Mesa Verde, Colorado—near what is now the junction among Utah, Colorado, New Mexico, and Arizona and known as the Four Corners—domesticated *M. gallopavo f. domestica* centuries before European contact. American paleontologist Stanley John Olsen (1919–2003) dated domestication no later than Pueblo I period (750–900 CE).[117]

Wild turkeys may have aided this transition by congregating among humans in hopes of eating leftovers. Reintroducing turkeys into Mesa Verde National Park in 1944, the U.S. Park Service witnessed their intrusiveness.[118] Park agents could not frighten them away with small explosives. Similar behavior may have led Ancestral Puebloans to herd turkeys, which benefited farmers by eating insects, slugs, and snails and consumers by furnishing flesh and eggs. In addition, Amerindians fashioned turkey bones into tools, used feathers for adornment, and sacrificed these birds during rituals.

The last two uses generated commentary. Relying on Spanish accounts, American anthropologist Corina M. Kellner and coauthors wrote that "turkeys were kept largely for their feathers at many pueblos."[119] American archaeologist and anthropologist Gordon F. M. Rakita and Mexican archaeologist Rafael Cruz noted that Mexicans in pre-Columbian Paquime in Chihuahua state interred headless turkeys with human corpses, speculating that decapitation occurred during burial

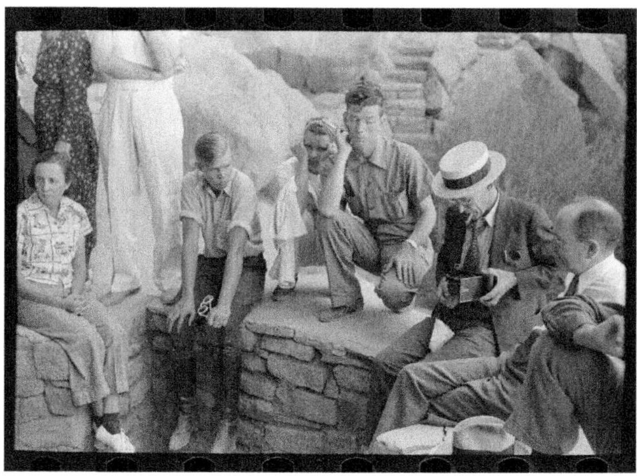

FIGURE 6.8 Mesa Verde National Park. (Photo courtesy of Library of Congress. https://www.loc.gov/pictures/item/2017740641/.)

rituals.[120] In the American Southwest, however, Rakita and Cruz identified consumption rather than religious uses.[121] Turkey intake increased as Southwestern populations grew and game dwindled.[122] "Turkeys might have been important sources of protein at certain Southwestern pueblos, part of a strategy to cope with relatively limited access to other types of meat," acknowledged Kellner and colleagues.[123]

Archaeologists and anthropologists may have overstated the extent of specialization. Raising turkeys for feathers did not preclude eating eggs or slaughtering birds for food when people were hungry or favored other types of ornamentation. Although killing turkeys during rituals and burying them afterward eliminated them as food, there is no reason to suppose that Amerindians eschewed eggs while hens matured to sizes deemed suitable for sacrifice. Plains Indians used all parts of bison, whose contributions to nutrition and health are in Chapter 4.[124] Similar behavior surely governed hungry tom and hen keepers.

This book emphasizes that anthropologists, archaeologists, biologists, and other scientists often infer animal consumption by counting bones in middens and bone fragments in coprolites. This method has the value of concreteness but is biased in favor of large, sturdy bones that tend to preserve better than small, light ones. As noted, however, bird bones fall into the second category. Absence from the archaeological record because of poor preservation does not preclude consumption unless evidence eliminates a food from diets. The problem of how to draw inferences from silence is central to an attempt to understand prehistory, when written records cannot be consulted for insights into any aspect of life.

Fortunately, the Southwest offers prehistorians an array of biofacts because aridity retarded deterioration. Readers may consult Chapter 15 for more information about climates favorable for preserving the past. Dryness yielded turkey bones and eggshells. Mesa Verde National Park's Mug House Ruin had over 1,074 bones from between 183 and 815 turkeys.[125] The park's Big Juniper House likewise possessed many bones. Other Southwest sites—including Poncho House in San Juan County, Utah, Betatakin Pueblo in Shonto, Arizona, Kiet Siel Pueblo near Kayenta, Arizona, Awatovi Ruins near Keams Canyon, Arizona, Arroyo Hondo near Taos, New Mexico, and Wupatki Pueblo near Flagstaff, Arizona—contained numerous turkey bones.[126] Cut marks—for example, on bones found at Pecos Pueblo in Pecos, New Mexico—evinced butchering.[127] There, turkey bones were more plentiful than those of any other bird, indicating dietary prominence. Bones represented turkeys at all stages of development, demonstrating that Amerindians ate them as hatchlings on up to maturity.[128] Bones' disarticulation—for example, at Gran Quivira in Salinas Pueblo Missions National Monument, New Mexico—indicated consumption of flesh in segments just as moderns eat chicken from legs or another part.[129] Bone fragments in coprolites at Cedar Mesa in San Juan County, Utah, prove ingestion.[130] Eggshells reveal that turkeys were tame enough to reproduce in captivity.

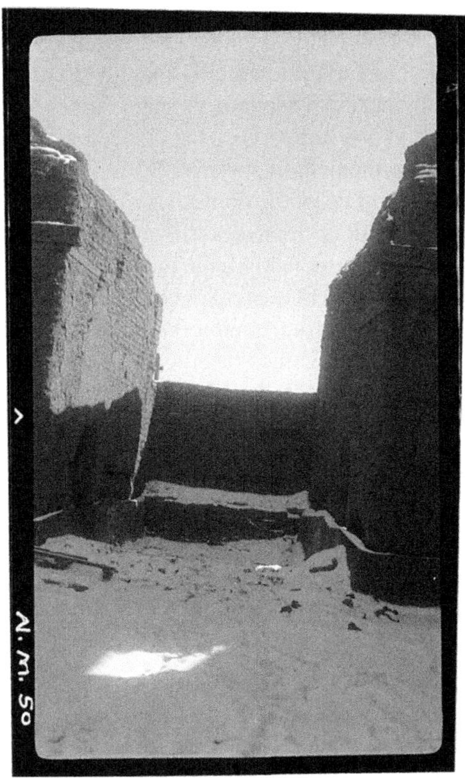

FIGURE 6.9 Pecos Pueblo. (Photo courtesy of Library of Congress. https://www.loc.gov/pictures/item/nm0044.photos.113783p/.)

Pecos Pueblo, inhabited from the thirteenth century CE to 1838 and excavated since the 1920s, has yielded nearly 2,000 partial and complete Amerindian skeletons.[131] This book repeatedly remarks that researchers have employed chemistry to study diets. Chapter 1 noted that plants use carbon dioxide (CO_2) in different ways. Transformation of it into the three-carbon compound phosphoglyceric acid ($C_3H_7O_7P$) is designated the C_3 pathway. All fruit trees and some plants that arose in the tropics—for example, sweet potatoes (*Ipomoea batatas*), tomatoes (*Solanum esculentum*), and beans (*Phaseolus vulgaris*, *P. lunatus*, *P. acutifolius*, and *P. coccineus*)—are C_3. In contrast, other tropical plants—for example, sugarcane (*Saccharum officinarum*), corn, millet, and sorghum (*Sorghum* species)—use carbon dioxide to make the four-carbon molecule oxaloacetic acid ($C_4H_4O_5$) by the C_4 pathway. These pathways use different carbon isotopes such that isotope ratios in animals, including humans, help determine what they ate.

Isotope proportions demonstrate that Pecos Puebloans ate mostly C_4 plants and animals that fed on these plants. For example, bison grazed C_4 grasses and were part of Pecos diets.[132] The pueblo's occupants were farmers more than hunter-gatherers and did not pursue bison, instead acquiring it through trade with Plains Indians. Conflicts—which Spaniards intensified upon entering the Southwest in the sixteenth century—disrupted trade, eliminating access to bison during these times. Yet isotope data indicate steady C_4-food intake. Uniformity resulted from consumption of C_4 staples such as corn and turkeys. Turkeys were especially important in this regard because Amerindians fed them corn. That is, domestic turkeys were a richer C_4 source than wild birds. This reasoning suggests not only that Pecos Puebloans depended on turkey but that they had fully domesticated the bird. In addition, Pecos Pueblo's denizens ate mule deer (*Odocoileus hemionus*), whose bones were numerous in middens.[133] This plentitude appears to contradict isotope results because these deer browsed C_3 plants.

In addition to biological and chemical evidence, art documented turkeys' prominence in the Southwest. At Awatovi, Hopi artists depicted them on kiva walls and pottery.[134] Between 1100 and 1300, the Navajo painted a mural of turkeys on a cliff roughly 20 meters (21.9 yards or 65.6 feet) aboveground at Canyon de Chelly National Monument near Chinle, Arizona.

Besides biology, chemistry, and art, numerous pens evinced turkeys' abundance. Thick layers of excrement confirmed pens' confinement of turkeys. Within homes, the structures concretized domestication in a fundamental way. The word "domesticate" derives from the Latin *domus*, meaning "home." The English noun "domicile" conveys this meaning. Domestication therefore was a process that made an animal or plant sufficiently tame and useful to merit its introduction into the home. What could not be brought into the home remained alien, and a source of unease, to civilization's order and stability. These pens thus confirmed turkeys' full integration into Southwestern life.

Additional evidence for domestication comes from feathers, whose color varies with diet. Wild turkeys, like humans, are omnivores. Their fondness for insects, slugs, snails, and worms gave them proteins with many amino acids. Turkeys must ingest the amino acid lysine to produce feathers with colors other than white. The feathers recovered from Mesa Verde have white tips, indicating insufficient lysine.[135] This coloration suggests turkeys' confinement and dietary restriction. They must have eaten just plants rather than the usual buffet of invertebrates and plants. Low in lysine, corn grown in the Southwest was probably the chief feed.

Surveying the evidence, Olsen judged turkey the primary animal in prehistoric Southwestern diets.[136] It fed natives in lands marginal for crops. Assailing the Southwest with repeated droughts, aridity endangered farming. The Medieval Warm Period (see Chapters 8, 9, and 16) between the ninth and thirteenth centuries did not benefit the Southwest as it did Europe. Between 1130 and 1180 drought desiccated lands west of the Mississippi River.[137] From 1276 to 1299, the Great Drought caused indigenes to abandon their homes.[138] Unpredictability magnified drought's threat as three wind patterns met at the Four Corner. The outcome of the tussle among the three varied, changing rainfall from year to year. Another danger came from the northwest, whose cold air descended on the region, shortening growing seasons.[139] Corn, the primary crop and a tropical grass in origin (see Chapter 12), suffered. Thirteenth-century harvests underfed populations. Such circumstances must have increased Amerindians' reliance on turkeys, eggs, and game.

Columbus and his crew were the first Europeans to see and taste turkey.[140] In 1502, on the fourth voyage, they landed on the coast of what is now Honduras. The native population brought the Spanish what they called "land chickens" and what scholars believe were turkeys.[141] The birds' terrestrial habits suggest that they could not fly. In 1519, Spanish conquistador Hernan Cortes (1485–1547) saw turkeys—which fed Aztecs absent large livestock—in Tenochtitlan, now Mexico City.[142] Visiting Mexico in 1529, Franciscan priest Bernardino de Sahagun (1499–1590) observed turkey eggs and flesh with chili pepper (*Capsicum* species) sauce, tomatoes, and squash (*Cucurbita* species) seeds in Aztec markets.[143] Between 1540 and 1542, Spanish conquistador Francisco Vasquez de Coronado (1510–1554) and his men ate turkeys while searching the Southwest for gold. One among them enthused about the "large numbers of native hens and cocks."[144] Although he did not name the bird, the adjective "native" implies turkey rather than chicken. Familiar with the latter, Europeans would not have designated it indigenous to the Americas. The turkey excited commentary because it was novel.

6.8.2 Turkeys, Amerindians, and Health

The aridity that preserved turkey bones and eggshells in the Southwest likewise perpetuated human remains. To be sure, conditions were imperfect. The extent of disarticulation complicated the tasks of reassembly and examination.[145] Coyotes (*Canis latrans*), foxes (*Vulpes macrotis* and *Urocyon cinereoargenteus*), bobcats (*Lynx rufus*), cougars (*Puma concolor*), or their combination worsened disorder by attempting to eat corpses, scattering bones in the process.[146] Amerindians contributed to disarray by reentering burial chambers over several generations, repositioning old remains to accommodate new ones.[147]

Despite this limitation, interest in Southwestern prehistory was as old as Spanish incursions. Early antiquarian curiosity began to yield to quantification around the turn of the twentieth century. Czech-American physician and anthropologist Ales Hrdlicka (1869–1943) aided this transition, not only measuring indigenes in the Southwest and northern Mexico between 1899 and 1902, but also examining every skeleton that might have illuminated when and by what route the first peoples entered the Americas.[148] Besides Hrdlicka, American anthropologist Earnest Albert Hooton (1887–1954) in 1930 published *The Indians of Pecos Pueblo: A Study of Their Skeletal Remains*. Examining 374 skeletons from what is now Pecos National Historical Park in Pecos, New Mexico, Hooton was among the first to quantify a population's health.[149] American anthropologist George John Armelagos (1936–2014), acknowledging the tendency to esteem the book as "the pivotal publication of the era," believed that its influence began only in the 1960s.[150] Since then, scientists and scholars have continued to cite it.[151]

Hooton expressed a dour view of the village, writing that "comparatively few of the Pecos Indians lived to old age" because of high mortality between ages thirty-five and fifty-four.[152] This language affirms my conviction, reiterated below, that premodern peoples led brief existences. Moreover, Pecos' inhabitants were shorter than modern Puebloans.[153] Stature shrank, and dental health declined over time.[154] Evincing life's physicality, osteoarthritis increased over the centuries but was never as widespread as in Mexico, Central America, or Peru. Although Hooton omitted specifics about diet, he rated it unbalanced and inadequate.[155]

As Hooton foresaw, *The Indians of Pecos Pueblo* was not the final word on Southwestern diet, nutrition, and health. American anthropologist and osteologist Ann Lucy Wiener Stodder and colleagues examined bones from at least 135 Ancestral Puebloans unearthed around 32.2 kilometers (20 miles) north of Mesa Verde National Park.[156] Reassembly yielded sixty-four skeletons complete enough for study. The individuals, occupying the northeasternmost range of Ancestral Puebloan settlement, lived between roughly 600 and 980 CE. The northern latitude and elevation produced short growing seasons with frost a danger in late spring and early autumn. Perhaps to deemphasize the scale of crop raising, the authors characterized the economy as horticulture rather than farming.[157] Crop production's unreliability must have increased Ancestral Puebloan reliance on turkeys and eggs.

Although onlookers might dismiss this area—now the town of Dolores, Colorado—as unsuitable for habitation, rainfall tended to be greater than elsewhere in the Southwest.[158] Around 600 CE, a warm interlude enticed Amerindians along Colorado and New Mexico's extension of the San Juan River north to Dolores. Despite warmth, rainfall diminished thereafter, and when the climate cooled again in the tenth century, people retreated to the river. Even while occupied, therefore, Dolores was a precarious location.

Unsurprisingly, skeletons revealed life's difficulties in a marginal environment. Setting aside those too incomplete to age, the remains included few young and old. Table 6.7 reveals that seventeen percent were estimated no older than eleven years, and only 3.8 percent reached their fifth decade.[159] The fact that nearly everyone perished before age forty aligns with data from Chapters 1 and 3 and with Hooton's findings. Deevey's computation in the above chapters that between Neanderthal prehistory and around 1900 CE, life expectancy at birth (e^0) seldom departed over five years from age twenty-five squares with Stodder and coauthors' e^0s for Southwestern sites Hawikku (21.5 years) near Zuni, New Mexico, and San Cristobal Pueblo (22.2 years) in San Cristobal, New Mexico.[160]

The authors omitted Dolores' e^0—perhaps because of the incomplete skeletons that could not be aged and the dearth of infants—though there is no reason to think it surpassed those for Hawikku and San Cristobal. As noted, Deevey also stated that roughly half of all children died before puberty, a pattern incompatible with pre-Columbian Dolores, whose remains registered 20.8

TABLE 6.7
Age range at death in Dolores CO c. 600–c. 980 CE

Age Range	# of Deaths	% of Deaths
<3 yr	3	5.7
3–7 yr	6	11.3
8–11 yr	0	0
12–15 yr	2	3.8
16–20 yr	11	20.8
21–26 yr	18	34
27–35 yr	5	9.4
36–40 yr	6	11.3
40+ yr	2	3.8
Total	53	100.1

percent of deaths before age sixteen.[161] This chapter entertains the possibility that not all juveniles were buried, that many child corpses did not persist into the present—especially given attention from carnivores—that birthrate was low, or that more than one factor was involved.

Whatever the explanation, Dolores' residents ailed. Forty percent of men, and double that of women, died between ages sixteen and twenty-six.[162] This decade overlapped women's reproductive years and may indicate high mortality during childbirth. Even so the disparity between women and men was large. Irrespective of sex, 78 percent of skeletons exhibited cribra orbitalia, defined in Chapter 1 as a mark of anemia, though only 9 percent betrayed porotic hyperostosis, also defined in Chapter 1. Osteoarthritis afflicted nearly everyone, even youths, suggesting life's arduousness.

Dolores' men averaged 162.3 centimeters (63.9 inches) and women were 156 centimeters (61.4 inches), whereas Mesa Verde's men between about 500 and 650 CE stood 162 centimeters (63.8 inches) and women 155.3 centimeters (61.1 inches), implying better nutrition at Dolores than Mesa Verde.[163] Dolores' mean heights also surpassed those at pre-Columbian Cuicuilco in Tlalpan borough, Mexico, Tikal in El Peten department, Guatemala, Cholula near Puebla, Mexico, and Yucatan peninsula dwellers after about 1520 CE.[164] Dolores' men stood taller than men in Jaina on Jaina Island, Mexico, but shorter than their counterparts in Teotihuacan 40 kilometers (25 miles) northeast of what is today Mexico City, in Tlatilco, which is today within Mexico City, and in Copan in Copan Ruinas, Honduras. Dolores' women were taller than those in Tlatilco, Teotihuacan, the Yucatan peninsula, Jaina, and Copan. Figure 8.8 tabulates Mesoamerican heights.

Dolores' mean heights were below averages for men and women in Tehuacan 254.4 kilometers (158.1 miles) southeast of Mexico City and for Maya in Copan.[165] Dolores' heights also trailed all Plains Indian averages in Table 4.7 calculated by German-American anthropologist Franz Uri Boas (1858–1942) and his assistants in the 1880s. Men averaged 172.2 centimeters (67.8 inches) and women 159.7 centimeters (62.9 inches).[166] The tallest were the Cheyenne, whose men were 176.7 centimeters (69.6 inches) and women 161.5 centimeters (63.6 inches). The shortest were the Comanche, whose men stood 168 centimeters (66.1 inches) on average. The mean for women was 156.7 centimeters (61.7 inches).

Even taller on average, northern European men between roughly 800 and 1300 CE (see Chapter 8) stood 173.4 centimeters (68.3 inches) according to military records.[167] Above these means were African Americans interred in Lafayette County, Arkansas' Cedar Grove Cemetery between 1881 and 1927. Skeletons of the fourteen men averaged 177.8 centimeters (70 inches), and the nineteen women were 162.8 centimeters (64.1 inches) on average.[168] Correlation between nutrition and height, discussed throughout this book, implies that Southwestern peoples were less nourished than Plains Indians, medieval northern Europeans, and Arkansas' rural African Americans. Comparisons between the Southwest on one hand and Central America and Mexico on the other yielded mixed results.

Health data also came from Hawikku, referenced earlier. Settled around 1425, habitation overlapped with Spanish incursion after 1539.[169] The Spanish brought Old World diseases to which Amerindians lacked immunities. With perhaps 4,000 to 7,000 occupants in 1538, Hawikku lost half its population to diseases in the sixteenth century, and deaths continued to mount through the next century. Skeletons revealed anemia in at least 84 percent of Zuni. The percentage must have been higher given that the condition must be severe and prolonged to mark bones. Ninety-four percent of individuals had teeth with enamel hypoplasia, which Chapter 1 defined as a sign of undernutrition, illness, parasitism, or their combination. Most hypoplasias formed between ages three and five, suggesting dietary stress, infections, parasites, or their combination after weaning.

San Cristobal, settled about 1350, suffered a similar fate when Coronado and his men arrived in 1540.[170] The Spanish stole Puebloan food, causing warfare between Amerindians and invaders. Diseases, droughts, and famines deepened conflict and instability. Ninety percent of skeletons exhibited anemia, and 85 percent had hypoplasia in at least one tooth.[171] Hypoplasia was commonest between ages 3 and 4.5. The few who reached age 45 lost on average 12.6 teeth. Life's brevity confined mean loss to 3.9 teeth per person.

Skeletons from other Southwestern sites tell similar stories. Judging from human remains, anemia afflicted 85 percent of Amerindians below age eleven in Black Mesa, Arizona, between 700 and 1100, 79 percent in Mesa Verde National Park between 700 and 1300, 72 percent in Canyon de Chelley in Canyon de Chelley National Monument, Arizona between 300 BCE and 700 CE, 68 percent in Chaco Canyon in Chaco Culture National Historical Park, New Mexico between 700 and 1100, and 45 percent in Pueblo Bonito also in Chaco Culture National Historical Park between 900 and 1100.[172] Table 6.8 tabulates anemia, bone lesions, and dental cavities among Southwestern peoples.

Yet skeletons from Grasshopper Pueblo in Coconino National Forest, Arizona, Pecos Pueblo, Arroyo Hondo, and Gran Quivira—all of which evinced turkey consumption—exhibited less anemia than other sites' remains. Hooton identified cribra orbitalia, porotic hypoplasia, or both in only 1.5 percent of Pecos Pueblo skeletons.[173] Kellner and colleagues reexamined the data, concluding

TABLE 6.8
Anemia Bone Lesions and Dental Caries in American Southwest

Place	Time	Anemia (#)	Bone Legions (#)	Caries (#)
Canyon de Chelley, AZ	c. 300 BCE–c. 700 CE	72	N/A	N/A
Dolores, CO	c. 600–c. 980 CE	78	12	71
Black Mesa, AZ	c. 700–c. 1100 CE	85	23	26
Chaco Canyon, NM	c. 700–c. 1100 CE	68	17	85
Pueblo Bonito, NM	c. 900–c. 1100 CE	45	N/A	N/A
Mesa Verde, CO	c. 700–c. 1300 CE	79	N/A	N/A
Grasshopper, AZ	c. 1245–c. 1400 CE	15	12	52
Tijeras, NM	c. 1300–c. 1425	N/A	3	23
Paako NM	c. 1300–c. 1600 CE	N/A	4	N/A
Arroyo Hondo, NM	c. 1300–c. 1600 CE	22	13	N/A
Gran Quivira, NM	c. 1300–c. 1520 CE	18	N/A	N/A
San Cristobal, NM	1350–c. 1520 CE	87	23	57
Hawikku, NM	1425–c. 1520 CE	74	36	53
Pecos Pueblo, NM	1425–1550 CE	N/A	N/A	48
Pecos Pueblo	1550–1600 CE	N/A	N/A	61

that the rate, between 2 and 4 percent overall, was worst among the youngest at 10.5 percent. The percentage for children under eleven years at Grasshopper was 15, at Gran Quivira 18, and at Arroyo Hondo 22.[174] This evidence suggests that Amerindians who appear to have eaten turkey in appreciable quantities were healthier than those who ate less or none.

Turkey may not deserve credit for little anemia, however, as measured by cribra orbitalia and porotic hypoplasia at Pecos Pueblo. First, this book emphasizes that anemia must be severe and sustained to affect bones. The condition's breadth was probably worse than bones imply. Second, earlier sections noted that turkey has less iron and vitamins B_9 and B_{12} than bison and venison by mass and that Pecos Puebloans ate all three. Even when bison was unavailable because warfare disrupted trade, these Amerindians could still rely on turkey and venison. If diet diminished anemia at Pecos Pueblo, venison and bison probably merited praise more than turkey.

Besides diet, Pecos Puebloans were fortunate to get water from a stream, whose movement likely prevented accumulation of pathogens and parasites, thereby reducing anemia.[175] Moreover, American ecologist Michele Elizabeth Morgan wrote that the village's occupants were active throughout life.[176] Walking and running appear to have been regular undertakings, especially for men. To be sure, there is no reason to suppose that other Southwestern peoples were inert. Activity differentiated Pecos Puebloans from moderns more than from contemporaries.

Despite comparatively little anemia at Pecos Pueblo, Grasshopper, Gran Quivira, and Arroyo Hondo, Stodder and coauthors ranked Southwestern health worse than that of South Carolina slaves.[177] In the late seventeenth century, Chapter 12 notes, rice (likely *Oryza glaberrima* followed by *O. sativa*) emerged as the plantation crop along South Carolina's coast. Rutgers University historians Nancy A. Hewitt and Steven Fred Lawson (b. 1945) described these farms as "virtual labor camps, where thousands of slaves worked under harsh conditions with no hope of improvement."[178] American historian Gary Baring Nash (b. 1933) and colleagues wrote that these slaves "working mostly on large plantations in swampy lowlands…endured the most life-sapping conditions on the continent."[179] American historian Henry Clay Dethloff (1934–2019) asserted that these plantations required the most "arduous and brutal" labor.[180]

Such commentary implies that rice plantations undermined health. South Carolina planter, soldier, and politician William Butler (1759–1821) blamed the air for harboring "so many diseases."[181] American historian Hayden Ros Smith acknowledged that these plantations trailed only sugar estates in mortality.[182] Thirty-seven African American skeletons from Paul Remley Plantation near Charleston, South Carolina—interred between roughly 1840 and 1870—exhibited anemia from childhood through adulthood.[183] Over 60 percent displayed cribra orbitalia, porotic hyperostosis, or both. American anthropologist Ted Allan Rathbun (b. 1942) and American economist Richard Hall Steckel (b. 1944) attributed these conditions to undernutrition and parasites. Obvious candidates were the malaria parasites *Plasmodium vivax* and *Plasmodium falciparum*, both of which reached South Carolina by the 1680s.[184] Deterioration of skeletons' joints indicated strenuous exertions.[185]

Stodder and colleagues also ranked Southwestern health below that of soldiers who died during the Civil War (1861–1865).[186] The deadliest U.S. conflict, the war witnessed over 600,000 deaths.[187] Although battlefield carnage was grisly, diseases were the principal killers, claiming nearly half a regiment in an average year.[188] Wounds that were not immediately fatal but that became infected made men corpses as surely as if artillery had destroyed them. By one estimate, diseases caused 413,458 of the Civil War's 617,528 (67 percent) deaths.

Stodder and coauthors blamed primarily contagion and secondarily inadequate diets for poor health in the Southwest.[189] Their argument that diseases were the chief bane and that Southwestern health was among the worst in the Americas necessitates that contagion was more lethal in the Southwest than elsewhere in the western hemisphere. This book disagrees, noting, first, that some of the authors' data came from pre-Columbian times, when Old World diseases were unknown in the Americas.

Second, these diseases were virulent throughout the New World, leaving no reason to suppose special ferocity in the Southwest. For example, perhaps 90 percent of Arawak indigenes died within seventy-five years of Columbus' 1492 arrival on Hispaniola.[190] These Indians are now extinct. Between roughly 1500 and 1650 native populations in Mexico and Central America plummeted from some 40 million to 3 million.[191] By 1569, about 90 percent of Mexico's Aztecs had perished from diseases.[192] From around 1530 to 1630, the Inca Empire contracted from some 10 million inhabitants to under 500,000. Entering California in 1542, the Spanish introduced smallpox, measles, cholera, and typhus.[193] Syphilis was also present, and malaria arrived with the gold rush (1848–c. 1855). The population, between roughly 310,000 and 705,000 natives about 1550, plunged by 1900 to around 15,000, though warfare, genocide, and starvation were also to blame.[194] In 1616 and 1619, bubonic plague killed some 90 percent of Amerindians from Maine to Cape Cod, Massachusetts.[195] In the 1630s, smallpox eradicated Massachusetts' Algonquin villages.[196] Between roughly 1630 and 1650 smallpox extirpated half the Hurons and Iroquois near the St. Lawrence River and Great Lakes. By 1759, smallpox had killed half the Cherokees and Catawbas in the Southeast.[197] Smallpox depopulated Puget Sound in what is today Washington state such that in 1792, British explorers found empty villages.[198] On the Great Plains in 1837, the disease killed over 95 percent of Mandan.[199] Chapter 5 noted that contagion exterminated Canada's Sadlermiut Inuit in 1903.[200]

If the Southwest suffered no more from diseases than elsewhere in the New World, then diets deserve attention. The issue may be less what Amerindians ate than amount. Earlier paragraphs noted the Southwest's unsuitability for farming. Droughts caused the food shortages that imperiled health. Beyond these considerations, reliance on corn—whose shortcomings Chapter 12 discusses—provided too few amino acids, fatty acids, vitamins, and minerals.

Confirmation of insufficiencies came from Grasshopper Pueblo, which Amerindians began to settle around 1275, having fled even harsher areas as aridity increased the difficulties of growing and finding enough food.[201] Protein, calorie, vitamin, and mineral intake appears to have diminished, and heights declined, before Grasshopper's abandonment around 1400.[202] Increases in consumption of C_4 foods may indicate reliance on corn. Although in his study of the village, American anthropologist Joseph Anthony Ezzo, Jr. (b. 1957) described turkeys as wild, the Southwest had already tamed them.[203] Of course, domestication would not have precluded consumption of wild turkeys, especially if domestic supply failed to feed everyone. If fed corn, the usual practice as noted, domestic turkeys constituted a C_4 source that aligned with isotope data. Whatever their status at Grasshopper, turkeys did not, and probably could not, protect Amerindians from the aridity that shrank food supplies.

Agriculture at Grasshopper and elsewhere in the Southwest was unreliable, and productivity decreased as droughts intensified. Amerindians who could not raise enough crops turned to turkeys, eggs, and game, though these foods did not offset life's rigors. Although overall Southwestern health was poor, turkey consumers appear to have enjoyed better nutrition and vigor than other Ancestral Puebloans.

NOTES

1 Carol Hand, *The Evolution of Birds* (Minneapolis, MN: Essential Library, 2019), 9–10.
2 Ibid.
3 Ibid., 5–6.
4 Ibid., 7–8.
5 Stanley A. Rice, *Encyclopedia of Evolution* (New York: Facts on File, 2007), 99.
6 Hand, 16.
7 "See Some of the Most Fantastic Birds in the World," *Wildfoot*, accessed July 18, 2019, https://www.wildfoottravel.com/antarctica/information/wildlife-plants/birds.
8 Stanley J. Ulijaszek, Neil Mann, and Sarah Elton, *Evolving Human Nutrition: Implications for Public Health* (Cambridge, UK: Cambridge University Press, 2012), 77.
9 Robert Jurmain, Lynn Kilgore, Wenda Trevathan, and Russell L. Ciochon. *Introduction to Physical Anthropology*, 2013–2014 ed. (Belmont, CA: Wadsworth Cengage Learning, 2014), 320.

10 Richard F. Johnston, "Pigeons," in *The Cambridge World History of Food*, vol. 1, ed. Kenneth F. Kiple and Kriemhild Conee Ornelas (Cambridge, UK: Cambridge University Press, 2000), 561.
11 Ibid.
12 Rosemary Luff, "Ducks," in *The Cambridge World History of Food*, vol. 1, ed. Kenneth F. Kiple and Kriemhild Conee Ornelas (Cambridge, UK: Cambridge University Press, 2000), 518.
13 Ibid.
14 Colin Barras, "How Humanity First Killed the Dodo, Then Lost It as Well," April 9, 2016, accessed August, 4, 2019, http://www.bbc.com/earth/story/20160408-how-humanity-first-killed-the-dodo-then-lost-it-as-well.
15 Eric Chaline, *Fifty Animals That Changed the Course of History* (New York: Firefly Books, 2011), 183.
16 Ibid., 182.
17 Barras.
18 Chaline, 183.
19 Barras.
20 David Quammen, *The Song of the Dodo: Island Biogeography in an Age of Extinctions* (New York: Scribner, 1996), 265–266; Stephen Jay Gould, *The Panda's Thumb: More Reflections in Natural History* (New York and London: Norton, 1980), 281.
21 Barras; Chaline, 183.
22 Barry Yeoman, "Why the Passenger Pigeon Went Extinct," *Audubon*, May-June 2104, accessed August 4, 2019, https://www.audubon.org/magazine/may-june-2014/why-passenger-pigeon-went-extinct.
23 Stephen Jay Gould, *Eight Little Piggies: Reflections in Natural History* (New York and London: Norton, 1993), 53.
24 Waverley Root and Richard de Rochemont, *Eating in America: A History* (Hopewell, NJ: Ecco Press, 1995), 69.
25 Gould, *Eight Little Piggies*, 53–54.
26 Elizabeth J. Reitz, "Temperate and Arctic North America to 1492," in *The Cambridge World History of Food*, vol. 1, ed. Kenneth F. Kiple and Kriemhild Conee Ornelas (Cambridge, UK: Cambridge University Press, 2000), 1297.
27 W. Stephen Damron, *Introduction to Animal Science: Global Biological, Social, and Industry Perspectives*, 3rd ed. (Upper Saddle River, NJ and Columbus, OH: Pearson/Prentice Hall, 2006), 395.
28 Annie Potts, *Chicken* (London: Reaktion Books, 2012), 150.
29 Damron, 21.
30 "Wholesale and Retail Prices for Chicken, Beef, and Pork," *National Chicken Council*, March 25, 2019, accessed August 1, 2019, https://www.nationalchickencouncil.org/about-the-industry/statistics/wholesale-and-retail-prices-for-chicken-beef-and-pork.
31 Potts, 153–163.
32 Damron, 19.
33 Ibid., 393–394.
34 Ibid., 17–18.
35 Ibid., 18.
36 Ibid., 19.
37 Ibid., 22.
38 Ibid., 421.
39 Ibid., 417.
40 J. R. Williams, J. M. Roseland, Q. V. Nguyen, J. C. Howe, K. Y. Patterson, P. R. Pehrsson, and L. D. Thompson, "Nutrient Composition and Retention in Whole Turkeys with and without Added Solution," *Poultry Science* 96, no. 10 (October 2017): 3586–3592, https://www.sciencedirect.com/science/article/pii/S003257911931572X?via%3Dihub.
41 "100 G Skinless Chicken Breast," *Fatsecret*, January 14, 2013, accessed August 1, 2019, https://www.fatsecret.com/calories-nutrition/generic/chicken-breast-skinless?portionid=4751539&portionamount=100.000.
42 Ibid.
43 Damron, 417; "Turkey, Whole, Breast, Meat Only, Cooked, Roasted," *USDA FoodData Central*, April 1, 2019, accessed February 10, 2020, https://fdc.nal.usda.gov/fdc-app.html#/food-details/171496/nutrients.
44 Damron, 9–10.
45 Ibid., 417; "Turkey, Whole, Breast, Meat Only, Cooked, Roasted."
46 Damron, 417; "Turkey, Whole, Breast, Meat Only, Cooked, Roasted;" Alexandra Schmid and Barbara Walther, "Natural Vitamin D Content in Animal Products," *Advances in Nutrition* 4, no. 4 (July 2013): 453–462, https://www.ncbi.nlm.nih.gov/pmc/articles/PMC3941824.

47 Damron, 389.
48 Ibid., 421.
49 Ibid.; Joseph Lamour, "Americans Eat on Average almost 300 Eggs a Year," *Kitchn*, March 1, 2019, accessed August 2, 2019, https://www.thekitchn.com/americans-eat-on-average-almost-300-eggs-a-year-267411.
50 Damron, 417.
51 Ibid.; "Eggs, Whole, Raw," *USDA FoodData Central*, April 1, 2019, accessed November 27, 2019, https://fdc.nal.usda.gov/fdc-app.html#/food-details/339003/nutrients; "Egg, Fresh, Raw, Whole," *Nutrition Facts*, 2019, accessed November 27, 2019, https://www.nutritionvalue.org/Egg%2C_fresh%2C_raw%2C_whole_nutritional_value.html; "FDA Vitamins and Minerals Chart," *FDA*, accessed April 24, 2019, https://www.accessdata.fda.gov/scripts/interactivenutritionfactslabel/factsheets/vitamin_and_mineral_chart.pdf.
52 Jerome C. Rose and Melissa Zabecki, "The Commoners of Tell el-Amarna," in *Beyond the Horizon: Studies in Egyptian Art, Archaeology and History in Honour of Barry J. Kemp*, ed. Salima Ikram and Aidan Dodson, vol 2 (Cairo: Supreme Council of Antiquities, 2009), 415.
53 Damron, 335, 417, 458; "FDA Vitamins and Minerals Chart;" "Turkey, Whole, Breast, Meat Only, Cooked, Roasted;" "FDA Vitamins and Minerals Chart;" "Game Meat, Bison, Top Sirloin, Separable Lean Only," 1; "Steak, Cooked, Broiled," *USDA FoodData Central*, April 1, 2019, accessed August 2, 2019, https://fdc.nal.usda.gov/fdc-app.html#/food-details/174423/nutrients; "Fish, Salmon, Atlantic, Wild, Raw," *USDA FoodData Central*, April 1, 2019, accessed August 2, 2019, https://fdc.nal.usda.gov/fdc-app.html#/food-details/173686/nutrients; "Game Meat, Deer, Tenderloin, Separable Lean Only, Cooked, Broiled," *USDA FoodData Central*, April 1, 2019, accessed August 2, 2019, https://fdc.nal.usda.gov/fdc-app.html#/food-details/174430/nutrients.
54 Potts, 7.
55 Stephen Jay Gould, *Hen's Teeth and Horse's Toes: Further Reflections in Natural History* (New York and London: Norton, 1983), 182–184.
56 Potts, 7.
57 Ibid., 8.
58 Ibid., 12; Damron, 394.
59 William J. Stadelman, "Chicken Eggs," in *The Cambridge World History of Food*, vol. 1, ed. Kenneth F. Kiple and Kriemhild Conee Ornelas (Cambridge, UK: Cambridge University Press, 2000), 500; Potts, 17.
60 Damron, 394.
61 Andrew Lawler, *Why Did the Chicken Cross the World? The Epic Saga of the Bird that Powers Civilization* (New York: Atria Books, 2014), 12.
62 Chaline, 91.
63 Potts, 12; Roger Blench and Kevin C. MacDonald, "Chickens," in *The Cambridge World History of Food*, vol. 1, ed. Kenneth F. Kiple and Kriemhild Conee Ornelas (Cambridge, UK: Cambridge University Press, 2000), 496.
64 Lawler, 13.
65 Ibid.
66 Blench and MacDonald, 496.
67 Chaline, 90–91.
68 Potts, 12.
69 Damron, 394; Chaline, 91.
70 Lawler, 28–29.
71 Ibid., 32.
72 Potts, 13.
73 Ibid.
74 Ibid.
75 Damron, 395.
76 Kristina Killgrove, "Ancient DNA Explains How Chickens Got to the Americas," *Forbes*, November 23, 2017, accessed August 3, 2019, https://www.forbes.com/sites/kristinakillgrove/2017/11/23/ancient-dna-explains-how-chickens-got-to-the-americas/#613e395256db.
77 Blench and MacDonald, 498.
78 Killgrove.
79 Blench and MacDonald, 498.
80 Luff, 517.
81 Ibid., 519.
82 Ibid., 517.

83 Ibid., 519.
84 Ibid.
85 Ibid.
86 Ibid., 520.
87 Damron, 410.
88 Ibid., 406.
89 Marc Oxenham, Nguyen Lan Cuong, and Nguyen Kim Thuy, "The Oral Health Consequences of the Adoption and Intensification of Agriculture in Southeast Asia," in *Bioarchaeology of Southeast Asia*, ed. Marc Oxenham and Nancy Tayler (Cambridge, UK: Cambridge University Press, 2006), 270–271.
90 Christopher A. King and Lynette Norr, "Paleodietary Change among Pre-State Metal Age Societies in Northeast Thailand: A Study Using Stable Isotopes," in *Bioarchaeology of Southeast Asia*, ed. Marc Oxenham and Nancy Tayler (Cambridge, UK: Cambridge University Press, 2006), 246.
91 Kathryn M. Domett, *Health in Late Prehistoric Thailand* (Oxford, UK: Archaeopress, 2001), 146–147.
92 King and Norr, 246, 248, 256.
93 Te-Tzu Chang, "Rice," in *The Cambridge World History of Food*, vol. 1, ed. Kenneth F. Kiple and Kriemhild Conee Ornelas (Cambridge, UK: Cambridge University Press, 2000), 139.
94 Oxenham, Cuong, and Thuy, 273.
95 Edward S. Deevey Jr., "The Human Population," *Scientific American* 203, no. 9 (September 1, 1960), 202.
96 Kate Domett and Nancy Tayles, "Human Biology from the Bronze Age to the Iron Age in the Mun River Valley of Northeast Thailand," in *Bioarchaeology of Southeast Asia*, ed. Marc Oxenham and Nancy Tayler (Cambridge, UK: Cambridge University Press, 2006), 225.
97 Domett, i, 38.
98 Ibid., i, 23, 42.
99 Ibid., i, 39.
100 Oxenham, Cuong, and Thuy, 270.
101 Ibid., 270, 273.
102 Domett and Tayles, 226.
103 John P. McKay, Bennett D. Hill, John Buckler, Clare Haru Crowston, Merry E. Wiesner-Hanks, and Joe Perry, *Understanding Western Society: A Brief History* (Boston and New York: Bedford/St. Martin's, 2012), 212.
104 Henri V. Vallois, "The Social Life of Early Man: The Evidence of Skeletons," in *Social Life of Early Man*, ed. Sherwood L. Washburn (Chicago: Aldine, 1961), 222.
105 Domett, 139.
106 Richard H. Steckel and Jerome C. Rose, "Introduction," in *The Backbone of History: Health and Nutrition in the Western Hemisphere*, ed. Richard H. Steckel and Jerome C. Rose (Cambridge, UK: Cambridge University Press, 2002), 6; Richard H. Steckel, Paul W. Sciulli, and Jerome C. Rose, "A Health Index from Skeletal Remains," in *The Backbone of History: Health and Nutrition in the Western Hemisphere*, ed. Richard H. Steckel and Jerome C. Rose (Cambridge, UK: Cambridge University Press, 2002), 72.
107 Oxenham, Cuong, and Thuy, 273.
108 Domett, 38–42.
109 Oxenham, Cuong, and Thuy, 273.
110 Domett, 16, 19.
111 Ibid., i.
112 Chaline, 130.
113 Ibid.
114 Stanley J. Olsen, "Turkeys," in *The Cambridge World History of Food*, vol. 1, ed. Kenneth F. Kiple and Kriemhild Conee Ornelas (Cambridge, UK: Cambridge University Press, 2000), 581.
115 Ibid., 582.
116 Colin Scanes, *Fundamentals of Animal Science* (Clifton Park, NY: Delmar Cengage Learning, 2011), 200.
117 Olsen, 579.
118 Ibid., 578–579.
119 Corina M. Kellner, Margaret Schoeninger, Katherine A. Spielmann, and Katherine Moore, "Stable Isotope Data Show Temporal Stability in Diet at Pecos Pueblo and Diet Variation among Southwest Pueblos," in *Pecos Pueblo Revisited: The Biological and Social Context*, ed. Michele E. Morgan (Cambridge, MA: Peabody Museum of Archaeology and Ethnology, Harvard University, 2010), 85.

120 Gordon F. M. Rakita and Rafael Cruz, "Organization of Production at Paquime," in *Ancient Paquime and the Casas Grandes World*, ed. Paul E. Minnis and Michael E. Whalen (Tucson: University of Arizona Press, 2015), 68–69.
121 Ibid., 69–70.
122 Ibid.; Kellner, Schoeninger, Spielmann, and Moore, 85.
123 Kellner, Schoeninger, Spielmann, and Moore.
124 J. Allen Barksdale, "American Bison," in *The Cambridge World History of Food*, vol. 1, ed. Kenneth F. Kiple and Kriemhild Conee Ornelas (Cambridge, UK: Cambridge University Press, 2000), 450–451.
125 Olsen, 581.
126 Ibid.; Kellner, Schoeninger, Spielmann, and Moore, 85.
127 Kellner, Schoeninger, Spielmann, and Moore.
128 Olsen, 579.
129 Kellner, Schoeninger, Spielmann, and Moore, 85.
130 Ibid., 86.
131 Ibid., 80; Lane Anderson Beck, "The Influence of Preservation on Observability of Pathology: A Case Study from Pecos," in *Pecos Pueblo Revisited: The Biological and Social Context*, ed. Michele E. Morgan (Cambridge, MA: Peabody Museum of Archaeology and Ethnology, Harvard University, 2010), 73.
132 Kellner, Schoeninger, Spielmann, and Moore, 83.
133 Ibid., 86.
134 Olsen, 581.
135 Ibid., 579.
136 Ibid., 581.
137 Donna M. Glowacki, *Living and Leaving: A Social History of Regional Depopulation in Thirteenth-Century Mesa Verde* (Tucson: University of Arizona Press, 2015), 39.
138 Ibid., 41.
139 Ibid., 39.
140 Olsen, 581.
141 Ibid.
142 Ibid.; Chaline, 131.
143 Sylvia A. Johnson, *Tomatoes, Potatoes, Corn, and Beans: How the Foods of the Americas Changed Eating around the World* (New York: Atheneum Books, 1997), 14, 43.
144 Ann L. W. Stodder, Debra L. Martin, Alan H. Goodman, and Daniel T. Reff, "Cultural Longevity and Biological Stress in the American Southwest," in *The Backbone of History: Health and Nutrition in the Western Hemisphere*, ed. Richard H. Steckel and Jerome C. Rose (Cambridge, UK: Cambridge University Press, 2002), 499.
145 Kerriann Marden, "Human Burials of Chaco Canyon: New Developments in Cultural Interpretations through Skeletal Analysis," in *Chaco Revisited: New Research on the Prehistory of Chaco Canyon, New Mexico*, ed. Carrie C. Heitman and Stephen Plog (Tucson: University of Arizona Press, 2015), 162.
146 Ibid., 172.
147 Ibid., 178–179.
148 Frank Spencer, "Hrdlicka, Ales," in *History of Physical Anthropology*, vol. 1: A-L, ed. Frank Spencer (New York and London: Garland Publishing, 1997), 503–504.
149 Katherine E. Weisensee and Richard L. Jantz, "Rethinking Hooton: A Reexamination of the Pecos Cranial and Postcranial Data Using Recent Methods," in *Pecos Pueblo Revisited: The Biological and Social Context*, ed. Michele E. Morgan (Cambridge, MA: Peabody Museum of Archaeology and Ethnology, Harvard University, 2010), 43–44; George J. Armelagos, "Paleopathology," in *History of Physical Anthropology*, vol 2: M-Z, ed. Frank Spencer (New York and London: Garland Publishing, 1997), 792.
150 Armelagos, 792.
151 Weisensee and Jantz, 43–44.
152 Earnest Albert Hooton, *The Indians of Pecos Pueblo: A Study of Their Skeletal Remains* (New Haven, CT: Yale University Press, 1930), 344.
153 Ibid., 346–347.
154 Ibid., 346, 348.
155 Ibid., 349.
156 Stodder, Martin, Goodman, and Reff, 487–488.
157 Ibid., 488.

158 Ibid.
159 Ibid., 489.
160 Deevey, 202; Stodder, Martin, Goodman, and Reff, 491.
161 Stodder, Martin, Goodman, and Reff, 489.
162 Ibid.
163 Ibid.
164 Ibid.; Lourdes Marquez Morfin, Robert McCaa, Rebecca Storey, and Andres Del Angel, "Health and Nutrition in Pre-Hispanic Mesoamerica," in *The Backbone of History: Health and Nutrition in the Western Hemisphere*, ed. Richard H. Steckel and Jerome C. Rose (Cambridge, UK: Cambridge University Press, 2002), 321.
165 Stodder, Martin, Goodman, and Reff, 489; Morfin, McCaa, Storey, and Del Angel, 321.
166 Joseph M. Prince and Richard H. Steckel, *Tallest in the World: Native Americans of the Great Plains in the Nineteenth Century* (Cambridge, MA: National Bureau of Economic Research, 1998), 29.
167 Richard H. Steckel, *Health and Nutrition in the Preindustrial Era: Insights from a Millennium of Average Heights in Northern Europe* (Cambridge, MA: National Bureau of Economic Research, 2001), i, 18.
168 James M. Davidson, Jerome C. Rose, Myron P. Gutmann, Michael R. Haines, Keith Condon, and Cindy Condon, "The Quality of African-American Life in the Old Southwest Near the Turn of the Twentieth Century," in *The Backbone of History: Health and Nutrition in the Western Hemisphere*, ed. Richard H. Steckel and Jerome C. Rose (Cambridge, UK: Cambridge University Press, 2002), 243.
169 Stodder, Martin, Goodman, and Reff, 490.
170 Ibid., 491.
171 Ibid., 492.
172 Ibid., 493.
173 Kellner, Schoeninger, Spielmann, and Moore, 82; Joseph A. Ezzo, *Human Adaptation at Grasshopper Pueblo, Arizona* (Ann Arbor, MI: International Monographs in Prehistory, 1993), 23.
174 Stodder, Martin, Goodman, and Reff, 493.
175 Kellner, Schoeninger, Spielmann, and Moore, 82.
176 Michele E. Morgan, "Conclusion," in *Pecos Pueblo Revisited: The Biological and Social Context*, ed. Michele E. Morgan (Cambridge, MA: Peabody Museum of Archaeology and Ethnology, Harvard University, 2010), 164.
177 Ibid., 498.
178 Nancy A. Hewitt and Steven F. Lawson, *Exploring American Histories: A Brief Survey with Sources* (Boston and New York: Bedford/St. Martin's, 2013), 87.
179 Gary B. Nash, Julie Roy Jeffrey, John R. Howe, Peter J. Frederick, Allen F. Davis, and Allan M. Winkler, *The American People: Creating a Nation and a Society*, vol. 1: to 1877, 2d ed. (New York: HarperCollins Publishers, 1990), 74.
180 Henry C. Dethloff, *A History of the American Rice Industry, 1685–1985* (College Station: Texas A & M University Press, 1988), 22.
181 Ibid., 23.
182 Hayden Ros Smith, "Rich Swamps and Rice Grounds: The Specialization of Inland Rice Culture in the South Carolina Lowcountry, 1670–1861." Ph.D. diss., University of Georgia, 2012, 10.
183 Ted A. Rathbun and Richard H. Steckel, "The Health of Slaves and Free Blacks in the East," in *The Backbone of History: Health and Nutrition in the Western Hemisphere*, ed. Richard H. Steckel and Jerome C. Rose (Cambridge, UK: Cambridge University Press, 2002), 214.
184 Jill Dubisch, "Low Country Fevers: Cultural Adaptations to Malaria in Antebellum South Carolina," *Social Science and Medicine* 21, no. 6 (February 1985): 643.
185 Rathbun and Steckel, 214.
186 Stodder, Martin, Goodman, and Reff, 498.
187 Stephan Thernstrom, *A History of the American People*, vol. 1: to 1877, 2d ed. (San Diego: Harcourt Brace Jovanovich, 1989), 379.
188 Ibid., 381.
189 Stodder, Martin, Goodman, and Reff, 483.
190 Thernstrom, 13.
191 Hewitt and Lawson, 18.
192 Nash, Jeffrey, Howe, Frederick, Davis, and Winkler, 24.

193 Phillip L. Walker and Russell Thornton, "Health, Nutrition, and Demographic Change in Native California," in *The Backbone of History: Health and Nutrition in the Western Hemisphere*, ed. Richard H. Steckel and Jerome C. Rose (Cambridge, UK: Cambridge University Press, 2002), 509, 520.

194 Ibid., 509–510.

195 Pauleena MacDougall, "Virgin Soil Epidemics in North America," in *World History Encyclopedia, Era 6: The First Global Age, 1450–1770*, vol. 11, ed. Alfred J. Andrea, Carolyn Neel, Dane A. Morrison, Alexander Mikaberidze, D. Harland Hagler, Jeffrey M. Diamond, and Monique Vallance (Santa Barbara, CA: ABC-CLIO, 2011), 105.

196 Timothy J. Watts, "Smallpox and Slavery—Demographic Catastrophe within the Americas," in *World History Encyclopedia, Era 6: The First Global Age, 1450–1770*, vol. 11, ed. Alfred J. Andrea, Carolyn Neel, Dane A. Morrison, Alexander Mikaberidze, D. Harland Hagler, Jeffrey M. Diamond, and Monique Vallance (Santa Barbara, CA: ABC-CLIO, 2011), 106.

197 MacDougall, 105.

198 Caroline Gallacci, "Driven to Extinction—The North American Fur Trade," in *World History Encyclopedia, Era 6: The First Global Age, 1450–1770*, vol. 11, ed. Alfred J. Andrea, Carolyn Neel, Dane A. Morrison, Alexander Mikaberidze, D. Harland Hagler, Jeffrey M. Diamond, and Monique Vallance (Santa Barbara, CA: ABC-CLIO, 2011), 64.

199 Raymond Pierotti, "Diseases, Animal," in *Berkshire Encyclopedia of World History*, vol. 2, ed. William H. McNeill, Jerry H. Bentley, David Christian, David Levinson, J. R. McNeill, Heidi Roupp, and Judith P. Zinsser (Great Barrington, MA: Berkshire Publishing Group, 2005), 555.

200 Jean L. Briggs, "Sadlermiut Inuit," The Canadian Encyclopedia, March 1, 2012, last modified March 4, 2015, accessed February 24, 2019, https://www.thecanadianencyclopedia.ca/en/article/sadlermiut-inuit.

201 Ezzo, 7, 77.

202 Ibid., 27, 65–67.

203 Ibid., 67.

7 Dairy

7.1 COMMON DAIRY PRODUCTS

7.1.1 Milk

Chapters 3 and 4 traced meat consumption's antiquity. Chapter 4 defined meat as mammalian flesh and discussed its derivation from game while humans were hunter-gatherers and from farm animals during the last 10,000 years. Animal husbandry's invention did not end hunting everywhere, though recent millennia witnessed a shift toward livestock. This transition permitted people to interact with animals at close quarters and thereby to tap a new source of nourishment in milk from cows (*Bos taurus*, *Bos indicus*, *Rangifer tarandus*, *Camelus dromedaries*, and *Bubalus bubalis*), ewes (*Ovis aries*), nannies (*Capra aegagrus hircus*), naks (*Bos grunniens*), mares (*Equus caballus*), and jennies (*Equus asinus*).

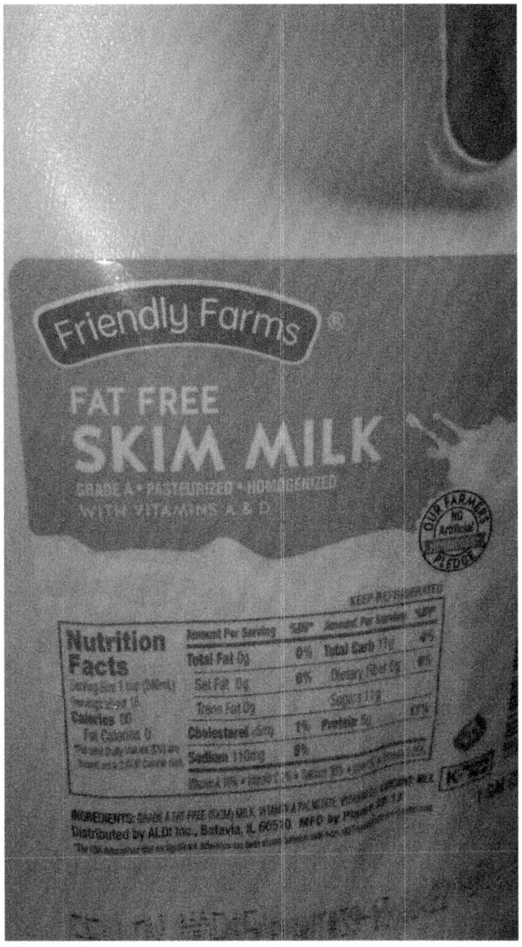

FIGURE 7.1 Skim milk. (Photo from author.)

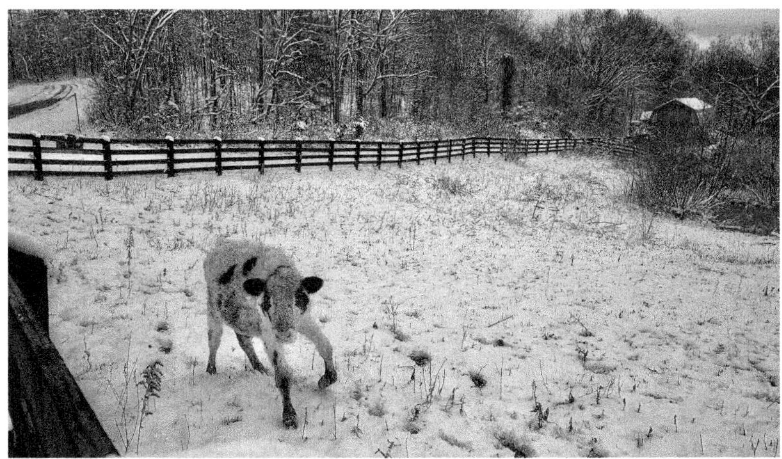

FIGURE 7.2 *Bos taurus*. (Photo courtesy of Jessica Vierling-West.)

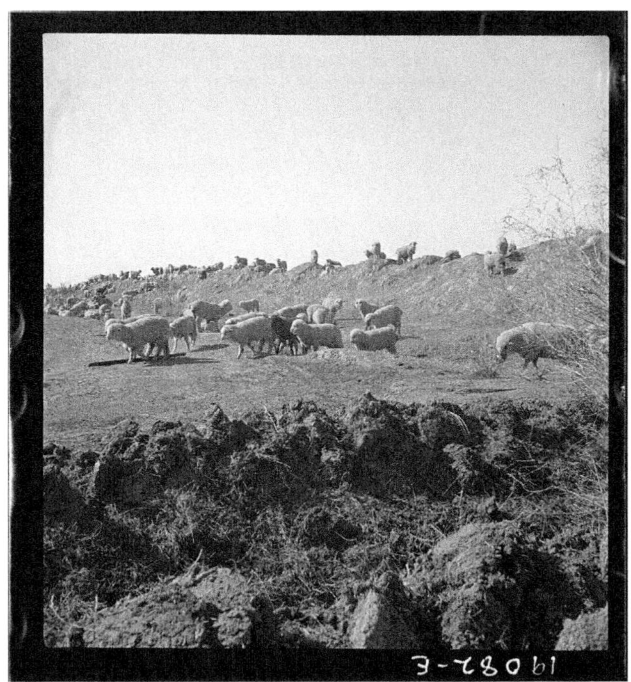

FIGURE 7.3 *Ovis aries*. (Photo courtesy of Library of Congress. https://www.loc.gov/pictures/item/2017771475/.)

This activity strikes people in nations with a dairy industry as more natural than it is. All mammalian mothers produce milk, but only for their young. Once weaned, almost all mammals forgo milk. Being mammals, human newborns and infants likewise nurse, but in some societies, weaning ends only ingestion of mother's milk. In its place, humans are the only animals that transition to milk from another mammal, a habit that may be lifelong. The association with milk does not end with the liquid because humans have learned to convert it into cheese, butter, ghee, yogurt, and other products.

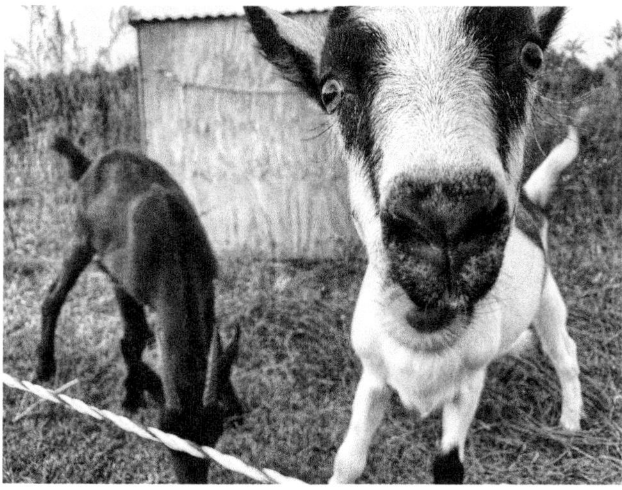

FIGURE 7.4 *Capra aegagrus hircus.* (Photo courtesy of Jessica Vierling-West.)

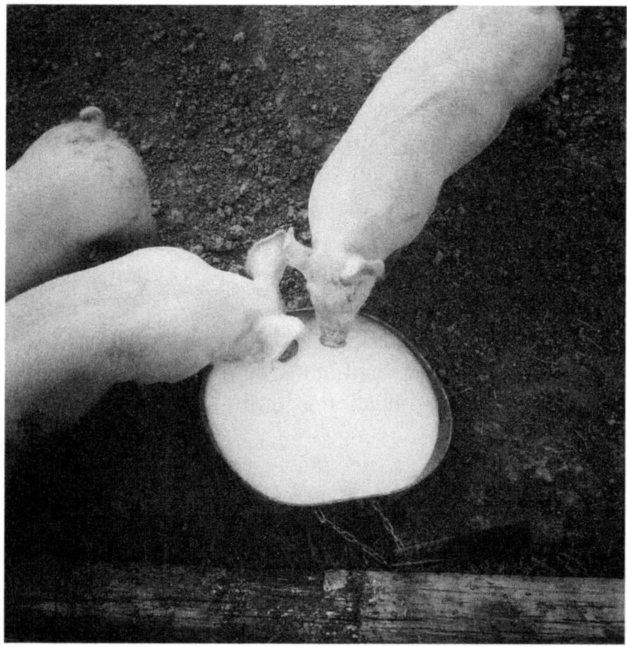

FIGURE 7.5 Pigs drinking goat's milk. (Photo courtesy of Jessica Vierling-West.)

Chapter 2 stated that milk has the disaccharide lactose, that its formula is ($C_{12}H_{22}O_{11}$), and that the body cannot digest it without lactase. People have not needed this enzyme beyond weaning absent dairying, the norm throughout much of the world and, as noted, among other mammals. The proportion of adults who cannot digest lactose may be between two-thirds and three-quarters worldwide.[1] Yet wherever dairying has a long history, lactase production is lifelong.

For this reason, the enzyme's prevalence in an adult population evinces longstanding milk intake. That is, lactase frequency among adults identifies dairying's extent if any. For example, since animal husbandry arose few Chinese have drunk milk, as discussed later, such that under 5 percent of adults produce lactase.[2] Table 7.1 lists the percentage of adults who produce lactase by ethnicity.[3]

TABLE 7.1
% Adult Lactase Producers by Ethnicity

Ethnicity	% Adult Lactase Producers
Swiss	94
U.S. White	81–98
English	78
Australian, White	80
Pakistani	70
Northern Indians	70
Southern Indians	33
Sri Lankan	33
African American	23–30
Ugandan	56–91
Bantu	10
Australian, Aborigine	10–20
Chinese, Japanese, Korean, Filipino	0–15
American Indian, Thai, New Guinean	c. 0

Japan, South Korea, North Korea, and the Philippines yield similar percentages that imply a link with China. Lactase is virtually nonexistent in adult Amerindians, Thais, New Guineans, and native Australians, indicating dairying's absence. None domesticated cows, sheep, or goats, though China tamed water buffalos, and it and Thailand now encourage milk consumption, especially among schoolchildren. West and Central Africans also exhibit low lactase frequencies in adulthood. But roughly one-quarter of African Americans produce the enzyme into adulthood, possibly because of exposure to milk in the western hemisphere, where they integrated into European colonial economies and adopted European habits.[4] Roughly 80 percent of Europeans—including 94 percent of Swiss—their Australian and American descendants, and at least 70 percent of Pakistanis and northern Indians produce lactase throughout life, underscoring milk's antiquity.[5] Movement south through the Indian subcontinent and into Sri Lanka, however, reduces the proportion to roughly one-third.[6] Similarly, Europe's lactase production is lowest in the south.

7.1.2 Cheese

Cheesemaking, mentioned in Chapter 2 and invented around 7500 BCE, separates curd and whey.[7] Because whey has most lactose, its removal yields cheeses suitable for lactase-deficient people. Because lactose is a sugar, as mentioned, brands with few sugars or carbohydrates in general have little of it. As a rule, the longer a cheese ages, the less lactose it has; hard cheeses have the least. For example, cheddar, parmesan, and swiss tend to contain under 0.5 grams of lactose per 30-gram (1-ounce) slice.[8] But other hand, lactose intolerant individuals should avoid fresh cheeses such as cottage, mozzarella, cream, and ricotta. Dieters should understand that hard cheeses have more calories than soft versions because moisture is low and fat high. A later section discusses calories, nutrients, and health.

Like the alcohol ethanol (C_2H_5OH), cheese is a microbial product. Whereas yeast fungi (*Saccharomyces cerevisiae*) make ethanol, bacteria produce cheese. These microorganisms, known as lactic-acid bacteria, convert lactose into lactic acid ($C_3H_6O_3$). Cheesemakers may add yeast or other microbes for flavor and color. For example, *Penicillium*—the mold genus that yielded the antibiotic penicillin—is used to create several types, including blue cheese from *Penicillium roqueforti* and brie and camembert from *Penicillium camemberti*. Rennet enzymes congeal the milk protein casein, making cheese solid rather than liquid. The primary enzyme in this process, chymosin, forms curds. Preferences govern the addition of salt, pepper (*Piper nigrum*), garlic (*Allium sativum*), chives (*Allium schoenoprasum*), or other ingredients. As implied earlier, cheese has few carbohydrates relative to fat and protein, though the use of skim milk reduces fat.

7.1.3 Butter and Ghee

Also with little lactose are butter and ghee. Among its constituents, whole milk has fat, solids, and water that vary by mammal. Focusing on fat, cow's milk is 4 percent by mass, though fat furnishes half its calories.[9] Milk from nannies has 56, and from humans 59, percent of calories as fat. Lighter than milk's other components, fat—known as butterfat—floats atop a container, where it may be removed to yield several products. Cream must have at least 18 percent butterfat by mass in the United States and at least 30 percent in the European Union (EU).[10] Butter is about 80 percent fat by mass with the rest water and solids.[11] Butter has so few carbohydrates that its lactose is minuscule and nutritionists tend to calculate its calories as entirely fat.[12] Clarification, the process that removes all or almost all water and solids, produces ghee, the fattiest dairy product. Over half the fat is saturated, a type that Chapter 2 defined. Ghee lacks carbohydrates and lactose; fat supplies all its calories. Butter and ghee satisfy low-carbohydrate proponents.

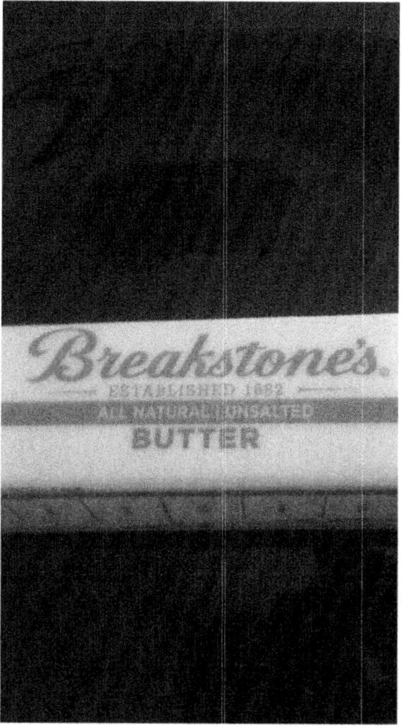

FIGURE 7.6 Butter. (Photo from author.)

7.1.4 Ice Cream

Cream may join milk, sugars, and flavorings to yield ice cream. Water in milk and cream becomes inflexible when frozen. Avoidance of this problem requires churning the ingredients to reduce ice crystals. Contents may vary, though the United States requires that ice cream have at least 10 percent fat and 20 percent milk solids. Low-fat brands are labeled accordingly. Concerns about the sugar sucrose ($C_{12}H_{22}O_{11}$) led manufacturers to substitute fruit, high fructose corn syrup (HFSC), or artificial sweeteners such as aspartame ($C_{14}H_{18}N_2O_5$). Chapter 2 defined and Chapter 11 evaluates the sweeteners sucrose, HFCS, and honey.

7.1.5 Yogurt

Yogurt, sometimes spelled yoghurt, may also have scant lactose. Like cheese and ethanol, its manufacture involves microbes. The responsible bacteria, known as yogurt cultures and in the genera *Lactobacillus*, *Streptococcus*, and *Bifidobacterium*, convert lactose into lactic acid, a process reminiscent of cheesemaking. During production, milk is heated to roughly 85 degrees Celsius (185 degrees Fahrenheit) to prevent curdling. Bacteria are added upon cooling to around 45 degrees Celsius (113 degrees Fahrenheit). Maintenance of this temperature at least four hours permits fermentation, during which bacteria degrade most lactose to yield a product that seldom upsets the stomach. The best yogurts for lactose sensitives have live bacteria. By killing them, pasteurization produces yogurts with more lactose. Yogurts with few carbohydrates supply little lactose. Greek yogurts have little whey and lactose.

7.2 CONSUMPTION OVER NINE MILLENNIA

7.2.1 Dairying's Origins

Dairying's origins are uncertain. Sub-Saharan Africa may be its cradle, but little is known about livestock taming for meat and milk there. Better attested is goats' domestication about 7000 BCE in southwestern Asia's Zagros Mountains.[13] Goat's milk was seldom consumed fresh but instead as cheese and butter. The Hittites in what are Anatolia (Asia Minor or Asian Turkey) and Iraq made cheese from goat, sheep, and cow's milk. During the seventh millennium BCE, India tamed *Bos indicus*, water buffalo, goat, and sheep.[14] Dairying concentrated in what are today northern India and Pakistan, which pastoralists occupied. The connection between cattle, buffalos, goats, and sheep on one hand and dairy foods on the other strengthened about 2000 BCE, when Central Asian horsemen invaded India, bringing their preference for milk, cheese, ghee, and Hinduism. The religion venerated cows as symbols of motherhood, nurturing, and Earth's bounty. These associations made dairy products, especially milk and ghee, sources of personal and national strength, vitality, and pride from an early date.

7.2.2 Dairying in Africa

Besides these developments, by 5000 BCE herders in what is now the Sahara Desert were milking cattle, goats, and sheep to derive cheese, butter, and yogurt.[15] The climate, wetter than today, supported grasslands suitable as pasture. By 4500 BCE, Egypt had imported goats and sheep from southwestern Asia and herded the now extinct auroch (*Bos primigenius*), all sources of milk.[16] From Egypt, dairying spread west throughout North Africa, today the nations of Libya, Tunisia, Algeria, and Morocco.

7.2.3 The Mediterranean and Europe

Throughout prehistory and history, Egypt and North Africa were more connected to Mediterranean lands, of which they were part than to sub-Saharan Africa. In Egypt and North Africa, Mediterranean olive (*Olea europaea*) oil competed with butter as a source of fat.[17] Competition also came from sesame (*Sesamum indicum*) oil produced locally and south of Egypt and North Africa.[18] Rome conquered North Africa during the second century BCE, adding Egypt in 30 BCE. Butter consumption declined as Rome intensified oleiculture, discussed in Chapter 10, though goats and sheep continued to supply milk for cheese. North Africa and Egypt depended on these ungulates, which were better adapted to the region's hot, dry climate than cows. Mediterranean farmers who owned cattle perceived them as work animals. For example, oxen (castrated bulls) pulled plows.

Northern Europe's cooler, wetter climate, however, favored cattle, which competed with sheep as sources of milk, cheese, and butter. Central Europeans drank milk, probably fermented into kefir, as early as 5900 BCE, a practice that spread to Britain by 4100 BCE.[19]

Before refrigeration, milk was too perishable for fresh consumption on a grand scale and was instead converted into cheese, butter, yogurt, ghee, and other durables. But none of these items permits indefinite storage even today. For example, ghee lasts about nine months if unopened and kept cool and away from light. Once opened, it endures about three months unrefrigerated and up to one year chilled.[20] Refrigerated butter goes rancid around two weeks after opening and one month if unopened. Six to nine months' storage is possible in the freezer. Yogurt should be consumed within three weeks of the sell-by date. Hard cheeses store longer than soft varieties.

Egypt identified goat and cow's milk as wholesome, feeding it to infants.[21] The Romans weaned infants with goat or sheep's milk. Greek physicians Soranus of Ephesus (c. 98–c. 138 CE) and Galen (c. 130–c. 210 CE) recommended goat's milk and honey for weaning, unwise advice given that goat's milk, deficient in iron, may have occasioned anemia. Moreover, honey that harbored the bacterium *Clostridium botulinum* caused botulism. If milk was hazardous, butter suited only barbarians, wrote Roman naturalist Pliny the Elder (23–79 CE).[22] Given milk's perishability and butter's crudity, the Mediterranean's poor relied on cheese for complete protein.[23] Goats were esteemed for cheese whereas sheep furnished both cheese and wool.[24] This situation reserved these ruminants for meat only when too old for other uses. Under Roman rule, the Aegean Sea's Cyclades Islands and southern Gaul (now southern France) attained renown for cheeses.

7.2.4 The Middle Ages

Cheese and butter persisted in medieval diets, though the poor afforded small amounts with bread.[25] Only the wealthy had cows and sheep to supply milk for cheese and butter. A destination for Eurasian migrants in prehistory, Ireland linked milk and butter to Christianity in the fifth century CE. Celtic goddess Brigid, who imbibed sacred milk, became St. Brigid (c. 451–c. 525 CE), who as a newborn drank milk from a white cow when her pagan mother could not lactate.[26] While managing the family's herds, she gave milk, cheese, and butter to the hungry, gifts that God replenished upon her prayers. Brigid became patroness of Ireland, milkmaids, cattle, and newborns.

In the ninth century, Vikings introduced cows and sheep into Iceland, where sheep became the primary dairy animal.[27] Vikings ate butter, yogurt, and cheese on Greenland in the tenth century, though fish—discussed in Chapter 5—and marine mammals became important before settlement's fifteenth-century demise. On continental Europe, the Black Death (1347–1351), discussed in Chapters 1 and 3, killed perhaps one-third the population, increasing wages amid scarce labor.[28] Europeans had more money for dairy and meat.[29]

7.2.5 Europe after the Middle Ages

Population growth eroded prosperity. Between 1500 and 1800 wages lagged prices as butter, cheese, and milk surpassed commoners' resources.[30] Ireland's reliance on milk and butter diminished in the eighteenth century as potatoes (*Solanum tuberosum*) sustained the masses. By 1800, only the wealthy had livestock for milk. In the late eighteenth century, Britain's rural poor drank on average 74 milliliters (2.5 ounces) of milk daily.[31] In the nineteenth century, the island's urban poor averaged 56 milliliters (1.9 ounces) per day. During this period, Vienna, Austria's poor averaged 100 grams (3.5 ounces) of cheese daily. Around 1800, dairy foods gave Belgians roughly 300 calories, 15 percent of the daily total.[32]

Switzerland emphasized dairying because its mountains suited livestock over crops.[33] From an early period, herders converted milk into butter and cheese. By the nineteenth century this lifeway, full of outdoor activity and sunshine, symbolized Swiss vitality. Originating in 1863, the Swiss Alpine Farming Association lauded cheese, butter, milk, meat, and exertion as paths toward personal and national strength. Manufacturers combined milk, chocolate, and sucrose, promoting milk chocolate as healthful. Emphasizing quality and flavor, dairies multiplied in the nineteenth century. A later section discusses Swiss emigres' role in dairying among Ohio's Amish.

7.2.6 The Caribbean and North America

The Amish were not alone in shaping the Americas. Although pre-Columbian peoples had few domestic animals and extracted milk from none, Italian-Spanish mariner Christopher Columbus (1451–1506) in 1493 introduced cattle, sheep, goats, and horses into Caribbean island Hispaniola, now Haiti and the Dominican Republic.[34] Humans milked all four, as noted, though Europeans favored cows, ewes, and nannies for dairy. From the Caribbean, Spaniards shipped cattle throughout the Gulf of Mexico, including Mexico and Florida. England, France, and the Netherlands brought cows to Virginia, New Jersey, New York, Massachusetts, Delaware, and New Hampshire. Those in Pennsylvania generated wealth and launched the career of caramel maker and chocolatier Milton Snavely Hershey (1857–1945). Colonial Americans added milk or cream to coffee (*Coffea* species), tea (*Camellia sinensis*), hot chocolate, and cider and combined butter, bread, and eggs at breakfast. Busy families ate bread and cheese for lunch and rated cheese versatile and flavorful enough to enhance any meal or serve as a snack.

7.2.7 Asia

Dairy products fed more than Europe and its colonies. An earlier section noted Central Asia's fondness for milk, cheese, and ghee. East of Central Asia, herds roamed Mongolia. Koumiss, fermented horse milk, has long been its principal beverage. Mongols' sixteenth-century conversion to Tibetan Buddhism accentuated dairy because the religion prohibited horsemeat and fish, both of which had been staples. Southeast of Central Asia and south of Mongolia, Tibet made butter and yogurt from yak's milk, which is 15–18 percent fat by mass compared to 4 percent, mentioned earlier, for cow's milk.[35] This extra fat yields 63 percent of yak milk's calories compared to the 59 percent for human milk, 56 percent for goat, and 50 percent for cow, all noted in the previous section. Yak milkfat makes flavorful butter rich in omega 3 fatty acids, which Chapter 2 defined. Yak yogurt sells in China, whose attitudes toward dairy are complex.

The traditional view that Chinese abhor dairy foods aligns with East Asian adult lactase infrequency, noted earlier, and with the story, perhaps apocryphal, of a northwestern Chinese man who pretended to be a Mongolian prince in Peking (now Beijing).[36] The city's elites celebrated his arrival with a series of feasts, though in time some officials began to doubt him. Crafting a test, they held a banquet full of koumiss, cheese, and butter. His refusal to eat or drink revealed him an imposter, and the man fled in shame.

Moreover, China's population was enormous from an early period. The imperative of feeding everyone commandeered land for crops. Little could be spared for pasture. With few cows, sheep, goats, or other large mammals, milk was uncommon. Moreover, China's rejection of dairy differentiated it from nomadic neighbors such as the Mongols and Tibetans who were disdained as uncouth.

Yet opinions about dairy fluctuated across class and time. Entering China in the third-century BCE, Buddhists regarded milk and its derivatives as wholesome, a perspective converts adopted.[37] Although the Han dynasty (206 BCE–220 CE) branded dairy as foreign and inferior, the herders who ruled China between roughly the third and tenth centuries encouraged consumption. The Mongols, controlling China between 1271 and 1368, amplified this enthusiasm. Although the countryside resisted this partiality, China's elites were open to foreign foods, including dairy. They owned dairies, whose existence texts corroborated between the sixth and nineteenth centuries. During the Tang dynasty (618–906), China and Mongolia allied as elites from both regions intermarried. Far from contempt, Chinese officials and intellectuals admired the Mongols during this period. In the thirteenth century, officials regulated and promoted koumiss and the restaurants that served it, cheese, and butter. Cosmopolitan urbanites sampled the best from Mongolian cuisine at these establishments. These perspectives and behaviors differentiated the middle and upper classes, who adopted foreign foods and habits, from peasants, who distrusted outsiders.

This urban-rural dynamic turned against dairy as nationalism and xenophobia intensified during the Ming dynasty (1368–1644).[38] Even then, however, texts documented butter consumption in cities. In the fifteenth century Taoists, and through the seventeenth-century Buddhists, used it. During the Qing dynasty (1644–1911), dairy reclaimed vogue. Adding milk to tea, the national beverage, urbanites stimulated demand for dairy. Qing texts noted dairy foods' consumption in eastern and central China. For example, butter and milk were popular in Zhejiang and Jiangsu provinces. In the twentieth century, Mongolia exported "huge amounts of butter" to Beijing.[39] Although some scholars asserted that the city did not use butter but instead reexported it, consumers somewhere must have wanted it enough to justify commercialization of large quantities.

In the subtropical south, Hong Kong supported cattle and water buffalos; their milk, cheese, and butter fed Indians and Europeans.[40] Chinese Christians emulated Europeans by giving infants and children cow's milk. The southwest's Yunnan province had dairies. Since the 1949 Maoist revolution, China has increased milk, powdered milk, cheese, butter, yogurt, and ice cream production, encouraging consumption in the belief that these foods promote growth and invigorate individuals, the economy, and the nation. In 1972, China counted nearly 1 million cows, and between 1990 and 2009 per person milk intake more than tripled.[41] As incomes rise, Chinese buy milk, yogurt, and ice cream—though less butter and cheese—and refrigerators and freezers for their storage. Eager for profits, European, Australian, New Zealand, and American investors fund Chinese dairies.

7.3 CHEESE AND HEALTH IN RURAL FRANCE

7.3.1 French Cheesemaking

An earlier section noted that what is today southern France gained prominence for cheese in Roman antiquity (c. 750 BCE – c. 500 CE). After Rome's decline, French monasteries preserved cheesemaking's lore and techniques, in the north producing *maroilles* from cow's milk in Picardy and Nord-Pas-de-Calais and *pont l'eveque* in Normandy, and in the east munster in Alsace, Lorraine, and Franche-Comte. During the thirteenth century, dairies spread throughout France, each targeting a local market. By then, monasteries faced competition from homemakers, who kept recipes and made cheese. Yet monasteries retained an advantage in being exempt from taxes while requiring secular cheesemakers to give them one-tenth (a tithe) of output. Cheesemakers who tithed cheese to monasteries and paid taxes with it resented the Catholic Church and government, nurturing grievances that would help ignite the French Revolution (1789–1799). Encouraging entrepreneurship, King Charles VI (1368–1422) in 1393 granted Roquefort, France, the right to produce and sell the ewe's milk cheese that bears its name. Subsequent monarchs likewise issued monopolies to cheesemakers. Able to choose from hundreds of types, consumers made cheese a national food by combining it with rye bread and wine.

7.3.2 Eighteenth-Century Poor Peasants

Longstanding tensions intensified in the 1760s as poor harvests increased food prices, causing French peasants to clash with landlords, tax collectors, and government officials.[42] The most vulnerable occupied under 1 hectare (2.5 acres), plots too small to support a family. Between 1700 and 1792, the number of these farms in Basse Auvergne in south-central France grew from 490 to 870 as rents tripled.[43] Peasants sought cash by migrating to large farms in search of employment or taking piece work from nascent industries.

7.3.3 Peasant Diets

In these precarious times, peasants relied on bread for carbohydrates and cheese for protein and fat. Twenty-three wills and marriage contracts—whose allotments are in Table 7.2—from Gevaudan, southern France, detailed diets among pensioners between 1754 and 1767.[44] Although this number

TABLE 7.2
Daily Rations per Pensioner

Pensioner	Bread (g)	Butter (g)	Cheese (g)	Chestnuts (g)
1	270.5	4.8	0	0
2	443	0	0	149
3	270.5	0	0	0
4	638	5.9	5.9	0
5	666.6	11.9	17.9	0
6	668.8	5.9	5.9	0
7	426.6	7.1	7.1	0
8	400	0	0	0
9	933.3	14.7	14.9	0
10	240	0	0	0
11	506.3	7.1	7.1	0
12	510.8	7.1	7.1	0
13	754.3	9	14.3	0
14	853.3	7.1	7.1	0
15	945.6	23.9	24.4	0
16	880.1	11.9	7.1	0
17	1,177.2	11.9	14.1	0
18	853.3	9	9	0
19	959.9	0	0	0
20	125.8	0	0	0
21	251.6	0	0	0
22	838.4	0	0	0
23	935.1	5.9	0	0

may seem too small for extrapolation, total recipients cannot have been large. Pensioners were too old, ailing, or disabled to care for themselves. Illness and disability truncated lives so that these unfortunates would not long have collected pensions. This book emphasizes that few premodern people surpassed age forty. Only a "small number" of eighteenth-century French reached sixty.[45] Life expectancy at birth (e^0) hovered around forty years, a number that this book judges unusually long or inaccurate.[46]

Poverty is evident from the fact that peasant bread was chiefly rye (*Secale cereale*) and barley (*Hordeum vulgare*), the second regarded as famine food. The masses afforded little wheat (*Triticum aestivum*). Fourteen pensions specified cheese as the only complete protein.[47] Only one pension provided another protein, namely chestnuts (*Castanea sativa*), discussed in chapter 9. The pensioner lived in Prevencheres, near Cevennes' chestnut forest in southern France. Fifteen pensions specified butter as the only other dairy product. Although appreciated for its fat, butter also has the mineral calcium and vitamins A, B_{12}, E, and K.[48] Chapter 2 discussed these and other nutrients.

Some diets were more diverse than bread, cheese, and butter. Thirteen pensions stipulated cabbage (*Brassica oleracea var. capitata*), turnips (*Brassica rapa spp. rapa*), and garden vegetables.[49] The last category is imprecise, though French gardens typically supplied onions (*Allium cepa*), carrots (*Daucus carota spp. sativus*), and celery (*Apium graveolens*). The number of pensioners who kept gardens must have been small given infirmities. Instead, they relied on family and neighbors for produce. Peasants grew the potato by the eighteenth century, though it usually fed more pigs than people.[50]

The most prevalent cheese was tomme—sometimes spelled tome—made from cow, sheep, or goat's milk. Removal of milkfat, needed for butter, before inoculation diminished tomme's fat. Gevaudan tomme, known as tomme de Lozere, contained ewe's milk and salt, an additive common in cheeses. Aged four to six months, tomme attracted houseflies (*Musca domestica*), which laid eggs in it. Peasants ate cheese and maggots.[51] Such behavior may discomfort us, though Chapter 3 noted entomophagy's antiquity among primates and prevalence among humans. Because Europeans and their descendants eschewed insects, however, readers might doubt that these peasants ate them.

Hunger overrode squeamishness, making the poor consume what was available. Three pensions totaled under 1,500 calories per day, and six incomplete pensions sank below 1,000 calories daily.[52] Only two surpassed the 2,400 calories thought adequate for daily existence in eighteenth-century France. Moreover, insectivory may have been acceptable. In 1827, French zoologist Georges Cuvier (1769–1832) described children's preference for grasshopper thighs.[53] Nature enthusiast Miles Olson described maggots as "a traditional superfood" with essential amino and fatty acids.[54] Although their contribution to eighteenth-century nutrition eludes quantification, maggots are 60 percent protein by mass.[55] One hundred grams more than doubled the recommended dietary allowance (RDA) for calcium and exceeded the RDA for phosphorus, zinc, and iron for children and adults including pregnant women.[56] Maggot-infested tomme must have been more nourishing than cheese alone.

The thirteen complete pensions allotted between 5.9 and 24.4 grams of cheese and between 4.8 and 23.9 grams of butter per day.[57] The mean of all thirteen for cheese is 10.9 grams daily and for butter 9.7 grams. These averages are almost equal, suggesting that the grantors valued both similarly. The larger cheese allocation implies that it was understood to be more nutritious, if only marginally. The greatest apportionments—between 125.8 and 1,177.2 grams daily—were for bread, reflecting its status as France's staple. The mean of all thirteen bread rations is 703.5 grams per day. These recipients would have done better to supplant bread with potatoes, which Chapter 13 judges the world's most nourishing food. The pensions specified exact amounts for only cheese, butter, bread, and chestnuts; other items cannot be pinpointed.

Considering the first three, the daily allotment averaged 724.1 grams of food, although the total must have been larger at least during summer, when cabbage, turnips, and other vegetables were available. Chestnuts, included only once, are omitted. Using 724.1 grams as the base, the mean cheese apportionment of 10.9 grams represented 1.5 percent of the total and butter, averaging 9.7 grams, was 1.3 percent. Neither was generous, though plentitude was improbable given poverty and hunger in eighteenth-century France. The 703.5 grams of bread, however, constituted slightly over fourteen slices per the U.S. Food and Drug Administration's (FDA) quantification of one slice (one serving) as 50 grams.[58]

7.3.4 Inadequate Nourishment and Health

French scholar R. J. Bernard judged the meager cheese and butter inadequate in calcium in absolute terms and relative to phosphorus and in vitamin D, calories, fat, and protein, though carbohydrates were adequate.[59] Additionally, he intimated deficiencies in "certain vitamins" without detailing them.[60] When in season, cabbage and other fresh vegetables supplied vitamin C, though deficiencies were widespread by winter's end in temperate lands.[61] Vitamins A, E, and K, all fat soluble and available in cheese, butter, or both, were inadequate given small quantities. Negligible fat implied inadequacies in these fat-soluble vitamins, discussed in Chapter 2. The remaining fat-soluble vitamin D—treated in Chapter 2—receives additional commentary below.

Bernard characterized the typical peasant bread as 40 percent rye, 40 percent barley, and the rest wheat.[62] These percentages made the daily 703.5 grams of bread 281.4 grams of rye and barley each and 140.7 grams of wheat. Because Chapter 12 examines grains' nutrition and health effects, details here are unnecessary. Our purposes are advanced by noting that whole rye flour has the minerals phosphorus, zinc, magnesium, iron, and potassium, B vitamins, vitamins E and K, protein, carbohydrates, fiber, and some fat.[63] Whole barley flour supplies carbohydrates, fiber, protein, the minerals copper, molybdenum, manganese, magnesium, selenium, phosphorus, and chromium and vitamins B_1 (thiamine or thiamin) and B_2.[64] Whole wheat flour furnishes iron, selenium, manganese, phosphorus, and copper, vitamins B_3, B_6 (pyridoxine), and B_9 (folate, folic acid, or pteroylmonoglutamic acid), carbohydrates, fiber, and protein.[65]

Providing the only complete protein, cheese must have protected against protein deficiency diseases like kwashiorkor. Yet residents from Gevaudan and nearby towns were the shortest, ricketiest early-nineteenth-century French conscripts.[66] This book correlates nutrition and height, indicating that shortness often reveals undernutrition. Inadequate vitamin D causes rickets. Considering diet, rickets' prevalence is unsurprising because unfortified dairy products, bread, and vegetables lack the vitamin.

Yet from youth, peasants worked outdoors and should have absorbed enough sunlight, at least during warm months, to avert a disease of vitamin D-deficient children. Depictions of eighteenth-century French peasants—for example, Figure 7.7—reveal, however, that their garments exposed little skin.[67] Broad hats shielded the face and neck. Only the hands were exposed, a practice that cannot have yielded enough vitamin D. As early as the second century CE, Galen reported the swaddling of infants, a habit that also caused rickets.[68] The condition is even older, retrogressing to Europe's Mesolithic Period (Middle Stone Age) between roughly 9000 and 7000 BCE.[69] Whatever rickets' cause among eighteenth-century French peasants, they were undernourished as rising food prices victimized many Europeans.

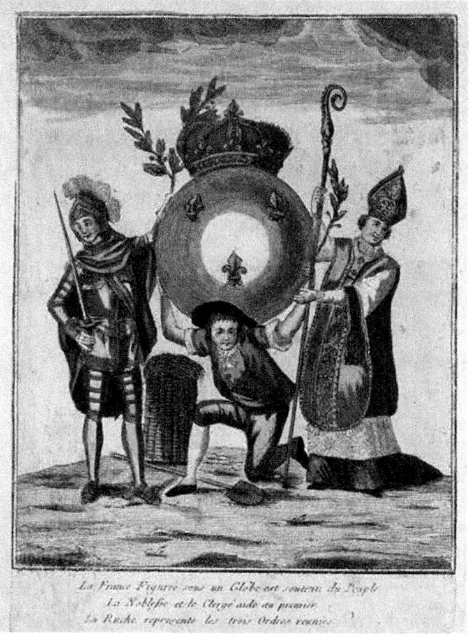

FIGURE 7.7 Eighteenth-century French peasant supporting nobility and church. (Photo courtesy of Library of Congress. https://www.loc.gov/pictures/item/2009633457/.)

7.4 URBANIZATION, INDUSTRIALIZATION, MILK, AND HEALTH

7.4.1 Raw Milk and Pathogens

Beginning about 1750, the Industrial Revolution made milk central to the quest for vitality. Europeans and Americans added the liquid to coffee and tea as they ingested caffeine to stay alert during long hours in factories. Working outside the home, women could not nurse newborns and infants, leaving the task to cow's milk. But raw milk could harbor pathogens, including *Escherichia coli* that causes diarrhea, Shiga toxins that cause dysentery, *Salmonella* bacteria that cause fever, cramps, diarrhea, and chills, *Mycobacterium tuberculosis* that causes tuberculosis, *Brucella* bacteria that cause brucellosis, and *Listeria monocytogenes* that causes listeriosis. These diseases were no abstractions given that almost one-fifth of Herculaneum's residents may have had brucellosis, for example, at Mount Vesuvius' 79 CE eruption.[70] Chapter 15 evaluates their diet, nutrition, and health.

During industrialization, milk producers amplified dangers by crowding cows, a practice that spread contagion. In 1815, deaths before age five totaled one-third of all Boston fatalities, but by 1839 the percentage had risen to 43.[71] In 1815, under one-third of deaths in Philadelphia and New York City occurred before age five, but by 1839, this cohort tallied half of all deaths. In the 1840s, nearly half of infants died before age five in Manhattan, New York.[72] In 1842, English American social reformer Robert Milham Hartley (1796–1881) blamed unsafe milk for these casualties.

Raw milk's dangers could not be pinpointed until microbiology and medicine developed new ideas. In 1857, French microbiologist and chemist Louis Pasteur (1822–1895) announced that microorganisms caused fermentation.[73] Six years later he enlarged this finding by demonstrating that they putrefied beverages and foods.[74] In 1876, German physician and bacteriologist Heinrich Hermann Robert Koch (1843–1910) linked microbes to diseases by identifying the bacterium *Bacillus anthracis* as anthrax's cause.[75] Spoilage could be avoided, and pathogens killed, with heat, a discovery Italian naturalist Lazzaro Spallanzani (1729–1799) had anticipated in 1765.[76]

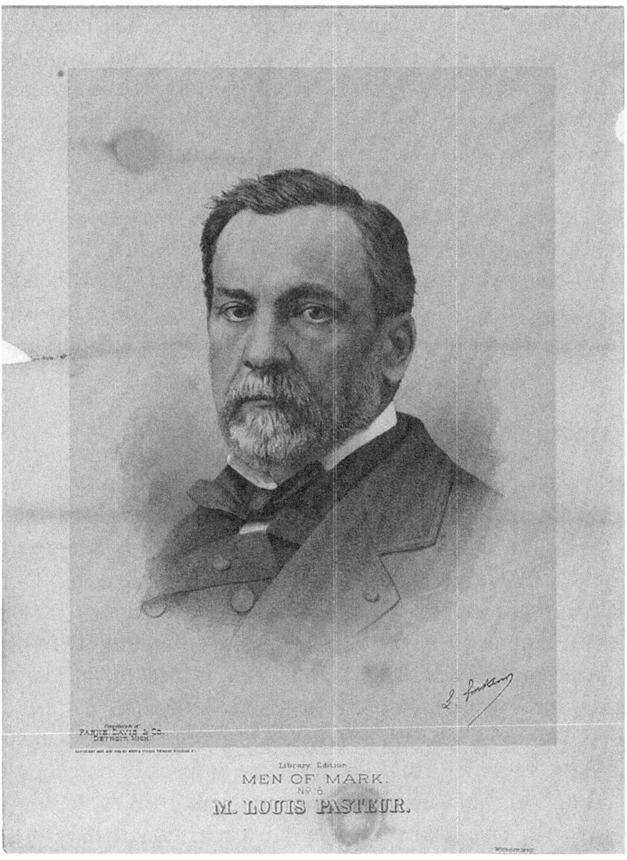

FIGURE 7.8 Louis Pasteur. (Photo courtesy of Library of Congress. https://www.loc.gov/pictures/item/2003680820/.)

7.4.2 Pasteurization

From these advances followed the insight that heating milk destroyed germs, a practice known as pasteurization. Pasteur invented it in 1863, though producers opposed it as an extra expense.[77] In 1908, Chicago became the first U.S. city to mandate pasteurization.[78] By 1917, forty-five cities imitated Chicago, and in 1947, Michigan was the first state to require the practice.[79] American veterinarian Russell W. Currier and American pediatrician John A. Widness credited it with halving infant mortality in Europe and the United States between 1850 and 1910.[80] British pediatrician, epidemiologist, and medical historian Thomas McKeown (1912–1988) attributed European and U.S. reduction in infant mortality between 1900 and 1931 to pasteurization.[81]

Yet as late as 1926, processors pasteurized only 1.5 percent of Britain's milk.[82] This year is too late to have reduced British mortality, a trend that began in the 1820s and accelerated after roughly 1870.[83] British historian and economist Roderick Castle Floud (b. 1942) credited improvements in "nutritional status"—the outcome of nutrition, public health initiatives, and efforts to eliminate or minimize childhood diseases—with decreasing death rate.[84] Increases in real income—wages rising faster than inflation—enhanced nutritional status and thereby decreased mortality, he believed. Efforts to sanitize hospitals after 1869 appear to have lessened mortality in London, England, and Paris, France, in the 1880s and must have contributed to general reductions in fatalities.[85] After 1905 in Lincoln, England, and after 1908 in Jersey City, New Jersey, use of chlorine—an element in the Periodic Table's group 17 (halogens) and a nutrient discussed in Chapter 2—to sanitize drinking water amplified this progress by eliminating waterborne diseases like cholera, dysentery, and typhoid.

These developments question McKeown's emphasis on pasteurization as dwindler of infant mortality between 1900 and 1931. For example, France required pasteurization only in 1935, and not until 1955 did it establish minimum standards for the procedure. Britain and France demonstrated that pasteurization made slow progress in parts of Europe. Moreover, mid-nineteenth-century mortality diminution, which Currier and Widness cited, owed nothing to pasteurization, which was then merely an idea. Besides pasteurization, water chlorination, and asepsis in hospitals, Oakland, California, businessmen in 1913 began manufacturing Clorox bleach.[86]

In this context, pasteurization is best conceived as part of a sanitary movement against germs in milk, water, hospitals, and homes. All reduced the infections that killed countless people over millennia. American physician and Rockefeller Foundation president John Hilton Knowles (1926–1979) summarized the situation, asserting in 1977 that pasteurization, clean drinking water, sewage treatment and disposal, and nutrition accounted for twentieth-century reductions in mortality.[87]

7.4.3 Milk as Wholesome

Hygienic milk came to symbolize wholesomeness. Early in the twentieth century, scientists and medical authorities announced that calcium made milk and other dairy foods indispensable in strengthening teeth and bones, increasing mass and density and thereby averting osteoporosis.[88] Cow's milk was thought valuable because its calcium surpassed that in human milk fourfold by mass, helping calf skeletons grow rapidly before weaning.[89] In addition to calcium, American biochemist Elmer Verner McCollum (1879–1967) in 1922 named vitamin D rickets' cure.[90] With ties to the dairy industry, he promoted milk, cheese, and butter as ideal foods. During the 1930s, manufacturers began to fortify milk with vitamin D.[91]

Milk penetrated the classroom. In the 1920s Newton, Massachusetts public schools typified the trend toward serving it, targeting children who were at least 10 percent underweight for their age and sex.[92] Some schools encouraged all students to drink milk while they listened to teachers espouse its benefits. As part of a national effort to improve nutrition, Britain in 1927 subsidized milk in schools, in 1934 reducing 151.2 grams (one-third pint) of milk—an amount thought adequate for children—to a halfpenny in elementary schools.[93] U.S. schools offered milk at breakfast and lunch, and the 1946 National School Lunch Act directed the federal government to reimburse them for it.[94]

As in Britain, milk and other dairy strengthened national security. Children who drank milk matured into adults fit for military duty when the nation demanded it. Congress subsidizes milk and cheese through the Special Supplemental Nutrition Assistance Program for Women, Infants, and Children (WIC), an outgrowth of the 1966 Child Nutrition Act.[95] The U.S. Department of Agriculture (USDA) food pyramid recommends two or three dairy servings daily. In the global arena, the United Nations Food and Agriculture Organization (FAO) in Rome, Italy—inaugurating World School Milk Day in September 2000—urges developing world schools to serve the beverage.[96]

7.5 DAIRY'S HEALTH EFFECTS SCRUTINIZED

7.5.1 Dairy, Bones, and Teeth

Despite the belief that dairy benefits teeth and bones, proof eludes scientists. Chapter 3 noted the trend toward diminishing robusticity during human evolution. Paleolithic hunter-gatherers lacked dairy but had stouter bones than we do. Chapter 4 indicated that Plains Indians had thick femurs without dairy. Their bones benefited from adequate nourishment absent dairy and from exposure to sunlight. Moreover, African Americans tend to eat less dairy than whites yet have more bone mass and fewer fractures.[97] East Asians, including those in the United States, eat less dairy and have less bone mass than white but fewer fractures. These realities indicate that dairy foods alone do not guarantee healthy bones. Other variables include genetics, exposure to sunshine, activity, mass, height, and intake of vitamin A, fluorine, sodium, potassium, fruits, vegetables, alcohol, and protein. Vitamin D may be the primary factor.

7.5.2 Western Diets and Calcium

To the extent that calcium is the concern, if some is beneficial, more is not always better. That human milk has four times less calcium than cow's, noted earlier, implies that cow's milk overdoses newborns and infants.[98] In this context, British cardiologist Stephen Seely in 2000 warned against the "excessively high calcium content of the Western diet."[99]

This caution mandates the mineral's examination. Besides calcium's role in teeth and bones, already mentioned, the body uses its cations (Ca^{2+}) as electrolytes, in the immune system, to regulate enzymes, and to help clot wounds. For these purposes, blood maintains the cations within a narrow range of concentrations. Ingestion of excess burdens the body with excreting what it cannot use. The kidneys put about 100 milligrams in urine daily.[100] Activity also helps because perspiration sheds calcium. The amount varies with sweat's volume but may approach 80 milligrams per day.

This book emphasizes, however, that people in developed countries tend to be inert. Those who ingest lots of calcium but perspire little tax the kidneys. This danger characterizes individuals whose incomes permit the consumption of animal products like dairy and whose lives center on the automobile and other machines. Several chapters criticize motorization and the inactivity it abets. Surplus calcium that the body cannot excrete may accumulate inside arteries, contributing to atherosclerosis as discussed in Chapter 4.

The body's calcium requirements vary throughout life and are greatest during growth. By age thirty-five, the skeleton has maximized mass and demand plateaus.[101] After age fifty, the skeleton dwindles, dumping the mineral in blood. With shrinking bones and extra calcium in blood, the body must work to rid superfluity. Calcium needs diminish accordingly.

7.5.3 Calcium Recommendations

These fluctuations led Seely to recommend daily calcium maximum intakes of 470 milligrams for active young adults and 290 for active elderly.[102] Inactivity reduces these limits to 390 milligrams

TABLE 7.3
Calcium (mg/d) Recommendations from U.S. National Academy of Sciences

Age	Intake (mg/d)
0–6 mo	210
6–12 mo	270
1–3 yr	500
4–8 yr	800
9–18 yr	1,300
19–50 yr	1,000
>50 yr	1,200
Pregnant or lactating, <19 yr	1,300
Pregnant or lactating, ≥19 yr	1,000

in young adulthood and 240 in senescence. The U.S. National Academy of Sciences in Washington, DC urges daily consumption, in Table 7.3, between 210 milligrams for newborns and 1,300 for pregnant or lactating women under age nineteen and for children between nine and eighteen.[103] The FDA recommends 1,000 milligrams daily above age three.[104] Austrian American physician and nutritionist Herta Spencer-Laszlo (1911–2007) put optimal adult ingestion at 1,200 milligrams daily.[105] American radiologist Stanley Boyd Eaton (b. 1938) and American biologist Stanley Boyd Eaton III, using hunter-gatherers as models, recommended 1,500 milligrams daily.[106] The European Union (EU) recommends 800 milligrams daily for anyone over eighteen years.[107] No one should exceed 1,500 milligrams per day. Doubtless aware of these differences, Scottish nutritionists Mike Lean and Emilie Combet acknowledged that optimal values "are difficult to determine."[108]

Uncertainty appears along national and hemispheric boundaries. The United States and Canada have higher RDAs for calcium at all ages than the World Health Organization (WHO) in Geneva, Switzerland, the United Kingdom (UK), and the EU.[109] Disagreement complicates attempts to quantify excess, though, as Chapter 2 mentioned, too much calcium impairs iron, phosphorus, and zinc absorption.[110] Surfeit causes kidney stones and atherosclerosis, as noted. Despite these findings, consumers who want calcium have options besides dairy. Fish, tofu, and dark green leafy vegetables also supply the mineral. Scientists and physicians have not demonstrated dairy's superiority to these alternatives.

Also unclear is preagricultural calcium intake. Chapter 3 emphasized that human diets and nutrients varied over time and space. Variability undermines attempts to generalize and to reach consensus. Seely believed that ancestral hunter-gatherers ate little calcium, for example, whereas American anthropologist Robert Jurmain and coauthors averred that they ingested over twice that in modern affluent diets.[111] Eaton and Eaton stated that modern hunter-gatherers consume more calcium than people in industrial nations and that the first group models preagricultural "lifeways."[112]

7.5.4 Dairy and Heart Disease

Whatever the differences between past and current calcium intakes, dairy correlates with heart disease. A 1988 study of fifty-two foods and food constituents found four of the six highest correlations between a dairy product and death from heart disease.[113] These items were whole milk, dairy protein without cheese protein, and milkfat with correlations of 0.91 and total dairy protein at 0.86. The highest correlation was for oats (*Avena sativa*) at 0.95. Seely identified calcium as common to oats and dairy.[114] Long vilified, sucrose ranked fifth at 0.90.[115]

TABLE 7.4
Calcium (mg) in Cheese (100 g)

Cheese	Ca (mg)	%DV
Cottage	73	7.3
Feta	360	36
Cheshire	560	56
Cream	98	9.8
Cheddar	720	72
Mozzarella	590	59
Parmesan	1,200	120
Gouda	740	74
Emmental	970	97
Ricotta	240	24
Brie	540	54
Queso Fresco	700	70
Camembert	350	35
Roquefort	530	53
Stilton	320	32
Cow's milk	120	12

Compared to these numbers, correlation between cheese or condensed milk and heart disease deaths was only 0.05.[116] Table 7.4 lists calcium in fifteen cheeses and *B. taurus*' milk.[117] By mass, thirteen cheeses have more calcium than milk, appearing to challenge the mineral's role in heart disease. Seely asserted that cheese may not contribute to heart disease because it has little lactose, noted earlier.[118] Lactose's absence or diminution eases calcium excretion. Substituting skim milk for cheese or condensed milk yielded a correlation of 0.61.[119] Butter was 0.77, and total dairy fat tallied 0.84.

The numbers complicate an attempt to pinpoint calcium and dairy's roles in heart disease. In general, associations were higher for fatty than low-fat foods, excepting nuts and lipid-rich fish, intimating but not proving a link between fat consumption and heart disease.[120] Chapter 10 examines the controversies surrounding fat. Overall, animal protein and fat correlate with death from heart disease whereas these macronutrients in plants appear to protect against it.

The foregoing indicates that more than dairy and calcium influence heart disease. The nations with the most heart disease fatalities per unit population were Finland, Ireland, the United Kingdom, and Sweden.[121] Other chapters mentioned that sunlight diminishes away from the equator. These four countries are north of 53 degrees latitude, but above 37 degrees the body makes enough vitamin D from sunshine only during summer.[122] Because this vitamin protects against atherosclerosis, its dearth during winter rather than dairy consumption may explain heart disease deaths at high latitudes.[123] Heart disease mortality decreases toward the equator, perhaps because perspiration, increasing with warmth, sheds calcium and because sunshine is more plentiful.[124] That is, latitude and heart disease mortality correlate.

Moreover, the relationship between sucrose and heart disease, already noted, demonstrates that calcium or another nutrient cannot be the only culprit. This link may implicate undernutrition rather than excess in heart disease. In this regard, correlation between beer and heart disease fatalities was 0.86.[125] Although Seely deemed this association "spurious," the beverage is not nutrient dense.[126] "Don't plan to get your nutrients from beer, or to drink beer…for health benefits," wrote American nutritionist and dietician Kathleen Manning Zelman.[127]

Finally, cardiovascular disease's causes are poorly understood, making premature attempts to blame dairy or calcium. For example, stroke correlates with low consumption of saturated fat.[128] As intake increases, stroke declines as a cause of death. Epidemiologists tracked this phenomenon in Japan since 1960. The inverse correlation between saturated fat and stroke baffles scientists and medical authorities because deposits, which should thicken with rising saturated fat intake, in the brain's blood vessels precipitate stroke. Equally puzzling, stroke mortality diminished in Japan despite "heavy smoking."[129] In passing, Seely mentioned that cardiovascular disease correlates with automobile ownership.[130] This book, especially Chapter 12, describes motorization's hazards in arguing that inactivity harms health.

7.5.5 Dairy and Stature

Concerns about dairy aside, it promotes growth, an unsurprising circumstance given that calves grow four times faster than infants, as implied earlier.[131] This fact was glimpsed in antiquity, when the Romans understood that dairy-eating Germans were taller than Mediterranean planteaters.[132] During the twentieth century, both stature and milk intake rose in the United States, Europe, and Japan.[133] Yet these peoples did not shrink with declining consumption after World War II. In this instance, milk is not the only variable because, as the next paragraph demonstrates, Americans are eating more cheese and yogurt while reducing milk.

7.5.6 Recent Trends

Milk's promotion comes amid declining per person consumption in the United States, Canada, Brazil, Mexico, Japan, and New Zealand between 1990 and 2009.[134] U.S. intake has fallen since World War II because Americans prefer soft drinks and other sugary beverages. Yet between 1909 and 2008, cheese consumption per American rose from 1.8 to 15 kilograms (4 to 33 pounds) per year.[135] Fatty cheeses are popular. Although Americans drink less total milk, they ingest more skim milk and yogurt.

In contrast to decreasing milk intake in the Americas, Japan, and New Zealand, China more than tripled per capita consumption from 1990 to 2009 despite lactose intolerance, noted earlier.[136] India and Australia have also registered gains. Indian producers aim to maximize output in hopes of affording the poor dairy. These circumstances indicate that India and Australia have not diminished ardor for dairy and that China has lessened its historic ambivalence.

7.6 THE AMISH

7.6.1 Amish Origins

From its first century CE origins, Christianity has been no monolith. Division arose in 1054, when the pope in Rome and the patriarch of Constantinople (now Istanbul, Turkey) expelled each other from what had formally been one church.[137] Thereafter, Western Europe was Catholic whereas Eastern Europe and the parts of Western Asia that remained Christian were Orthodox. By then the Catholic Church had grown wealthy and worldly. Critics charged it with abandoning early Christianity's simplicity, poverty, and piety. Criticisms intensified in the sixteenth century as Europeans who lost hope of reforming Catholicism formed rival churches. In 1525, infant baptism's opponents in Zurich, Switzerland, began to admit only adults as full members and to form their own theology.[138] Among these anabaptists, convert and leader Jakob Amman (c. 1656–c. 1730) urged Christians to reject sinful secular society.[139]

His followers, the Amish, emigrated to Canada, the United States, Argentina, and Bolivia after 1730.[140] Inhabiting thirty-one U.S. states, they maintain their largest community—roughly 35,000 adherents—in Holmes County, Ohio.[141] Partitioning modest parcels into smallholdings of roughly 4 hectares (10 acres) per family, the Amish transitioned from grains to vegetables, though dairying undergirded the economy since the nineteenth century.[142]

7.6.2 Dairying among Amish

Holmes County boasts two cheese factories, both in the county seat Millersburg. The older originated in Swiss immigrant and cheesemaker John Dauwalder's work at Bunker Hill Cheese Co-op, which he bought in 1935, transforming it into Heini's Cheese Chalet.[143] The facility uses milk from over 200 nearby farms.[144] Millersburg's Amish invited a second Swiss cheesemaker, Alfred Guggisberg (1914–1985), to purchase property, which in 1950 became Guggisberg Cheese Factory.[145] In 1967 he made a cheese with small holes that wife Margaret dubbed baby swiss. Its success helped the company become the largest U.S. swiss cheese producer.

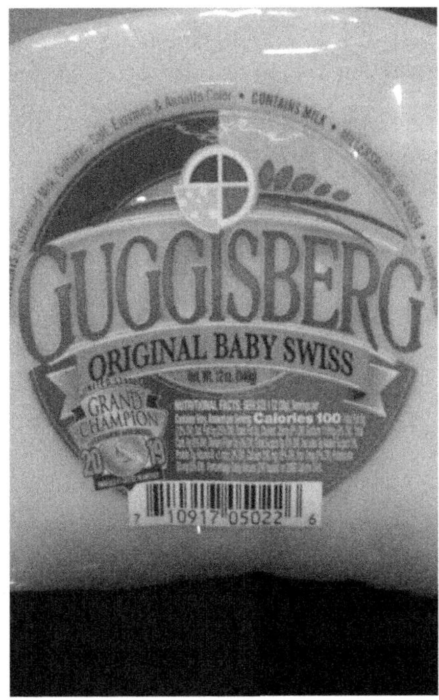

FIGURE 7.9 Guggisberg baby swiss. (Photo from author.)

Holmes County's small businesses sell cheese, butter, ice cream, pudding, and custard. For example, Fox's Pizza Den in Millersburg, ostensibly wedded to cheese, meats, and dough, sells twenty-four ice cream flavors.[146] Broad Run Cheesehouse in Dover retails over thirty cheeses, whereas Guggisberg has twice the selection.[147] Ashery Country Store in Fredericksburg and Walnut Creek Cheese in Walnut Creek sell cheese and custard.[148] Millersburg's Chalet in the Valley serves cheese fondue, and Troyer Country Market makes cheeseballs and ice cream on site.[149]

Cheese—including the cottage cheese *schmierkase*—custard, pudding, butter, milk, and ice cream characterize a diet of animal products.[150] Amish pizza follows tradition in featuring cheese. Children and adults drink raw milk, believing it healthful.[151] Even families that do not sell milk often keep a cow for their needs. Amish eat butter noodles, cheeseburgers, milk chocolate, crème pie, and cheesy Mexican fare.

7.6.3 Amish Foods besides Dairy

Other items include beef, pork, lunchmeats, venison, poultry, eggs, potatoes, bread, pancakes, cabbage, corn (*Zea mays*) and cornmeal, carrots, beets (*Beta vulgaris*), cucumbers (*Cucumis sativus*) and pickles, squashes (*Cucurbita* species), celery, rhubarb (*Rheum rhabarbarum*), tomatoes

(*Solanum esculentum*), peas (*Pisum sativum*), beans (*Phaseolus vulgaris* and *P. lunatus*), peanuts (*Arachis hypogaea*) and peanut butter, pretzels, lard, sucrose, molasses, strawberries (*Fragaria x ananassa*), blackberries (*Rubus* species), raspberries (*Rubus idaeus*), grapes (*Vitis vinifera*), apples (*Malus domestica*), blueberries (*Vaccinium angustifolium*, *V. corymbosum*, and related species), peaches (*Prunus persica*), pears (*Pyrus* species), cantaloupes and muskmelons (both *Cucumis melo*), watermelons (*Citrullus lanatus*), and plums (*Prunus* species). The Amish tend to eat more whole, fresh, organic foods and less junk than many other Americans. This differentiation may lessen as young Amish, unable to profit from farming, enter construction and other occupations that take them out of the community and into mainstream America's fast-food establishments.

7.6.4 Demographic Interest in the Amish

A 2012 paper examined Old Order Amish, the largest group in Holmes County, which an earlier paragraph designated the biggest U.S. Amish community.[152] This order's members are the most numerous among North American Amish and consider themselves the original practitioners, using a prayer book thought to have been published in 1564, forty-seven years after the Protestant Reformation began.[153] The Amish, Old Order or otherwise, interest demographers because of detailed genealogies that retrogress centuries. Amish populations also merit investigation because they eschew automobiles and so retain lifestyles that counter modernity's idleness. That is, like pre-twentieth-century peoples, the Amish illuminate how food and exertion influence health. This book emphasizes that diet alone cannot produce vitality. Activity is also necessary.

7.6.5 Amish Longevity

The 2012 publication compared longevity of 2,108 Amish born from 1890 to 1921 with that of their contemporaries who participated in the Framingham Heart Study.[154] All Framingham participants and the Amish had European ancestry, facilitating comparisons between both. American epidemiologist Braxton D. Mitchell and coauthors examined only Amish and Framingham participants above age twenty-nine, eliminating youth mortality from consideration and neutralizing differences in childhood immunizations, which Amish tended to avoid. A 1984 study, for example, calculated that only 63 percent of U.S. Amish vaccinated their children compared to 85 percent among non-Amish.[155] To be sure, vaccination was not widespread for those born in 1890, the earliest year of Mitchell and coauthors' data. But by the terminal year 1921, immunizations were becoming standard in the United States, the U.S. Supreme Court in 1905 having affirmed state's authority to compel vaccination.[156] By the 1920s, vaccines were available for diphtheria, tuberculosis, tetanus, whooping cough, and smallpox.

Dairy and other animal products may explain higher cholesterol and blood pressure for Amish than for Framingham subjects.[157] Inbreeding among Amish may have exacerbated these problems. Such conditions usually entail drug therapies; yet only 3.7 percent of Amish with high cholesterol and only 6.2 percent with high blood pressure ingested medicine. Although many more Framingham participants with these conditions took medication, Amish men on average outlived non-Amish by three years, and no difference existed between women. Greatest lifespan did not vary, with Amish reporting a maximum of 103 years compared to 104 years among Framingham participants. Average longevity favored the Amish even though Framingham subjects visited physicians and hospitals whereas Amish seldom did. Amish reliance on dairy and other animal foods neither shortened lifespan nor predisposed them to heart attack, stroke, or type 2 diabetes.

But because many people eat dairy, eggs, and meat while suffering these afflictions, these items alone cannot be decisive. If diet is a factor, Amish preference for whole foods over junk may provide an advantage. American nutritionist Thomas Colin Campbell (b. 1934), introduced in Chapter 1, advocated consumption of foods "as close to their natural state as possible."[158]

Although he favored plants, this advice should apply to all victuals. In addition to whole foods, Amish ate organic produce, which over 400 articles judged more nutritious than agribusiness' edibles.[159]

Mitchell and colleagues went beyond diet, crediting exertion as chief contributor to Amish longevity and vitality.[160] Not only is work arduous, but, absent automobiles, many Amish ride bicycles for transportation. These authors inversely correlated activity and obesity. Although exertion conferred vigor, it did not lengthen maximum lifespan, as noted. Physicians who treated Amish observed that lifelong exertion gave them osteoarthritis, slowing them in their 50s.[161] As they became less mobile, their mass increased, and by their seventh decade they had many of inactivity's ailments. Besides exertion, fewer Amish than Framingham subjects smoked or drank alcohol.[162] Finally, Michell and coauthors speculated that communal ties improved longevity and quality of life, noting that Amish cared for elderly at home rather than consigned them to nursing homes.[163] Religion strengthened community, providing cohesion and meaning.

7.7 FINLAND

7.7.1 Settlement and Economy

Like other chapters, this one notes that geography influences diet, especially absent long-distance trade. In northern Europe, Finland straddles the Arctic Circle. Distant from the equator, as noted, the Nordic nation needs the Gulf stream and Baltic Sea for warmth. Forests, covering some three-quarters of Finland, limit agriculture.[164] Since 9000 BCE migrants from what are today Estonia, Latvia, Poland, and Russia settled Finland and about 2500 BCE began milking cows, though many continued to forage or combined pastoralism, farming, hunting, fishing, and gathering.[165] Short growing seasons led Finns to emphasize livestock raising for dairy and meat.

Over one-third of Finnish farms yield milk, cheese, butter, and yogurt, with dairy totaling two-thirds of agrarian income.[166] The average Finn drinks 130 liters (34.3 gallons) of milk annually, the most worldwide.[167] Popular are buttermilk and fermented milk, known as *piima* and *rahka* respectively. Breakfast is incomplete without milk, which may be added to oats, rye, barley, or a combination of grains. Finnish cheeses include emmental—a type of swiss—*kotijuusto*, and *leipajuusto*. Emmental enters domestic and export markets. Finns deem the fermented yogurt *viili* a national food.[168] Dairy with little or no lactose satisfies wary consumers, though few Finns fail to produce lactase throughout life. Health enthusiasts prefer high-protein dairy.

Dairy alone has not sustained Finns. Ancient farmers grew oats, rye, and barley for domestic consumption. Rye bread remains popular at meals. Turnips have long been part of diets, though since the seventeenth century potatoes have rivaled them. As implied, the first Finns were hunter-gatherers, and game like deer (*Odocoileus* species), moose (*Alces alces*), and rabbits (*Oryctolagus cuniculus*) furnish protein and other nutrients. Reindeer (*Rangifer tarandus*), duck (*Anas platyrhynchos*), pork, beef, salmon (*Oncorhynchus* species), herring (*Clupea herengus*), and whitefish (*Coregonus* species) also supply complete protein. Crayfish (species in the families Astacidae, Parastacidae, and Austraostracidae) are available between July and September. Wild mushrooms like chanterelles (*Cantharellus cibarius*) and morels (*Morchella esculenta*) are added to the soup *korvasienikeitto*, a practice borrowed from Russia. To the west, Sweden heightened Finns' preference for smoked salmon, salami, cheeses, and salads.

7.7.2 Finnish Health

Into the 1960s health was not paramount. Finland paid dairy farmers by milkfat, and Finns exhibited the world's worst heart disease.[169] By 1974, Finland's death rate was nearly one-third higher than in Italy and Spain.[170] High in saturated fat, dairy elevated cholesterol and blood pressure. Comparison among Finland, the United States, Italy, Spain, South Africa, Japan, and what was then Yugoslavia—now Bosnia and Herzegovina, Croatia, Montenegro, Macedonia, Serbia, and Slovenia—documented the highest cholesterol in Finns.[171] Finnish diets featured whole milk and bread with butter while minimizing vegetables, fruits, and fiber. Inactivity and smoking increased cancer rates, especially lung.

Chapter 4 noted that menarche, correlating with calories, protein, iron, zinc, calcium, and vitamin B_9, may gauge nutrition and health.[172] This event may not reflect optimal nutrition, however, because junk foods or too many calories in general may hasten menarche. Additionally, poor girls tend to enter puberty early independent of other factors, indicating that nutrition may play a secondary role.[173] Whatever the mechanisms involved, Finnish menarche fell from 16.5 years in 1850 to thirteen in 1983.[174]

The abundant food that sped puberty also increased population. Finland began counting citizens in the 1750s, when the number was under 500,000.[175] It grew to 800,000 in 1800, 1.8 million in 1870, over 2.5 million in 1915, 4 million in 1945, and 5.5 million in 2016. Travel writer Tan Chung-Lee and comparative-literature scholar Elizabeth Schmermund credited medicine with these gains, though Finland's experience resembled Ireland's, both of which adopted the potato. Chapter 13 examines it in northern Europe. Particularly relevant is Finland and Ireland's population enlargement upon its introduction. Finland began growing potatoes in the seventeenth century, as mentioned and as Chapter 13 discusses, after which population increased.

As noted, Finnish health compared poorly with other nations. A 1952–1974 study of Finland, the United States, Italy, Spain, South Africa, Japan, Bosnia and Herzegovina, Croatia, Montenegro, Macedonia, Serbia, and Slovenia, already mentioned, found that over half the participants smoked irrespective of nationality.[176] Yet Finnish smokers died youngest. Even Finns who quit had twice the mortality of nonsmokers in the other countries. Whether smokers or not, rural Finns had twice as many heart attacks as rural Italians at ages forty-five and fifty-five.[177] "In the 1970s, we held the world record for heart disease," admitted Finland's National Institute of Public Health director Pekka Puska in 2005.[178]

Between the 1970s and 2005, however, Finland cut deaths from heart disease and lung cancer by 65 percent.[179] Diet aided this reversal, as government paid dairy farmers by milk protein rather than fat and encouraged skim milk's consumption. Finland promoted low sodium foods to reduce blood pressure and subsidized cultivation of berries—like blackberries, raspberries, cranberries (*Vaccinium oxycoccos*), cloudberries (*Rubus chamaemorus*), strawberries, lingonberries (*Vaccinium vitis-idaea*), bilberries (*Vaccinium myrtillus*), and redcurrants (*Ribes rubrum*)—suited to short growing seasons.[180] Consumers add cheese, cream, and sucrose to cloudberries. Finns supplement these items by picking wild berries. Fruit and vegetable intake more than doubled between 1978 and 2008.[181]

Besides diet, Finland discouraged smoking by banning all tobacco advertising. Between the 1970s and 2005, Finnish smokers fell from half to under one-third the population.[182] No less important was activity. Following government mandates, general practitioners prescribed exercise for many conditions. Only when it proved inadequate did they dispense drugs. Government loaned bicycles to those who could not afford one and built paths for cyclists and walkers. Finland set aside parks for cross-country skiing and dug swimming pools.

Emphasis on exertion battled factories that produced record numbers of cars in the 1980s, exacerbating obesity.[183] Yet efforts to improve diets, increase activity, and minimize smoking have extended lifespan. By 2005 Finnish men lived seven more years on average, and women six, than in the 1970s. Green League—the second largest party in the capital Helsinki—sought to expand health initiatives in 2017 by banning automobiles in the city.[184] The attempt failed, though Finns cycle, walk, and use public transit to reduce dependence on cars. In 2018 Finland's e^0 ranked fortieth at 80.2 years.[185] The next year, Bloomberg Global Health Index ranked Finland the world's fifteenth healthiest nation.[186] Finland demonstrates, as this book reiterates, that diet alone does not bestow vitality. Activity and avoidance of tobacco are essential.

NOTES

1 Andrea S. Wiley, *Re-Imagining Milk* (New York and London: Routledge, 2011), 28–29.
2 Marco Ceresa, "Milk and National Identity in China," in *Food and Identity in the Ancient World*, ed. Cristiano Grottanelli and Lucio Milano (Padova: Sargon, 2004), 10.
3 Ibid., 10; Wiley, 19; Nicholas Scott Cardell and Mark Myron Hopkins, "The Effect of Milk Intolerance on the Consumption of Milk by Slaves in 1860," *Journal of Interdisciplinary History* 8, no. 3 (Winter 1978): 509.
4 Cardell and Hopkins, 509.
5 Ceresa, 10; Cardell and Hopkins, 509; Wiley, 19.
6 Wiley, 19.
7 Colin Scanes, *Fundamentals of Animal Science* (Clifton Park, NY: Delmar Cengage Learning, 2011), 466.
8 Melanie Pinola, "The Best Cheeses to Eat If You're Lactose Intolerant," *Life Hacker*, April 15, 2014, accessed March 8, 2019, https://lifehacker.com/the-best-cheeses-to-eat-if-youre-lactose-intolerant-1563386663.
9 Wiley, 10; "Milk, Goat, Fluid, with Added Vitamin D," *USDA FoodData Central*, April 1, 2019, accessed February 10, 2020, https://fdc.nal.usda.gov/fdc-app.html#/food-details/171278/nutrients.
10 "Cream—Types of Cream and Their Uses," *The Epicentre*, accessed March 9, 2019, http://theepicentre.com/ingredient/cream-types-of-cream-and-their-uses.
11 Fred Decker, "Butter Fat vs. Milk Fat," *SFGate*, last modified November 19, 2018, accessed March 9, 2019, https://healthyeating.sfgate.com/butter-fat-vs-milk-fat-11424.html.
12 "Is Clarified Butter Healthy?" *Nutritious Life*, accessed March 9, 2019, https://nutritiouslife.com/eat-empowered/clarified-butter-healthy.
13 Shawn Bubel, "Plant and Animal Domestication in the Ancient Near East," in *World History Encyclopedia, vol. 2, Era 1: Beginnings of Human Society*, ed. Mark Aldenderfer (Santa Barbara, CA: ABC-CLIO, 2011), 134–135.
14 Parth Chauhan, "Early Food Producers in the Indus Valley," in *World History Encyclopedia, vol. 2, Era 1: Beginnings of Human Society*, ed. Mark Aldenderfer (Santa Barbara, CA: ABC-CLIO, 2011), 140.
15 Stephanie Pappas, "Once-Green Sahara Hosted Early African Dairy Farms," Live Science, June 20, 2012, accessed March 12, 2019, https://www.livescience.com/21070-green-sahara-hosted-african-dairy-farms.html.
16 A. M. Mannion, "Plant Cultivation and Animal Use in the Nile Valley," in *World History Encyclopedia, vol. 2, Era 1: Beginnings of Human Society*, ed. Mark Aldenderfer (Santa Barbara, CA: ABC-CLIO, 2011), 135–136.
17 Delphine Roger, "The Middle East and South Asia," in *The Cambridge World History of Food*, vol. 2, ed. Kenneth F. Kiple and Kriemhild Conee Ornelas (Cambridge, UK: Cambridge University Press, 2000), 1146
18 Peter Garnsey, *Food and Society in Classical Antiquity* (Cambridge, UK: Cambridge University Press, 1999), 14.
19 Wiley, 38.
20 "Does Ghee Expire?" *The Times of India*, last modified August 21, 2019, accessed November 12, 2019, https://timesofindia.indiatimes.com/life-style/health-fitness/photo-stories/does-ghee-expire/photostory/60308368.cms.
21 Wiley, 40.
22 Mark Kurlansky, *Milk!: A 10,000-Year Food Fracas* (New York: Bloomsbury Publishing, 2018), 26.
23 Beatrice Caseau, "Byzantium," in *A Companion to Food in the Ancient World*, ed. John Wilkins and Robin Nadeau (Malden, MA: Wiley Blackwell, 2015), 365.
24 Christopher Chandezon, "Animals, Meat, and Alimentary By-Products: Patterns of Production and Consumption," in *A Companion to Food in the Ancient World*, ed. John Wilkins and Robin Nadeau (Malden, MA: Wiley Blackwell, 2015), 136–137.
25 Wiley, 41.
26 Kurlansky, 38.
27 Ibid., 47.
28 John P. McKay, Bennett D. Hill, John Buckler, Clare Haru Crowston, Merry E. Wiesner-Hanks, and Joe Perry, *Understanding Western Society: A Brief History* (Boston and New York: Bedford/St. Martin's, 2012), 324, 327.
29 Wiley, 41.
30 Ibid.

31 Ibid., 42.
32 Ibid., 41.
33 Ibid., 42–43.
34 W. Stephen Damron, *Introduction to Animal Science: Global, Biological, Social, and Industry Perspectives*, 6th ed. (New York: Pearson, 2018), 303, 413, 446.
35 "Gateway to Dairy Production and Products," *Food and Agriculture Organization of the United Nations*, 2019, accessed March 13, 2019, http://www.fao.org/dairy-production-products/products/milk-composition/en.
36 Ceresa, 1.
37 Ibid., 4–5.
38 Ibid., 6.
39 Ibid., 7.
40 Ibid.
41 Ibid., 8; Wiley, 86.
42 Olwen Hufton, "Social Conflict and the Grain Supply in Eighteenth-Century France," *Journal of Interdisciplinary History* 14, no. 2 (Autumn 1983): 319.
43 Ibid., 308.
44 R. J. Bernard, "Peasant Diet in Eighteenth-Century Gevaudan," in *European Diet from Pre-Industrial to Modern Times*, ed. Elborg Forster and Robert Forster (New York: Torchbooks, 1975), 20–21, 24, 33.
45 Ibid., 36.
46 Ibid., 35–36.
47 Ibid., 24–27.
48 "Butter, without Salt," *USDA FoodData Central*, April 1, 2019, accessed February 10, 2020, https://fdc.nal.usda.gov/fdc-app.html#/food-details/173430/nutrients; Atli Arnarson, "Butter 101: Nutrition Facts and Health Effects," *Healthline*, November 3, 2014, accessed March 13, 2019, https://www.healthline.com/nutrition/foods/butter.
49 Bernard, 24–27.
50 Ibid., 29.
51 Ibid., 32.
52 Ibid., 35.
53 Gene R. De Foilart, "Chapter 9: Western Attitudes toward Insects as Food: Europe, the United States, Canada," in *The Human Use of Insects as a Food Resource: A Bibliographic Account in Progress*, last modified September 29, 2002, accessed March 13, 2019, http://labs.russell.wisc.edu/insectsasfood/files/2012/09/Book_Chapter_9.pdf.
54 Miles Olson, "11 Edible Bugs and How to Eat Them," *Mother Earth News*, May 30, 2013, accessed March 13, 2019, https://www.motherearthnews.com/real-food/edible-bugs-zebz1305znsp.
55 Thijs Westerbeek, "Geert Bruggeman—Maggots: The Perfect Protein Source," *Youris.com*, European Research Media Center, April 1, 2014, accessed March 13, 2019, http://www.youris.com/bioeconomy/interviews/geert-bruggeman--maggots-the-perfect-protein-source.kl.
56 Daniel Calder, "Insect Harvesting: Edible Flies and Fly Larvae (Maggots) Pack a Nutritional Punch," *The Dietician's Guide to Eating Bugs*, 2018, accessed March 13, 2019, https://www.secretsofsurvival.com/survival/insect-harvesting-flies.html.
57 Bernard, 33.
58 "Is a Serving of Bread One Slice or Two Slices?" *Fooducate*, November 24, 2014, accessed March 13, 2019, https://www.fooducate.com/community/post/Is%20a%20Serving%20of%20Bread%20One%20Slice%20or%20Two%20Slices%3F/547323C3-A80E-1665-430F-AD0A7EE040F5.
59 Bernard, 37–40.
60 Ibid., 40.
61 Donald J. Ortner and Gretchen Theobald, "Paleopathological Evidence of Malnutrition," in *The Cambridge World History of Food*, vol. 1, ed. Kenneth F. Kiple and Kriemhild Conee Ornelas (Cambridge, UK: Cambridge University Press, 2000), 37.
62 Bernard, 28.
63 Annie Price, "Improve Your Waistline and Heart Health with Rye Flour," *Dr. Axe*, April 2, 2016, accessed March 13, 2019, https://draxe.com/rye-flour.
64 Alina Petre, "9 Impressive Health Benefits of Barley," *Healthline*, September 18, 2018, accessed March 13, 2019, https://www.healthline.com/nutrition/barley-benefits.
65 Atli Arnarson, "Wheat 101: Nutrition Facts and Health Effects," *Healthline*, February 25, 2015, accessed March 13, 2019, https://www.healthline.com/nutrition/foods/wheat.

66 Hufton, 308.
67 "Fashion History Timeline, 1790–1799," State University of New York, 2020, accessed March 9, 2020, https://fashionhistory.fitnyc.edu/1790-1799.
68 Garnsey, 47; Ortner and Theobald, 36.
69 Ortner and Theobald, 36–37.
70 Robert Sallares, "Ecology," in *The Cambridge Economic History of the Greco-Roman World*, ed. Walter Scheidel, Ian Morris, and Richard Saller (Cambridge, UK: Cambridge University Press, 2007), 34.
71 Kurlansky, 164.
72 Ibid., 163.
73 Gerald L. Geison, "Pasteur, Louis," in *Dictionary of Scientific Biography*, vol. 10, ed. Charles Coulston Gillispie (New York: Charles Scribner's Sons, 1981), 362.
74 Ibid., 364.
75 Anne Rooney, *The History of Medicine* (New York: Rosen Publishing, 2013), 62.
76 Claude E. Dolman, "Spallanzani, Lazzaro," in *Dictionary of Scientific Biography*, vol. 12, ed. Charles Coulston Gillispie (New York: Charles Scribner's Sons, 1981), 555.
77 Scanes, 467.
78 Wiley, 50.
79 Kurlansky, 186; Wiley, 50.
80 Russell W. Currier and John A. Widness, "A Brief History of Milk Hygiene and Its Impact on Infant Mortality from 1875 to 1925 and Implications for Today: A Review," *Journal of Food Protection* 81, no. 10 (October 2018): 1713–1722, https://jfoodprotection.org/doi/full/10.4315/0362-028X.JFP-18-186.
81 Robert William Fogel, "Nutrition and the Decline in Mortality since 1700: Some Preliminary Findings," in *Long-Term American Economic Growth*, ed. Stanley L. Engerman and Robert E. Gallman (Chicago and London: University of Chicago Press, 1986), 441.
82 P. J. Atkins, "The Pasteurization of England: The Science, Culture and Health Implications of Food Processing, 1900–1950," *Academia*, accessed March 22, 2019, https://www.academia.edu/3161171/The_pasteurization_of_England_the_science_culture_and_health_implications_of_food_processing_1900-1950, 6.
83 Jacques Vallin, "Mortality in Europe from 1720 to 1914: Long-Term Trends and Changes in Patterns by Age and Sex," in *The Decline of Mortality in Europe*, ed. R. Schofield, D. Reher, and A. Bideau (Oxford: Clarendon Press, 1991), 44.
84 Roderick Floud, "Medicine and the Decline of Mortality: Indicators of Nutritional Status," in *The Decline of Mortality in Europe*, ed. R. Schofield, D. Reher, and A. Bideau (Oxford: Clarendon Press, 1991), 155–156.
85 Jean Noel Biraben, "Pasteur, Pasteurization, and Medicine," in *The Decline of Mortality in Europe*, ed. R. Schofield, D. Reher, and A. Bideau (Oxford: Clarendon Press, 1991), 226–227, 230.
86 "The Facts about Bleach," *Clorox*, 2015, accessed March 23, 2019, http://factsaboutbleach.com/clorox_history.html.
87 John H. Knowles, "The Responsibility of the Individual," *Daedalus* 106, no. 1 (Winter 1977): 57.
88 Wiley, 53.
89 Ibid.; Stephen Seely, "The Cardiovascular System, Coronary Artery Disease, and Calcium: A Hypothesis," in *The Cambridge World History of Food*, vol. 1, ed. Kenneth F. Kiple and Kriemhild Conee Ornelas (Cambridge, UK: Cambridge University Press, 2000), 1117.
90 Elmer Verner McCollum, *A History of Nutrition: The Sequence of Ideas in Nutrition Investigations* (Boston: Houghton Mifflin, 1957), 276.
91 Wiley, 54.
92 Ibid., 55.
93 Walter Gratzer, *Terrors of the Table: The Curious History of Nutrition* (Oxford and New York: Oxford University Press, 2005), 8.
94 Wiley, 57–58.
95 Wiley, 1–2.
96 "School Milk," *FAO*, 2019, accessed March 14, 2019, http://www.fao.org/economic/est/est-commodities/dairy/school-milk/en.
97 Wiley, 80.
98 Seely, 1117.
99 Ibid.
100 Ibid.

101 Ibid.
102 Ibid., 1117–1118.
103 Julian E. Spallholz, L. Mallory Boylan, and Judy A. Driskell, *Nutrition Chemistry and Biology*, 2nd ed. (Boca Raton, FL: CRC Press, 1999), 292.
104 "FDA Vitamins and Minerals Chart," *FDA*, accessed April 24, 2019, https://www.accessdata.fda.gov/scripts/interactivenutritionfactslabel/factsheets/vitamin_and_mineral_chart.pdf.
105 Herta Spencer, "Calcium," in *The Cambridge World History of Food*, vol. 1, ed. Kenneth F. Kiple and Kriemhild Conee Ornelas (Cambridge, UK: Cambridge University Press, 2000), 789.
106 S. Boyd Eaton and Stanley B. Eaton III, "Hunter-Gatherers and Human Health," in *The Cambridge Encyclopedia of Hunters and Gatherers*, ed. Richard B. Lee and Richard Daly (Cambridge, UK: Cambridge University Press, 1999), 454.
107 Sarah Brewer, *Nutrition: A Beginner's Guide* (London: Oneworld, 2013), 94.
108 Mike Lean and Emilie Combet, *Barasi's Human Nutrition: A Health Perspective*, 3rd ed. (Boca Raton, FL: CRC Press, 2017), 85.
109 Wiley, 65.
110 Naim Maalouf, "How Much Calcium Is Too Much?" *UT Southwestern Medical Center*, February 2, 2015, accessed March 15, 2019, https://utswmed.org/medblog/calcium.
111 Seely, 1117; Robert Jurmain, Lynn Kilgore, Wenda Trevathan, and Russell L. Ciochon. *Introduction to Physical Anthropology*, 2013–2014 ed. (Belmont, CA: Wadsworth Cengage Learning, 2014), 446–447.
112 Eaton and Eaton, 449, 453.
113 Seely, 1116.
114 Ibid., 1117.
115 Ibid., 1116.
116 Ibid.
117 "Calcium & pH," *Cheese Science Toolkit*, 2019, accessed November 16, 2019, https://www.cheesescience.org/calcium.html.
118 Seely, 1118.
119 Ibid., 1116.
120 Ibid.
121 Ibid., 1115.
122 *World Atlas* (United States: Hammond Publications, 1999), 6, 18; "Time for More Vitamin D," *Harvard Medical School*, September 2008, accessed November 16, 2019, https://www.health.harvard.edu/staying-healthy/time-for-more-vitamin-d.
123 Brewer, 88.
124 Seely, 1119.
125 Ibid., 1115.
126 Ibid.
127 Kathleen M. Zelman, "The Truth about Beer," *WebMD*, 2014, accessed November 16, 2019, https://www.webmd.com/food-recipes/features/truth-about-beer.
128 Seely, 1113.
129 Ibid.
130 Ibid., 1115.
131 Ibid., 1117.
132 Nikola C. G. Kopke, "Regional Differences and Temporal Development of Nutritional Status in Europe from the 8th Century B.C. until the 18th Century A.D." PhD diss., Universitat Tubingen, 2008, 139.
133 Wiley, 68.
134 Ibid., 86.
135 Ibid., 60–61.
136 Ibid., 86.
137 William C. Placher, *A History of Christian Theology: An Introduction* (Philadelphia: Westminster Press, 1983), 88.
138 Steven M. Nolt, *A History of the Amish*, rev. ed. (Intercourse, PA: Good Books, 2003), 11–12.
139 "Welcome," *Ohio Amish Country Map and Visitors' Guide, 2019*, 1.
140 Nolt, 63, 116.
141 "Amish Studies," *The Young Center*, accessed March 14, 2019, https://groups.etown.edu/amishstudies; "Welcome," 1.
142 "When to Visit Ohio's Amish Country," *Touring Ohio*, 2019, accessed March 14, 2019, http://touringohio.com/ohio-amish.html.

143 "About Us," *Bunker Hill Cheese*, 1935–2019, accessed March 14, 2019, https://bunkerhillcheese.com/about-us-en-2.html.
144 *Heini's*, Millersburg, OH.
145 "The History of Guggisberg Cheese," *Guggisberg Cheese*, 2019, accessed March 14, 2019, https://www.babyswiss.com/history.
146 "About Us," *Fox's Pizza Den*, accessed March 14, 2019, http://www.foxspizza.com/locations/oh/millersburg/millersburg-oh-119/index.html.
147 "Attractions, Shops and Artisans," *Ohio Amish Country Map and Visitors' Guide, 2019*, 9, 11.
148 "Food Stores," *Ohio Amish Country Map and Visitors' Guide, 2019*, 25–26.
149 "Dining," *Ohio Amish Country Map and Visitors' Guide, 2019*, 29; Olivia Bloom, "The Great Taste of Amish Country," *Ohio's Amish Country*, Winter 2018, 23.
150 "United States Amish and Pennsylvania Dutch," *Food in Every Country*, 2019, accessed March 14, 2019, http://www.foodbycountry.com/Spain-to-Zimbabwe-Cumulative-Index/United-States-Amish-and-Pennsylvania-Dutch.html.
151 "What Do Amish Eat?" *Amish America*, accessed March 14, 2019, http://amishamerica.com/what-do-amish-eat.
152 Braxton D. Mitchell, Woei-Jyh Lee, Magdalena I. Tolea, Kelsey Shields, Zahra Ashktorab, Laurence S. Magder, Kathleen A. Ryan, Toni I. Pollin, Patrick F. McArdle, Alan R. Shuldiner, and Alejandro A. Schaffer," Living the Good Life? Mortality and Hospital Utilization Patterns in the Old Order Amish," *Plos One* 7, no. 12 (December 19, 2012), https://journals.plos.org/plosone/article?id=10.1371/journal.pone.0051560; "Welcome," 1.
153 Dave Tabler, "Old Order Amish," *Appalachian History*, November 21, 2017, accessed March 15, 2019, http://www.appalachianhistory.net/2017/11/old-order-amish.html; Albrecht Powell, "Amish Origin, Beliefs, and Lifestyle," *Trip Savvy*, last modified December 26, 2018, accessed March 15, 2019, https://www.tripsavvy.com/guide-to-the-amish-lifestyle-2707217.
154 Mitchell, Lee, Tolea, Shields, Ashktorab, Magder, Pollin, McArdle, Shuldiner, and Schaffer.
155 Charles E. Hurst and David L. McConnell, *An Amish Paradox: Diversity and Change in the World's Largest Amish Community* (Baltimore: Johns Hopkins University Press, 2010), 228.
156 *Jacobson v. Massachusetts*, 197 U.S. 11 (1905).
157 Mitchell, Lee, Tolea, Shields, Ashktorab, Magder, Pollin, McArdle, Shuldiner, and Schaffer.
158 T. Colin Campbell, *Whole: Rethinking the Science of Nutrition* (Dallas, TX: Ben Bella Books, 2013), 7.
159 Michell, Lee, Tolea, Shields, Ashktorab, Magder, Pollin, McArdle, Shuldiner, and Schaffer; Brewer, 169–170.
160 Mitchell, Lee, Tolea, Shields, Ashktorab, Magder, Pollin, McArdle, Shuldiner, and Schaffer.
161 Hurst and McConnell, 232.
162 Ibid., 233; Mitchell, Lee, Tolea, Shields, Ashktorab, Magder, Pollin, McArdle, Shuldiner, and Schaffer.
163 Mitchell, Lee, Tolea, Shields, Ashktorab, Magder, Pollin, McArdle, Shuldiner, and Schaffer.
164 Geri Clark, *Finland: Enchantment of the World* (North Mankato, MN: Scholastic, 2019), 25.
165 Tan Chung-Lee and Elizabeth Schmermund, *Finland* (New York: Cavendish Square, 2017), 19.
166 Ibid., 44.
167 James O'Sullivan, "Demystifying Finnish Dairy Food," *This Is Finland*, March 2015, accessed March 17, 2019, https://finland.fi/life-society/demystifying-finnish-dairy-food; "Countries Who Drink the Most Milk," *World Atlas*, 2019, accessed March 17, 2019, https://www.worldatlas.com/articles/countries-who-drink-the-most-milk.html.
168 Clark, 122.
169 "Fat to Fit: How Finland Did It," *The Guardian*, January 15, 2005, accessed March 17, 2019, https://www.theguardian.com/befit/story/0,15652,1385645,00.html; Gretel H. Pelto and Pertti J. Pelto, "Diet and Delocalization: Dietary Changes since 1750," *Journal of Interdisciplinary History* 14, no. 2 (Autumn 1983): 520.
170 Ancel Keys, *Seven Countries: A Multivariate Analysis of Death and Coronary Heart Disease* (Cambridge, MA and London: Harvard University Press, 1980), 317.
171 Ibid., 323.
172 Ashraf Soliman, Vincenzo De Sanctis, and Rania Elalaily, "Nutrition and Pubertal Development," *Indian Journal of Endocrinology and Metabolism* 18 (November 2014), https://www.ncbi.nlm.nih.gov/pmc/articles/PMC4266867.
173 "Poorer Girls over Twice as Likely to Start Period by 11," *Economic and Social Research Council*, October 12, 2016, accessed February 10, 2019, https://esrc.ukri.org/news-events-and-publications/news/news-items/poorer-girls-over-twice-as-likely-to-start-period-by-11.

174 Pelto and Pelto, 525.
175 Chung-Lee and Schmermund, 63.
176 Keys, 325–326.
177 Ibid., 321.
178 "Fat to Fit."
179 Ibid.
180 Chapter 2 discussed sodium as an electrolyte, constituent of bones, and contributor to high blood pressure. Chapter 5 indicated that English peers' longevity increased as sodium intake diminished.
181 Allison Van Dusen and Ana Patricia Ferrey, "World's Healthiest Countries," April 8, 2008, accessed March 18, 2019, https://www.forbes.com/2008/04/07/health-world-countries-forbeslife-cx_avd_0408health_slide.html?thisspeed=25000#168589b943c5.
182 "Fat to Fit."
183 Ibid.
184 Gordon F. Sander, "An Offer Finns Can't Refuse? Helsinki Woos Car Owners to Give up Their Autos," *Christian Science Monitor*, June 23, 2017, accessed March 17, 2019, https://www.csmonitor.com/World/Europe/2017/0623/An-offer-Finns-can-t-refuse-Helsinki-woos-car-owners-to-give-up-their-autos.
185 "The World: Life Expectancy (2018)," *geoba.se*, 2019, accessed January 26, 2019, http://www.geoba.se/population.php?pc=world&type=015&year=2018&st=country&asde=&page=1.
186 "Healthiest Countries 2019," *World Population Review*, accessed March 18, 2019, http://worldpopulationreview.com/countries/healthiest-countries.

8 Legumes

8.1 TERMINOLOGY AND DESCRIPTION

In the Fabaceae or Leguminosae family, legumes comprise roughly 650 genera and 18,000 species, several feeding humanity for millennia.[1] Their classification, popular and scientific, creates confusion. The public and American olericulturists Vincent Rubatzky and Mas Yamaguchi make vegetables an overbroad category by including legumes.[2] This book disagrees, considering them here and vegetables in Chapter 15. Chapter 12 notes that some agronomists call legumes that feed humans "grain legumes."[3] This expression emphasizes that people eat the seeds rather than other plant parts, useful information given that livestock eat legumes like alfalfa (*Medicago sativa*) and clover (*Trifolium species*), which this book omits, in their entirety. Yet the adjective "grain" risks conflating legumes and cereal grains, which Chapter 12 treats.

Also prevalent is the tendency to designate seed legumes "pulses," though the American Pulse Association, Pulse Canada, and USA Dry Pea and Lentil Council define only dried legume seeds as such.[4] These organizations exclude fresh seeds, peanuts (*Arachis hypogaea*), and soybeans (*Glycine max*). This parsing is pointless because all are legumes with similar, though nonidentical, nutrients. For example, peanuts and soybeans have more fat and calories than beans (*Phaseolus vulgaris, P. lunatus, P. acutifolius, and P. coccineus*) and peas (*Pisum sativum*).

American historian Ken Albala (b. 1964) grouped all seed legumes under the term "bean," language that aligns with chickpeas' designation as garbanzo beans.[5] But such terminology blurs the ancient tendency to separate peas and beans. For example, in the second century BCE, Roman statesman and agriculturist Cato the Elder (234–149 BCE) differentiated broad beans (*Vicia faba*), also known as fava or faba beans, from chickpeas (*Cicer arietinum*).[6] Between the first century BCE and the fourth century CE, Roman scholar Marcus Terentius Varro (116–27 BCE), Roman soldier and agriculturist Lucius Junius Moderatus Columella (4–70 CE), Roman naturalist Pliny the Elder (23–79), and Roman agricultural writer Rutilius Taurus Aemilianus Palladius were not content to designate all edible legumes as beans, distinguishing among peas, lentils (*Lens culinaris*), chickpeas, lupines (*Lupinus* species), and broad beans.

The difference between pea and bean, if one must be specified, is partly linguistic because people have long used the term "pea" to mean the garden pea—or the pea, chickpea, and cowpea (*Vigna unguiculata*)—whereas the name "bean" is broadly applied to many legumes. Another difference concerns preparation. Peas may be eaten uncooked, but beans should be soaked in water and boiled to make them palatable. Although the seed is the unit of consumption, people eat seeds and pods as green beans or snap peas.

Egyptians and Romans observed that legumes improved soil fertility without understanding why. In 1886, German chemists Hermann Hellriegel (1831–1895) and Hermann Wilfarth (1853–1904) supplied the answer by describing nitrogen fixation.[7] *Rhizobium* bacteria and legumes interact symbiotically. The bacteria infect legume root filaments, known as hairs, forming nodules. Nodules shelter these bacteria, which convert the soil's nitrogen gas (N_2) into ammonium cations (NH_4^+). Plants, and in turn herbivores and omnivores, depend on this transformation because roots cannot absorb nitrogen gas but can take up ions as nourishment. Ammonium benefits not only legumes. Unabsorbed surplus remains available for next year's crops.

No chapter can discuss all legumes that sustain humankind. Our efforts focus on four genera—*Phaseolus*, *Arachis*, *Glycine*, and *Pisum*—that have nourished people since prehistory. Being 20–40 percent protein by weight, legumes fed the poor with little access to meat, fish, poultry, eggs, or dairy.[8] Beans nourished North and South America, spreading throughout the Old World after

1500 CE. Peas helped fuel the Neolithic Revolution in southwestern Asia, dispersing worldwide during prehistory and history. Peanuts contribute to American, African, and Asian diets. A Chinese domesticate, soybeans feed the world's peoples and livestock. Many items have soybean oil or protein as an additive.

8.2 CALORIES, NUTRIENTS, AND HEALTH

8.2.1 Nutrient Density

"Of all the foods, legumes most adequately meet the recommended dietary guidelines for healthy eating," wrote New Zealand nutritionist Bernard Venn.[9] "They are high in carbohydrates and dietary fiber, mostly low in fat, and supply adequate protein while being a good source of minerals and vitamins, although lacking in vitamin B_{12}." Chapter 13 amasses evidence that potatoes (*Solanum tuberosum*) rather than legumes are most nutritious, though his opinion is germane to our investigation here.

8.2.2 Peanuts' Nutrients

Of this chapter's legumes, raw peanuts have the most calories at 567 per 100 grams.[10] Most come from the 49.24 grams of fat per 100 grams of dry-roasted peanuts. At 9.4 calories per gram of fat (see Chapter 2), peanuts' 49.24 grams of fat in 100 grams total supply 462.86 of 567 calories as lipids. Of total fat per 100 grams, 6.9 grams are saturated. The rest are monounsaturated and polyunsaturated in roughly a 5:3 ratio. The 104.14 calories not from fat are carbohydrates; 8.5 grams per 100 grams of raw peanuts are fiber, cannot be digested (see Chapter 2), and supply few calories. Table 8.1 lists calories and nutrients in peanuts, peas, soybeans, and green beans.[11]

This book does not demonize calories. The issues are whether calories exceed, balance, or trail requirements and whether foods have empty energy, as with processed junk, or many nutrients. Table 8.1 shows that peanuts occupy the second category, with 100 grams having 25.8 grams of protein, 96.5 percent of the U.S. Food and Drug Administration's (FDA) daily value (DV) for manganese, 57 percent for copper, 42 percent for magnesium, 25.4 percent for iron, 21.8 percent for zinc, 20.1 percent for potassium, 60.4 percent for vitamin B_3 (niacin or nicotinic acid), 60 percent for vitamin B_9 (folate, folic acid, or pteroylmonoglutamic acid), 55.5 percent for vitamin E, and 42.6 percent for vitamin B_1 (thiamine or thiamin).[12]

Referencing Chapter 4's Table 4.1 and Chapter 5's Table 5.3, peanuts have more protein at 25.8 grams per 100 grams total than wild salmon (*Oncorhynchus* species) at 19.84 grams, wild catfish at 16.38 grams, farm catfish at 15.23 grams, and bison (*Bison bonasus* and *B. bison*) at 20.23 per 100 grams total but less than beef, pork, mutton, goat, and venison at 36.1, 27.8, 33.43, 27.1, and 36.08 grams, respectively.[13] By mass, peanuts have more vitamin E than salmon, trout (species in genera *Oncorhynchus*, *Salmo*, and *Salvelinus*), avocados (*Persea americana*), red peppers (*Capsicum annuum*), Brazil nuts (*Bertholletia excelsa*), turnip greens (*Brassica rapa ssp. rapa*), and mangos (*Mangifera indica*), and more manganese than sunflower seeds (*Helianthus annuus*), cashews (*Anacardium occidentale*), almonds (*Amygdalus communis*), potatoes, onions (*Allium cepa*), bananas (*Musa x paradisiaca*), and carrots (*Daucus carota ssp. sativus*).[14]

8.2.3 *Phaseolus* Beans' Calories and Fat

Peanuts are just one of several nourishing legumes. Readers concerned about fat intake may appreciate that *Phaseolus* beans have little. Table 8.2 shows that 100 grams (half a cup) of red kidney, pink, great northern, and cranberry beans have 0.4 grams of fat.[15] The same quantity of black beans has 0.5 grams of fat and of navy and pinto beans 0.6 grams. This dearth translates into few calories, with a range between 104 for 100 grams of great northern and 127 for an equal amount of navy beans.

TABLE 8.1
Nutrients in Legumes 100 g

Nutrient	Peanut	%DV	Green Bean	%DV	Pea	%DV	Raw Soybean	%DV
Calories	567	N/A	31	N/A	81	N/A	416	N/A
Protein (g)	25.8	N/A	1.83	N/A	5.42	N/A	36.49	N/A
Fat (g)	49.24	N/A	0.22	N/A	0.4	N/A	19.94	N/A
Carbs (g)	16.13	N/A	6.97	N/A	14.45	N/A	30.16	N/A
Fiber (g)	8.5	N/A	2.7	N/A	5.7	N/A	4.96	N/A
Minerals								
Ca (mg)	92	9.2	37	3.7	25	2.5	277	27.7
Fe (mg)	4.58	25.4	1.03	5.7	1.47	8.2	15.7	87.2
Mg (mg)	168	42	25	6.3	33	8.3	280	70
P (mg)	37.6	3.8	38	3.8	108	10.8	704	70.4
K (mg)	705	20.1	211	6	244	7	1,797	51.3
Na (mg)	18	0.75	6	0.3	5	0.2	2	0.08
Zn (mg)	3.27	21.8	0.24	1.6	1.24	8.3	4.89	32.6
Cu (mg)	1.14	57	0.07	3.5	0.18	9	1.66	83
Mn (mg)	1.93	96.5	0.29	14.5	0.41	20.5	2.52	126
Se (mcg)	7.2	10.3	0.6	0.9	1.8	2.6	17.8	25.4
Vitamins								
A (IU)	0	0	700	14	765	15.3	24	0.5
B_1 (mg)	0.64	42.6	0.08	5.3	0.27	18	0.87	58
B_2 (mg)	0.14	8.2	0.1	5.9	0.13	7.6	0.87	51.2
B_3 (mg)	12.07	60.4	0.73	3.7	2.09	10.5	1.62	8.1
B_5 (mg)	1.77	17.7	0.07	0.7	0.1	1	0.79	7.9
B_6 (mg)	0.35	17.5	0.14	7	0.17	8.5	0.38	19
B_9 (mcg)	240	60	33	8.3	65	16.3	375.1	93.8
B_{12} (mcg)	0	0	0	0	0	0	0	0
C (mg)	0	0	12.2	20.3	40	66.7	6	10
D (IU)	0	0	0	0	0	0	0	0
E (mg)	8.33	55.5	0.41	2.7	0.13	0.9	0.85	5.7
K (mcg)	0	0	43	53.8	24.8	31	47	58.9

TABLE 8.2
Calories and fat in *Phaseolus vulgaris* 100 g

Bean	Calories	Fat (g)
Black	114	0.5
Cranberry	120	0.4
Great Northern	104	0.4
Navy	127	0.6
Pink	126	0.4
Pinto	122	0.6
Red Kidney	112	0.4

8.2.4 Soybeans' Nutrients

The next section discusses peas, though soybeans' aliment is considered here. Their preparation—to which a U.S. Department of Agriculture (USDA) handbook devoted twenty-three pages—affects calories and nutrients.[16] Rather than treat all, this section examines roasted soybeans, tofu, soy sauce, and *tempeh* given their antiquity, popularity, and nutriment. Additionally, tofu deserves attention because it is eaten "everywhere" in China, the world's most populous country.[17]

Roasted soybeans may be the oldest preparation and appear to have sustained China's poor during famines since at least the first century CE. Tradition credited Chinese nobleman and alchemist Liu An (179–122 BCE) with inventing tofu or soybean curd, though scholars doubt this claim.[18] American anthropologist Christine M. Du Bois (b. 1962) suspected that tofu arose serendipitously when someone seasoned soybean porridge or gruel with sea salt, whose magnesium chloride ($MgCl_2$) solidified soy proteins.[19] This process resembles cheesemaking, which Chapter 7 described. American anthropologist Sidney Wilfred Mintz (1922–2015) characterized soy sauce as "the most widespread fermented legume product on earth."[20] Being a microbial process, fermentation required bacteria, fungi, mold, or their combination. Preferences dictated addition of ingredients like grain and brine. Wheat (*Triticum monococcum, T. dicoccon, T. aestivum*, and *T. durum*) was popular because it complemented soybeans as a northern Chinese crop. After fermentation, compression of the mixture yielded the liquid known as soy sauce. Indonesians may have invented *tempeh* or *tempe* around 1000 CE, though no text mentioned it before the eighteenth century.[21] The mold *Rhizopus oligosporus* ferments soaked, cooked beans into *tempeh*, a savory cake with meaty texture and flavor.

Table 8.3 tabulates calories and nutrients in 100 grams of roasted soybeans, tofu, soy sauce, and *tempeh*. *Tempeh*'s 14 percent of DV for vitamin B_{12} (cobalamin) is noteworthy because few plant foods supply it.

8.2.5 Legumes' Non-Nutrients

Despite legumes' nutriment, they may have been comparatively late additions to diets. American botanist Lawrence Kaplan (1926–2018) asserted that hunter-gatherers first targeted tubers, roots, leaves, insects, and game.[22] Only later did they turn to seeds like legumes and grains. Many legumes would have been unappealing raw given toxins and chemicals—such as phytic acid discussed elsewhere—that retard nutrient absorption. Peas, however, are free from this hazard. Fire's control and use for cooking (see Chapter 3) destroyed many of these substances, permitting legumes' consumption. Once in the food supply, they grew to dominate diets such that humans use more Fabaceae species than those in any other family.[23] For example, people worldwide eat more soybeans, discussed later, than any other plant, doubtless because countless foods contain soy protein or oil.[24] American journalist and food writer Michael Kevin Pollan (b. 1955) estimated that two-thirds of processed items have one or both.[25]

8.2.6 Legumes as Inexpensive Protein

Since domestication, legumes have given commoners inexpensive protein.[26] Their value since antiquity (c. 3000 BCE–c. 500 CE) is difficult to overstate for people who ate them at nearly every meal.[27] The previous section noted that they may be up to 40 percent protein by mass, but the body cannot absorb it as well as animal protein. Legume protein is better assimilated when combined with whole grains, meat, fish, poultry, eggs, or dairy. Beans, however, are seldom consumed with animal products because of separate trajectories. As early as 1930, the U.S. Census Bureau documented an inverse correlation between bean consumption and income.[28] The poor eat beans whereas the affluent eat meat and kindred foods. This reality affirms Chapter 4's remark that meat has long signaled privilege.

TABLE 8.3
Nutrients in Soy Foods 100 g

Nutrient	Roasted Soybeans	%DV	Tofu	%DV	Soy Sauce	%DV	Tempeh	%DV
Calories	471	N/A	76	N/A	53	N/A	199	N/A
Protein (g)	35.2	N/A	8	N/A	5.2	N/A	19	N/A
Fat (g)	25.4	N/A	4.8	N/A	0.1	N/A	7.68	N/A
Carbs (g)	33.6	N/A	1.9	N/A	8.5	N/A	17.03	N/A
Fiber (g)	4.6	N/A	0.08	N/A	0	N/A	1.4	N/A
			Minerals					
Ca (mg)	138	13.8	105	10.5	17	1.7	93	9.3
Fe (mg)	3.9	21.7	5.36	29.8	2.02	11.2	2.26	12.6
Mg (mg)	145	33.6	103	25.8	34	8.5	70	17.5
P (mg)	363	36.3	97	9.7	110	11	206	20.6
K (mg)	1,470	42	121	3.5	180	5.1	367	10.5
Na (mg)	163	6.8	7	0.3	5,715	238.1	6	0.3
Zn (mg)	3.14	20.9	0.8	5.3	0.37	2.5	1.81	12.1
Cu (mg)	0.83	41.4	0.19	9.5	0.12	5.8	0.67	33.5
Mn (mg)	2.16	108	0.61	30.5	1.02	60	1.43	71.5
Se (mcg)	19.3	27.6	8.9	12.7	0.5	0.7	0	0
			Vitamins					
A (IU)	200	4	85	1.7	0	0	686	13.7
B_1 (mg)	0.1	6.7	0.08	5.4	0.05	3.3	0.13	8.7
B_2 (mg)	0.15	8.5	0.05	2.9	0.13	7.6	0.11	6.5
B_3 (mg)	1.41	7	0.2	1	3.36	16.8	4.63	23.2
B_5 (mg)	0.45	4.5	0.07	0.7	0.32	3.2	0.36	3.6
B_6 (mg)	0.21	10.4	0.01	0.5	0.17	8.5	0.3	15
B_9 (mcg)	211	52.8	15	3.8	15.5	3.9	52	13
B_{12} (mcg)	0	0	0	0	0	0	0.84	14
C (mg)	2.2	3.7	0.1	0.2	0	0	0	0
D (IU)	0	0	0	0	0	0	0	0
E (mg)	N/A	N/A	0.01	0.07	0	0	N/A	N/A
K (mcg)	37	46.3	2.4	3	0	0	N/A	N/A

8.2.7 Legumes and Mortality

Returning to Venn's judgment, a 2004 paper documented an 8 percent decline in mortality among Japanese, Swede, Greek, and European-Australian septuagenarians for every 20 grams (0.7 ounces) of legumes eaten daily.[29] No other food matched this improvement, though fish and shellfish and a high ratio of unsaturated to saturated fat also lessened mortality. Among legumes, the authors cited *Phaseolus* beans, peas, chickpeas, lentils, and soybeans as whole beans, tofu, natto, and miso. Like *tempeh* and soy sauce already mentioned, natto and miso are fermented.

8.3 EASTERN HEMISPHERE ORIGINS

8.3.1 *Pisum sativum*

Most scholars believe that farming and livestock raising arose first in southwestern Asia. Prehistorians have focused on grains, though this region also appears to have pioneered legume cultivation. Between about 7000 and 3000 BCE, farmers there domesticated peas, chickpeas, lentils, and broad beans.[30] All have fed humans, though among the four, this chapter treats just peas in the conviction that they are a world food whereas the others are regional items. Attention on southwestern Asia should not obscure the possibility that pea farming and consumption may have originated in India, Myanmar, or Thailand. Interesting is evidence of 11,000-year-old peas on the border between what are today Myanmar and Thailand.[31] This find proves consumption even if peas were not domesticated then.

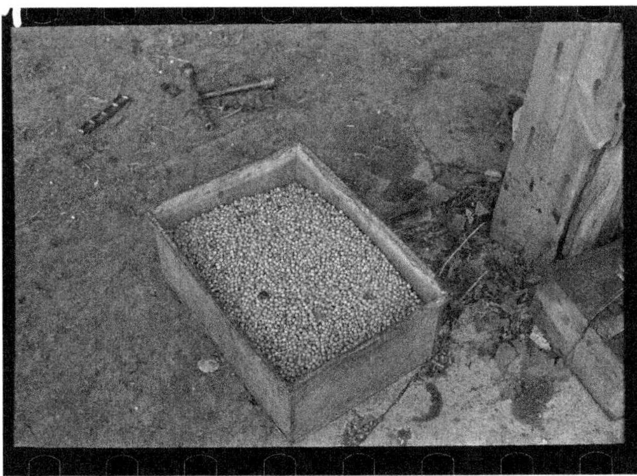

FIGURE 8.1 Peas. (Photo courtesy of Library of Congress. https://www.loc.gov/pictures/item/2017735605/.)

From southwestern Asia, peas traveled south to Egypt's Nile delta around 4500 BCE, moving south along the river through Upper Egypt during the next millennium. Chapter 4 described Egypt's geography, climate, and early history. Peas may have attracted notice there because they mature rapidly and tolerate aridity. From southwestern Asia, peas moved north into Georgia in the fifth millennium BCE and east into Afghanistan, Pakistan, and northern India—assuming origin in southwestern Asia and not India—by 2000 BCE. During the second millennium BCE, peas migrated south through India. They entered Eastern Europe from Georgia by 2000 BCE, and during prehistory spread south into Greece, west into Switzerland and France, and northwest into Britain. Northern Europe's cool climate suited the legume. Quick maturation permitted biannual crops, one in spring and another in autumn.

Because peas are nearly 80 percent water, what could not be eaten fresh was dried to prevent deterioration.[32] Once dried, peas fortified soups and stews. The rhyme "pease porridge hot, pease porridge cold, pease porridge in the pot nine days old," possibly dating to the high (c. 1000–c. 1300 CE) or late (c. 1300–c. 1500) Middle Ages, suggests that people ate the legume day after day.[33] Such monotony was unlikely voluntary but instead reflected meat's expensiveness. Peas and other legumes—dubbed "poor man's protein" or "poor man's meat"—permitted survival despite infrequent access to animal products.[34] Peas' protein sustained medieval commoners, most of whom "never tasted meat," wrote American Egyptologist Robert Brier (b. 1943) and American philosopher A. Hoyt Hobbs.[35] This dependence intensified when grains were unavailable or expensive.[36] In this vein, Kaplan stated that the legume was "food of primary importance for the European peasantry of the Middle Ages."[37] By the eleventh century, for example, Britons ate chiefly peas.[38]

Between roughly 500 and 1500 CE, the Middle Ages spanned too vast a period for easy evaluation of health. The Black Death (1347–1351)—which killed around one-third of Europeans—and the macabre art and literature that followed it enshrouded the era in gloom, making tempting the assertion that Europe was an unhealthy place.[39] Chapter 3 listed the long series of recurrent famines before and after this catastrophe, heightening the perception that deprivation, disease, and death haunted the Middle Ages.

Military records, revealing a mean stature of 173.4 centimeters (68.3 inches) for northern European men between roughly 800 and 1300, challenge this negativity.[40] This average surpassed mean heights, discussed in Chapter 4, of nineteenth-century Assiniboine, Blackfoot, Comanche, Kiowa, and Sioux men on the Great Plains.[41] Only Arapaho, Cheyenne, and Crow males stood taller in the nineteenth century, and these peoples were the world's tallest.[42] Crow men stood just 2 millimeters above those from medieval northern Europe, a trivial difference. Because nutrition and height correlate, as noted throughout this book, medieval northern Europeans were well nourished on peas even without meat and grains.

Peas were not the lone advantage. Food supply expanded as agriculture benefited from a warm climate between about 800 and 1300.[43] Warmth lengthened the growing season three or four weeks yearly. This interval's end corresponded with the tallest Europeans. In addition to farm productivity, medieval Europe's population, at least in the countryside, was sparse enough to reduce infectious diseases. Economic backwardness and meager trade further isolated Europe from contagion.[44] After 1300, the climate cooled, agriculture shrank, cod (*Gadus morhua* and *G. macrocephalus*) migrated to warmer waters, and European stature diminished.[45] These changes precipitated famines and the Black Death.

Besides the underclass, peas fed elites. Rome's wealthy Piso family took its name from peas, declaring that its ancestors had been pea farmers who embodied the rural virtues of thrift, diligence, piety, and self-reliance.[46] Gourmet Marcus Gavius Apicius (c. 25 BCE–c. 37 CE) was among several Romans who devised high-end pea recipes.[47] Medieval cookbooks expanded this focus to create dishes of peas, almonds, and spices.

In the eighth century, Frankish King Charlemagne (742–814), enjoying fresh peas, ordered peasants to plant them for his armies as they marched through the empire.[48] Scandinavians ate peas and pork. Peas soup, known as *aertsoppa* in Sweden, *gula aerter* in Denmark, *harnekeitto* in Finland, and *arwtensoap* in the Netherlands, nourished northern Europeans.[49] Sweden's nobility, including King Eric XIV (1533–1577), favored it. Fondness for peas doomed the king, whose brother killed him by putting arsenic in his soup. In Florence, Italy, the wealthy Medicis ate fresh peas. In 1533, Catherine de Medici (1519–1589), having married French King Henry II (1519–1559), brought new pea varieties to France.[50] They must not have made converts because in 1695 King Louis XIV (1638–1715) had to be persuaded to sample them.[51] Delighted with the flavor, he commanded his gardener to plant them in royal greenhouses. Unlike beans, therefore, peas dodged being stigmatized as ordinary.

From their Asian origins, Italian-Spanish mariner Christopher Columbus (1451–1506) in 1493 planted peas on Caribbean island Hispaniola, now Haiti and the Dominican Republic.[52] Sixteenth-century Spain introduced peas to Mexico and Florida. In 1608, one year after the colony's founding, the English brought peas to Jamestown, Virginia. In 1629, probably in a separate introduction, the Massachusetts Bay Colony began growing them. In the 1670s, food shortages in the Carolinas reduced each colonist to subsisting daily on half a liter (one pint) of peas.[53] The ration prevented starvation, implying that the legume preserved health. Third U.S. President Thomas Jefferson (1743–1826) declared peas his favorite vegetable—Chapter 15 defines vegetables—cultivating them as early as 1767 at Monticello. Planting thirty varieties, he competed with neighbors to harvest the earliest peas.

Some seventeenth century Americans ate peas thrice daily. First Lady Martha Dandridge Custis Washington's (1731–1802) *Booke of Cookery*, which circulated in manuscript, included recipes for pease porridge and pea soup with mint (*Mentha* species). American author Amelia Simmons' *American Cookery* (1796) advised bakers to substitute peas for apples (*Malus domestica*) and other fruits in pies. *The Virginia Housewife: Or Methodical Cook* (1824) recommended that peas be cooked with butter and mint (*Mentha* species) and detailed recipes for pea soup with celery (*Apium graveolens*) and pease pudding with pork. In 1841, American author and editor Sarah Josepha Hale's (1788–1879) *The Good Housekeeper* recommended soups of peas and spinach (*Spinacia oleracea*) or lettuce (*Lactuca sativa*). New Englanders ate peas with corned beef, thyme (*Thymus vulgaris*), and marjoram (*Origanum majorana* and *O. onites*). Cooks used pearl ash to soften old peas.

Today the French eat peas with lettuce, onions, and butter.[54] Cooks add peas to stir-fries and Thai curries, often combining them with shrimp (species in the infraorder Caridea). Spaniards consume peas, meat, and baked eggs. The Portuguese prefer peas with eggs. Iranians enjoy peas with lamb (*Ovis aries*). Germans make stew with peas, bacon, carrots, and celery. Pea soups are popular in Denmark, the Netherlands, and the United States besides Sweden. Peruvians eat peas and shrimp stew. Brazilians pair peas with chicken (*Gallus gallus domesticus*). Indians combine the legume with potatoes or paneer cheese. Like peanuts in the United States, roasted, salted peas are a snack in Japan, China, Taiwan, Thailand, and Malaysia. Pea leaves are a Chinese delicacy. Greeks and Turks, including those on Mediterranean island Cyprus, enjoy pea, meat, and potato stew.

Although one anecdote may not warrant extrapolation, in 1999, American journalist and food writer Raymond Sokolov (b. 1941) recounted an attempt to lose weight by eating only peas, drinking coffee (*Coffea* species) and diet sodas, and ingesting vitamin and mineral tablets.[55] With few calories, little fat, and no cholesterol, peas satisfied his criteria for wholesomeness. Sokolov calculated that a daily allocation of 1.1 kilograms (2.5 pounds) provided just 882 calories, a value near the USDA computation of 891 calories.[56] Table 8.4 tabulates this spartan fare's calories and nutrients.[57]

TABLE 8.4
Nutrients in Peas 1.1 kg

Nutrient	Peas	%DV
Calories	891	N/A
Protein (g)	59.6	N/A
Fat (g)	4.4	N/A
Carbs (g)	158.95	N/A
Fiber (g)	62.7	N/A
	Minerals	
Ca (mg)	275	27.5
Fe (mg)	16.2	90
Mg (mg)	363	91
P (mg)	1,188	297
K (mg)	2,684	77
Na (mg)	55	2.3
Zn (mg)	13.6	91
Cu (mg)	1.9	95
Mn (mg)	4.5	225
Se (mcg)	19.8	28
	Vitamins	
A (IU)	8,415	168.3
B_1 (mg)	2.9	193.3
B_2 (mg)	1.5	88
B_3 (mg)	23	115
B_5 (mg)	1.1	11
B_6 (mg)	1.9	95
B_9 (mcg)	715	178.9
B_{12} (mcg)	0	0
C (mg)	440	733.3
D (IU)	0	0
E (mg)	1.43	10
K (mcg)	272.8	341

TABLE 8.5
Nutrients in Peas 141.6 g

Nutrient	Peas	%DV
Calories	114	N/A
Protein (g)	7.7	N/A
Fat (g)	0.57	N/A
Carbs (g)	20.46	N/A
Fiber (g)	8.07	N/A
	Minerals	
Ca (mg)	35.4	3.5
Fe (mg)	2.08	11.6
Mg (mg)	46.73	11.7
P (mg)	152.93	15.3
K (mg)	345.5	9.9
Na (mg)	7.08	0.3
Zn (mg)	1.76	11.7
Cu (mg)	0.25	12.7
Mn (mg)	0.58	29
Se (mcg)	2.55	3.6
	Vitamins	
A (IU)	1,083.24	21.7
B_1 (mg)	0.38	25.5
B_2 (mg)	0.18	10.8
B_3 (mg)	2.96	14.8
B_5 (mg)	0.14	1.4
B_6 (mg)	0.24	12
B_9 (mcg)	92.04	23
B_{12} (mcg)	0	0
C (mg)	56.64	94.4
D (IU)	0	0
E (mg)	0.18	1.2
K (mcg)	35.12	43.9

Combined with coffee's caffeine, Sokolov claimed enough nourishment and pep from peas for an hour's vigorous workout each day.

This regimen recalls Carolina colonists' subsistence on half a liter of peas per day. Making the appropriate conversions, this volume of peas has a mass of 141.6 grams, or just 12.9 percent of Sokolov's ration.[58] Reducing energy and nutrients accordingly, each colonist had only 114 calories and 7.7 grams of protein daily. Table 8.5 summarizes this quantity's calories and nutrients. Absence of deaths from starvation suggests that this austerity was brief and that colonists supplemented peas with whatever could be hunted or collected, though American food writer Meredith Sayles Hughes asserted that they ate little beyond peas.[59]

Sokolov's confession that the "pea diet is barbarous" implies preference for an alternative.[60] Had he substituted 1.1 kilograms of McDonald's hamburger for peas, Table 8.6 shows that Sokolov would have consumed 2,904 calories; 142 grams of protein; 111 grams of fat; 14.3 grams of fiber; over the DV for calcium, iron, phosphorus, zinc, and vitamins B_1, B_2, B_3, and B_{12}; 60 percent for potassium; 58 percent for magnesium; and 11 percent for vitamin C.[61] The burger would have more than tripled peas' calories while supplying less magnesium, phosphorus, potassium, and vitamins

TABLE 8.6
Nutrients in McDonald's Hamburger 1.1 kg

Nutrient	McDonald's Hamburger	%DV
Calories	2,904	N/A
Protein (g)	142	N/A
Fat (g)	111	N/A
Carbs (g)	333.08	N/A
Fiber (g)	14.3	N/A
	Minerals	
Ca (mg)	1,397	139.7
Fe (mg)	31.57	175.4
Mg (mg)	231	58
P (mg)	1,177	117.7
K (mg)	2,112	60
Na (mg)	5,434	226.4
Zn (mg)	21.45	143
Mn (mg)	3.54	177.1
Se (mcg)	288.2	411.7
	Vitamins	
A (IU)	605	121
B_1 (mg)	2.72	181.1
B_2 (mg)	2.63	154.6
B_3 (mg)	49.98	249.9
B_5 (mg)	N/A	N/A
B_6 (mg)	N/A	N/A
B_9 (mcg)	704	176
B_{12} (mcg)	9.13	152.2
C (mg)	6.6	11
D (IU)	N/A	N/A
E (mg)	N/A	N/A
K (mcg)	N/A	N/A

B_1 and C. By mass, peas have over sixty-six times more vitamin C than the burger. Despite peas' merits, Sokolov's language demonstrates the folly of ignoring palatability and variety. Anything eaten to the exclusion of all else provokes backlash. Chapter 13 emphasizes that if one food must be favored, the potato supplies the most nutrients per unit mass. The tuber aside, this chapter lauds peas for furnishing ample nutriment at a fraction of convenience foods' calories.

8.3.2 *Glycine max*

Asia's vastness is evident in the many kilometers between peas in the southwest and soybeans in northern China. Millennia separated peas' entrance into diets at least 11,000 years ago and soybeans' domestication around 2800 BCE.[62] From the outset, soybeans—"the meat without bones"—added protein to plant diets.[63] American agronomist Theodore Hymowitz (b. 1934) remarked that the legume "has been the cornerstone of east Asian nutrition" for centuries.[64] Early evidence of health comes from Manchuria, an area in northeastern China where these beans have a long history.[65] During prehistory and antiquity, lands between Manchuria's Liao and Heilongjiang rivers produced most of the world's crop.[66]

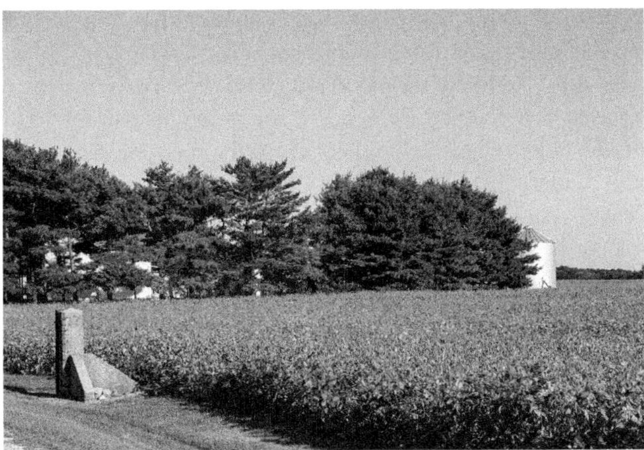

FIGURE 8.2 Soybeans. (Photo courtesy of Library of Congress. https://www.loc.gov/pictures/item/2016631548/.)

Five tombs in central Manchuria's Jilin province date about 3000 BCE, around when soybeans were domesticated. Even if these burials predated domestication, consumption of wild beans is likely.[67] Fish, ox (*Bos taurus*), horse (*Equus caballus*), and dog (*Canis lupus familiaris*) bones indicate animal consumption, though Chapters 1 and 3 noted that such remains overstate reliance on fish and meat because bones persist longer than plant residues. Emphasis on a fish or meat diet does not square with the fact that calories and nutrients have long come mostly from plants in China, Korea to Manchuria's south, and Japan to the east.[68] Moreover, oxen, horses, and dogs, needed for work, may not have been eaten.

Returning to the burials, two of the five graves had more than one person.[69] Of the eight deceased, four were assigned ages: eleven, sixteen, forty, and fifty-five years. Their mean, 30.5 years, implies a moderate lifespan by premodern standards. To be sure, four skeletons are too slender a thread to support weighty generalizations. Nonetheless, they align with American ecologist and limnologist Edward Smith Deevey Jr.'s (1914–1988) calculation, introduced in Chapter 3, that between Neanderthal prehistory and 1900 CE, e^0 seldom departed over five years either way of twenty-five years.[70] The four skeletons' mean age of death, if deemed approximations of e^0, occupied this range's ceiling.

Tradition credited first Chinese emperor Shen Nung, whose historicity is questionable, with listing soybeans among five "sacred foods" in the third millennium BCE.[71] The other four were barley, rice, millets (species in Eragrostideae tribe), and wheat. A fifth century BCE text deemed soybeans one of China's "five sacred grains," without which civilization could not exist.[72] The reference was probably not meant to conflate soybeans with cereals, only to identify seeds as the edibles. Inexplicably, the list totals seven crops: soybeans, wheat, barley, sesame (*Sesamum indicum*), millets, rice, and adzuki beans (*Vigna angularis*).

By 2207 BCE, soybeans were important enough to warrant discussion in an agronomy treatise.[73] This date approached some 800 burials between roughly 2000 and 1500 BCE in Liaoning, Manchuria.[74] This sample, larger than the first, allows greater confidence that e^0s are not anomalies. The mean age of demise was between twenty and thirty years, encompassing the first sample's e^0 and affirming Deevey.[75] Moreover, this range matches e^0s for Egyptian and Roman antiquity (c. 750 BCE–c. 500 CE) mentioned in Chapters 4 and 10.[76] Such agreement strengthens confidence that Liaoning and Jilin fit a pattern beyond East Asia and suggests that Manchurian foodstuffs, including soybeans, were on par with what fed the ancient Mediterranean as discussed in Chapters 4, 10, and 15. Under 10 percent of Liaoning's interred died in life's sixth decade, approximating Europe's mortality into the Middle Ages, noted in Chapters 1 and 3, and with French anthropologist and paleontologist Henri Victor Vallois's (1889–1981) judgment in Chapter 3 that "few individuals passed forty years, and it is only quite exceptionally that any passed fifty."[77]

During the Shang (c. 1600–1046 BCE) and Zhou (1046–256 BCE) dynasties, soybeans spread throughout China. An eleventh century BCE poem recommended boiling soybeans before consumption. The ancients ate beans whole and did not crush them for oil. Another poem endorsed soybean leaves as food and fodder. Texts attributed to Chinese philosopher Confucius (551–479 BCE) restricted the big five to soybeans, wheat, sorghum (*Sorghum bicolor*), foxtail millet (*Setaria italica*), and hemp (*Cannabis sativa*). Another list whose attribution is contested retained the Confucian crops except for hemp, which yielded to rice. Chinese farmers aimed to plant 2 hectares (5 acres) of soybeans for each household member.[78]

From China, soybeans migrated to Korea no later the first century CE.[79] Land and oceanic trade took the legume to Japan, Indonesia, the Philippines, Vietnam, Thailand, Malaysia, Myanmar, Nepal, and India between the first and sixteenth centuries.[80] Bangladeshis ate beans roasted and in biscuits and fed them to chickens, importing meal from India and, in the twentieth century, oil from South America. Before then, soybeans were part of East, South, and Southeast Asian foodways. Paralleling combinations of beans and corn in the Americas and beans and rice in Africa and the Americas, both discussed in the next section, Asians paired soybeans with rice, thereby improving nutrition.

The legume's healthfulness in Japan and Korea is unclear. Japanese consumption of soybeans in soup and as soy sauce appears to have increased between the seventeenth and mid-nineteenth centuries to judge from the large number of recipes then; e^0 began to rise, however, only between the 1870s and 1890s.[81] Soybeans, at least as sauce and soup, cannot have caused this gain. South Korean ingestion of soybeans as soymilk has grown since the 1960s.[82] By 2008, South Koreans drank it between and during meals. Yet e^0 began to lengthen in the 1910s, half a century before soymilk's introduction.[83] Again, soybeans appear not to have influenced modern lifespan.

Seventeenth century Europe imported soy sauce from Indonesia and likely soybeans from South, Southeast, or East Asia. Tradition credited German physician and naturalist Englebert Kaempfer (1651–1716) in 1712 with giving Europe soybeans, which he must have identified while in India, Southeast Asia, and Japan between 1683 and 1693.[84] If he had acquired beans then, they would not have been viable in 1712, implying that he must have planted them on his 1693 return to Europe.

In 1737, Swedish naturalist Carl von Linne (1707–1778)—better known as Carolus Linnaeus—published the plant's description.[85] Two years later, missionaries in China sent soybeans to Paris, France's Jardin des Plantes, though farmers grew few before 1855.[86] In 1790, Britain's Royal Botanic Garden in Kew planted them.[87] In 1804, soybeans fed chickens and possibly people in what are today Bosnia and Herzegovina, Croatia, Macedonia, Montenegro, Serbia, and Slovenia. Europe's demand outstripped production by 1910, when Germany, Denmark, and the Netherlands began importing the legume from Manchuria. In 1934, Germany sought imports from Romania and Bulgaria. After World War II, soybeans came from the United States, Canada, Argentina, and Brazil. Europe has never been a large producer but into the twenty-first century continued to import soybeans.

Africa was a latecomer. In 1896, France planted soybeans in Algeria, then its principal North African colony. As this instance suggests, European colonists, usually French and British, promoted soybean foodways in Africa. These Europeans looked to China—including Manchuria—Korea, and Japan for oil-rich varieties to plant in Africa, whose harvest was meant for the mother country. In 1908, Nigeria and the next year Gambia and Ghana—all in West Africa—produced their first crop. Colonialism's collapse after World War II retarded efforts to grow soybeans in Africa. Only in 1981 did West Africa's Guinea-Bissau begin growing the legume. Cote d'Ivoire farmers complained of low yields. African smallholders completed poorly against U.S., Brazilian, and Argentinian agribusiness.

Previous paragraphs intimated North and South America's ascent as soybean producers. In 1765, British sailor Samuel Bowen gave soybeans to surveyor Henry Yonge, who planted them on his Georgia farm to make vermicelli (noodles) and soy sauce.[88] In 1769, Philadelphia, Pennsylvania's American Philosophical Society began advocating soybeans as crop and food. The next year American scientist, inventor, and statesman Benjamin Franklin (1706–1790), while in Britain, sent them to John Bartram (1699–1777), arguably America's most distinguished botanist then.[89] Bartram planted the beans in his garden near Philadelphia as a curiosity. By 1804, Pennsylvania had enough hectares to entice physician and amateur botanist James Mease (1771–1846) to tour farms in hopes of learning more about them.[90] In 1829, Cambridge, Massachusetts' botanical garden planted the legume.[91]

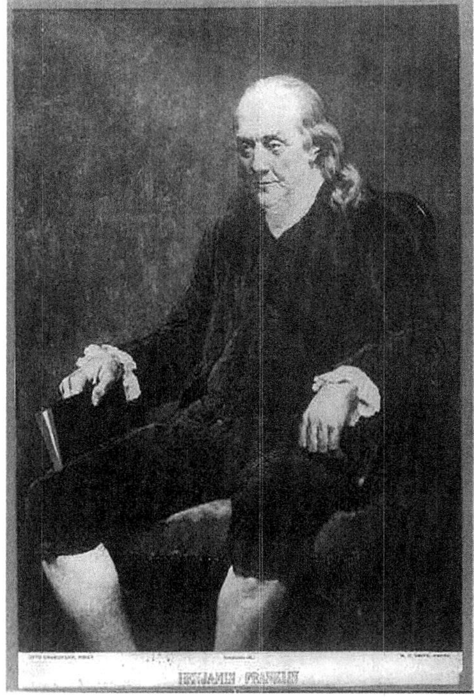

FIGURE 8.3 Benjamin Franklin. (Photo courtesy of Library of Congress. https://www.loc.gov/pictures/item/2004679607/.)

Scientific interest motivated these efforts, though around 1850 midwestern farmers began to grow soybeans as fodder. Illinois planted the legume in 1851, Iowa and Ohio in 1852, and the rest of the Midwest's corn belt in subsequent years.[92] To encourage cultivation, in 1854 the U.S. Patent Office began distributing free seeds to any farmer who requested them.[93] In 1873, missionaries in China collected the variety Mammoth Yellow, the first to be grown throughout the United States. It was especially popular in the South, though other varieties proved suitable in the North and West. In 1898, the USDA began collecting Asian varieties for introduction into the United States.[94] By 1931, the USDA had amassed 4,500 varieties from China—including Manchuria—Japan, Korea, Indonesia, and India.

Parallel to these efforts, Hellriegel and Wilfarth discovered how legumes increase usable nitrogen in soils, discussed earlier. Responding to this news, the Massachusetts Agricultural Experiment Station in Amherst urged soybeans' cultivation to improve soils.[95] In 1904 African American agricultural chemist George Washington Carver (1864–1943) planted soybeans at what is today Tuskegee University in Tuskegee, Alabama.[96] Satisfied with their protein and oil, he promoted them as food and fodder. In 1907, the USDA joined Carver in efforts to expand soybean agriculture.

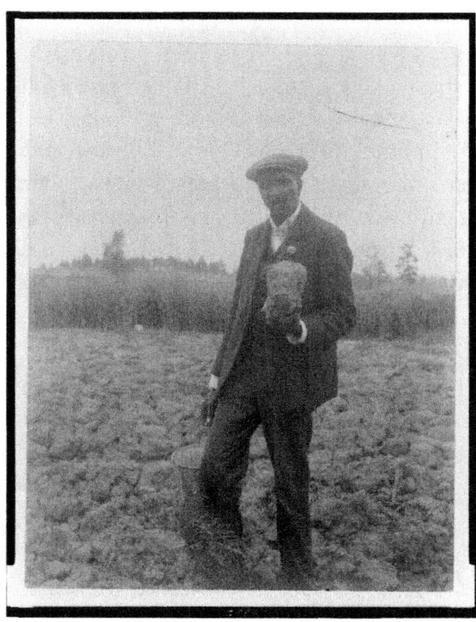

FIGURE 8.4 George Washington Carver. (Photo courtesy of Library of Congress. https://www.loc.gov/pictures/item/95507555/.)

A decade later American physician John Harvey Kellogg (1852–1943), a proponent of vegetarianism, championed soybeans as ideal for diabetics.[97] After 1921, he urged Americans to substitute tofu, soymilk, soy sauce, and soybean sprouts for meat as protein. Kellogg persuaded U.S. automaker Henry Ford (1863–1947) to grow the legume near his Michigan factories.[98] Ford ate soybeans, derived plastic from them for automobiles, and funded research on soy culinary and industrial uses.[99]

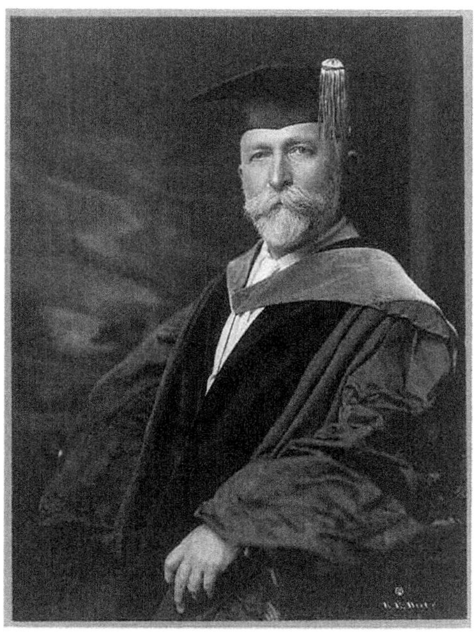

FIGURE 8.5 John Harvey Kellogg. (Photo courtesy of Library of Congress. https://www.loc.gov/pictures/item/2002715785/.)

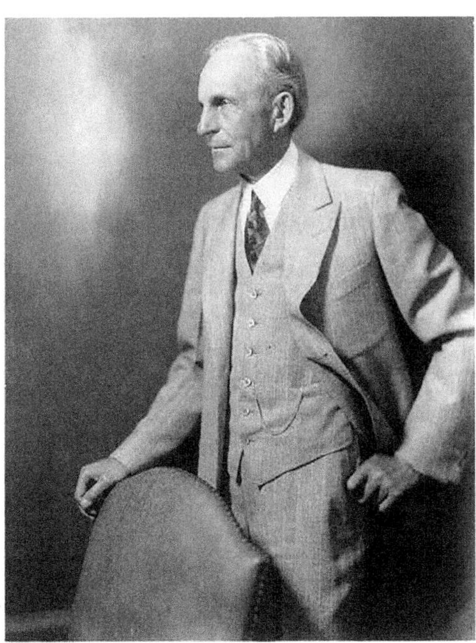

FIGURE 8.6 Henry Ford. (Photo courtesy of Library of Congress. https://www.loc.gov/pictures/item/2002706165/.)

Another factor, the boll weevil (*Anthonomus grandis*) crossed the Rio Grande north into the United States in 1892, devastating cotton.[100] The ensuing shortage of cottonseed oil prompted farmers to plant soybeans for oil.[101] As noted later, others switched from cotton to peanuts. After 1910, the tractor replaced horses, prompting transition from oats that had fed them to soybeans.[102] The 1930s' dust bowl revealed soybeans' greater drought tolerance than grain, leading farmers to plant them.[103] Moreover, Congress combatted the Great Depression (1929–1939) by paying farmers not to plant cotton and other crops that glutted the market. Because Congress did not extend this provision to soybeans, farmers abandoned cotton for them, collecting government payments and harvesting a crop that generated income on its own.[104]

As soybean hectarage rose, farmers learned that the legume complemented corn in rotation by restoring nitrogen that the grass depleted from soils.[105] Eager to encourage cultivation, U.S. and Canadian scientists bred 274 new soybean varieties between 1939 and 1988.[106] Before World War II, soybean plants fed livestock or were a cover crop. Afterward, interest in the whole plant declined as demand for oil led farmers to favor varieties with fatty seeds. Chapter 10 discusses soybean oil in evaluating fat's health effects. Summarizing these developments, Vincent Rubatzky and Mas Yamaguchi—mentioned earlier—asserted in 1997 that "as a major source of plant protein and edible oil, soybeans are without doubt the world's most important food legume."[107] Similarly, French author Maguelonne Toussaint-Samat (1926–2018) and American historian of science and medicine Lois N. Magner (b. 1943) described soybeans as the world's "most widely eaten plant."[108]

8.4 WESTERN HEMISPHERE ORIGINS

8.4.1 *Phaseolus vulgaris, P. lunatus, P. acutifolius,* and *P. coccineus*

English speakers typically call *Phaseolus vulgaris*' seeds "beans" and *Phaseolus lunatus*' seeds "lima beans," a tendency that stems from geography and familiarity. Sixteenth century Spaniards encountered beans in South America, distinguishing *P. lunatus*—domesticated about 8000 BCE—from other beans by naming lima beans after Peru's capital.[109] Having originated in Mexico and South America, *Phaseolus* beans were grown and eaten throughout the Americas before European contact. The Latin *vulgaris*, meaning "common," acknowledges these beans' ubiquity. Domestication occurred independently in Peru around 6000 BCE and in Mexico a millennium later.[110] Peruvians ate beans before they added corn to diets whereas Mexicans reversed this sequence.

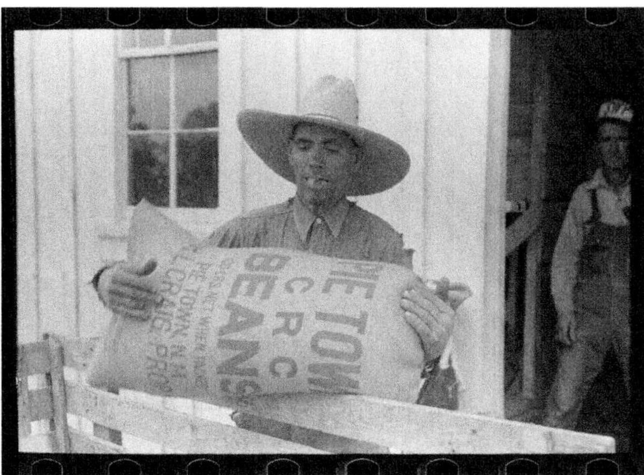

FIGURE 8.7 *Phaseolus vulgaris*. (Photo courtesy of Library of Congress. https://www.loc.gov/pictures/item/2017742359/.)

Mexican anthropologist Lourdes Marquez Morfin and colleagues identified bean eaters in two of five central Mexican societies between 1600 BCE and 1521 CE.[111] The earliest of the five and the first to grow beans, Tlatilco, existed from roughly 1600 BCE to 300 CE as a group of agricultural villages, each with a "few hundred inhabitants."[112] Excavations yielded almost 500 skeletons, 343 complete enough for inspection.[113] Their e^0, thirty-seven years, nearly doubled ancient Egypt's longevity—mentioned in Chapters 3 and 4—and surpassed Deevey's earlier estimate of thirty years as e^0's upper bound before roughly 1900 CE.[114] Table 8.7 lists e^0 in four precontact Mexican populations.

Onlookers might wonder whether Tlatilco's exceptional e^0 resulted from low birthrate, discussed in Chapter 1, which would likely have produced fewer aggregate infant deaths, thereby raising e^0 even if people were not especially healthy or well nourished. Yet Morfin and coauthors described the society as dynamic, with high fertility increasing population.[115] In this context, an e^0 of thirty-seven years is remarkable and may represent healthfulness. Alternatively, the skeletons may underreport Tlatilco's mortality. A population that does not bury dead newborns and infants, a problem discussed in Chapter 1, creates a cemetery that inflates e^0. Even when these dead are interred, their delicate bones tend to decay quicker than adult remains, again exaggerating e^0.

TABLE 8.7
E^0 in Precontact Mexico

Place	Time	E^0 (yr)
Tlatilco	c. 1600 BCE–c. 300 CE	37
Cuicuilco	c. 800–c. 600 BCE	40
Teotihuacan	c. 300 BCE–c. 1 CE	21
Cholula	c. 900 BCE–1521 CE	20

TABLE 8.8
Stature in Precontact Mesoamerica

Place	Time	Men (cm)	Women (cm)
Tehuacan	<c. 250 CE	167.2	158.5
Tlatilco	<c. 250 CE	162.8	153.8
Cuicuilco	<c. 250 CE	161.7	150.4
Teotihuacan	c. 250–c. 900 CE	166	153
Cholula	>c. 1520 CE	160.6	151.8
Tikal	<c. 250 CE	161.7	144.4
Yucatan	<c. 250 CE	164.4	151.2
Tikal	c. 250–c. 900 CE	155.2	148.5
Jaina	c. 250–c. 900 CE	160.6	151
Copan	c. 250–c. 900 CE	162.8	155.5
Yucatan	>c. 1520 CE	161.5	148.4

Another health index—the best according to Dutch historian Willem Marinus Jongman as quoted in Chapter 4—is stature. Table 8.8 shows that of ten Mexican societies, Tlatilco's women were third tallest at a mean 153.8 centimeters (60.6 inches).[116] Its men tied for fourth at 162.8 centimeters (64.1 inches).

Tlatilco's inhabitants were not tall in an absolute sense. All nineteenth century CE Plains Indians in Table 4.7 were taller on average than Tlatilco's people.[117] This result is unsurprising given American anthropologist Joseph M. Prince and American economist Richard Hall Steckel's (b. 1944) remark that Plains Indians were then the world's tallest.[118]

Moreover, military records from roughly 800 to 1800 CE indicate that northern European men were taller than their Tlatilcoan counterparts.[119] Even the shortest European averages surpassed Tlatilcoan men by almost three centimeters. This outcome is unsurprising if height increases with distance from the equator because Tlatilco, at 19.5 degrees North, was within the tropics whereas Sweden, the source of the best data on northern European heights, was at 60.1 degrees North.[120] But the relationship between height and latitude is uncertain, Chapter 4 stated, and adequately nourished people, partitioned by sex, tend to be roughly the same height irrespective of geography.[121]

Stature implies that northern Europeans were healthier than prehistoric Mexicans. Chapters 4, 5, 6, and 7 indicated that northern Europeans ate meat, fish, poultry, and dairy whereas Tlatilco's indigenes favored plants like beans, corn, squashes (*Cucurbita* species), and peppers, though supplements included fish, rodents, deer (*Odocoileus* species), peccary (species in genera *Tayassu*, *Catagonus*, and *Pecari*), and rabbit (*Oryctolagus cuniculus*).[122] This comparison suggests that animal products were more nourishing than plants in premodern times, though readers should not conclude that they should swap beans for meat. All data predated 1800 CE, when scarcity prevailed over abundance. This environment demanded caloric foods such as meat. Today, however, plentitude has replaced deprivation in affluent nations, mandating parsimony rather than gluttony. This chapter joins the rest of this book in emphasizing that context should inform food choices.

Bone deformations constitute a third health gauge. Chapter 1 defined porotic hyperostosis and cribra orbitalia as evidence for anemia, which may result from iron deficiency alone or insufficient iron and vitamin B_9 or B_{12}. When both iron and a B vitamin are involved, neither shortage need be marked to produce the malady. Yet diet is not the only factor. Chapter 1 noted that parasites or pathogens can cause anemia even when diet is adequate. In this respect and as Chapter 1 remarked, anemia may have evolved as a defense against invaders.[123] Because many parasites and pathogens need iron to grow and reproduce, the body's ability to put it in the spleen, liver, and bone marrow—causing anemia in the process—inhibits invaders.

TABLE 8.9
Porotic Hyperostosis and Cribra Orbitalia in Precontact Mexico

Place	Tlatilco		Cuicuilco		Teotihuacan		Cholula	
Time	c. 1600 BCE–c. 300 CE		c. 800–c. 600 BCE		c. 300 BCE–c. 1 CE		c. 900 BCE–1521 CE	
Porotic Hyperostosis	# examined	%	# examined	%	# examined	%	# examined	%
Women 15+yr	128	10	29	38	4	0	57	9
Men 15+yr	88	14	33	36	13	8	43	5
Boys and girls <15 yr	51	10	10	20	17	6	62	19
Cribra Orbitalia Women 15+yr	96	19	24	38	4	0	43	21
Cribra Orbitalia Men 15+yr	66	23	29	31	11	18	31	19
Cribra Orbitalia boys and girls <15 yr	42	43	8	25	16	13	43	54

Mindful that anemia does not always evince dietary distress, Table 8.9 indicates that Tlatilco's inhabitants below age fifteen had the second lowest proportion of porotic hyperostosis—but the second highest of cribra orbitalia—of the five Mexican societies.[124] Although it may have been a well-nourished community compared to other prehistoric Mexican settlements, Tlatilco, readers may recall, was the earliest of the five. Population was sparser than in later sites. Low population density minimized contagion, and little waste reduced habitats for insects, pathogens, parasites, and rodents. Whatever anemia's cause, beans' phytic acid retards iron absorption, though Amerindians would have destroyed some or most phytic acid by soaking and cooking them. Moreover, consumption of peppers, rich in vitamin C, would have aided iron assimilation.

The second central Mexican bean eaters inhabited Teotihuacan between roughly 300 BCE and 1 CE.[125] Again, growth was rapid, with population doubling about every generation. Tlatilco and Teotihuacan enlargement suggests that beans supplied adequate calories and nutrients. Teotihuacan diets resembled those in Tlatilco, featuring beans, corn, squashes, eggs, and small game. Teotihuacan's over 200 skeletons yielded fifty complete enough for examination.[126] These revealed 42 percent of deaths under age twenty and an e^0 of twenty-one years, numbers that typified prehistory and history, as this book emphasizes, and that countered Tlatilco's unusually generous e^0.[127]

Other measures were less dismal. Table 8.9 shows that Teotihuacan skeletons betrayed little porotic hyperostosis and cribra orbitalia.[128] Its women ranked fourth in height at an average of 153 centimeters (60.2 inches) and its men were second tallest on average at 166 centimeters (65.4 inches). Larger and more populous than Tlatilco, Teotihuacan probably suffered more pathogens, parasites, insects, and rodents, all undermining health. Under these circumstances, beans should not be faulted for brief lives, especially because minimal bone deformities and tall men imply adequate nutrition.

About 300 BCE, Mexicans cultivated a third species, *Phaseolus acutifolius* (tepary bean), which tolerates aridity.[129] Around 800 to 1000 CE, the bean migrated to Arizona. Noting their diet, Spaniards named Arizona's Papago "bean people."[130] Returning to an earlier time, *P. vulgaris* spread north through eastern North America by 2500 BCE. Beans sustained dense Mississippian settlements. In the southeast, Cherokee made bread from beans and corn. Near Lake Ontario, Iroquois favored the three sisters: beans, corn, and squashes.

Boiled beans and corn, known as succotash, were popular throughout North America. Today lima beans are standard in the dish. Chapter 12 mentions the Amerindian preference for pairing beans and corn in several ways. In parts of North and South America, the three sisters, as intimated, defined foodways. Richard Steckel and coauthors stated that American Indians who ate this trio were less healthy than their hunter-gatherer predecessors.[131]

Steckel and colleagues' judgment must be evaluated against the dissimilarities that complicated comparisons between hunter-gatherers and farmers. Agriculture and animal husbandry supported larger populations, than were possible among hunter-gatherers, increasing crowding, contagion, insects, parasites and rodents in sedentary societies. These ills worsened health and truncated lives. Problems intensified as settled peoples created commercial networks that brought microbes and pests from foreign lands. Consequently, urban mortality usually exceeded rural death rates.[132]

Returning to beans, they were sun dried after being shelled. Alternatively, Amerindians dried and cooked them in the pod, shelling them before consumption. Like the Cherokee, Maya in Mexico and Central America made bread from beans and corn. At other times they ate beans, squash seeds, and onions or paired beans with chili peppers (*Capsicum* species). Mayan descendants consumed black beans, onions, and the herb epazote (*Dysphania ambrosioides*). In the Aztec capital Tenochtitlan, street vendors sold beans. Reaching Mexico in 1529, Franciscan priest Bernardino de Sahagun (1499–1590) counted twelve bean varieties in cultivation.[133]

In first millennium CE Peru, the Moche painted lima bean images on pottery.[134] Images of men and women holding beans in one hand and corn in the other may suggest that these foods were eaten together, a practice that earlier paragraphs mentioned as common in the Americas. Images of women and beans may imply that cultivation and preparation were female tasks. Images of soldiers with lima bean bodies may indicate that beans sustained Peruvian armies.

In 1492, Columbus encountered beans on Caribbean island Cuba.[135] In 1519, Spanish conquistador Hernan Cortes (1485–1547) came upon beans in Mexico.[136] During the 1520s, Spanish explorer Alvar Nunez Cabeza de Vaca (1490–1559) reported bean cultivation and consumption in Texas, New Mexico, and Florida. A decade later, French explorer Jacques Cartier (1491–1557) found the legumes north in Canada and New York's Saint Lawrence River.[137]

Caribbean cuisine featured kidney beans, coconut (*Cocos nucifera*), and thyme. Jamaicans combined these beans with rice and coconut milk. Copying Spain, Cubans made black beans with rice and pork. In the Caribbean, Mexico, Brazil, South Carolina, and Georgia, slaves ate variants of rice and legumes. Although not our primary focus, cowpeas—also known as black-eyed peas—had been a West African staple since about 3000 BCE.[138] Portugal gave West Africa beans in the sixteenth century, adding another legume. Slaves employed these possibilities in the Americas, eating black beans and rice in the Caribbean whereas New Orleans, Louisiana, specialized in red kidney beans and rice. Cowpeas and rice fed South Carolinian and Georgian slaves. On the Sea Islands off the coast of South Carolina, Georgia, and Florida, the preferred cowpea was the sea island red pea.

Whole grain rice and legumes complement each other. Like other grains, rice has little essential amino acid lysine, which legumes like beans furnish.[139] Beans lack the essential amino acid methionine, which rice supplies. White or parboiled rice lacks fiber, which legumes provide. Beans, peas, lentils, and other legumes contribute potassium, iron, manganese, magnesium, and vitamin B_9. More nourishing, beans are also more expensive than rice throughout much of the world, causing the poor to skimp on them while eating more rice and reducing nutrients in the process.[140] Improvements might include substituting brown rice for white to increase fiber and nutrients. Inclusion of tomatoes (*Solanum esculentum*) or peppers adds vitamin C. A side of carrots or spinach boosts vitamins A (as beta carotene) and C.

At the intersection of American and African cuisine is Hoppin' (or Hopping) John, which used cowpeas, though introduction of *Phaseolus* beans into Africa permitted their substitution. Purists do not deviate from cowpeas. Recipes add cowpeas or beans to rice, onions, peppers, celery, cloves (*Syzygium aromaticum*), and thyme. The dish may be served with bacon, ham, or another type of pork, collard (*Brassica oleracea var. acephala*) or turnip greens, tomatoes, and cornbread.

On their own, beans' nutrients depend on type. For example, 100 grams of white kidney beans have 9 grams of protein.[141] The same amount of black, cranberry, pinto, pink, navy, and red kidney beans have 8 grams, great northern beans have 7, and red beans have 6. One hundred grams of cowpeas has 6.6 grams of protein.[142] Beans and cowpeas also furnish fiber, iron, potassium, phosphorus, copper, magnesium, manganese, and vitamins B_1, B_2, B_6, and B_9. One hundred grams of cranberry beans provide 46 percent of vitamin B_9.[143] The same quantity of cowpeas furnishes 44.5 percent of it.[144]

Hopping John's other ingredients augment nutriment. Onions have fiber, vitamins B_9 and C, calcium, and iron. Peppers supply potassium, carotenoids (vitamin A precursors), and vitamins B_9, C, E, and K. Celery has fiber, carotenoids, molybdenum, manganese, copper, calcium, potassium, phosphorus, magnesium, and vitamins B_2, B_5, B_6, B_9, C, and K. Cloves are not nutrient rich but have small amounts of fiber, calcium, magnesium, manganese, and vitamins C, E, and K. Thyme has fiber, carotenoids, iron, copper, manganese, calcium, phosphorus, zinc, potassium, and vitamins B_2, B_6, B_9, and C.

Of the remaining ingredients, Table 4.1 listed pork's nutrients. Chapter 12 discusses corn's merits and drawbacks. Collard greens have protein, omega 3 fatty acids, iron, copper, magnesium, phosphorus, potassium, and vitamins B_1, B_3, B_5, B_6, B_9, and E. Turnip greens provide fiber, protein, carotenoids, calcium, copper, manganese, and vitamins B_6, B_9, C, E, and K. Tomatoes furnish potassium, the antioxidant lycopene, and vitamins B_9, C, and K. These details indicate that hopping John has more than beans or cowpeas to recommend it.

Beans entered American lore during the first Thanksgiving in 1621. This mythology avers that Native Americans taught the English to make baked beans, a tradition retained in the United States.[145] New Englanders soaked navy beans in water, then baked them with onions and deer fat. Saturday dinners featured the dish. Bostonians substituted lard for deer fat and added brown sugar (from *Saccharum officinarum* or *Beta vulgaris*). Saturday mornings, bakers gathered pots of beans from each house, baking them in the community oven in time for dinner. This practice earned Boston the moniker Beantown.[146] Religious prohibitions against Sunday work led women to bake beans on Saturday for consumption next day.

Referenced earlier, *American Cookery* paired beans with lamb. *Miss Leslie's Complete Cookery* (1851) recommended that green beans and scarlet runner beans (*Phaseolus coccineus*) be boiled at least one hour to tenderize them. *The Improved Housewife* (1853) urged cooks to bake beans overnight. In 1875, American company Burnham and Morrill pioneered the manufacture and sale of canned baked beans. *Mrs. Rorer's Philadelphia Cookbook* (1886) combined beans, lemon (*Citrus limon*), and hard-boiled eggs. That year American seed company W. Atlee Burpee marketed a scarlet runner bean with a tender pod, the Golden Wax Flageoler. In 1895, American food company H. J. Heinz advertised canned baked beans.

Outside the Americas, Columbus took beans to Spain in 1493.[147] Thinking *P. vulgaris* resembled familiar broad beans, lentils, peas, cowpeas, and chickpeas Europeans adopted it more quickly than unfamiliar potatoes, treated in Chapter 13, and tomatoes.[148] In 1528, Italy acquired *P. vulgaris* from Spain, adding white kidney beans to minestrone and pasta e fugioli (pasta and beans), known in the United States as pasta fazool. France paired beans—green beans being popular throughout the country—with meat to make cassoulet.[149] In the late sixteenth century, English naturalist and barber surgeon John Gerard (c. 1565–1612) grew scarlet runner beans, named for their red flowers and valued as ornamental and food. Today farmers grow *P. vulgaris* in more countries than any other legume, though the global soybean harvest is larger.[150]

8.4.2 *Arachis hypogaea*

Despite its name, the peanut is neither pea nor nut, though it is related to peas because both are legumes. Reference to peanuts as groundnuts emphasizes that pods and seeds develop underground. Indigenous to South America, the legume is thought to have originated in Brazil, Argentina, Paraguay, or Bolivia; the last—having the largest number of *Arachis* species—was peanuts' probable cradle.[151] Around 3000 BCE, peanuts were cultivated and consumed throughout Brazil and the Caribbean.[152] Between 1200 and 800 BCE, Peru adopted the legume. Like modern Americans, Peruvians snacked on groundnuts. In the first millennium CE, Peru's Nazca and Chimu emblazoned pottery with peanut images.[153] As grave goods, groundnuts were likely intended to feed the dead in the afterlife. In the second millennium, peanuts nourished Inca, Aztecs, and Bahamians.

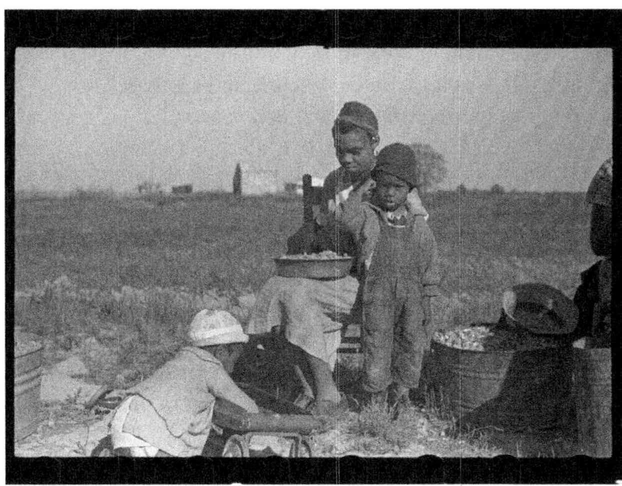

FIGURE 8.8 Peanuts. (Photo courtesy of Library of Congress. https://www.loc.gov/pictures/item/2017716923/.)

Like *Phaseolus* beans, pineapple (*Ananas comosus*), tobacco (*Nicotiana tabacum*), squashes, corn, sweet potatoes (*Ipomoea batatas*), and cassava (*Manihot esculenta*), the Caribbean islands mediated Europe's encounter with peanuts. Arriving on Hispaniola in 1502, Spanish priest Bartolome de las Casas (1484–1566) was probably the first European to see the legume, comparing it to peas and chickpeas.[154] Although de las Casas praised the flavor as superior to hazelnuts (*Corylus avellana*) and walnuts (*Juglans regia*), Spanish historian Gonzalo Fernandez de Oviedo y Valdes (1478–1557), who in 1527 published the first description of peanuts, dismissed them as suitable only for slaves, children, commoners, or people "who do not have a fine taste."[155]

From Brazil, Portugal gave Africa peanuts before 1560.[156] Roughly 26 percent protein by mass compared to 14 percent for soybeans and 6–9 percent for beans and peas, peanuts were essential to the masses, who seldom afforded animal products.[157] Wherever diets were threadbare, peanuts provided abundant nutrients and calories. Forty-seven percent fat by mass, 0.5 kilograms (1 pound) of peanuts have as many calories as 1 kilogram (2 pounds) of beef, 0.7 kilograms (1.5 pounds) of cheddar cheese, or thirty-six medium eggs.[158]

West Africans paired peanuts with leafy green vegetables or added them to soups and stews of yams (*Dioscorea* species), tomatoes, and okra (*Abelmoschus esculentus*). Ghanaians ate peanut stew with cassava, yams, or bananas (*Musa x paradisiaca*). Senegal and Mali's Bombara combined peanut stew with chicken, okra, tomatoes, or sweet potatoes. Fried peanut cakes are popular in Mali. Like Americans, Zimbabweans snacked on roasted, salted peanuts.[159] Kenyans made peanut and bean stew, eating it with corn pudding. Malawians and Zambians ate peanuts with tomatoes. Mozambicans prepared pudding with peanuts, egg yolks, and sucrose ($C_{12}H_{22}O_{11}$), a sugar discussed in Chapters 2 and 11. Africans and Asians favored peanut oil for frying because it does not overpower other flavors and because it does not smoke at high temperatures.

Besides Africa, Portugal brought peanuts to India while Spain carried them to the Philippines before 1600. From these islands, the legume migrated to China, Japan, Malaysia, and Indonesia. Like Africa, peanuts have been indispensable in Asia, where population threatened to surpass the land's capacity to feed it. Mainland Southeast Asians make sauce from peanuts, chili peppers, coconut milk, and lime (*Citrus aurantifolia*) juice, using the sauce to flavor rice, meat, chicken, and vegetables. Indonesians and Thais add peanut sauce to meat and rice. Indonesians apply a sauce of peanuts, ginseng (*Panax ginseng*), chili peppers, shallot (*Allium cepa var. aggregatum*), and garlic (*Allium sativum*) to vegetables and shrimp. They shape chopped peanuts into wafers, add them to salads, and boil peanuts with chili sauce. Javanese fry rice in peanut oil. Thais pair peanuts, which season many dishes, and papaya

(*Carica papaya*). Malaysians top vegetables with coconut milk and peanut sauce. Combinations of the legume and root vegetables feed Vietnamese, whose children eat boiled peanuts at breakfast. Chinese add peanuts to stir fries and make candy with the legume and sucrose. Southwestern China's Sichuan and Yunnan provinces stir-fry peanuts, chili peppers, and vegetables. Indians eat trail mix of peanuts, chickpeas, and other legumes. Peanut curry is popular in southern India.

Returning to the western hemisphere, the most direct route should have moved peanuts north from South America, the Caribbean, and Mexico into the United States. Instead they crossed the Atlantic Ocean to Africa, returning during the slave trade as ships' leftovers.[160] Slaves and Amerindians were the first to cultivate and consume peanuts in the American colonies, combining them with beans, corn or cornbread, collard greens, turnip greens, and other vegetables. Peanuts were ubiquitous in slave gardens. Because they stored well, peanuts sustained slaves during winter's privations. Deeming the legume inferior because of its association with Africans and indigenes, whites hesitated to eat it but instead let pigs (*Sus scrofa domesticus*), cattle (*Bos taurus*), chickens, and turkeys (*Meleagris gallopavo f. domestica*) devour the entire plant.[161] Before the Civil War, peanuts were grown and eaten in Alabama, Georgia, Louisiana, Mississippi, the Carolinas, Florida, Arkansas, Tennessee, Texas, and Virginia.

The Civil War (1861–1865) elevated the legume from a regional and an ethnic item into a national food. As in previous wars, soldiers lived off the land when supplies were inadequate. Union troops in the South ate what farms provided. In this way, the war introduced many northerners to the peanut. They returned home with the desire to make it a regular part of diets.[162] To meet demand, the United States tripled the peanut harvest between 1865 and 1870.[163] About 1870, American entertainer Phineas Taylor (P. T.) Barnum (1810–1891) sold roasted, salted peanuts to circus goers, fueling demand for them as a snack.[164]

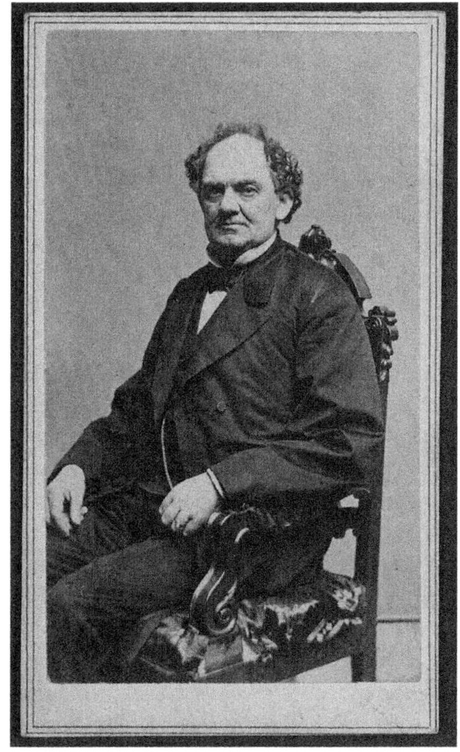

FIGURE 8.9 P. T. Barnum. (Photo courtesy of Library of Congress. https://www.loc.gov/pictures/item/2013648325/.)

The South benefited from peanuts' stardom. By 1880, South Carolina's harvest was large enough to distribute throughout the United States and overseas. The boll weevil prompted cotton growers in Alabama, Georgia, North Carolina, and South Carolina to plant the legume. By 1917, Coffee County, Georgia, once cotton territory, led the United States in peanut production.[165] In Alabama, a white woman who had jettisoned cotton for peanuts asked George Washington Carver for help marketing her crop.[166] He transcended the traditional advice of feeding them to pigs by creating over 300 peanut products, including flour, cake, candies, gingerbread, milk, cheese, feed, shoe polish, ink, varnish, pickles, salad dressing, margarine, paint, rubber, coffee, vinegar, punch, cough syrup, and face cream.[167] Carver even floated the idea that topical applications of peanut oil might treat polio, a claim that displeased many physicians.[168]

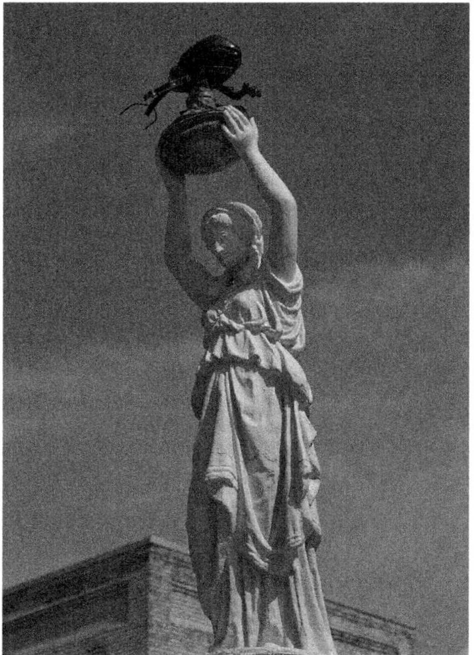

FIGURE 8.10 Boll weevil. (Photo courtesy of Library of Congress. https://www.loc.gov/pictures/item/2010638568/.)

Carver was not alone in envisioning new uses for peanuts. In 1898, John Harvey Kellogg patented peanut butter.[169] Despite this assertion of novelty, he was not the inventor because Aztecs had created it around the first century CE, and Carver had also developed an early version.[170] Believing that nutrition underpinned health, Kellogg promoted peanut butter as ideal nourishment for people unable to chew tough foods. It became popular among children as a mainstay of the lunchtime sandwich or snack. In 1903, American physician Ambrose Straub (1842–1912) patented a machine to make peanut butter. In 1922, American businessman Joseph Louis Rosefield (1888–1958) added partially hydrogenated oils to prevent peanut oil's separation from the solids.[171] The result was a product that spread easily. In 1932, he created Skippy, now part of American company Hormel Foods.

Furthering the legume as snack, in 1901, American inventors F. V. Mills and H. S. Mills devised a machine that dispensed roasted peanuts for a penny.[172] Before 1910, the United States had some 30,000 dispensers. Paralleling this development, confectioners began mass producing peanut candies. In 1906, Italian American entrepreneurs Amedeo Obici (1877–1947) and Mario Peruzzi (1875–1955) founded Planters Nut and Chocolate Company in Wilkes-Barre,

Pennsylvania, now a global peanut seller.[173] The company's Mr. Peanut, debuting in 1981, is recognizable worldwide.[174]

Before World War I (1914–1918), the United States was a net importer. Disrupting trade, the war forced American farms to meet domestic demand, prompting Texas, Alabama, Georgia, Louisiana, Oklahoma, and Mississippi to expand peanut hectarage. The Red Cross declared it among soldiers' four most nourishing foods. With wheat (*Triticum aestivum*) funneled to servicemen and allies, Americans extended bread with peanut flour. The National Emergency Board Garden Commission urged gardeners to plant peanuts for sustenance. One Floridian made headlines by living entirely on peanuts during the war.[175] Patriotic organizations urged Americans to forego meat and instead eat peanuts and other protein-rich plants.

World War II (1939–1945) again spotlighted the legume. In 1941, Congress declared peanuts an essential crop and food, and the U.S. harvest leapt between 1940 and 1945.[176] Under USDA guidelines, farmers sold part of the crop to the federal government, guaranteeing them income, and marketed the rest to satisfy domestic demand.[177] The appetite for peanuts continued to expand after the war, and by 1990, Americans consumed most peanuts as peanut butter. Nowadays, one-fifth of the harvest is eaten roasted and salted and another one-quarter goes to candies.[178] Many people find irresistible the combination of peanuts and chocolate. An early peanut candy, Reese's Peanut Butter Cups cost a penny per cup in 1938.[179] Others followed, including popular Baby Ruth and Snickers. In various forms, peanuts have become ubiquitous at sporting events and on airplanes.

Yet concerns have arisen that peanuts are too caloric for affluent nations' inactive inhabitants. Moreover, reports of allergies and even deaths led administrators to remove peanuts and peanut butter from school lunches.[180] Between 1982 and 2002, amid weak domestic demand, Mexican and South American imports reduced U.S. farm income. Since 2002, Weight Watchers and the American Diabetic Association combated these trends, emphasizing peanuts' healthfulness. What peanuts Americans do not eat are sold abroad, making the United States the largest exporter. It sells three-fifths of the harvest to the European Union (EU), with the United Kingdom (UK), the Netherlands, and Germany being principal buyers.[181] The United States exports peanut butter to Saudi Arabia, Canada, Japan, Germany, and South Korea.[182] Among candy bars, Snickers is Russia's favorite.

From its inception in 1862, the USDA promoted peanuts' wholesomeness.[183] The land-grant colleges and agricultural experiment stations, founded in subsequent years, agreed. Central to these efforts and part of the agricultural-science establishment, Carver championed the legume. In 1923, he touted peanuts as more nourishing than steak, emphasizing them as inexpensive protein and other nutrients.[184] His contemporary, American chemist Walter Hollis Eddy (1877–1959), declared peanuts "virtually a nutritive goldmine."[185]

Their value was evident to the Floridian, mentioned above, who in 1917 subsisted on 226.8 grams (0.5 pounds) of them daily plus an unspecified amount of corn.[186] As noted about the pea diet, one anecdote may not merit extrapolation; nonetheless, his story concretizes peanuts' adequacy when other foods are unaffordable or unavailable. Peas and peanuts' examples underscore legumes' prehistoric and historic role in feeding the downtrodden. Chapter 13 cites potatoes as another inexpensive staple. Such essentials gave the masses the nutrients and energy to be productive despite oppression, thereby perpetuating unequal economic, social, and political systems.

Ignoring corn given absence of amount, Table 8.10 lists calories and nutrients in 226.8 grams of peanuts.[187] This list indicates that peanuts supply ample nutrients while leaving room for other foods to reach the current benchmark of 2,000 calories daily.[188]

Twentieth century medical authorities and nutritionists recruited peanuts against protein deficiency. Chapter 12 mentions that Jamaican physician Cicely Delphine Williams (1893–1992) sounded the alarm in 1933, naming the deficiency disease kwashiorkor.[189] In 1950, the United Nations Food and Agriculture Organization (FAO) in Rome, Italy designated it the world's most prevalent disease. Two years later the World Health Organization (WHO) in Geneva, Switzerland

TABLE 8.10
Nutrients in Peanuts 226.8g

Nutrient	Peanut	%DV
Calories	1,286	N/A
Protein (g)	58.5	N/A
Fat (g)	111.6	N/A
Carbs (g)	36.5	N/A
Fiber (g)	19.3	N/A
	Minerals	
Ca (mg)	209	20.9
Fe (mg)	10.38	57.7
Mg (mg)	381.02	95.3
P (mg)	853	85.3
K (mg)	1,598.94	45.7
Na (mg)	40.82	1.7
Zn (mg)	7.42	49.4
Cu (mg)	2.59	129.3
Mn (mg)	4.38	218.9
Se (mcg)	16.33	23.3
	Vitamins	
A (IU)	0	0
B_1 (mg)	1.45	96.8
B_2 (mg)	0.32	18
B_3 (mg)	27.37	136.9
B_5 (mg)	4.01	40.1
B_6 (mg)	0.79	39.7
B_9 (mcg)	544.32	136.08
B_{12} (mcg)	0	0
C (mg)	0	0
D (IU)	0	0
E (mg)	18.89	125.9
K (mcg)	0	0

blamed insufficient protein as the cause and noted kwashiorkor's ubiquity among tropical and subtropical poor. A 1954 recommendation that ailing lactase producers, discussed in Chapter 7, drink milk for protein confronted the reality that many in developing countries lacked the beverage. This realization spurred the search for protein-laden plants.

In this effort, the U.S. Agency for International Development (USAID) in Washington, DC in 1965 funded Virginia Polytechnic Institute and State University's program to encourage peanuts' cultivation and consumption in the Philippines.[190] Concurrently, the university sought to minimize the legume's contamination by the fungus *Aspergillus flavus*, which emitted a possible liver carcinogen. Studying both peanuts and the fungus, American nutritionist Thomas Colin Campbell (b. 1934)—then at Virginia Polytechnic—discovered that Filipino children who ate the most protein were at greatest risk of liver cancer.[191] Protein rather than the fungus was to blame, he concluded. Although this finding appeared to disqualify peanuts—which have plentiful protein as noted—from fighting undernutrition and poverty, Campbell blamed animal rather than plant protein for these cancers.[192] International agencies and researchers continue to fight undernutrition in developing countries with peanuts and their products, including peanut butter.[193]

8.5 LEGUMES, SLAVES, AND HEALTH

8.5.1 Legumes in Slave Diets

Perhaps no subject provokes such debate and emotion among historians as New World slavery. Although the practice is ancient, its fusion with racism was a modern European invention that continues to plague the Americas. Controversies taint every facet of slaves' existence, including diets, nutrition, and health. Historians studied corn and pork's contributions to slave diets in the American colonies and their successor nation, the United States, though eyewitnesses and food historians described diverse diets that included legumes.

American food historian Andrew Francis Smith (b. 1946), for example, remarked that the peanut fed slaves before Amerindians and Europeans adopted it in the American colonies.[194] Moreover, he argued that slaves introduced peanuts into the colonies and were responsible for bringing them to wider attention. Eighteenth-century travelers through the South and the Caribbean mentioned slaves' cultivation and consumption of the legume.

American historian Marcie Cohen Ferris deemed peanuts "ubiquitous" in colonial South Carolina and Georgia, and peas and beans popular in North and South Carolina.[195] Peas fed slaves and Europeans from an early date. British naturalist Mark Catesby (1683–1749) stated while touring the American Southeast and Caribbean in the eighteenth century that kidney beans were a "strong, hearty food" for slaves.[196] Besides these legumes, an earlier section noted, and Chapter 12 mentions, that in coastal South Carolina, Georgia, and the Sea Islands, slaves ate cowpeas, often coupled with rice as hopping John. Ferris mentioned peas as a substitute for cowpeas in this dish.[197] American economist, historian, and 1993 Nobel laureate in economics Robert William Fogel (1926–2013) and American economist and historian Stanley Lewis Engerman (b. 1936) listed peas among slaves' eleven primary foods.[198]

8.5.2 Slaves' Health

Given this variety, examination of slaves' nutrition and health permits evaluation of peas, beans, peanuts, and cowpeas. These qualities were awful for the youngest, but legumes deserve no blame. Owners worked pregnant women to within days of delivery. Arduous field labor, much of it while stooped, harmed mother and fetus. Richard Steckel calculated that newborns averaged just 2.3 kilograms (5.1 pounds).[199] Such low masses exacerbated infant mortality of at least 35 percent. Conditions did not improve during early childhood's meager diets. Undernutrition made children lethargic and docile, exactly what owners wanted.

Diets improved only when juveniles were old enough to toil in the fields such that "working-age slaves were remarkably well off."[200] In *Time on the Cross*—arguably the twentieth century's seminal book on slavery—Fogel and Engerman calculated that slaves consumed nearly 4,200 calories daily, exceeding recommendations for protein, iron, calcium, and vitamin C.[201] The authors emphasized that "the high slave consumption of meat, sweet potatoes, and peas goes a long way toward explaining" why "the slave diet was not only adequate, it actually exceeded modern (1964) recommended daily levels of the chief nutrients."[202] Amplifying this point, previous sections and tables noted that legumes have plentiful protein, minerals, vitamins, and, in the case of peanuts and soybeans, fat. Readers may recall that peanuts are an excellent source of copper, manganese, and vitamins B_3, B_9, and E. Peas and beans are rich in phosphorus, manganese, iron, copper, magnesium, zinc, potassium, and vitamins A (equivalents), B_1, B_2, B_3, B_6, B_9, C, and K. These nutrients made legumes valuable in slave diets and advanced Fogel and Engerman's contention that slaves were as well, or perhaps better, nourished than free people.[203] Among their conclusions, the two debunked "the belief that the typical slave was poorly fed", writing that it "is without foundation in fact."[204] *Time on the Cross* angered historians who believed the book implied that slavery was not entirely loathsome.

Echoing Fogel and Engerman, American chef April McGreger remarked that "there is shockingly little evidence of nutritional diseases among slaves."[205] Given Steckel's above data, she must have had adults in mind.

Slavery must be repudiated while attempting to examine slaves' nutrition and health. Slave girls reached puberty no later than age 14.5, two years or more before European girls.[206] That is, slave teens must have been well enough nourished to mature quickly. Yet strenuous exertions depleted calories and nutrients such that slave men were over 2.5 centimeters (1 inch) shorter than free American men.[207] Nonetheless, U.S. slaves were taller than British and Russian workers and Caribbean and Brazilian slaves. This book correlates nutrition and height.

Beyond these data, slave birthrates—despite appalling newborn and infant mortality—exceeded deaths in the American South but not in the Caribbean, Mexico, Central America, and South America, implying that slaves ate better in the United States than elsewhere.[208] By 1720, the U.S. slave birthrate surpassed the number of imports, a circumstance otherwise unknown in the Americas.[209] Fogel and Engerman calculated e^0 for U.S. slaves in 1850—in Table 8.11—at thirty-six years, a duration longer than the average for free residents of New York City, Boston, and Philadelphia in 1830, the occupants of Manchester, England in 1850, Austrians in 1875, Italians in 1885, and Chileans in 1920.[210]

Diet cannot fully explain these differences. The American colonies and United States were healthier than slave societies elsewhere in the western hemisphere because tropical diseases killed fewer slaves in temperate North American than in Brazil, the Caribbean, and other lands nearer the equator.[211] Additionally, tropical plantations specialized in sugarcane (*Saccharum officinarum*), which required strenuous labor in hot, humid climates and which Chapter 11 discusses. Such an environment was enervating in leisure and crippling under duress.

8.5.3 Comparisons between Slaves and Free People

This book acknowledges the limitations of comparing slaves and free people. Toil undermined nutrition and health by sapping calories and nutrients. American historian Richard Slator Dunn (b. 1928) blamed overwork among other factors for truncating Caribbean slaves' lives in the seventeenth and early eighteenth centuries.[212] Masters were no less ruthless in the American South, forcing pregnant women to pick cotton (*Gossypium hirsutum*) as late as the week of delivery.[213] Compulsion began earlier in childhood and required more hours per week and days per year for slave than free.[214] So strenuous was this routine that children and women halved their workload upon emancipation.[215] Whippings and other punishments enforced discipline, indicating that slaves

TABLE 8.11
E^0 for Slaves and Free Peoples

Group	Place	Time	E^0 (yr)
Slave	United States	1850	36
White	NYC	1830	24
White	Boston	1830	24
White	Philadelphia	1830	24
White	Manchester, England	1850	24
Latino/a	Chile	1920	31
White	Austria	1875	31
White	Italy	1885	35
White	France	1854–1856	36
White	Netherlands	1850–1859	36
White	England, Wales	1838–1854	40
White	United States	1850	40

had no choice but to outwork free laborers. Unsurprisingly, slaves were roughly one-third more productive than free labor.[216]

Such exertions exacted costs. For example, a rice plantation near Charleston, South Carolina, yielded thirty-six skeletons, buried between 1840 and 1870, with osteoarthritis, spinal degeneration, and large slots where tendons had attached to bones, all indicating arduous toil.[217] Skeletons at Sugar Land, Texas, exhibited bones distorted by intense exertions, revealing how difficult labor was on sugarcane plantations.[218] Although Sugar Land's remains came from people who lived after slavery's putative abolition, the Thirteenth Amendment—ratified in 1865—permitted it and "involuntary servitude"…"as punishment for a crime."[219] Another index of strenuousness is the estimate, stated earlier, that slaves consumed on average around 4,200 calories daily just to maintain their mass.

Yet comparisons are valid when and where wage labor was harsh, justifying British poet William Blake's (1757–1827) 1804 description of factories as "dark Satanic mills."[220] About 1830 U.S. factories mandated an average workday of 11.5 hours, which summer's extra daylight lengthened.[221] In 1890, blast furnaces mandated eighty-four-hour weeks.[222] Although, an eight-hour day became standard during World War I, the assembly line's adoption around then intensified work by requiring employees to keep pace with the movement of parts. A woman complained to Henry Ford that "the chain system you have is a slave driver!... My husband has come home and thrown himself down and won't eat his supper—so done out!"[223] As this quote suggests, onlookers likened factories to plantations and prisons.[224] Farm work remains exhausting absent mechanization. For example, California migrants weed potato fields in 41.7 degrees Celsius (107 degrees Fahrenheit) heat.[225] Constant stooping disfigures them.

NOTES

1 Lawrence Kaplan, "Legumes in the History of Human Nutrition," in *The World of Soy*, ed. Christine M. Du Bois, Chee-Beng Tan, and Sidney W. Mintz (Urbana and Chicago: University of Illinois Press, 2008), 27.
2 Vincent E. Rubatzky and Mas Yamaguchi, *World Vegetables: Principles, Production, and Nutritive Values*, 2nd ed. (New York: Chapman and Hall, 1997), 474.
3 Ibid.
4 Ibid; Georgina Pearman, "Nuts, Seeds, and Pulses," in *The Cultural History of Plants*, ed. Ghillean Prance and Mark Nesbitt (New York and London: Routledge, 2005), 142; "What Are Pulses?" American Pulse Association, Pulse Canada, and USA Dry Pea and Lentil Council, accessed April 21, 2019, https://pulses.org/nap/what-are-pulses.
5 Ken Albala, *Beans: A History* (Oxford and New York: Berg, 2017), 75.
6 K. D. White, *Roman Farming* (Ithaca, NY: Cornell University Press, 1970), 198.
7 H. Schadewaldt, "Hellriegel, Hermann," in *Dictionary of Scientific Biography*, vol. 6, ed. Charles Coulston Gillispie (New York: Charles Scribner's Sons, 1981), 237.
8 Pearman, 142.
9 Bernard Venn, "Legumes," in *Essential of Human Nutrition*, ed. Jim Mann and A. Stewart Truswell, 5th ed. (Oxford: Oxford University Press, 2017), 277.
10 David B. Haytowitz and Ruth H. Matthews, *Composition of Foods: Legumes and Legume Products: Raw, Processed, Prepared* (Washington, DC: U.S. Department of Agriculture, 1986), 129; "Peanuts, All Types, Raw," *USDA FoodData Central*, April 1, 2019, accessed December 9, 2019, https://fdc.nal.usda.gov/fdc-app.html#/food-details/172430/nutrients.
11 Haytowitz and Matthews, 112, 129; "Peanuts, All Types, Raw;" "Peas, Green, Raw," *USDA FoodData Central*, April 1, 2019, accessed January 23, 2020, https://fdc.nal.usda.gov/fdc-app.html#/food-details/170419/nutrients; "Soybeans, Mature Seeds, Raw," *USDA FoodData Central*, April 1, 2019, accessed January 23, 2020, https://fdc.nal.usda.gov/fdc-app.html#/food-details/174270/nutrients; "Beans, String, Green, Raw," *USDA FoodData Central*, April 1, 2019, accessed January 23, 2020, https://fdc.nal.usda.gov/fdc-app.html#/food-details/342596/nutrients; "Green Beans," *The World's Healthiest Foods*, January 20–26, 2020, accessed January 23, 2020, http://www.whfoods.com/genpage.php?tname=foodspice&dbid=134.
12 "FDA Vitamins and Minerals Chart," *FDA*, accessed October 14, 2019, https://www.accessdata.fda.gov/scripts/interactivenutritionfactslabel/factsheets/vitamin_and_mineral_chart.pdf.

13 "Peanuts, All Types, Raw."
14 Atli Arnarson, "20 Foods That Are High in Vitamin E," *Healthline*, May 24, 2017, accessed May 11, 2019, https://www.healthline.com/nutrition/foods-high-in-vitamin-e; "Manganese," *The World's Healthiest Foods*, May 6–12, 2019, May 11, 2019, http://www.whfoods.com/genpage.php?tname=nutrient&dbid=77.
15 Julie Garden-Robinson and Krystle McNeal, "All about Beans: Nutrition, Health Benefits, Preparation and Use in Menus," North Dakota State University, February 2018, accessed April 27, 2019, https://www.ag.ndsu.edu/publications/food-nutrition/all-about-beans-nutrition-health-benefits-preparation-and-use-in-menus#section-0; "Top Measurements: Beans, Dry Beans, Whole," *Cookit Simply*, 2003–2010, accessed April 27, 2019, http://www.cookitsimply.com/measurements/cups/dry-beans-whole-0070-02g5.html.
16 Haytowitz and Matthews, 129–152.
17 Chee-Beng Tan, "Tofu and Related Products in Chinese Foodways," in *The World of Soy*, ed. Christine M. Du Bois, Chee-Beng Tan, and Sidney W. Mintz (Urbana and Chicago: University of Illinois Press, 2008), 99.
18 Albala, 213.
19 Christine M. Du Bois, *The Story of Soy* (London: Reaktion Books, 2018), 29–30.
20 Sidney W. Mintz, "Fermented Beans and Western Taste," in *The World of Soy*, ed. Christine M. Du Bois, Chee-Beng Tan, and Sidney W. Mintz (Urbana and Chicago: University of Illinois Press, 2008), 60.
21 Albala, 220; Myra Sidharta, "Soyfoods in Indonesia," in *The World of Soy*, ed. Christine M. Du Bois, Chee-Beng Tan, and Sidney W. Mintz (Urbana and Chicago: University of Illinois Press, 2008), 201.
22 Kaplan, "Legumes in the History of Human Nutrition," 28.
23 Ibid., 27.
24 Lois N. Magner, "Korea," in *The Cambridge World History of Food*, vol. 2, ed. Kenneth F. Kiple and Kriemhild Conee Ornelas (Cambridge, UK: Cambridge University Press, 2000), 1185.
25 Michael Pollan, *The Omnivore's Dilemma: A Natural History of Four Meals* (New York: Penguin Press, 2006), 35.
26 Sylvia A. Johnson, *Tomatoes, Potatoes, Corn, and Beans: How the Foods of the Americas Changed Eating around the World* (New York: Atheneum Books, 1997), 28.
27 Ibid., 27.
28 Lawrence Kaplan and Lucille N. Kaplan, "Beans of the Americas," in *Chilies to Chocolate: Food the Americas Gave the World*, ed. Nelson Foster and Linda S. Cordell (Tucson and London: University of Arizona Press, 1992), 75.
29 Irene Darmadi-Blackberry, Mark L. Wahlqvist, Antigone Kouris-Blazos, Bertil Steen, Widjaja Lukito, Yoshimitsu Horie, and Kazuyo Horie, "Legumes: The Most Important Dietary Predictor of Survival in Older People of Different Ethnicities," *Asia Pacific Journal of Clinical Nutrition* 13, no. 2 (2004): 219.
30 "Legumes," in *The Cambridge World History of Food*, vol. 2, ed. Kenneth F. Kiple and Kriemhild Conee Ornelas (Cambridge, UK: Cambridge University Press, 2000), 1799.
31 Meredith Sayles Hughes, *Spill the Beans and Pass the Peanuts: Legumes* (Minneapolis, MN: Lerner Publications, 1999), 44.
32 Peas, Green, Raw."
33 Hughes, 44.
34 Mariam Alireza, "Legumes: The Poor Man's Protein," *Arab News*, December 8, 2004, accessed April 27, 2019, http://www.arabnews.com/node/259264; Naomi F. Miller and Wilma Wetterstrom, "The Beginnings of Agriculture: The Ancient Near East and North Africa," in *The Cambridge World History of Food*, vol. 2, ed. Kenneth F. Kiple and Kriemhild Conee Ornelas (Cambridge, UK: Cambridge University Press, 2000), 1135; Jennifer A. Woolfe, *Sweet Potato: An Untapped Food Resource* (Cambridge, UK: Cambridge University Press, 1992), 119; Peter Garnsey, *Food and Society in Classical Antiquity* (Cambridge, UK: Cambridge University Press, 1999), 15.
35 Bob Brier and Hoyt Hobbs, *Ancient Egypt: Everyday Life in the Land of the Nile* (New York: Sterling, 2009), 119.
36 Beryl Brintnall Simpson and Molly Conner Ogorzaly, *Economic Botany: Plants in Our World*, 3rd ed. (Boston: McGraw Hill, 2001), 145.
37 Kaplan, "Legumes in the History of Human Nutrition," 37.
38 Jack Staub, *The Illustrated Book of Edible Plants* (Layton, UT: Gibbs Smith, 2017), 132.
39 John P. McKay, Bennett D. Hill, John Buckler, Clare Haru Crowston, Merry E. Wiesner-Hanks, and Joe Perry, *Understanding Western Society: A Brief History* (Boston and New York: Bedford/St. Martin's, 2012), 324.
40 Richard H. Steckel, *Health and Nutrition in the Preindustrial Era: Insights from a Millennium of Average Heights in Northern Europe* (Cambridge, MA: National Bureau of Economic Research, 2001), i, 18.

41 Joseph M. Prince and Richard H. Steckel, *Tallest in the World: Native Americans of the Great Plains in the Nineteenth Century* (Cambridge, MA: National Bureau of Economic Research, 1998), 29.
42 Ibid., 1, 29.
43 Steckel, 18.
44 Ibid., 19.
45 Ibid., 20.
46 Albala, 66.
47 Ibid, 37–38.
48 Ibid., 38.
49 Ibid., 66–67.
50 Hughes, 47.
51 Maguelonne Toussaint-Samat, *A History of Food*, expanded ed., trans. Anthea Bell (Chichester, UK: Wiley-Blackwell, 2009), 39.
52 Hughes, 48.
53 Ibid.
54 Ibid., 52.
55 Raymond Sokolov, "Culture and Obesity," *Social Research* 66, no. 1 (Spring 1999): 33.
56 Ibid; "Peas, Green, Raw."
57 "Peas, Green, Raw;" "FDA Vitamins and Minerals Chart," https://www.accessdata.fda.gov/scripts/interactivenutritionfactslabel/assets/InteractiveNFL_Vitamins&MineralsChart_March2020.pdf; "Vitamin E Fact Sheet for Consumers," *NIH*, last modified May 9, 2016, accessed April 24, 2019, https://ods.od.nih.gov/factsheets/VitaminE-Consumer.
58 "Food Weight to Volume," *AVCalc*, 2019, accessed May 7, 2019, https://www.aqua-calc.com/calculate/food-weight-to-volume/substance/peas-coma-and-blank-green-coma-and-blank-frozen-coma-and-blank-unprepared-blank--op-includes-blank-foods-blank-for-blank-usda-quote-s-blank-food-blank-distribution-blank-program-cp-.
59 Hughes, 48.
60 Sokolov, 35.
61 "McDonald's, Hamburger," *USDA FoodData Central*, April 1, 2019, accessed February 11, 2020, https://fdc.nal.usda.gov/fdc-app.html#/food-details/170717/nutrients.
62 C. Wayne Smith, *Crop Production: Evolution, History, and Technology* (New York: Wiley, 1995), 350.
63 Hughes, 70.
64 Theodore Hymowitz, "Soybeans: The Success Story," in *Advances in New Crops: Proceedings of the First National Symposium New Crops, Research, Development, Economics, Indianapolis, Indiana, October 23–26, 1988*, ed. Jules Janick and James E. Simon (Portland, OR: Timber Press, 1990), 159.
65 Sarah M. Nelson, "Conclusion," in *The Archaeology of Northeast China: Beyond the Great Wall*, ed. Sarah Milledge Nelson (London and New York: Routledge, 1995), 251–252.
66 Te-k'un Cheng, *The World of the Chinese: A Struggle for Human Unity* (Hong Kong: Chinese University Press, 1980), 7; Tan, 100.
67 Liu Zhen-hua, "Recent Neolithic Discoveries in Jilin Province," in *The Archaeology of Northeast China: Beyond the Great Wall*, ed. Sarah Milledge Nelson (London and New York: Routledge, 1995), 112.
68 Francoise Sabban, "China," in *The Cambridge World History of Food*, vol. 2, trans. Elborg Forster, ed. Kenneth F. Kiple and Kriemhild Conee Ornelas (Cambridge, UK: Cambridge University Press, 2000), 1166; Magner, 1184; Naomichi Ishige, "Japan," in *The Cambridge World History of Food*, vol. 2, ed. Kenneth F. Kiple and Kriemhild Conee Ornelas (Cambridge, UK: Cambridge University Press, 2000), 1175–1176.
69 Zhen-hua, 111–112.
70 Edward S. Deevey Jr., "The Human Population," *Scientific American* 203, no. 9 (September 1, 1960), 202.
71 Hughes, 59.
72 "Lecture on Soybeans and Their Products," accessed April 27, 2019, https://www.chefshalhoub.com/Soybeanlecture.htm.
73 C. Wayne Smith, 350.
74 Guo Da-shun, "Lower Xiajiadian Culture," in *The Archaeology of Northeast China: Beyond the Great Wall*, ed. Sarah Milledge Nelson (London and New York: Routledge, 1995), 147, 169.
75 Ibid., 169.
76 Garnsey, 59; Walter Scheidel, "Demography," in *The Cambridge Economic History of the Greco-Roman World*, ed. Walter Scheidel, Ian Morris, and Richard Saller (Cambridge, UK: Cambridge University Press, 2007), 38.

77 McKay, Hill, Buckler, Crowston, Wiesner-Hanks, and Perry, 212; H. V. Vallois, "The Social Life of Early Man: The Evidence of Skeletons," in *Social Life of Early Man*, ed. S. L. Washburn (Chicago: Aldine, 1961), 222.
78 C. Wayne Smith, 351.
79 Thomas Sorosiak, "Soybean," in *The Cambridge World History of Food*, vol. 1, ed. Kenneth F. Kiple and Kriemhild Conee Ornelas (Cambridge, UK: Cambridge University Press, 2000), 423.
80 Hymowitz, 159.
81 Erino Ozeki, "Fermented Soybean Products and Japanese Standard Taste," in *The World of Soy*, ed. Christine M. Du Bois, Chee-Beng Tan, and Sidney W. Mintz (Urbana and Chicago: University of Illinois Press, 2008), 151; James C. Riley, *Low Income, Social Growth, and Good Health: A History of Twelve Countries* (Berkeley: University of California Press, 2008), 53.
82 Katarzyna J. Cwiertka and Akiko Moriya, "Fermented Soyfoods in South Korea: The Industrialization of Tradition," in *The World of Soy*, ed. Christine M. Du Bois, Chee-Beng Tan, and Sidney W. Mintz (Urbana and Chicago: University of Illinois Press, 2008), 165.
83 Riley, 53.
84 Sorosiak, 423.
85 Hymowitz, 160.
86 Hughes, 60; C. Wayne Smith, 351.
87 Hughes, 60.
88 Theodore Hymowitz and Jack R. Harlan, "Introduction of the Soybean to North America by Samuel Bowen in 1765," *Economic Botany* 37, no. 4 (October 1983): 373–374.
89 Ibid., 375.
90 Hymowitz, 160.
91 C. Wayne Smith, 352.
92 A. H. Probst and Robert W. Judd, "Origin, United States History and Development, and World Distribution," in *Soybeans: Improvement, Production, and Uses*, ed. Billy E. Caldwell, Robert W. Howell, Robert W. Judd, and Herbert W. Johnson (Madison, WI: American Society of Agronomy, 1973), 11.
93 Hymowitz, 161.
94 Christine M. Du Bois, "Social Context and Diet: Changing Soy Production and Consumption in the United States," in *The World of Soy*, ed. Christine M. Du Bois, Chee-Beng Tan, and Sidney W. Mintz (Urbana and Chicago: University of Illinois Press, 2008), 209–210.
95 C. Wayne Smith, 352.
96 Hughes, 63.
97 Albala, 192.
98 Ibid., 193.
99 Du Bois, "Social Context and Diet," 214.
100 C. Wayne Smith, 297–298.
101 Andrew B. Jacobson, "Age of Industrialization and Agro-industry," in *The Cultural History of Plants*, ed. Ghillean Prance and Mark Nesbitt (New York and London: Routledge, 2005), 364–365.
102 Du Bois, "Social Context and Diet," 212.
103 C. Wayne Smith, 353, 356.
104 Du Bois, "Social Context and Diet," 213.
105 Hughes, 64.
106 C. Wayne Smith, 353.
107 Rubatzky and Yamaguchi, 509.
108 Toussaint-Samat, 46; Magner, 1185.
109 Johnson, 28; Linda Civitello, *Cuisine and Culture: A History of Food and People*, 3rd ed. (Hoboken, NJ: Wiley, 2011), 7.
110 "Beans," in *The Cambridge World History of Food*, vol. 2, ed. Kenneth F. Kiple and Kriemhild Conee Ornelas (Cambridge, UK: Cambridge University Press, 2000), 1729.
111 Lourdes Marquez Morfin, Robert McCaa, Rebecca Storey, and Andres Del Angel, "Health and Nutrition in Pre-Hispanic Mesoamerica," in *The Backbone of History: Health and Nutrition in the Western Hemisphere*, ed. Richard H. Steckel and Jerome C. Rose (Cambridge, UK: Cambridge University Press, 2002), 312–315.
112 Ibid., 313.
113 Ibid., 310.
114 Ibid., 319; Ann E. M. Liljas, "Old Age in Ancient Egypt," March 2, 2015, accessed January 18, 2019, https://blogs.ucl.ac.uk/researchers-in-museums/2015/03/02/old-age-in-ancient-egypt.

115 Morfin, McCaa, Storey, and Del Angel, 317.
116 Ibid., 321.
117 Prince and Steckel, 29.
118 Ibid., 1.
119 Steckel, i.
120 Ibid.; *World Atlas* (United States: Hammond Publications, 1999), 18, 151.
121 Lars G. Sandberg and Richard H. Steckel, "Soldier, Soldier, What Made You Grow So Tall? A Study of Height, Health, and Nutrition in Sweden, 1720–1881," *Economy and History* 23, no. 2 (1980): 92.
122 Morfin, McCaa, Storey, and Del Angel, 312–313.
123 Susan Kent, "Iron Deficiency and Anemia of Chronic Disease," in *The Cambridge World History of Food*, vol. 1, ed. Kenneth F. Kiple and Kriemhild Conee Ornelas (Cambridge, UK: Cambridge University Press, 2000), 922.
124 Morfin, McCaa, Storey, and Del Angel, 320, 322.
125 Ibid., 315.
126 Ibid., 311.
127 Ibid., 318–319.
128 Ibid., 321.
129 Lawrence Kaplan, "Beans, Peas, and Lentils," in *The Cambridge World History of Food*, vol. 1, ed. Kenneth F. Kiple and Kriemhild Conee Ornelas (Cambridge, UK: Cambridge University Press, 2000), 275.
130 Hughes, 57.
131 Richard H. Steckel, Jerome C. Rose, Clark Spencer Larsen, and Phillip L. Walker. "Skeletal Health in the Western Hemisphere from 4000 BC to the Present." *Evolutionary Anthropology* 11, no. 4 (August 13, 2002): 149–150.
132 Scheidel, 39.
133 Johnson, 30.
134 Ibid., 29.
135 Waverly Root and Richard de Rochemont, *Eating in America: A History* (Hopewell, NJ: Ecco Press, 1995), 44.
136 Johnson, 8.
137 Albala, 113.
138 J. G. Vaughan and C. A. Geissler, *The New Oxford Book of Food Plants: A Guide to the Fruit, Vegetables, Herbs and Spices of the World*, rev. ed. (Oxford: Oxford University Press, 1997), 48.
139 Jimmy Louie, "Breads and Cereals," in *Essentials of Human Nutrition*, 5th ed., ed. Jim Mann and A. Stewart Truswell (Oxford, UK: Oxford University Press, 2017), 274; Venn, 277.
140 Sarah Zielinski, "Man Cannot Live on Rice and Beans Alone (But Many Do)," *NPR*, May 3, 2012, accessed June 23, 2019, https://www.npr.org/sections/thesalt/2012/05/03/151932410/man-cannot-live-on-rice-and-beans-alone-but-many-do.
141 "Bean Nutrition Overview," The Bean Institute, 2019, accessed April 27, 2019, http://beaninstitute.com/bean-nutrition-overview; "Top Measurements: Beans, Dry Beans, Whole."
142 "Cowpeas Facts and Health Benefits," *Health Benefits Times*, accessed April 27, 2019, https://www.healthbenefitstimes.com/cowpeas.
143 Garden-Robinson and McNeal.
144 "Cowpeas Facts and Health Benefits."
145 Hughes, 69.
146 Ibid.
147 Johnson, 31–32.
148 Albala, 116.
149 Vaughan and Geissler, 40.
150 Simpson and Ogorzaly, 149.
151 C. Wayne Smith, 409; Hughes, 12; Rubatzky and Yamaguchi, 503.
152 Hughes, 13.
153 Ibid., 13.
154 C. Wayne Smith, 408–409.
155 Ibid., 409; R. O. Hammons, "The Origin and History of the Groundnut," in *The Groundnut Crop: A Scientific Basis for Improvement*, ed. J. Smartt (London: Chapman and Hall, 1994), 26–27.
156 Andrew F. Smith, *Peanuts: The Illustrious History of the Goober Pea* (Urbana and Chicago: University of Illinois Press, 2002), 8–9.

157 Venn, 277; Johnson, 56.
158 Venn, 277; C. Wayne Smith, 408.
159 Hughes, 25.
160 C. Wayne Smith, 411; Andrew F. Smith, 12–13; Johnson, 58.
161 C. Wayne Smith, 411.
162 Hughes, 16.
163 C. Wayne Smith, 412.
164 Johnson, 61.
165 Stephen Yafa, *Big Cotton: How a Humble Fiber Created Fortunes, Wrecked Civilizations, and Put America on the Map* (New York: Viking, 2005), 235.
166 Andrew F. Smith, 88.
167 Ibid., 91–94; Hughes, 17.
168 Andrew F. Smith, 96–98.
169 C. Wayne Smith, 412.
170 Hughes, 28.
171 Andrew F. Smith, 42.
172 C. Wayne Smith, 412.
173 Andrew F. Smith, 50.
174 C. Wayne Smith, 414.
175 Andrew F. Smith, 89.
176 C. Wayne Smith, 422.
177 Ibid., 425–426.
178 Andrew F. Smith, 133.
179 Ibid., 83.
180 Ibid., 120.
181 Ibid., 131.
182 Ibid., 132.
183 Ibid., 87.
184 Ibid., 117, 205, 210; Michael Burgan, *George Washington Carver: Scientist, Inventor, and Teacher* (Minneapolis, MN: Compass Point Books, 2007), 69.
185 Andrew F. Smith, 117.
186 Ibid., 89.
187 "Peanuts, All Types, Raw."
188 Alfred E. Harper, "Recommended Dietary Allowances and Dietary Guidelines," in *The Cambridge World History of Food*, vol. 2, ed. Kenneth F. Kiple and Kriemhild Conee Ornelas (Cambridge, UK: Cambridge University Press, 2000), 1617.
189 J. D. L. Hansen, "Protein-Energy Malnutrition," in *The Cambridge World History of Food*, vol. 1, ed. Kenneth F. Kiple and Kriemhild Conee Ornelas (Cambridge, UK: Cambridge University Press, 2000), 980–982.
190 T. Colin Campbell, *Whole: Rethinking the Science of Nutrition* (Dallas, TX: BenBella Books, 2013), xi.
191 Ibid, xi–xii; T. Colin Campbell and Thomas M. Campbell II, *The China Study*, rev. ed. (Dallas, TX: BenBella Books, 2016), 27–28.
192 Campbell, 31.
193 "Peanut Butter May Help Overcome Malnutrition in Developing World," *Voice of America*, October 29, 2009, accessed July 2, 2019, https://www.voanews.com/archive/peanut-butter-may-help-overcome-malnutrition-developing-world-2002-03-20; Nathan Collins, "Are Peanuts the Answer to Preventing Malnutrition in Africa?" February 10, 2016, accessed July 2, 2019, https://psmag.com/social-justice/is-preventing-malnutrition-in-africa-as-easy-as-peanuts.
194 Andrew F. Smith, 13–15.
195 Marcie Cohen Ferris, *The Edible South: The Power of Food and the Making of an American Region* (Chapel Hill: University of North Carolina Press, 2014), 12, 14.
196 Ibid, 12.
197 Ibid.
198 Robert William Fogel and Stanley L. Engerman, *Time on the Cross: The Economics of American Negro Slavery* (New York and London: Norton, 1995), 111–113.
199 Richard H. Steckel, "Birth Weights and Infant Mortality among American Slaves," *Explorations in Economic History* 23, no. 2 (April 1986): 174.
200 Ibid., 175.

201 Fogel and Engerman, 112–113.
202 Ibid., 113, 115.
203 Ibid., 113.
204 Ibid., 109.
205 April McGreger, *Sweet Potatoes* (Chapel Hill: University of North Carolina Press, 2014), 6.
206 Jeremy Atack and Peter Passell, *A New Economic View of American History*, 2d ed. (New York and London: Norton, 1994), 345.
207 Ibid., 343.
208 Fogel and Engerman, 25.
209 Ibid., 29.
210 Ibid., 125.
211 Richard S. Dunn, *Sugar and Slaves: The Rise of the Planter Class in the English West Indies, 1624–1713* (Chapel Hill: University of North Carolina Press, 1972), 301.
212 Ibid., 302–317.
213 Atack and Passell, 348.
214 Ibid., 381.
215 Ibid., 382.
216 Ted A. Rathbun and Richard H. Steckel, "The Health of Slaves and Free Blacks in the East," in *The Backbone of History: Health and Nutrition in the Western Hemisphere*, ed. Richard H. Steckel and Jerome C. Rose (Cambridge, UK: Cambridge University Press, 2002), 221.
217 Ibid., 214, 220.
218 Jessica Campisi and Brandon Griggs, "Nearly 100 Bodies Found at a Texas Construction Site Were Probably Black People Forced into Labor—after Slavery Ended," July 19, 2018, accessed January 18, 2019, https://www.cnn.com/2018/07/18/us/bodies-found-construction-site-slavery-trnd/index.html.
219 U.S. Const. amend. XIII.
220 Brian Duignan, ed., *Economics and Economic Systems* (New York: Britannica, 2013), 84.
221 Atack and Passell, 542.
222 Nancy A. Hewitt and Steven F. Lawson, *Exploring American Histories: A Brief Survey with Sources* (Boston and New York: Bedford/St. Martin's, 2013), 531.
223 Joshua Freeman, Nelson Lichtenstein, Stephen Brier, David Bensman, Susan Porter Benson, David Brundage, Bret Eynon, Bruce Levin, and Bryan Palmer, *Who Built America?: Working People and the Nation's Economy, Politics, Culture, and Society, vol. 2: From the Gilded Age to the Present* (New York: Pantheon Books, 1992), 280.
224 Hewitt and Lawson, 529.
225 David Bacon, *In the Fields of the North* (University of California Press, 2016), 36.

9 Nuts

9.1 DEFINITION

Modern taxonomy's originator, Swedish naturalist Carl von Linne (1707–1778)—better known as Carolus Linnaeus—defined a nut as a seed with rigid skin.[1] Among botanists, this idea has yielded to the definition of a nut as a fruit within a shell. Chapter 14 defines a fruit as a flower's fertilized ovary, which develops to hold seeds. A nut, therefore, has an additional structure—a shell that encases a fruit—and so is more than a fruit by itself and more than Linnaeus' seed inside unyielding skin. The botanical definition of a nut, in excluding mere seeds within shells, rejects naming almonds (*Amygdalus communis*), pecans (*Carya illinoinensis*), and walnuts (*Juglans regia*) as nuts. Some edibles that are branded nuts—for example, coconuts (*Cocos nucifera*), peanuts (*Arachis hypogaea*), pine nuts (*Pinus* species), Brazil nuts (*Bertholletia excelsa*), and Grape nuts—are also not nuts. Grape nuts flagrantly misuse language, being neither grapes (*Vitis vinifera*) nor nuts.

As is true of vegetables (see Chapter 15), confusion obscured the attempt to separate true nuts from imposters. To clarify the issue, American food historian Ken Albala (b. 1964) crafted a definition that satisfies much of what the public thinks about nuts and borrows from Linnaeus. Albala stipulated first that nuts grow on trees, a requirement that affirms popular opinion by including walnuts, pecans, and almonds, and that at the same time rejects the commonplace that peanuts are nuts.[2] Yet this first condition does not exclude tree fruits such as apples (*Malus domestica*), oranges (*Citrus sinensis* and *C. aurantium*), grapefruits (*Citrus paradisi*), apricots (*Prunus armeniaca*), plums (*Prunus domestica*), peaches (*Prunus persica*), pears (*Pyrus communis*), cherries (*Prunus avium, P. cerasus*, and *P. serotina*), figs (*Ficus carica*), dates (*Phoenix dactylifera*), pomegranates (*Punica granatum*), and many more. The second stipulation, asserting the Linnaean criterion of a shell, disqualifies tree fruits. Even fruits with rind, like citrus, can be pealed and so lack a rigid exterior. Third, Albala defined nuts as edibles, a requirement that retains items, like acorns, that need processing (discussed later) before consumption. Finally, nuts must be crunchy rather than soft, another concession to popular sentiment.

9.2 PREHISTORY AND HISTORY

Because little besides shells persists in the archaeological record, nut consumption's origin is uncertain.[3] Albala suspected that humanity's ancestors ate nuts, though the first to do so is unknown. Early hominids must have favored them because cooking was unnecessary whereas it was desirable or essential for meat and tough roots and tubers. Fire's control about 1 million years ago, discussed in Chapter 3, allowed humans to boil nuts, but the practice neither enhanced flavor nor eased chewing.[4] Nuts must have frustrated attempts to skewer and roast, though baking them with meat or vegetables might have appealed to hunter-gatherers. Writing's invention around 3300 BCE permitted the preservation of recipes—the first for nuts appeared about 1600 BCE—on clay or papyrus.[5]

This chronology notes that scientists and scholars know little about nuts' prehistory. Paucity of knowledge invites speculation and contrary opinions, a problem Chapter 1 identified in the current debate over diet, nutrition, and health. Swedish family physician Andreas Eenfeldt (b. 1972) and American neurologist David Perlmutter (b. 1954)—introduced in Chapter 1—joined Albala in averring that preagricultural peoples ate nuts, though no such claim came from American nutritionist and exercise physiologist Loren Cordain (b. 1950), who favored game, fish, fruits, and vegetables as staples.[6] Concentration on nuts permitted Perlmutter to suppose that humanity's ancestors derived three-quarters of calories from fat, an assertion that the next chapter disputes.[7] Situating nuts at the dawn of humankind reinforces belief in their naturalness, a conviction that allows contrast between hunter-gatherer purity and agrarian taint. These opposites place our ancestors in Eden and denigrate agriculture as a fall from grace, an oversimplification dispelled in Chapter 3.

This book cannot determine whether nuts deserve acclaim as among the first foods. Our aim is to gauge their health effects in prehistory and history. Not all nuts can or should receive scrutiny because only a few were staples. In this group, chestnuts (*Castanea* species) and acorns (*Quercus* species) nourished Amerindians, Europeans, and Asians. The best data on chestnuts come from the study of eighteenth-century French peasants examined in Chapter 7 and on acorns from research on prehistoric Californians. Later sections treat both.

9.3 CONSUMPTION AND NUTRITION

9.3.1 Nuts as Energy

Because most have plentiful fat, nuts furnished energy amid the food shortages that characterized all but recent times. This dearth made them as valuable for oil as for consumption whole.[8] By mass, most nuts range between 45 and 75 percent fat, though chestnuts have only 2.7 percent according to Australian dietician Margaret Allman-Farinelli and between 1 and 3 percent, wrote French historian Antoinette Fauve-Chamoux (b. 1945).[9] At the upper bound, macadamia nuts (*Macadamia ternifolia* and *M. tetraphylla*) are 77.6 percent fat by mass, though the U.S. Department of Agriculture (USDA) puts the percentage at 75.77.[10] Using the USDA figure, 100 grams of macadamia nuts contain 75.77 grams of fat. At 9.4 calories per gram of fat (see Chapter 2), these nuts supply 712.24 of their 718 calories (99.2 percent) per 100 grams as oil. Nut oils tend to be unsaturated rather than saturated, earning praise from nutritionists, dieticians, and medical practitioners. Macadamia nuts have abundant monounsaturated fatty acids, which Chapter 2 defined. Among polyunsaturated acids, walnuts have omega 3 and omega 6, both essential and discussed in Chapter 2. In addition to fat, nuts' energy density derives from low water content.

For these reasons, nuts are among the most caloric foods. The previous paragraph listed 718 calories in 100 grams of macadamia nuts. Other caloric nuts per 100 grams include pecans at 687.8 calories, Brazil nuts at 652.6 calories, pine nuts at 629, walnuts at 617.3, almonds at 600, cashews (*Anacardium occidentale*) at 582, and pistachios (*Pistacia vera*) at 564.4.[11] These numbers contrast with vegetables like cabbage (*Brassica oleracea var. capitata*) at 17.6 calories per 100 grams, iceberg lettuce (*Lactuca sativa var. capitata*) at 14.1, spinach (*Spinacia oleracea*) at 24.7, and carrots (*Daucus carota ssp. sativus*), celery (*Apium graveolens*), broccoli (*Brassica oleracea var. italica*), and brussels sprouts (*Brassica oleracea var. gemmifera*) at 35.2.[12] Tables 9.1 and 9.2 aid comparison between these nuts and vegetables by listing their calories and fat.

TABLE 9.1
Calories and Fat in Selected Nuts 100g

Nut	Calories	Fat (g)
Macadamia	718	75.77
Pecan	687.8	70.5
Brazil	652.6	67
Walnut	617.3	60
Pine nut	823.1	82.3
Almond	600	52.9
Cashew	582	49.4
Pistachio	564.4	45.9

TABLE 9.2
Calories and Fat in Selected Vegetables 100 g

Vegetable	Calories	Fat (g)
Cabbage	17.6	0
Celery	35.2	0
Iceberg lettuce	14.1	0
Spinach	24.7	0
Carrot	35.2	0
Brussels sprout	35.2	0
Broccoli	35.2	0
Onion	44.1	0

9.3.2 Nuts as Nutrient Packages

This book emphasizes that calories alone are an inadequate gauge of food. A better measure is nutrient density. Although macro and micronutrients may differ by species, most nuts supply fiber, protein, iron, zinc, potassium, calcium, magnesium, and vitamins B_1 (thiamine or thiamin), B_2 (riboflavin), B_3 (niacin or nicotinic acid), and E.[13] Protein varies between 2 and 25 percent by mass. Unlike animal products, nuts do not supply all essential amino acids, discussed in Chapter 2. Like grains, they lack lysine.[14] Chapter 8 referenced legumes as good sources of this amino acid; their combination with nuts yields complete protein.

9.3.3 Chestnut Nutrients

With an eye toward later sections, this paragraph introduces chestnuts, whose value depends partly on whether they are fresh or dried. Fauve-Chamoux judged 100 grams of fresh chestnuts as 40–60 percent water, 30–50 percent carbohydrates, 1–3 percent fat, and 3–7 percent protein.[15] Differences in climate and soils affect nutrients, especially minerals. Drying concentrates calories by removing water but may reduce nutrients, especially water-soluble vitamins. For example, drying increases calories in 100 grams of chestnuts from roughly 200–370. Although essential to health, water is sometimes omitted from nutritional considerations.

The USDA furnishes data for fresh and dried chestnuts from *Castanea sativa* and unspecified Chinese and Japanese species. Rather than ponder all possibilities, this section considers dried *C. sativa* nuts to permit comparison with dried acorns, the next paragraphs' topic. Concentration on the European chestnut *C. sativa* anticipates later treatment of French peasants, who ate this species' nuts. Table 9.3 shows calories and nutrients in 100 grams.[16] Dried and fresh chestnuts are notable sources of vitamin C, 100 grams of fresh *C. sativa*, boiled and steamed, having 44.5 percent.[17] Attention may focus on this vitamin, which chestnuts supply abundantly in contrast to other nuts. Apparently ignoring chestnuts, Allman-Farinelli erred by stating that "Nuts and seeds contain no vitamin C."[18]

9.3.4 Acorns' Tannins

Discussed more fully in a later section, acorns vary in the amount of tannins, toxins that prevent protein absorption, inhibit many enzymes, cause fatigue, and impair growth.[19] Defining the cupule as an acorn's top, tannins concentrate at the bottom. For this reason, insects, squirrels (species in the family Sciuridae), blue jays (*Cyanocitta cristata*), and grackles (*Quiscalus* and *Macroagelaius* species, *Hypopyrrhus pyrohypogaster*, and *Lampropsar tanagrinus*) eat the top and middle, consuming little if any of the bottom.[20] Another way to minimize tannins is to eat the least bitter acorns—sometimes

TABLE 9.3
Nutrients in Dried *Castanea sativa* 100 g

Nutrient	Chestnuts	%DV
Calories	374	N/A
Protein (g)	6.39	N/A
Fat (g)	4.45	N/A
Carbs (g)	77.31	N/A
Fiber (g)	11.7	N/A
Minerals		
Ca (mg)	67	6.7
Fe (mg)	2.38	13.2
Mg (mg)	74	18.5
P (mg)	175	17.5
K (mg)	986	28.2
Na (mg)	37	1.5
Zn (mg)	0.35	2.3
Cu (mg)	0.65	32.5
Mn (mg)	1.3	65
Se (mcg)	1.8	2.6
Vitamins		
A (IU)	0	0
B_1 (mg)	0.3	20
B_2 (mg)	0.36	21.2
B_3 (mg)	0.85	4.3
B_5 (mg)	0.9	9
B_6 (mg)	0.66	33
B_9 (mcg)	109	27.3
B_{12} (mcg)	0	0
C (mg)	15	25
D (IU)	0	0
E (mg)	N/A	N/A
K (mcg)	N/A	N/A

designated sweet—because bitterness correlates with tannin content. Deciduous *Quercus* species have between 3.2 and 6.7 percent tannins whereas evergreen species range between 1.2 and 2.5 percent.[21]

Humans solved the problem of tannins by soaking bitter acorns in water before consumption to leach tannins.[22] American agronomist Jack Rodney Harlan (1917–1998) deemed treatment unnecessary for sweet acorns, though the Japanese soaked all acorns.[23] With or without this practice, the nuts were often ground and dried to make a flour substitute. Table 9.4 lists calories and nutrients in 100 grams of dried acorns.[24]

9.3.5 Comparison of Chestnuts and Acorns

The foregoing implies that both nuts benefit consumers, though neither has all nutrients. Chestnuts are the lone source of vitamin C and have more carbohydrates, calcium, iron, phosphorus, potassium, selenium, and vitamins B_1 and B_2 by mass whereas acorns have more calories, protein, fat, fiber, magnesium, zinc, copper, manganese, and vitamins A, B_3, B_5, B_6, and B_9, and no sodium. Neither has vitamins B_{12} and D, though both have minerals, some B vitamins, carbohydrates, fat, and protein. The fact that humans cannot rely on one nut, or one food, for complete nourishment—though

TABLE 9.4
Nutrients in Dried Acorns 100 g

Nutrient	Acorns	%DV
Calories	509	N/A
Protein (g)	8.1	N/A
Fat (g)	31.41	N/A
Carbs (g)	53.66	N/A
Fiber (g)	14.3	N/A
	Minerals	
Ca (mg)	54	5.4
Fe (mg)	1.04	5.8
Mg (mg)	82	20.5
P (mg)	103	10.3
K (mg)	709	20.3
Na (mg)	0	0
Zn (mg)	0.67	4.5
Cu (mg)	0.82	41
Mn (mg)	1.36	68
Se (mcg)	0	0
	Vitamins	
A (IU)	39	0.8
B_1 (mg)	0.15	10
B_2 (mg)	0.15	8.8
B_3 (mg)	2.41	12.1
B_5 (mg)	0.94	9.4
B_6 (mg)	0.7	35
B_9 (mcg)	115	28.8
B_{12} (mcg)	0	0
C (mg)	0	0
D (IU)	0	0
E (mg)	10.78	71.9
K (mcg)	N/A	N/A

Chapter 13 indicates that potatoes (*Solanum tuberosum*) come close—underscores the wisdom of a balanced diet. Premodern peoples, too often under threat or actuality of shortage, could not always eat a variety of foods.

9.4 CHESTNUTS

9.4.1 Origins and Antiquity

In the Fagaceae family, *Castanea* species yielded the chestnuts that nourished Asians, North Africans, Europeans, and Amerindians since prehistory. The generic name may derive from Kastana in northern Greece or Kastanis, Turkey.[25] *C. sativa* is the symbol of Castanea, Italy, another candidate for the generic name's origin. Alternatively, these regions may have been named after the chestnut. The link between *Castanea* and these lands suggests the Mediterranean basin as an area of domestication. Researcher Georgina Pearman at the Eden Project in Cornwall, England, favored domestication in Turkey and between the Black and Caspian Seas, with later dispersal west throughout the Mediterranean.[26]

East Asia originated four species: *Castanea crenata* in Japan and Korea, and the Chinese chestnut (*Castanea mollissima*), the dwarf Chinese chestnut (*Castanea seguini*), and the Chinese chinquapin (*Castanea henryi*) in China. Southwestern Asia and northwestern Africa—an area known as the Maghreb—have *Castanea sativa*. North America was the cradle of the American chestnut (*Castanea dentata*) and the Alleghany chinquapin (*Castanea pumila*).

Greek physicians Pedanius Dioscorides (c. 40–90 CE) and Galen (130–210 CE) noted chestnuts' importance as food throughout the Mediterranean, warning that excessive consumption caused flatulence.[27] Because these doctors treated the wealthy, their concern indicated that elites ate the nuts, though from early times they fed principally the poor.

9.4.2 Pedology and Geography

Trees were numerous in mountains, hills, and soils unsuitable for grains, whose absence left chestnuts as sustenance. Mountains and hillsides tended to have soils—sandy or rocky but not clay, for example—that drained well, a necessity for chestnut roots, which rotted when wet. Where conditions dictated, transition to agriculture favored *C. sativa* rather than wheat (*Triticum monococcum*, *T. dicoccon*, *T. aestivum*, and *T. durum*), barley (*Hordeum vulgare*), millet (species in Eragrostideae tribe), grapes (*Vitis vinifera*), olives (*Olea europaea*), broad beans (*Vicia faba*), or other Mediterranean crops.

Beyond pedological matters, geography determined chestnuts trees' utility. Because they seldom fruited above 52 degrees north, growers who wanted more than timber had to live below much of Canada, northern Europe, and Russia.[28] Although trees survive without human assistance, plentiful nut production requires grafting and pruning. Without both, nuts tend to be small and trees are usually more vulnerable to the diseases that devastated American and European species after roughly 1850.

9.4.3 Chestnuts in North America

Before chestnut blight fungus *Cryphonectria parasitica* reached North America around 1900, the continent may have had 4 billion chestnut trees.[29] Native to what is today southern Ontario, Canada, and the eastern United States, *C. dentata* was among the most numerous members of the region's deciduous forests. One account held that before the fungus' arrival, a squirrel could travel from Maine to Georgia without touching the ground, so ubiquitous were chestnut trees.[30] Up to 40 meters (130 feet) tall, the species was conspicuous as "the king of trees," "the queen of trees," and the "redwood of the east."[31]

Another label, "the farmer's friend," acknowledged rural reliance on the tree's nuts and wood.[32] American forester Harold Scofield Betts mythologized the chestnut's "close association with the early home life of this country."[33] Dependence was evident in Appalachia, where *C. dentata* may have totaled one-quarter of trees.[34] As elsewhere, Appalachia's hillsides suited chestnut trees rather than grains. The region's small farmers relied on the nuts for food and cash, selling them for transit to cities, where residents bought them from street vendors.[35] In good years, chestnuts fetched more income than cattle (*Bos taurus*) in parts of Appalachia. Growers filled attics with the harvest's remainder, eating nuts during winter.

This dependence predated European contact. For example, Iroquois near the Great Lakes ate chestnuts raw, boiled them, and added them to cornbread.[36] Southeastern Cherokee created chestnut orchards by killing competing flora. *C. dentata*'s small nuts disappointed Europeans, who planted *C. sativa*. Third U.S. President Thomas Jefferson (1743–1826) raised *C. sativa* at his home in Charlottesville, Virginia.[37] At the continent's western end, American horticulturist Luther Burbank (1849–1926) used *C. crenata* to breed new chestnut varieties. By 1886, his nursery had some 10,000 chestnut hybrids.[38]

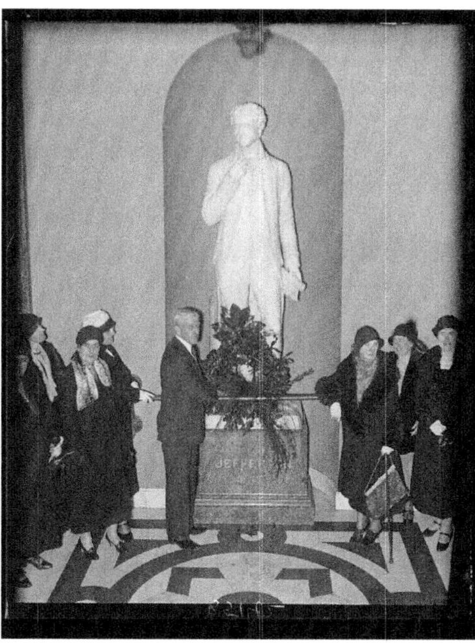

FIGURE 9.1 Thomas Jefferson. (Photo courtesy of Library of Congress. https://www.loc.gov/pictures/item/2016879561/.)

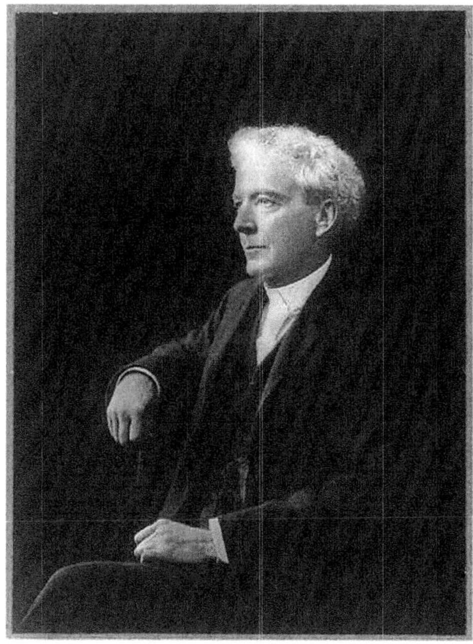

FIGURE 9.2 Luther Burbank. (Photo courtesy of Library of Congress. https://www.loc.gov/pictures/item/2016879561/.)

So important were chestnuts that they sustained North America's fauna. Not only humans, but also bears (*Ursus americanus*), elk (*Cervus canadensis*), squirrels (*Sciurus carolinensis*), raccoons (*Procyon lotor*), mice (*Peromyscus leucopus* and *Mus musculus*), wild turkeys (*Meleagris gallopavo*), and passenger pigeons (*Ectopistes migratorius*) ate the nuts. Chestnut blight's destruction of *C. dentata* may have hastened wild turkeys' extinction.[39] Besides these animals, European introduction of livestock into the Americas added another layer of chestnut consumers. Rather than feed them, stockmen expected pigs (*Sus scrofa domesticus*) to forage for nuts. The result was tender pork, though the flavor was stronger than meat from cornfed hogs and counter to American and Canadian preferences.[40] Where chestnuts were adequate for livestock, farmers did not need land for pasture.

9.4.4 Chestnuts in Europe

Across the Atlantic Ocean, *C. sativa* grew from Portugal and Spain in the west to Iran in the east.[41] During the first millennium BCE, Europeans began cooking chestnuts, likely by roasting.[42] Romans ground chestnuts into flour to mix with barley, wheat, rye (*Secale cereale*), or another grain to extend bread, a custom that persists in southern Europe. Rome planted chestnut trees wherever they would grow in the provinces as part of an effort to integrate disparate peoples into the empire; its dissolution in the fifth century CE did not diminish reliance on the nuts.[43] In the sixteenth century, French anatomist and physician Charles Estienne (1504–1564) and French agronomist and physician Jean Liebault (1535–1596) wrote that "an infinity of people live on nothing else but this fruit [the chestnut]".[44] Dependence extended to hilly Tuscany, Italy, where a nineteenth-century Italian agronomist stated that "the fruit of the chestnut tree is practically the sole subsistence of our highlanders."[45] In 1879, French economist Pierre Guillaume Frederic le Play (1806–1882) remarked that "chestnuts almost exclusively nourish entire populations for half a year."[46]

This duration was not hyperbole. With less fat than other nuts, chestnuts were slow to turn rancid. They lasted about three months fresh and two or three years dried.[47] Collected in October, fresh chestnuts endured through mid-January, sustaining peasants during winter's lean months. Because farmers ate most of what they gathered, few nuts entered trade. For example, in 1872, Paris imported only around 5.4 million kilograms (6,000 tons) of France's 453.6 million-kilogram (500,000-ton) harvest. Because *C. sativa* did not drop nuts at once, the harvest typically lasted over three weeks and involved an entire family. Ten hours' exertions yielded from 50 to 150 kilograms (110.2 to 330.7 pounds) of nuts. A family sold the largest, fed the smallest—about one-fifth of the harvest—to pigs or poultry, and kept the rest.

Two hectares (4.9 acres) of *C. sativa* carpeted the ground with 4,989.5 kilograms (5.5 tons) of nuts, according to an estimate that omitted planting density.[48] Allotting 175 trees per hectare (seventy per acre), British agronomist and economist Arthur Young (1741–1820) wrote that 0.4 hectares (1 acre) of trees produced enough chestnuts to feed one man for fourteen months.[49] Judging this arrangement too dense, Fauve-Chamoux estimated thirty-five to one hundred trees per hectare (fourteen to twenty-five trees per acre) and a harvest of roughly 2,800 kilograms (6,172.9 pounds) of chestnuts. At 2 kilograms (4.4 pounds) of nuts per person, this produce would have fed a family of five for nearly seven months with enough left for one or two pigs. Chestnuts were eaten raw, in porridge or soup, or as bread or pancakes.

9.4.5 Chestnuts' Problems

Although important in diets, chestnuts waned in the eighteenth century. Europe's frigid 1709 winter killed countless trees.[50] As the century progressed, opinion held that the nuts had few nutrients and were fit only for pigs. Economists, sure that cash crops alone generated wealth, decried chestnuts as a remnant of subsistence and a waste of land. Between 1823 and 1832, Italy uprooted around 43,000 chestnut trees south of the Alps in an area known as Piedmont. France's chestnut hectarage declined from 578,224 in 1852 to 309,412 in 1892, to 167,940 in 1929, and to about 32,000 in 1975.

Exacerbating these woes, the fungus *Phytophthora cambivora* struck Italy's chestnut trees in 1842, spreading to Portugal in 1853 and France in 1860.[51] Around 1904 *C. parasitica*, mentioned earlier, entered the New York Zoological Park (now the Bronx Zoo) in New York City, where several trees ailed.[52] By 1911, the park had only two live trees, both of which later died. Between 1904 and 1954, the fungus spread from Canada to the Gulf of Mexico and from New York City to California, Oregon, and Washington.[53] By 1920, New Jersey had just twenty-five living chestnut trees, none of which survived. Up to 4 billion Canadian and U.S. trees succumbed to blight during the twentieth century.[54]

This destruction brought East Asia to prominence. The world's leading chestnut grower, China harvested over 80 percent of the global total in 2016, though success came centuries earlier.[55] Northeast of what is today Beijing, Miyun District emerged as China's primary producer before Jesus' birth. Its farmers raised more chestnuts than any other commodity, exporting the surplus to Japan, Korea, and Southeast Asia. What is not sold abroad feeds China's cities. Beyond China, Turkey and South Korea ranked third and fourth worldwide in chestnut metric tonnage in 2016, and Japan and North Korea were ninth and tenth. Outside Asia, Bolivia ranked second. Resuscitating arboriculture, Italy, Greece, Portugal, and Spain also occupied the top ten.

9.4.6 Chestnuts and Health in France

Chapter 7 examined diets, nutrition, and health among rural poor in eighteenth-century Gevaudan, southern France. Evidence came from twenty-three wills and marriage contracts that detailed pensioners' diets, in Table 7.2, between 1754 and 1767. These documents listed one ration of chestnuts: 90 liters or 54.4 kilograms (119.9 pounds) annually for a recipient in Prevencheres, near Cevennes' chestnut forest in southern France.[56] This amount allotted a daily average of just 149 grams (5.3 ounces) of chestnuts, well below Fauve-Chamoux's estimate of 1–2 kilograms (2.2–4.4 pounds) throughout history.[57] Greater is her approximation of 2 kilograms per person daily in the nineteenth century.[58] Even the low figure of 1 kilogram surpasses 149 grams nearly sevenfold. The pensioner's meager quantity underscored his or her poverty, as Chapter 7 acknowledged.

The pensioner was not alone. Mass impoverishment characterizes history, as the coterie of elites increased their wealth by extracting more blood from innumerable tiny turnips metaphorically representing commoners. A problem throughout the past has been the growth of population beyond the land's capacity to feed it. In agrarian France, families divided property among offspring, a practice that shrank hectarage per person whenever birthrate rose faster than mortality.[59] This difficulty arose as population rebounded after the Black Death (1347–1351), mentioned in Chapters 1 and 3. In this context, dietary information between 1754 and 1767 came at a crucial juncture given unabated land division between roughly 1750 and 1770.[60] All else equal, small holdings yielded less than large ones, impoverishing the land's tillers.

The poorest occupied less than 1 hectare (2.5 acres), too little to support a family.[61] Between 1700 and 1792, the number of these farms in Basse Auvergne in south-central France grew from 490 to 870 as rents tripled. Peasants tried to earn cash by migrating to large farms in search of employment or taking piece work from nascent industries. These efforts did not mitigate "chronic undernutrition."[62]

Conditions were dismal in the mountains, where chestnuts fed peasants. French historian Emmanuel Bernard Le Roy Ladurie (b. 1929) described their "low living standard and deplorable state of health."[63] Work earned them little beyond chestnuts and fatty pork.[64] Even prosperous landlords added only wheat and wine to this duo.

The pensioner who relied on chestnuts was thus no anomaly. The daily 149 grams were not the sole sustenance because his or her allotment also listed rye, probably as bread.[65] Striking, however, is absence of any other food in this pension. Setting aside rye, this inquiry would benefit from knowing whether 149 grams of chestnuts per day were typical in mid-eighteenth-century France. Fauve-Chamoux's estimate of 1–2 kilograms daily, already noted, implies that the pensioner was atypical. Ladurie specified no amounts, though he gave the impression that they were large by recounting bucolic scenes of sixteenth-century girls passing winter around the fireplace eating roasted chestnuts until they could stomach no more.[66] Even if this language is accurate, what characterized the sixteenth century may not have typified the mid-eighteenth century.

Without a guide, this section assumes a low of 149 grams of chestnuts per day in the mid-eighteenth century and a maximum of 2 kilograms, Fauve-Chamoux's upper bound. The mean of these numbers is 1,074.5 grams (1.0745 kilograms or 37.9 ounces) daily and, absent a better estimate, serves as the typical ration. This quantity's calories and nutrients depend on whether chestnuts were fresh or dried. Ladurie's imagery of roasted chestnuts does not help because they need not have been dried beforehand. Neither does this section benefit from knowing that he chose winter for the fireplace scene because, as noted, Fauve-Chamoux stated that chestnuts gathered in autumn stored until mid-January without drying. Because winter lingers until about March 20, it seems fair to assume that at least some chestnuts were dried before ingestion. Moreover, year-round consumption necessitated drying given collection only in autumn. Rather than try to fabricate a proportion of fresh versus dry, this section simplifies calculations by assuming that all chestnuts were dried before consumption even as it acknowledges that this scenario is likely to be fiction to a greater or lesser extent.

Returning to the USDA database, 1,074.5 grams of dried *C. sativa* nuts have 4,018.6 calories, an amount near Fauve-Chamoux's 4,000-calorie estimate.[67] This rough equivalence confirms the appropriateness of our surmise that 1,074.5 grams of chestnuts typified mid-eighteenth-century daily consumption in France. Table 9.5 lists nutrients in this quantity.[68]

TABLE 9.5
Nutrients in Dried *Castanea sativa* 1074.5 g (1.0745 kg)

Nutrient	Chestnuts	%DV
Protein (g)	68.66	N/A
Fat (g)	47.82	N/A
Carbs (g)	830.7	N/A
Fiber (g)	125.72	N/A
	Minerals	
Ca (mg)	719.92	72
Fe (mg)	25.57	142.1
Mg (mg)	795.13	198.8
P (mg)	1,880.38	188
K (mg)	10,594.57	302.7
Na (mg)	397.57	16.6
Zn (mg)	3.76	25.1
Cu (mg)	6.98	349.2
Mn (mg)	13.97	698.4
Se (mcg)	19.34	27.6
	Vitamins	
A (IU)	0	0
B_1 (mg)	3.22	214.9
B_2 (mg)	3.87	227.5
B_3 (mg)	9.13	45.7
B_5 (mg)	9.67	96.7
B_6 (mg)	7.09	354.6
B_9 (mcg)	1,171.2	292.8
B_{12} (mcg)	0	0
C (mg)	161.18	268.6
D (IU)	0	0
E (mg)	N/A	N/A
K (mcg)	N/A	N/A

These amounts indicate that aside from fat-soluble vitamins A, D, E, and K, 1,074.5 grams of chestnuts approached or exceeded current recommendations for daily nutrient intake.

These data support Fauve-Chamoux's assertion that "chestnuts provide a balanced diet" and question British historian Olwen H. Hufton's (b. 1938) claim that roughly 30–70 percent of eighteenth-century French were undernourished.[69] Ladurie's estimate that about one-third of Frenchmen subsisted on under 1,800 calories per day in the 1780s more than halves this section's calculation of 4,018.6—and Fauve-Chamoux's 4,000—calories. Today 4,000 calories daily all but guarantee obesity. This book emphasizes, however, that current standards are inappropriate for the past given widespread inactivity among people dependent on automobiles and other machines since roughly the 1920s. Summarizing modernity's sloth, British-American nutritionist Peter L. Pellett (1928–2018) wrote in 2000 that "Average physical activity in Western society is now considered to be undesirably low."[70]

Today's indolence contrasted with eighteenth-century French rural poor's exertions. Ladurie described the toil of erecting and repairing walls on steep mountainsides and grafting and pruning chestnut trees.[71] Although these comments applied to the sixteenth century, technology did not change to lessen strenuousness two centuries later. This book notes that before mechanization, people had little besides muscles to accomplish an employer's dictates. This reality needs no belaboring except that modern life differs so radically from past arduousness.

The issue, then, is whether 4,018.6 calories daily were adequate for eighteenth-century French peasants. This intake compares with American economist, historian, and 1993 Nobel laureate in economics Robert William Fogel (1926–2013) and American economist and historian Stanley Lewis Engerman's (b. 1936) estimate, mentioned last chapter, that nineteenth-century U.S. slaves ingested nearly 4,200 calories daily.[72] Early twentieth-century allotments gave U.S. soldiers 3,851 calories daily and sailors almost 5,000.[73] Agreement among these numbers is close but imperfect, leading this section to seek additional corroboration.

One attempt along these lines approximates energy metabolized to determine whether intake and expenditure aligned. Expenditures cannot be pinpointed and must have varied with the day's demands. Absent precision, an estimate must suffice and can be determined in at least two ways. First, the United Nations Food and Agriculture Organization (FAO) in Rome, Italy, tabulated values for physical activity level (PAL) that varied with exertions' intensity.[74] Values corresponded to decimals: 1.55 for light activity for a man, 1.8 for moderate activity, and 2.1 for heavy exertions. FAO also supplied decimals for boys, girls, and women, though these numbers are omitted for brevity. An estimate of daily caloric needs comes from multiplying the appropriate decimal by basal metabolism (basal metabolic rate or BMR), the energy necessary for a person at rest. Victoria, Australia's Department of Health and Human Services approximated an average man's BMR at 7,100 kilojoules (1,696.9 calories) daily.[75]

As noted, eighteenth-century farm work varied in intensity, and its classification as light, moderate, or heavy may be subjective. For example, American physiologist Ancel Benjamin Keys (1904–2004) wrote that farm labor with nothing besides plow, hoe, and sickle could be sustained "hour after hour, all day long."[76] His language implied that the work was not especially taxing, an opinion that must seem strange to anyone who has toiled at physical tasks. Against Keys, Chapter 6 expressed the consensus that work on antebellum South Carolina rice plantations was exhausting, a judgment that informs this section's classification of eighteenth-century French farm work as heavy, earning a rating of 2.1 and daily expenditure around 3,563.5 calories.

This number invites comparison with calories expended as the second method of estimating how many calories these peasants needed. In 2009, United Kingdom (UK) pharmacologist Paul Clayton and historian Judith D. Rowbotham (b. 1952), both introduced in Chapter 1, estimated that the arduousness of life and work about 1850 led British men to burn between 3,000 and 4,500 calories per day, a range that encompasses the above estimate.[77] Our approximation also nears four nineteenth-century estimates for calories expended in heavy labor: 3,370 calories per day by German physiologist Carl von Voit (1831–1908), 3,644 by German physiologist Max Rubner (1854–1932), 3,750 by

British scientist and nobleman Lyon Playfair (1818–1898), and 4,060 by American chemist Wilbur Olin Atwater (1844–1907).[78]

Comparison may also be made with other demanding occupations. Early twentieth-century estimates put daily energy expenditures at 3,053 calories for British tailors, 3,194 for German carpenters, 3,436 for Swedish laborers, 3,590 for Massachusetts glassblowers, 3,622 for Canadian factory workers, 3,675 for Russian laborers, 4,117 for British blacksmiths, 4,428 for Massachusetts mechanics, and 4,641 for German brickmakers.[79]

The mean of these thirteen, from Voit's 3,370 to German brickmakers' 4,641, is 3,736.9 calories metabolized and may approximate average daily energy expenditure for hard labor. It seems reasonable to suppose, then, that eighteenth-century French peasants burned about 3,736.9 calories for every 4,018.6 ingested. These numbers suggest that average daily intake of 1,074.5 grams of dried *C. sativa* nuts provided at least adequate energy. But calorie consumption might have been lower because some chestnuts, surely eaten fresh, had less energy because of a greater proportion of water. On the other hand, inclusion of additional foods in diets would have increased total calories, though, as noted, the Italian agronomist, Estienne, Liebault, and le Play emphasized chestnuts as sole sustenance in many cases. Whatever the exact calories, Hufton's description of these peasants as "puniest" indicated that they did not overeat and were neither overweight nor obese.[80]

Absence of excess bodyfat did not guarantee health. The poorest rural tenants subsisted on chestnuts at least two or three months per year and were the ricketiest early-nineteenth-century French conscripts.[81] Table 9.3 showed that chestnuts lack vitamin D and so must have abetted the disease. Yet these nuts cannot bear full blame given that sunlight supplies most vitamin D for most people.[82] Because diet seldom fulfills the body's vitamin D needs, chestnuts cannot be singled out for criticism. Rickets' prevalence in France, therefore, was first a problem of insufficient sun exposure and only second a dietary issue. Chapter 7 noted that French peasants clothed nearly the entire body and wore hats, preventing absorption of enough ultraviolet light to meet the body's vitamin D requirement. Chapter 2 discussed the relationship among vitamin D, calcium, and other minerals to highlight the vitamin's importance to health.

Another health gauge involves goiter's prevalence among France's mountaineers, the people whom readers may remember as dependent on chestnuts.[83] Discussing cassava, Chapter 13 identifies iodine deficiency as the cause. In their recitation of chestnuts' nutrients, neither USDA nor Fauve-Chamoux mentioned iodine, permitting the inference that overreliance on them may have contributed to goiter. More generally, deficiency diseases like goiter underscore the danger of narrow diets and the need for variety.

Beyond these considerations, Ladurie and Hufton characterized French peasants as underfed.[84] Undernutrition likely explained why France's chestnut eaters were the shortest army recruits in the early nineteenth century.[85] Given chestnuts' plentiful nutrients, already noted, the temptation is to blame poverty for these peasants' undernutrition and shortness. This explanation's weakness lies in the reality that so many eighteenth-century Frenchmen were desperately poor and hungry. Hufton, for example, estimated that undernutrition beset up to 70 percent of farmers and laborers in some areas.[86] Although an earlier paragraph questioned this figure because chestnuts are nourishing, this section does not doubt impoverishment and misery. Widespread poverty and undernutrition counter the premise that chestnut consumers were poorer or hungrier than other commoners.

Absent evidence that chestnut eaters were especially poor by eighteenth-century standards, the inference that the nuts did not promote full adult stature among the poor may be warranted. This possibility does not suppose that chestnuts lack nutrients; the opposite is true. Yet Chapter 1 mentioned that such attainment requires adequate calories, protein, vitamin A, and zinc.[87] Table 9.3 demonstrated that chestnuts lack vitamin A and have scant zinc. Even 1,074.5 grams of chestnuts, in Table 9.5, have just 25.1 percent of the U.S. Food and Drug Administration's (FDA) daily value (DV) for zinc.[88] Besides inadequate vitamin A and zinc, strenuous labor likely weakened peasants from youth, stunting growth.

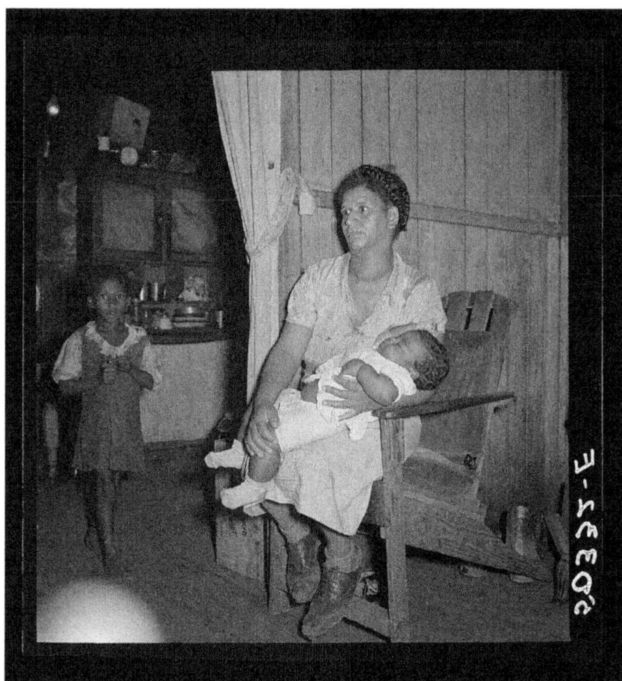

FIGURE 9.3 Woman with goiter. (Photo courtesy of Library of Congress. https://www.loc.gov/pictures/item/2017799592/.)

9.5 ACORNS

9.5.1 Antiquity

Like chestnuts—and aligning with Albala's definition discussed earlier—acorns come from trees. All populate the genus *Quercus*, whose 400–800 species inhabit Asia, Africa, Europe, North America, South America, and Oceania.[89] Widespread in the northern hemisphere, oaks occupy diverse habitats, including rainforests in Malaysia and on the island of Borneo; on Costa Rica's coast along the Caribbean Sea; in Mexico's Sierra Madre; throughout hardwood forests in China, Japan, and the eastern United States; in the Mediterranean south through North Africa; on mountains in Texas, Arizona, and the Pacific Northwest; near California's coast; and in its central valley, the last treated in the last treated in subsequent sections.

Ancient is the perception that acorns, and nuts generally, were a natural food more nourishing than grains and other domesticates.[90] As such, acorns occupied a mythology in which the first people inhabited a pristine world of plentitude without effort.[91] Chapter 3 characterized such distortions as Garden of Eden nostalgia. Genesis aside, this thinking pervaded European accounts of the earliest humans—the balanophagoi (acorn eaters) or Arcadians (sometimes spelled Arkadians)—who visited oaks for acorns on the ground and honey in beehives perched on branches.[92]

This idyll enabled people to "flourish continually with good things," wrote Greek poet Hesiod (c. 750–c. 700 BCE).[93] British artist and botanist Frederick Edward Hulme (1841–1909) expressed this sentiment over 2,000 years later, describing a past when "Heroes on earth once lived, men good and great, Acorns their food, – thus fed they flourished, And equaled in their age the long lived oak."[94] Poetic contentment with, and repeated references to, acorns as early sustenance may intimate folk memories of a time when Eurasians depended on these nuts as their primary food.[95]

But acorns' primacy is difficult to verify. Roman poet Ovid (43 BCE–17 CE) held that humans first ate leaves and grasses, transitioning to acorns only when goddess Ceres gave them nuts.[96]

Affirming the notion of acorns as secondary sustenance was their portrayal as famine food. In this tradition, Galen recounted a famine that compelled farmers to eat their pigs, which ordinarily would have grown fat on acorns.[97] Hunger still extreme, farmers consumed what acorns pigs had not devoured. Albala detected no hint from Galen that acorns were second-rate, though this opinion may be doubted because people ate them only after exhausting the first option. Additional evidence of acorns' nonelite status came from American naturalist Clinton Hart Merriam (1855–1942), who in 1918 described British, French, and Italian resort to acorns only when other edibles were scarce.[98]

The notion of acorns as primeval sustenance persisted into the sixteenth century when French scholar and food writer Jean-Baptiste La Bruyere-Champier speculated that primordial peoples inhabited caves and ate primarily acorns.[99] In this context, an onlooker might identify these nuts as the original paleo diet. Even if acorns were not the first food, they fed entire communities in Israel over 19,000 years ago and in Syria 14,000 years ago.[100] These dates suggest Paleolithic acorn consumption. Early in the Neolithic Period or New Stone Age (c. 7000–c. 5800 BCE), people in the village Catal Huyuk in what is today Turkey ate acorns, whose remains were found near hearths as though ready for roasting.[101] The nuts also appeared in the archaeological record from Neolithic Achilleion and Sesklo, Greece. Bronze Age (c. 3750–c. 2900 BCE) Bulgarians ground acorns into flour, combining it with barley and einkorn (*Triticum monococcum*).

9.5.2 Acorns and Livestock

Early identification of acorns may not prove human consumption because many peoples fed them to livestock, especially pigs.[102] Roman agriculturist Cato the Elder (234–149 BCE) noted the practice of feeding acorns to oxen (castrated bulls). In the twentieth century, Turks fed them to goats (*Capra aegagrus hircus*), and rural Spanish markets sold the nuts as pig feed. Even so, acorn collection for this purpose must have been laborious when it was easier to let animals forage in nearby woods.

9.5.3 Acorns in Eastern and Western Hemispheres

Like chestnuts, people who occupied mountains and hillsides consumed acorns because such lands were suitable for little else.[103] For example, Greek geographer and historian Strabo (c. 64 BCE–c. 23 CE) wrote that the nuts sustained northern Spain's mountain dwellers. Southern Greece's mountains likewise yielded acorns. In the Middle Ages, Europe, the American Midwest, and California depended on them. In the nineteenth century, they constituted about one-fifth of rural Italian and Spanish diets.[104] Other nineteenth-century consumers were Portuguese, Greeks, Arabs, and Algerians.[105] By then, acorns were the chief food of California Indians, whose health is the next section's topic.[106]

In 1918, Merriam wrote that acorns constituted one-fifth of diets among Spain and Italy's poor and were widely eaten in Mexico, Algeria, and Morocco.[107] He declared that some Spaniards preferred acorns to chestnuts. In the 1940s, acorns remained the staple in southeastern Turkey, where shepherds still snack on them.[108] A 1952 estimate, differing from Merriam's opinion, put consumption among Italy and Spain's poor around one-quarter of daily intake.[109] Sardinians also ate numerous acorns at mid-century.[110] As late as 1985, the nuts fed South Koreans, Iraqis, and Moroccans.[111] Koreans throughout the peninsula continue to eat acorns in gruel and as noodles.[112]

9.5.4 Acorns and Health in California

Acknowledging that debate continues, Chapter 3 estimated that humans entered North America some 15,000 years ago. They first settled what is today California between roughly 10,000 and 8000 BCE, congregating near lakes to target waterfowl and thirsty mammals.[113] Perhaps to access the most calories and nutrients per kill, these hunters sought the largest game. Plants supplemented diets. Few skeletons exist of the founder populations, precluding attempts to pinpoint health, though

American anthropologist Phillip Lee Walker (1947–2009) and Cherokee-American anthropologist Russell Thornton (b. 1942) suspected that early populations had ample food and were too sparse to sustain many pathogens and parasites.[114] But surpluses may have been irregular, and storage may have been limited, causing hunger during scarcity.

Rainfall began to diminish around 7500 BCE, drying lakes that had lured birds and mammals.[115] Amerindians compensated by broadening plant gathering. Between around 3000 and 2000 BCE mortars and pestles appeared in the archaeological record. Anthropologists interpreted them as evidence of acorns, which were ground, in diets. These dates may not mark the origins of balanophagy (acorn eating) because earlier tools might have removed shell and cupule. This possibility may put acorn consumption before 3000 BCE, though British-American anthropologist Brian Murray Fagan (b. 1936)—mentioned in Chapter 5—dated its beginning around 2000 BCE in response to increasing populations' need for more food.[116] Canadian anthropologist Aubrey Cannon believed that the second date marked acorn eating's intensification rather than genesis.[117] California then was wetter and cooler than today, hindering grasses whose seeds Amerindians ate. Acorns filled the void, and by roughly 1 CE, they sustained peoples in the region that now encompasses Oregon in the north and California to the Mojave and Colorado deserts in the southeast.[118]

Belief that acorns were eaten only after climate change reduced the hunt's bounty contradicts Merriam's 1918 pronouncement that in California "the acorn is, and always has been, the staff of life."[119] He emphasized that this dependence persisted into the twentieth century, when Amerindians made cornbread with one part acorn flour to four parts cornmeal.[120] Absent gluten, cornmeal does not cohere to form dough. Despite gluten's absence, acorn flour coheres when wet, enabling cornbread to be made. Merriam described acorns as native sustenance from Canada to the Gulf of Mexico in eastern North America.[121] In Canada's Quebec and Ontario provinces, the Algonquin made acorn bread and combined the nuts with fish or game. Louisiana's Choctaw likewise ate acorn bread. In 1841, American geologist James Dwight Dana (1813–1895)—while in California with the United States Exploring Expedition (1838–1842)—sampled the bread, remarking that "the taste, though not very pleasing, is not positively disagreeable."[122] Other indigenes combined acorns with potatoes and squashes (*Cucurbita* species). As late as 1972, California Amerindians added acorns to bread and soup.[123]

Trading with Southwestern peoples millennia earlier, these Californians knew about farming but chose to remain hunter-gatherers because a few weeks in autumn yielded a year's acorns, according to Fagan.[124] American anthropologist Stephen Le estimated that such efforts furnished acorns for two or three years.[125] Amerindians' teeth recorded intensification of collecting and consuming acorns; their carbohydrates caused cavities uncommon among fish and game eaters.[126] Although previous sections indicated worldwide balanophagy, nowhere were acorns as important as in California. "By 500 CE, thousands of California Indians depended heavily on the immense acorn harvest," wrote Fagan.[127] Sixteenth-century Europeans in the region observed that acorns constituted up to half Amerindian diets. By then the annual harvest totaled around 60,000 metric tons (66,000 tons).

Like all estimates, this one disguises fluctuations. If a good year yielded about 784 kilograms per hectare (691.2 pounds per acre)—a quantity that exceeded ancient grain yields and approximated medieval production—a year or two of smaller harvests might follow.[128] Writing about southwestern Spain, British archaeologist Sarah Louise Rhoda Mason estimated acorn production between 500 and 700 kilograms per hectare (440.8 and 617.1 pounds per acre).[129]

Adversity depressed output, especially because the Medieval Warm Period between the ninth and thirteenth centuries, discussed in Chapters 6 and 8, diminished rainfall in North America.[130] Droughts caused fires that killed oaks. Moreover, frail trees were especially vulnerable to insects. Although droughts' effects on prehistoric acorn production cannot be pinpointed, estimation is possible given that between 1986 and 1992 perhaps one-tenth of central California oaks perished from insufficient rainfall. Although plentiful, reliable production might have supported fifty to sixty times more people in prehistoric California, subpar yields kept population below the hypothetical maximum.

These risks were not unique to acorn eaters because, this book emphasizes, uncertainty characterized food acquisition and production for almost everyone until recent times. Earlier chapters noted the prevalence of famine, which plagued the decades before and after the Black Death and the decades before the Irish Potato Famine, treated in Chapters 1 and 3. Beyond discussing famine throughout the past, Chapter 3 quoted French historian Fernand Paul Braudel (1902–1985) that it "recurred so insistently for centuries on end that it became incorporated into man's biological regime and built into his daily life."[131]

Focusing on central California—defined as the middle third of the state—as a region of oaks and acorns, American anthropologists David N. Dickel, Peter D. Schulz, and Henry Malcolm McHenry (b. 1944) divided habitation into three periods: an early phase between roughly 2000 and 1000 BCE, the middle around 1000 BCE to 1000 CE, and the late covering subsequent centuries.[132]

A previous paragraph mentioned that California's earliest inhabitants enjoyed abundance. Central California, our immediate concern, had ample edible plants, game, fish, and shellfish.[133] Insects furnished additional nutrients and calories.[134] The coast supplied seafood and marine mammals, notably seals (species in the families Phocidae and Otariidae), sea otters (*Enhydra lutris*), and an occasional beached whale (species in infraorder Cetacea). These resources may have deterred plant and animal domestication, though humans managed the environment, for example, by igniting fires to drive insects from oaks and to kill competing vegetation.[135] Such efforts safeguarded central California's "balanophagous" economies.[136]

Early research documented these acorn eaters' vitality. In 1966, American anthropologist Alice Mossie Brues (1913–2007) lamented that they "were so healthy that it is somewhat discouraging to work with them [their skeletons]."[137] Two years later, American anthropologist Bert Alfred Gerow (1915–2001) noted skeletal pathologies' near absence.[138] In a study unpublished as of 1984, Dickel and Schulz remarked that "cribra orbitalia and cranial porotic hyperostosis are so rare that meaningful comparisons across age, sex, and temporal samples were not possible."[139] Chapter 1 defined these deformities.

In 1984, Dickel, Schulz, and McHenry reassessed over 900 skeletons.[140] This number belies the rarity of sizable cemeteries given that these Amerindians preferred cremation, a practice that increased over time.[141] Cremation complicated research because native Californians may have reserved the practice for elites, especially prominent men.[142] Under this circumstance, skeletons revealed the poor's health—which this book emphasizes as usually worse than the wealthy's—and indicated nothing about the affluent. This stipulation is important because this book affirms that the poor far outnumbered the rich such that skeletons, even if only of paupers, furnished information about almost everyone. Consequently, this book contends that cremation, and elimination as evidence, of the few elites did not weaken skeletons as representations of the population and therefore as evidence about prehistoric Californians' diet, nutrition, and health.

Burials' chronology and number demonstrated that populations increased over time. In the sixteenth century, density may have been between 3.4 and 4.4 people per square kilometer (km^2).[143] Even these estimates may underreport crowding, which may have rivaled farm communities.[144] Chapter 6 mentioned that when Europeans entered California in 1542, Amerindians totaled between roughly 310,000 and 705,000.[145] Like farmers, these Californians were sedentary because food was abundant and reliable enough to end nomadism, though they never adopted agriculture and animal husbandry. Emphasizing sedentism, Fagan supposed that by roughly 900 CE, most natives never ventured beyond 8 kilometers (5 miles) from home.[146]

Population expansion's pace is difficult to quantify. When number of settlements is plotted over time in Graph 9.1 growth looks exponential in accelerating through time.[147]

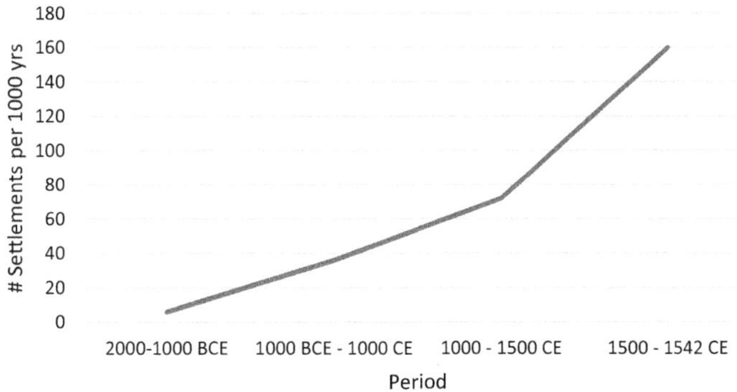

GRAPH 9.1 # of precontact settlements in central California. Courtesy of Dietra Cumo.

But the number of burials increased most rapidly in the early phase, slowing during middle and late periods.[148] The second curve—Graph 9.2—suggests an early spurt as humans had ample food and reproduced quickly.[149] As population approached the land's carrying capacity, growth slowed.

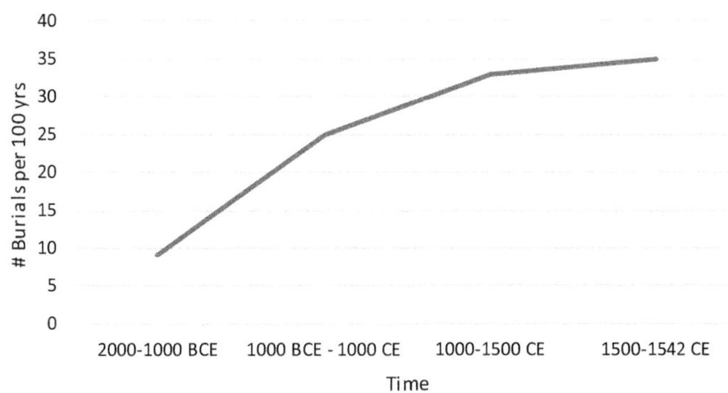

GRAPH 9.2 # of precontact burials in central California. Courtesy of Dietra Cumo.

But both scenarios cannot be true. Perhaps cremation increased over time, reducing the number of burials even as population enlarged from early to late phases. This claim is unconvincing if Amerindians reserved cremation for elites, who were too small a group to affect the curve. For example, an August 20, 2019, estimate that the world has around 7.7 billion people would not change with the addition or subtraction of several thousand people.[150] That is, inclusion or exclusion of Vatican City and places like it from the total would modify the count in only the tiniest way.

Whatever the growth rate, population increases only when births exceed deaths. Other chapters emphasize that premodern mortality was high. Such a situation demanded exceptional fertility, which necessitated adequate food to permit early menarche, reduce the interval between births, and feed more mouths. For example, Chapter 15 states that the average woman who reached menopause had to birth between 4.5 and 6.5 children just to replace the losses from antiquity's mortality.[151] Expansion required still greater fertility.

An earlier paragraph indicated that California diets varied over time. The initial emphasis on hunting left people little time to fish and collect acorns and other plant foods.[152] Before roughly 1000 BCE, native Californians ate fewer acorns than afterward. Even during the early phase, however, tools near what is today San Francisco processed acorns.[153] People without these technologies may not have eaten acorns because aridity reduced the number of oaks.[154] After about 1000 BCE, rainfall and acorn intake increased, prompting Dickel, Schulz, and McHenry to report that these nuts "presumably played a prominent role in the increase of population densities."[155]

Density depended on overall population and sedentism. Oaks affected these factors by providing a reliable harvest and by being stationary. That is, Amerindians did not need to migrate in pursuit of trees as they had done when hunting game. Dropping acorns in autumn, oaks supplied food for immediate needs and for storage against winter's lean months.

Adequate food during winter lessened seasonal shortages that had undermined health. When aridity made acorns scarce during the early phase, 80 percent of central California interments were in winter.[156] Later burials, however, cannot be pinpointed by season, preventing evaluation of the hypothesis that acorns lessened winter deaths. But Harris lines on bones, signaling temporary growth cessation, were traced through time. Bones may have stopped lengthening because of insufficient food, too many pathogens, parasites, or both, or synergy among too little food, diseases, and parasites. Harris lines became less frequent over time, with the greatest decrease between early and middle phases. As noted, the transition between these periods witnessed increases in acorn consumption. The inverse relationship between acorn intake and Harris lines strengthens the inference that acorns lessened seasonal shortages and undernutrition by supplying food for winter.

Yet nature never guaranteed the harvest. As noted, Amerindians could not expect uniform production over time, as two Yokut Indian cemeteries in central California's San Joaquin Valley revealed. Burials around 1 CE—when acorns were a staple—had skeletons with stout femurs and few pathologies, evincing adequate nutrition.[157] Skeletons dating roughly 850 years later exhibited more disease, lighter femurs, and shorter lifespan, betraying undernutrition and illness, likely because drought reduced acorn output.

Besides skeletal information, enamel hypoplasia—defined in Chapter 1—supplied additional health data, diminishing from early to middle phases but increasing thereafter, according to Dickel, Schulz, and McHenry.[158] Reduction from early to middle periods correlated with growing reliance on acorns, but late phase increases occurred as acorn intake continued to enlarge. If acorns improved nutrition early, reducing hypoplasia, this effect should have persisted throughout California prehistory. Yet as populations expanded over time, settlements grew crowded; contagion and parasites spread, undermining health even amid nourishing food. Problems multiplied during the late phase when Europeans introduced Old-World pathogens and parasites into California, a tragedy mentioned in Chapter 6.

But this explanation may be doubted. Because the same stresses caused Harris lines and enamel hypoplasia, they should have exhibited the same pattern. Both declined from early to middle phases, but from middle to late periods Harris lines diminished whereas enamel hypoplasia worsened, as noted, according to Dickel, Schulz, and McHenry. This divergence, if real, has no ready resolution. Yet, Dickel and coauthors' data may be incorrect because Walker and Thornton asserted that hypoplasia decreased with increases in acorn intake between roughly 600 BCE and 1250 CE.[159] Their view entails an inverse relationship between acorn consumption on one hand and Harris lines and hypoplasia on the other. If correct, Walker and Thornton's stance strengthens confidence in acorns' healthfulness.

Related to diseases and parasites is longevity, which "may have decreased as acorn specialization increased."[160] This reversal merits scrutiny given emphasis on longevity as health index, Chapter 1 noted. This perspective holds that if acorns, or any food, enhanced vitality, then people should have lived longer. But Chapter 1 described another interpretation. Increases in food raised birthrate, as observed earlier, causing the number of newborns and infants to enlarge more rapidly than adults. But a large youth population yields appreciable juvenile deaths even without ghastly child mortality. These fatalities diminish life expectancy at birth (e^0) even amid satisfactory diet and nutrition, causing e^0 to understate nutrition and health. The problem with this explanation is that over time California Indian mortality increased most between ages twenty and forty-five.[161] Such deaths, unconnected to juvenile mortality, prevent this section from generalizing about acorns' effect on longevity.

Retaining a focus on youths, prepubescent mortality diminished from early to middle phases, thereafter plateauing.[162] This trend implies adequate nutrition during childhood, when growth demands calories and nutrients. Survival gains came after age four, diminishing overall youth mortality. This improvement should not obscure that deaths before age two increased throughout all phases. Dickel, Schulz, and McHenry specified no age at weaning, leaving unknown whether deaths rose then. If so, acorns and other edibles were inadequate first solid foods.

Beyond these considerations, longevity data came from California natives who probably fished more than gathered acorns, complicating the relationship between acorns and lifespan.[163] Where acorns were the staple, men lived shorter lives over time whereas women's lifespans lengthened from early to middle phases but decreased thereafter. Dissimilar survival should eliminate acorns, and food generally, from consideration given the implausibility that men and women ate different diets during early and middle phases, when survivability diverged, but the same in the late period when longevity fell for both. If practiced more later and more often for prominent men than women, cremation might explain worse male longevity because over time burials would have disproportionately preserved poor men's skeletons, thereby magnifying the contributions of inadequate diets, nutrition, and health to the late phase. Again, this explanation is unpersuasive because elites were few.

Another health gauge is height, which this book describes as dependent on nutrition. As elsewhere, this section emphasizes that nutrition involves more than food because diseases and parasites worsen what might be termed net nutrition by forcing the body to expend calories and nutrients to combat them. That is, a nourishing diet may not avail when pathogens and parasites are prevalent.

Adult stature decreased between the early and middle phases, though Dickel, Schulz, and McHenry rated the magnitude insignificant.[164] Additional data concerned the Pacific Ocean's Channel Islands, west of what are today Santa Barbara, Ventura, and Los Angeles and southwest of central California, which may be remembered as Dickel, Schulz, and McHenry's focus. On these islands, men and women shrank gradually from roughly 600 BCE to 1250 CE.[165] These reductions, beginning at least 1,400 years after mortars and pestles appeared, were probably unrelated to acorn consumption. Moreover, islanders also ate seafood, excluding acorns as sole stature determiner even had nut intake and height reduction coincided.[166]

Diseases may have amplified the trend toward shortness, with nonvenereal syphilis present as early as 2600 BCE and worsening over time.[167] Other diseases in prehistoric California included streptococcal infections, staphylococcal infections, and coccidioidomycosis. Another factor may have been warfare, with conflicts escalating after bow and arrow replaced club about 500 CE. Over one-tenth of burials between then and 1250 had skeletons with arrow wounds.[168]

Stature comparisons reveal that northern Californians were taller than those in the south, represented by the islanders.[169] To the extent that diet contributed to this contrast, northerners concentrated on acorns whereas seafood sustained the south.[170] The generalization that acorns were more nourishing than fish and shellfish is gratuitous, however, because diet and nutrition may not have been the crucial factors. Different waves of northeast Asians peopled north and south during the last ice age, raising the possibility that genetic differences between them contributed to height disparities. Moreover, southern skeletons betrayed more arrow wounds and other evidence of violent deaths than those in the north.[171] Warfare and instability marred health, exacerbating height differences. In any event, native nutrition was unlikely to have been excellent given that Europeans who entered California in the eighteenth century averaged almost 8 centimeters (3.1 inches) taller than indigenes.

The best stature statistics came from measurements of thirty-six groups of California Indians between roughly 1905 and 1925.[172] Omitting tribes that supplied under eleven men or women as too small a sample reduces the list from thirty-six to eight. Of them and as Table 9.6 shows, the Mojave had the tallest mean at 171 centimeters (67.3 inches) for men and 158 centimeters (62.2 inches) for women.[173] Below them, male means ages nineteen to sixty were 169 centimeters (66.5 inches) for the Luiseno, 168 centimeters (66.1 inches) for the Cupeno and Yokuts, 167 centimeters (65.7 inches)

TABLE 9.6
California Indian Heights

Affiliation	# Men Sampled	Mean (cm)	# Women Sampled	Mean (cm)
Yurok	11	164	13	153
Hupa	32	166	14	152
Yuki	20	157	25	148
Yokut	16	168	15	155
Luiseno	52	169	42	157
Cupeno	14	168	20	156
Cahuilla	28	167	25	158
Mojave	45	171	25	158
Mean	27.25	166.3	22.38	154.6

for the Cahuilla, 166 centimeters (65.4 inches) for the Hupa, 164 centimeters (64.6 inches) for the Yuroks, and 157 centimeters (61.8 inches) for the Yuki.

In descending order beneath Mojave and Cahuilla women at 158 centimeters, female means ages seventeen to sixty were 157 centimeters for the Luiseno, 156 centimeters (61.4 inches) for the Cupeno, 155 centimeters (61 inches) for the Yokuts, 153 centimeters (60.2 inches) for the Yuroks, 152 centimeters (59.8 inches) for the Hupa, and 148 centimeters (58.3 inches) for the Yuki. The means of these averages are 166.3 centimeters (65.4 inches) for men and 154.6 centimeters (60.9 inches) for women and are thought typical of early-twentieth-century California natives. This book cannot determine whether these averages represent earlier populations because publications about them did not pinpoint their stature. The important point is that these means described stature among peoples for whom acorns were still the staple, as Merriam stated in 1918.

Comparison between these averages and those of other Amerindians suggests that California men were taller than Southwestern men at Mesa Verde, Colorado, from around 500–650 CE and at Delores, Colorado, between about 600 and 980.[174] California men also stood above men at prehistoric Tlatilco, Cuicuilco, Tlajinga, and Cholula, Mexico and in Maya communities at Tikal, Guatemala, Jaina, Mexico, Copan, Honduras, and the Yucatan Peninsula in Mexico, Guatemala, and Belize but shorter than men at precontact Tehuacan, Mexico.[175] California women were taller on average than women at Tlatilco, Cuicuilco, Tlajinga, Cholula, Tikal, Jaina, and the Yucatan but shorter than those at Tehuacan and Copan.

These comparisons imply that indigenous Californians were healthier on average than their counterparts in many precontact Southwestern, Mexican, and Central American communities and that acorns may have provided nutrition superior to the turkeys that sustained the Southwest and the corn (*Zea mays*), beans (*Phaseolus vulgaris, P. lunatus, P. acutifolius,* and *P. coccineus*), and squashes that fed pre-Columbian Mesoamerica. Chapter 6 detailed diets, nutrition, and health in the Southwest. Chapters 8 and 12 discuss beans and corn's health effects, respectively. Chapter 14 omits squashes, which are fruits, for brevity.

These considerations aside for the moment, California height reductions, gradual and protracted, implied incremental health diminution. Walker and Thornton documented that the region's prehistoric fish and shellfish consumers had as much anemia as corn growers throughout the Americas.[176] Chapter 5 noted that seafood is nutrient dense whereas Chapter 12 discusses corn's nutritional shortcomings and association with anemia among other maladies. In this context, seafood eaters should not have suffered anemia at the same rate as corn consumers. Diet being an unsatisfactory explanation, Walker and Thornton faulted sedentism and attendant buildup of pathogens, parasites, insects, and rodents. This rationale squares with their inference that acorn eaters were healthier than corn growers, both sedentary, but sicker than hunter-gatherers who remained nomads.

Besides these health indicators, Europeans disclosed their impressions about California natives. In 1579, English cleric Francis Fletcher remarked that one Coast Miwok Indian, in what are today Marin and southern Sonoma counties, had the strength of two or three white men.[177] Unnamed observers labeled these indigenes "muscular" and "strong."[178] In 1877, American journalist Stephen Powers (1840–1904), though declaring acorns and the like inferior to "bread and beans," praised California Indians as excellent athletes who enjoyed long, healthy lives.[179] He stated that they could shoot an arrow 0.4 kilometers (0.25 miles) and hold their breath twice whites' duration while retrieving mussels. He referenced one who ran 80.5 kilometers (50 miles) in under twelve hours and another who covered 19.3 kilometers (12 miles) in slightly over an hour. An especially swift runner was reputed to have completed 321.9 kilometers (200 miles) in a single day. A Mojave needed 3.5 hours to run 33.8 kilometers (21 miles).

Some of these assertions may be fanciful. The record distance over twenty-four hours is 303.5 kilometers (188.6 miles) for men and 252.2 kilometers (156.7 miles) for women.[180] Even if the possibility is granted that the 321.9 kilometers took longer than 24 hours, the runner would still have displayed extraordinary stamina to achieve what no one else appears to have duplicated. Such claims of prowess are unusual enough to elicit doubt. Similarly, 0.4 kilometers for a native archer seems improbable given the record 0.34 kilometers (0.21 miles) for an arrow shot with a longbow, a weapon unknown to Amerindians and more powerful than the standard bow and arrow.[181]

Such anecdotes suggest that Europeans envied natives' strength and endurance enough to exaggerate them but are otherwise unhelpful. Tests of hand strength measured by grip intensity and published in the early twentieth century, however, indicated that these Indians surpassed whites and Southwestern Amerindians.[182] Northern Californians exhibited the greatest strength, and those from central California ranked third. Between the two were Apache in Oklahoma, Texas, Arizona, and New Mexico. Whites scored below all but Arizona's Papago, Chapter 8's "bean people."[183]

These data do not permit unequivocal judgments about California indigenes' health. American archaeologist Robert Fleming Heizer (1915–1979) and colleague ascribed their superior strength and stamina to a vigorous lifestyle rather than to diet and nutrition.[184] Noteworthy is these authors' assertion that the Indians were more active than Americans before 1920. Afterward, fitness declined because, Chapter 12 emphasizes, Americans became inert and overweight upon purchase of automobiles. Other chapters, notably 16, discuss this deterioration.

Seeking greater clarity about native Californian health, this section considers an aspect of society that Dickel, Schulz, and McHenry mentioned in passing: Stratification increased through time.[185] Chapter 4 indicated that premodern societies tended to bifurcate into haves and have nots. A middle class was absent or minuscule in all but recent times. This bifurcation concentrated wealth among elites. Impoverishment undermined commoners' health in central California and may have magnified decreases in height and lifespan and increases in enamel hypoplasia, if Dickel, Schulz, and McHenry's statistics are right.

NOTES

1 Ken Albala, *Nuts: A Global History* (London: Reaktion Books, 2014), 11.
2 Ibid.
3 Ibid., 41.
4 Ibid.; Robert Jurmain, Lynn Kilgore, Wenda Trevathan, and Russell L. Ciochon. *Introduction to Physical Anthropology*, 2013–2014 ed. (Belmont, CA: Wadsworth Cengage Learning, 2014), 321.
5 Albala, 41.
6 Andreas Eenfeldt, *Low Carb, High Fat Food Revolution: Advice and Recipes to Improve Your Health and Reduce Your Weight*, trans. Viktoria Lindback (New York: Skyhorse Publishing, 2014), 18; David Perlmutter, *Grain Brain: The Surprising Truth about Wheat, Carbs, and Sugar—Your Brain's Silent Killers*, rev. ed. (New York: Little, Brown Spark, 2018), 49; Loren Cordain, *The Paleo Diet: Lose Weight and Get Healthy by Eating the Foods You Were Designed to Eat*, rev. ed. (Hoboken, NJ: Wiley, 2011), 9.

7 Perlmutter, 35.
8 Margaret Allman-Farinelli, "Nuts and Seeds," in *Essentials of Human Nutrition*, 5th ed., ed. Jim Mann and A. Stewart Truswell (Oxford, UK: Oxford University Press, 2017), 279.
9 Ibid., 279–280; Antoinette Fauve-Chamoux, "Chestnuts," in *The Cambridge World History of Food*, vol. 1, ed. Kenneth F. Kiple and Kriemhild Conee Ornelas (Cambridge, UK: Cambridge University Press, 2000), 360.
10 Allman-Farinelli, 280; "Nuts, Macadamia Nuts, Raw," *USDA FoodData Central*, April 1, 2019, accessed January 23, 2020, https://fdc.nal.usda.gov/fdc-app.html#/food-details/170178/nutrients.
11 Allan Borushek, *The CalorieKing Calorie, Fat, and Carbohydrate Counter* (Huntington Beach, CA: Family Health Publications, 2019), 130; "Nuts, Pine Nuts, Pinyon, Dried," *USDA FoodData Central*, April 1, 2019, accessed January 24, 2020, https://fdc.nal.usda.gov/fdc-app.html#/food-details/170592/nutrients.
12 Borushek, 158–160; Meika Foster, "Vegetables," in *Essentials of Human Nutrition*, 5th ed., ed. Jim Mann and A. Stewart Truswell (Oxford, UK: Oxford University Press, 2017), 284.
13 Allman-Farinelli, 280.
14 Ibid.; Jimmy Louie, "Breads and Cereals," in *Essentials of Human Nutrition*, 5th ed., ed. Jim Mann and A. Stewart Truswell (Oxford, UK: Oxford University Press, 2017), 274.
15 Fauve-Chamoux, 360.
16 "Nuts, Chestnuts, European, Dried, Unpeeled," *USDA FoodData Central*, April 1, 2019, accessed December 1, 2019, https://fdc.nal.usda.gov/fdc-app.html#/food-details/170576/nutrients.
17 "Nuts, Chestnuts, European, Boiled and Steamed," *USDA FoodData Central*, April 1, 2019, accessed January 23, 2020, https://fdc.nal.usda.gov/fdc-app.html#/food-details/170168/nutrients; "FDA Vitamins and Minerals Chart," https://www.accessdata.fda.gov/scripts/interactivenutritionfactslabel/factsheets/vitamin_and_mineral_chart.pdf.
18 Allman-Farinelli, 280.
19 Stephen Le, *100 Million Years of Food: What Our Ancestors Ate and Why It Matters Today* (New York: Picador, 2016), 22.
20 Ibid., 22–23.
21 Toshio Matsuyama, "Nut Gathering and Processing Methods in Traditional Japanese Villages," in *Affluent Foragers: Pacific Coasts East and West*, ed. Shuzo Koyama and David Hurst Thomas (Osaka, Japan: National Museum of Ethnology, 1979), 133–134.
22 Le, 23.
23 Jack R. Harlan, *Crops and Man*, 2nd ed. (Madison, WI: American Society of Agronomy, Crop Science Society of America, 1992), 21; Matsuyama, 133–134.
24 "Nuts, Acorns, Dried," *USDA FoodData Central*, April 1, 2019, accessed February 12, 2020, https://fdc.nal.usda.gov/fdc-app.html#/food-details/170565/nutrients; "FDA Vitamins and Minerals Chart."
25 Ernest Small, *North American Cornucopia: Top 100 Indigenous Food Plants* (Boca Raton, FL: CRC Press, 2014), 61.
26 Georgina Pearman, "Nuts, Seeds, and Pulses," in *The Cultural History of Plants*, ed. Ghillean Prance and Mark Nesbitt (New York and London: Routledge, 2005), 136.
27 Fauve-Chamoux, 359.
28 Ibid., 359–360.
29 Small, 62.
30 Ibid., 61.
31 Ibid., 62.
32 Ibid., 63.
33 H. S. Betts, *Chestnut* (Washington, DC: U.S. Department of Agriculture, 1945), 1.
34 Small, 61.
35 Ibid., 65.
36 Ibid., 64–65.
37 Susan Freinkel, *American Chestnut: The Life, Death, and Rebirth of a Perfect Tree* (Berkeley: University of California Press, 2007), 16.
38 Ibid., 68.
39 Small, 63.
40 Ibid., 65.
41 Fauve-Chamoux, 359.
42 Pearman, 136.
43 Fauve-Chamoux, 359.

44 Ibid.
45 Ibid.
46 Frederic le Play, *Les ouvriers europeens*, vol. 1 (Tours, France: A. Mame, 1879), 310.
47 Fauve-Chamoux, 361–362.
48 Ibid., 361.
49 Ibid., 362.
50 Ibid., 362–363.
51 Ibid., 363.
52 Freinkel, 28–29.
53 Jesse D. Diller, *Chestnut Blight* (Washington, DC: U.S. Department of Agriculture, 1965), 1–2.
54 Freinkel, 82.
55 "Chestnut Production," *World Mapper*, 2019, accessed August 17, 2019, https://worldmapper.org/maps/chestnut-production-2016.
56 R. J. Bernard, "Peasant Diet in Eighteenth-Century Gevaudan," in *European Diet from Pre-Industrial to Modern Times*, ed. Elborg Forster and Robert Forster (New York: Torchbooks, 1975), 24, 28.
57 Fauve-Chamoux, 360.
58 Ibid., 361.
59 Ralph E. Giesey, "Rules of Inheritance and Strategies of Mobility in Prerevolutionary France," *American Historical Review* 82, no. 2 (April 1977): 271.
60 Emmanuel Le Roy Ladurie, *The Peasants of Languedoc*, trans. John Day (Urbana: University of Illinois Press, 1974), 5.
61 Olwen Hufton, "Social Conflict and the Grain Supply in Eighteenth-Century France," *Journal of Interdisciplinary History* 14, no. 2 (Autumn 1983): 308.
62 Ladurie, 295.
63 Ibid., 70.
64 Ibid., 67.
65 Bernard, 24.
66 Ladurie, 66.
67 "Nuts, Chestnuts, European, Dried, Unpeeled;" Fauve-Chamoux, 363.
68 "Nuts, Chestnuts, European, Dried, Unpeeled."
69 Fauve-Chamoux, 363; Hufton, 305.
70 Peter L. Pellett, "Energy and Protein Metabolism," in *The Cambridge World History of Food*, vol. 1, ed. Kenneth F. Kiple and Kriemhild Conee Ornelas (Cambridge, UK: Cambridge University Press, 2000), 896.
71 Ladurie, 67–68.
72 Robert William Fogel and Stanley L. Engerman, *Time on the Cross: The Economics of American Negro Slavery* (New York and London: Norton, 1995), 112–113.
73 Pellett, 898.
74 Ibid., 897.
75 "Metabolism," Victoria State Government, 2018, accessed August 26, 2019, https://www.betterhealth.vic.gov.au/health/conditionsandtreatments/metabolism.
76 Ancel Keys, *Seven Countries: A Multivariate Analysis of Death and Coronary Heart Disease* (Cambridge, MA: Harvard University Press, 1980), 214.
77 Paul Clayton and Judith Rowbotham, "How the Mid-Victorians Worked, Ate and Died," *International Journal of Environmental Research and Public Health* 6, no. 3 (March 2009): 1235–1253. https://www.ncbi.nlm.nih.gov/pmc/articles/PMC2672390.
78 Pellett, 898.
79 Ibid.
80 Hufton, 308.
81 Ibid., 307–308.
82 Rathish Nair and Arun Maseeh, "Vitamin D: The 'Sunshine' Vitamin," *Journal of Pharmacology and Pharmacotherapeutics* 3, no. 2 (April-June 2012): 118–126, https://www.ncbi.nlm.nih.gov/pmc/articles/PMC3356951.
83 Ladurie, 68.
84 Ibid.; Hufton, 305, 307–308.
85 Hufton, 308.
86 Ibid., 305.

87 Alan H. Goodman and Debra L. Martin, "Reconstructing Health Profiles from Skeletal Remains," in *The Backbone of History: Health and Nutrition in the Western Hemisphere*, ed. Richard H. Steckel and Jerome C. Rose (Cambridge, UK: Cambridge University Press, 2002), 20.
88 "FDA Vitamins and Minerals Chart."
89 "Acorn," in *The Cambridge World History of Food*, vol. 2, ed. Kenneth F. Kiple and Kriemhild Conee Ornelas (Cambridge, UK: Cambridge University Press, 2000), 1714; Peter Young, *Oak* (London: Reaktion Books, 2013), 7.
90 Albala, 15–16.
91 Ibid.; Sarah Mason, "Acornutopia?: Determining the Role of Acorns in Past Human Subsistence," in *Food in Antiquity*, ed. John Wilkins, David Harvey, and Mike Dobson (Exeter, UK: University of Exeter Press, 1995), 12.
92 Albala, 15–16.
93 Ibid.
94 Le, 17.
95 Mason, 12.
96 Ibid., 13.
97 Albala, 16–17.
98 C. Hart Merriam, "The Acorn, a Possibly Neglected Source of Food," *National Geographic Magazine* 34, no. 1 (August 1918): 136.
99 Albala, 17.
100 Mason, 14; Brian Fagan, *The Great Warming: Climate Change and the Rise and Fall of Civilizations* (New York: Bloomsbury Press, 2008), 123.
101 Mason, 14.
102 Ibid., 15–16.
103 Ibid., 13.
104 Fagan, 123.
105 Le, 23.
106 Pearman, 133.
107 Merriam, 134, 136.
108 Pearman, 134.
109 Mason, 22.
110 Pearman, 134.
111 Le, 23.
112 Pearman, 134.
113 Phillip L. Walker and Russell Thornton, "Health, Nutrition, and Demographic Change in Native California," in *The Backbone of History Health and Nutrition in the Western Hemisphere*, ed. Richard H. Steckel and Jerome C. Rose (Cambridge, UK: Cambridge University Press, 2002), 508; Liz Sonneborn, *California Indians* (Chicago: Heinemann Library, 2012), 42.
114 Walker and Thornton, 508.
115 Ibid.
116 Fagan, 121–122.
117 Aubrey Cannon, "Archaeology of North American Hunters and Gatherers," in *The Cambridge Encyclopedia of Hunters and Gatherers*, ed. Richard B. Lee and Richard Daly (Cambridge, UK: Cambridge University Press, 2004), 33.
118 Fagan, 121–122.
119 Merriam, 129.
120 Ibid., 129–130.
121 Ibid., 132–134.
122 Ibid., 130.
123 Waverley Root and Richard de Rochemont, *Eating in America: A History* (Hopewell, NJ: Ecco Press, 1995), 18.
124 Fagan, 122.
125 Le, 23.
126 Fagan, 122.
127 Ibid., 123.
128 Ibid., 124–125; Mason, 13.
129 Mason, 13.

130 Fagan, 124–125.
131 Fernand Braudel, *Capitalism and Material Life, 1400–1800*, trans. Miriam Kochan (New York: Harper Colophon Books, 1973), 38.
132 David N. Dickel, Peter D. Schulz, and Henry M. McHenry, "Central California: Prehistoric Subsistence Changes and Health," in *Paleopathology at the Origins of Agriculture*, ed. Mark Nathan Cohen and George J. Armelagos (Orlando, FL: Academic Press, 1984), 441.
133 Ibid., 439.
134 Sonneborn, 13.
135 Dickel, Schulz, and McHenry, 439; Cannon, 32.
136 Dickel, Schulz, and McHenry, 440.
137 Alice M. Brues, "Discussion," in *Human Palaeopathology*, ed. Saul Jarcho (New Haven, CT and London: Yale University Press, 1966), 108.
138 Dickel, Schulz, and McHenry, 444.
139 Ibid.
140 Ibid., 453.
141 Ibid.; Walker and Thornton, 507.
142 Dickel, Schulz, and McHenry, 453.
143 Ibid., 450.
144 Ibid., 440; Walker and Thornton, 507.
145 Walker and Thornton, 509.
146 Fagan, 124.
147 Dickel, Schulz, and McHenry, 451.
148 Ibid., 452.
149 Ibid.
150 "Current World Population," *Worldometers*, accessed August 20, 2019, https://www.worldometers.info/world-population.
151 Walter Scheidel, "Demography," in *The Cambridge Economic History of the Greco-Roman World*, ed. Walter Scheidel, Ian Morris, and Richard Saller (Cambridge, UK: Cambridge University Press, 2007), 41.
152 Dickel, Schulz, and McHenry, 441.
153 Ibid., 442.
154 Ibid., 442–443.
155 Ibid., 452.
156 Ibid., 444.
157 Fagan, 126.
158 Dickel, Schulz, and McHenry, 446.
159 Walker and Thornton, 520.
160 Dickel, Schulz, and McHenry, 453.
161 Ibid., 454.
162 Ibid.
163 Ibid.
164 Ibid., 448.
165 Walker and Thornton, 511.
166 Ibid., 512–513.
167 Ibid., 514.
168 Ibid., 515.
169 Ibid., 516.
170 Ibid., 520.
171 Ibid., 517.
172 Edward Winslow Gifford, "Californian Anthropometry," in *University of California Publications in American Archaeology and Ethnology*, ed. A. L. Kroeber and Robert H. Lowie (Berkeley: University of California Press, 1965), 223, 232.
173 Ibid., 232–233.
174 Ann L. W. Stodder, Debra L. Martin, Alan H. Goodman, and Daniel T. Reff, "Cultural Longevity and Biological Stress in the American Southwest," in *The Backbone of History: Health and Nutrition in the Western Hemisphere*, ed. Richard H. Steckel and Jerome C. Rose (Cambridge, UK: Cambridge University Press, 2002), 488–489.

175 Lourdes Marquez Morfin, Robert McCaa, Rebecca Storey, and Andres Del Angel, "Health and Nutrition in Pre-Hispanic Mesoamerica," in *The Backbone of History: Health and Nutrition in the Western Hemisphere*, ed. Richard H. Steckel and Jerome C. Rose (Cambridge, UK: Cambridge University Press, 2002), 321.
176 Walker and Thornton, 518–519.
177 Robert F. Heizer and Carol Treanor, "Observations on Physical Strength of Some Western Indians and 'Old American' Whites," in *Two Papers on the Physical Anthropology of California Indians* (Berkeley, CA: Archaeological Research Facility, 1974), 49.
178 Ibid., 50.
179 Ibid.
180 Runtastic Team, "11 Incredible Running Records that Will Knock Your Socks off," *Runtastic*, May 17, 2015, accessed September 19, 2019, https://www.runtastic.com/blog/en/11-incredible-running-records-that-will-knock-your-socks-off.
181 "How Far Could an English War Bow Shoot?" *History Stack Exchange*, accessed September 19, 2019, https://history.stackexchange.com/questions/8022/how-far-could-an-english-war-bow-shoot.
182 Heizer and Treanor, 50–55.
183 Meredith Sayles Hughes, *Spill the Beans and Pass the Peanuts: Legumes* (Minneapolis, MN: Lerner Publications, 1999), 57.
184 Heizer and Treanor, 53–54.
185 Dickel, Schulz, and McHenry, 440.

10 Fat

10.1 FAT AS DIETARY COMPONENT

Chapter 2 categorized fat among the three macronutrients—the others being carbohydrates and protein—and described its structure and function. Fat enticed the human lineage when primates' forerunners—discussed in Chapter 3—began eating insects, which may be half fat by mass, around 65 million years ago.[1] Chapters 3 and 4 noted that anthropologists accord meat, whose nutrients include fat, a central role in our evolution. Besides flesh from terrestrial and aquatic mammals, fish, and poultry, humans ingested fat from nuts and seeds. Amid the food scarcity of all but recent times, fat supplied badly needed energy. Hunger led a seventeenth-century CE peasant to remark that "If I were a king, I'd eat nothing but fat."[2] Our long association with fat underscores its importance.

From its inception as a science, nutrition has labored to determine what and how much should be eaten. Emulating physics' experimentalism, nutritionists and physiologists fed laboratory animals, usually rodents, various foods in hopes of pinpointing the necessities. In 1881, Russian pediatrician Nikolai Ivanovich Lunin (1853–1937) demonstrated that mice could not survive on just casein (milk protein), lard (pig fat), the disaccharide sucrose ($C_{12}H_{22}O_{11}$), water, and minerals.[3] Whole milk, however, permitted normal development.

His work prompted others to undertake similar experiments, and in 1907, American nutritionist Elmer Verner McCollum (1879–1967) began feeding cows (*Bos taurus*) an assortment of foods. Turning his attention to rats (*Rattus* species), he showed that they languished on the milk sugar lactose (also $C_{12}H_{22}O_{11}$)—discussed in Chapter 7—protein, lard or olive oil, and minerals. Addition of butterfat or egg yolk restored vigor, leading him in 1912 to posit the existence of "fat-soluble factor A," now known as vitamin A.[4] McCollum's demonstration that vitamin A was essential and that it stored only in fat proved fat indispensable to health. Subsequent research identified vitamins D, E, and K—all discussed in Chapter 2—as also fat soluble, furnishing more evidence of fat's necessity.

This work implied, however, that not all fat was necessary; otherwise, lard or olive oil should have produced better results. Independent of McCollum, American chemist Ava Josephine McAmis (1897–1991) and colleagues showed that cod liver oil and peanut oil had essential fats.[5] Among peanut oil's polyunsaturated fats is linoleic acid ($C_{18}H_{32}O_2$), an omega 6 fatty acid. In 1929, American biochemists and spouses George Oswald Burr (1896–1990) and Mildred M. Burr demonstrated that even small amounts of linoleic acid invigorated undernourished rats. Later studies identified other omega 6 fatty acids and omega 3 fatty acids—cod liver oil, for example, has the latter—necessary for vitality.

Chapter 2 noted that the body manufactures fat from fatty acids ingested from foods or made from other substances. The forgoing research demonstrated that the body cannot synthesize two classes of fatty acids—omega 3 and omega 6—making them essential. Chapter 2 described how chemists name fatty acids. Chapter 3 indicated that modern diets supply too many omega 6 fatty acids and too few omega 3 compared with preagricultural diets and that this misalignment harms the body.[6] Prominent among medical authorities, American radiologist Stanley Boyd Eaton (b. 1938) and coauthors maintained since 1985 that hunter-gatherers ate a 1:1 ratio of omega 6 to omega 3 and that modern diets must restore parity to improve health.[7] Greek American endocrinologist Artemis P. Simopoulos (b. 1933) reached similar conclusions, arguing that insufficient omega 3 and excess omega 6 cause heart disease, cancers, inflammation, and autoimmune diseases.[8]

Chapter 2 also mentioned that fat is more than energy. It constitutes the membrane of all the body's cells and is especially conspicuous in the central nervous system (CNS), where it forms neural membranes and the myelin sheath that surrounds each neuron's axon. Comprising neurons, the brain is roughly 70 percent fat.[9] Cells and the CNS, including the brain, could neither exist as discrete units nor function without fat. Even bacteria have fatty membranes, evidence that fat has been essential to life since its origin nearly 4 billion years ago. These facts must be evident to American neurologist David Perlmutter (b. 1954)—introduced in Chapter 1—whose specialty is the CNS and whose ideas receive attention next.

10.2 SPECULATION ABOUT THE AMOUNT OF FAT IN PREAGRICULTURAL DIETS

10.2.1 Proponents of High Fat Intake

Advocating high-fat, low-carbohydrate diets, Perlmutter asserted in *Grain Brain* (2018) without evidence or sources that preagricultural diets were 75 percent fat, 20 percent protein, and 5 percent carbohydrates.[10] Because humans hunted game and collected wild plants far longer than they have farmed, evolution shaped them to consume mostly fat, if Perlmutter is right. But people in developed nations are out of step with their past because their diets are 60 percent carbohydrates, 20 percent fat, and 20 percent protein, claimed Perlmutter.[11]

American science writer Gary Taubes (b. 1956) sketched this rationale in 2011, mentioning but not citing the 1919 recollections of American cardiologist Blake F. Donaldson.[12] Concerned about his obese patients, wrote Taubes, Donaldson wanted to prescribe a healthful diet. Reasoning that the best regimen would mimic humanity's past, he asked unnamed anthropologists what our ancestors ate, learning that they preyed upon "'the fattest meat they could kill,' with some minimal roots and berries for variety."[13]

Taubes' account is misleading. Although he accurately quoted part of Donaldson's recollections of a visit to New York City's American Museum of Natural History, Taubes implied that the cardiologist learned that day of humanity's preoccupation with meat and fat. Contrary to this characterization, Donaldson emphasized humanity's omnivory and eclecticism: Mongols ate rice (*Oryza sativa*) and soybeans (*Glycine max*), North Africans consumed grains and chili peppers (*Capsicum annuum*), Italians and Amerindians favored corn (*Zea mays*), Central Americans ingested bananas (*Musa x paradisiaca*), central Africans hunted hippopotami (*Hippopotamus amphibius*), and Inuit targeted walruses (*Odobenus rosmarus*).[14] This variety led Donaldson to conclude that "All over the globe eating habits vary depending upon the availability of food."[15] This book echoes Donaldson's conclusion and describes omnivory and eclecticism as strategies that permitted humans to occupy diverse ecosystems worldwide.

10.2.2 Criticism of These Proponents' Speculation

Perlmutter and Taubes' contrast between prehistory and modernity is simple, stark, and incorrect. This book disagrees that a chasm separated preagricultural and agricultural diets. For example, Chapter 12 notes that southwestern Asians ate wild grains millennia before domesticating them.[16] The same applies to legumes, roots and tubers, and many other foods. The transition to farming continued and intensified preagricultural habits and preferences rather than repudiated them. Moreover, agriculture and animal husbandry did not immediately end hunting and gathering. Chapter 16 states that as late as 1921, for example, American home economist Helen Woodard Atwater (1876–1947) reported game in U.S. rural diets.[17] In other words, Perlmutter and Taubes created a false dichotomy.

The foregoing suggests that their scheme oversimplifies prehistory. Chapter 3 indicated that humanity's lineage stretches many millions of years into the past. Restricting this time to roughly the last 150,000 years, when anatomically modern peoples arose in Africa, still leaves a vast period when humans ate the same proportion of macronutrients according to Perlmutter and Taubes. During roughly the last 50,000 years modern peoples colonized every continent but Antarctica, occupying diverse biomes, climates, and topographies; yet these authors want readers to suppose that despite such diversity, humans insisted upon the same high-fat diet everywhere.

Belief that diversity yielded uniformity is untrue. Discussing archaic *Homo sapiens*' diets in Chapter 3, Israeli American anthropologist Ofer Bar-Yosef (1937–2020) echoed Donaldson, remarking that people have always eaten what their environment furnished.[18] But environments varied. Chapters 4 and 5 noted that at high latitudes, short summers precluded year-round reliance on plants. Hunter-gatherers adapted by eating game and fish. At the other extreme, Africa and Asia's tropics, rich in florae, gave prehistoric peoples over 60 percent of calories from plants, estimated Bar-Yosef.[19] Observing today's hunter-gatherers, Eaton and colleagues asserted that preagricultural diets supplied over 30 percent of calories as protein and below one-quarter as fat.[20] Using African herbivores as proxies for game that our ancestors scavenged and hunted, Eaton and American anthropologist Melvin Joel Konner (b. 1946) estimated paleolithic meat under 4 percent fat by mass compared to livestock at "25 to 30 percent fat or even more."[21] American nutritionist and exercise physiologist Loren Cordain (b. 1950) put Paleolithic or Old Stone Age (c. 70,000–c. 9000 BCE) fat consumption between 28 and 47 percent of calories.[22]

None of these schemes matches Perlmutter's figures, an unsurprising outcome given that human variability complicates, if not derails, attempts to encapsulate behavior over many millennia in a single set of numbers. Chapter 3 treated humans' dietary diversity, sketching the variety of plants and animals consumed in pre-Columbian North America alone. Such diversity multiplied on a global scale as people filled innumerable niches. Despite humankind's flexibility and adaptability, Perlmutter and Taubes redefined us as rigid and unimaginative. In effect, they put humanity on a dietary Procrustean bed. Such an approach rids the past of subtlety.

Besides these flaws, Perlmutter and Taubes unrealistically supposed that hunter-gatherers loaded up on fat from wild animals.[23] They have fat, though the amount varied with their fortunes. During flush times, animals ate their fill and accumulated fat, but scarcity made them lean and hungry. Chapter 3 introduced the phenomenon of rabbit starvation, a type of protein toxicity, whereby people died from eating exceptionally lean animals like rabbits (*Oryctolagus cuniculus*).[24] Such game furnished insufficient fat, carbohydrates, vitamins, minerals, or their combination. Rabbit starvation implies that wild animals were leaner than Perlmutter imagined, especially during privation.

Fat's quantification in prehistoric game is impossible, a circumstance that invites speculation from Perlmutter and others. Belief that it was very fat seems implausible given that Table 4.1 tabulated 100 grams of bison (*Bison bison* and *B. bonasus*) and venison at 7.21 grams and 3.93 grams of fat, respectively. The mean of these numbers is 5.57 grams, or 52.36 calories at 9.4 calories per gram of fat, as Chapter 2 mentioned. Table 4.1 listed 146 calories in 100 grams of bison and 190 calories in the same amount of venison. The mean is 168 calories in 100 grams. These numbers imply that wild animals supplied 31.2 percent of calories as fat. Even if this percentage is doubled to appease Perlmutter, preagricultural peoples would have derived 62.4 percent of calories from fat, not his 75 percent.

New Zealand chemist and food consultant Laurence Eyres regarded game as so lean that he omitted it as a source of fat for hunter-gatherers.[25] American historian Kenneth Franklin Kiple (1939–2016) estimated that such animals by mass had only 10–14 percent the fat in livestock, writing that even where preagricultural diets approached 80 percent of calories from game, only one-fifth of those calories were fat.[26] To be fair, Kiple's numbers—like Perlmutter's—are speculation, underscoring the difficulty of pinpointing prehistoric fat consumption.

Rather than game, Eyres wrote that preagricultural fat came from fish, nuts, and seeds.[27] But if bison, deer (*Odocoileus* species), and other wild mammals were unlikely to have had ample fat, fish might not have yielded much more. Like mammals, fish are too diverse to permit generalizations. Chapter 5's Table 5.1 listed 0.96 grams of fat and 86 calories in 100 grams of tuna (*Thunnus* species), 1.7 grams of fat and 96 calories in the same amount of tilapia (species in the family Cichlidae), 0.41 grams of fat and 56 calories in pollock (*Pollachius pollachius* and *P. virens*), 0.67 grams of fat and 82 calories in cod (*Gadus morhua* and *G. macrocephalus*), and 11.91 grams of fat and 189 calories in mackerel (species in genera *Rastrelliger* and *Scomber*). The means of these numbers are 3.13 grams of fat and 101.8 calories. This quantity of fat has 29.42 calories, yielding 28.9 percent of calories from fat as the average among tuna, tilapia, pollock, cod, and mackerel. Again, doubling this percentage to 57.8 fails to reach Perlmutter's 75 percent threshold. Citing another example, shellfish fed coastal peoples and have little fat, Chapter 5 and Table 5.2 noted.

Comparisons may be enlarged to include aquatic mammals, birds, and eggs, but these possibilities are no easier to quantify. For example, the U.S. Department of Agriculture (USDA) collects no information about fat and other nutrients in wild eggs. An impression may be formed from eggs laid by pasture-raised hens (*Gallus gallus domesticus*), which have access to the outdoors. They eat what they find, though owners provide feed and may limit time outside. These conditions do not duplicate existence in the wild, though they may simulate some aspects of it. The nonprofit George Mateljan Foundation tabulated that pasture-raised eggs furnish 64.1 percent of calories as fat, an amount near but still beneath Perlmutter's boundary.[28] These examples suggest that preagricultural peoples ingested under 75 percent of calories from fat.

In evoking prehistory, Perlmutter and Taubes apparently sought evolutionary support for high-fat consumption. The word "evolution" is shorthand for species' adaptation to their environment over time. Since British naturalist Charles Robert Darwin (1809–1882) published *On the Origin of Species* in 1859, biologists have described adaptation in reproductive terms. Organisms best adapted to their environment are most likely to survive long enough to populate the world with their offspring. Because progeny tend to resemble parents, organisms with advantageous traits often pass these advantages to the next generation. Over time, organisms with such traits dominate an environment, in this way fitting species to it.

Applying this process (natural selection) to Perlmutter and Taubes' version of prehistory, hunter-gatherers should have become efficient at digesting and metabolizing fat because they supposedly consumed 75 percent of calories from it and only 5 percent from carbohydrates over many millennia. In other words, a preponderance of fat in diets should have favored the survival and reproduction of people who best digested and metabolized it, ensuring over time that efficient fat burners dominated environments. These fat specialists, seldom consuming carbohydrates, should have been inefficient at digesting and metabolizing them. Because these adaptations to a putatively fat-rich environment enabled our ancestors to populate the world, we must have inherited their advantageous characteristics and so must be most efficient at digesting and metabolizing fat.

Yet physiology rebuts this view because our cells are most efficient at digesting and metabolizing carbohydrates, which the body prefers as energy.[29] For example and as Chapter 2 mentioned, the body absorbs between 97 and 99 percent of carbohydrates it ingests, but 95 percent of fat and 92 or 93 percent of protein.[30] Like other cells, those in the brain metabolize the sugar glucose ($C_6H_{12}O_6$)—Chapter 2 described its manufacture, structure, and metabolism—a carbohydrate. In this context, American nutritionist and dietician Stephanie Green estimated that the brain requires between 50 and 100 grams of carbohydrates daily.[31] Only inadequacy compels it to metabolize fat. Because the body is less efficient at metabolizing fat or protein, the body prefers to metabolize carbohydrates rather than store them while doing the reverse with fat. Endurance athletes apply this knowledge when they consume carbohydrate-rich foods, a practice known as carbohydrate loading, before competition.[32] The outcome of this metabolic bias in favor of carbohydrates is the body's small supply of glycogen relative to adipose when calories are in excess.[33] Moreover and as Chapter 2 noted, fat metabolism's inefficiency is evident in that the body requires more oxygen to metabolize a gram of fat than a gram of carbohydrates. From an evolutionary perspective, humans must have adapted to an environment that supplied carbohydrates, not fat or protein, as the primary macronutrient.

American nutritionist Barry Michael Popkin (b. 1944) echoed this judgment, characterizing humanity's ancestral diet rich in carbohydrates, including fiber, and low fat.[34] Saturated fat was especially meager. More active than moderns, paleolithic hunter-gatherers were seldom overweight or obese.

Additionally, Perlmutter and Taubes' opinion contradicts American botanist Lawrence Kaplan's (1926–2018) belief that hunter-gatherers first targeted tubers, roots, leaves, insects, and game.[35] Chapter 13 indicates that tubers and roots tend to have little fat. Like tubers and roots, leaves are vegetables, most of which Chapter 15 describes as having scant fat. Previous paragraphs debunked the idea that game had much adipose.

Process of elimination leaves insects, which Chapter 3 identified as good sources of several nutrients including fat. Dutch entomologist Arnold van Huis (b. 1946) and coauthors characterized insects' fat content as "high" while acknowledging their nutrients as "highly variable."[36] Sampling species in Cameroon, Africa, the authors calculated between 9 and 67 percent fat by mass.[37] They assigned the highest value (67 percent) to the grasshopper *Ruspolia differens*, but Kenyan food scientists John N. Kinyuru and colleagues quoted lower amounts of 46.2–48.2 percent.[38] These numbers underscore the difficulties of determining fat content today. The problems become insurmountable upon retrogressing millennia into the past. In this regard, conflict between Perlmutter and Taubes' judgment on one hand and Kaplan's on the other may be insoluble given inability to pinpoint preagricultural diets' macro- and micronutrients.

Because the specifics of the preagricultural era faded with time, researchers have used modern hunter-gatherers to approximate the past. Rebutting Perlmutter and Taubes, Eaton and colleague wrote in 1999 that these moderns ate "much less total fat" than developed nations' denizens.[39] Even traditional Inuit diets, treated in Chapter 5, had less fat than today's U.S. fare. Moreover, Inuit consumed less saturated fat than Americans. These contrasts led Eaton and coauthor to recommend fat intake not above 20 percent of calories and avoidance of saturated and hydrogenated fat.[40]

Grain Brain's incongruity is that the quest for fatty foods yields the best results for domesticated animals and plants rather than wild ones. Referencing Table 4.1 again, 100 grams of beef and pork supply 5.8 and 15.3 grams of fat, respectively. Readers may recall that the same amount of venison has 3.93 grams of fat. Chapter 8 and Table 8.1 noted that 100 grams of raw peanuts (*Arachis hypogaea*) total 462.86 of 567 calories, or 81.6 percent, as fat. That is, peanuts, the seeds of a domesticated legume, surpass Perlmutter's 75 percent threshold whereas game, fish, and eggs fall short. Cashews (*Anacardium occidentale*), a nut from a domesticate, furnish 74.8 percent of calories as fat, an amount within an eyelash of Perlmutter's boundary.[41] Pistachios (*Pistacia vera*) exceed it at 75.5 percent of calories as fat.[42] At 99.5 percent of calories as fat, macadamia nuts (*Macadamia integrifolia*) also come from a domesticated tree.[43] Australian geneticist Catherine Jane Nock and coauthors credited Europeans with domesticating the tree in the nineteenth century.[44] This list need not be extended to demonstrate that Perlmutter and Taubes are searching the wrong side of the Neolithic divide for abundant fat.

Moreover, an appeal to nuts as fatty foods erroneously supports belief that past diets supplied ample fat because oily nuts seldom sustained populations. Chapter 9 identified as staples acorns (*Quercus* species) in prehistoric California, Asia, Africa, Europe, and Oceania, and chestnuts (*Castanea* species) in North America, Europe, Asia, and North Africa. Tables 9.3 and 9.4 listed 100 grams each of dried chestnuts and dried acorns at 4.45 and 31.41 grams of fat, respectively. Calories totaled 374 and 509 per 100 grams of each nut. Repeating earlier calculations, dried chestnuts and dried acorns furnish 11.2 and 58 percent of calories as fat. Once more, these numbers fall below Perlmutter's 75 percent.

Turning to animals and their products, Chapter 4 remarked that during the Neolithic Revolution, humans domesticated the pig (*Sus scrofa domesticus*), cow, sheep (*Ovis aries*), and goat (*Capra aegagrus hircus*). Pigs supply lard whereas cows, sheep, and goats furnish fat known as tallow. Chapter 7 noted that domestication permitted humans to milk livestock. After animal husbandry arose, people favored milk from cows, sheep, and goats rather than pigs. Chapter 7 indicated that milk and its derivatives contain fat in varying quantities. Whereas fish, nuts, and seeds provided unsaturated fat, dairy foods added saturated fat to the diet, sometimes in sizable amounts. For example, 100 grams of parmesan cheese have 25 grams of fat, 14.9 of them (59.6 percent) saturated.[45] Saturated fat supplies 35.7 percent of parmesan cheese's calories. Parmesan cheese's saturated and unsaturated fats furnish 59.9 percent of total calories.

Besides meat and dairy, the Neolithic supplied cocoa butter—being 65 percent saturated by mass—from cacao (*Theobroma cacao*) seeds.[46] Lipids from oil palm (*Elaeis guineenis*) seeds, known as palm kernel oil, rank higher at 90 percent saturated. Coconut (*Cocos nucifera*) oil is an even richer source at 92 percent saturated.[47] By contrast, palm oil comes from fruit rather than seed and is 49.3 percent saturated by mass.[48] Less may be obtained from cottonseed (*Gossypium hirsutum* and *G. herbaceum*), peanut, soybean, and olive (*Olea europaea*) oils, which are 26, 19, 15, and 14 percent saturated, respectively, by mass.[49]

By supplying saturated fat, animal husbandry and agriculture altered the nutrition and diets of people whose preagricultural predecessors had consumed primarily unsaturated lipids. Beginning to collect nutrition and health data in 1952, American physiologist Ancel Benjamin Keys (1904–2004) correlated early deaths with diets high in saturated fat, which increased cholesterol and blood pressure and heightened the risk of heart disease and stroke.[50] Smoking and sucrose consumption also exacerbated these dangers. Keys' work was compelling because of breadth and thoroughness, deriving information over decades from Finland, the United States, Italy, Spain, South Africa, Japan, Bosnia and Herzegovina, Croatia, Montenegro, Macedonia, Serbia, and Slovenia. Table 10.1 encapsulates farming and livestock raising's effects on dietary proportions of saturated and unsaturated fats by listing eleven lipids.[51]

TABLE 10.1
Fat % by Type in Selected Lipids

Lipid	Saturated (%)	Monounsaturated (%)	Polyunsaturated (%)
Butter	64	33	3
Canola	7	63	30
Coconut	92	6	2
Cottonseed	26	22	51
Olive	14	76	10
Palm	51	39	10
Peanut	19	45	36
Safflower	9	14	77
Soybean	15	23	62
Sunflower	11	23	66
Tallow	50	47	3

10.2.3 The Controversy over Fat Intake

In 1957, the American Heart Association targeted not just saturated fat, advocating a reduction in total fat intake. Although medical authorities emphasized the link between fat and disease, dieters who cut the macronutrient did so to diminish calories in hopes of regaining a slim, youthful figure. This approach leveraged the fact, mentioned in Chapter 2, that by mass fat more than doubles the calories in carbohydrates or protein. A current proponent of lean diets, American nutritionist Thomas Colin Campbell (b. 1934)—introduced in Chapter 1—recommended consumption of 10 percent of calories from fat and protein each, and the rest from carbohydrates.[52]

Parallel to these developments, fat enthusiasts co-opted the message of trimness. American cardiologist Robert Coleman Atkins (1930–2003), introduced in Chapter 4, advocated liberal ingestion of fat and protein, not carbohydrates, as the path toward a slender physique.[53] His *Dr. Atkins' Diet Revolution: The High Calorie Way to Stay Thin Forever* (1972) promoted the illusion that indulgence yielded leanness, permitting the reader to "eat as *much* as you want, as *often* as you want."[54]

Atkins evoked a now-familiar past during which humanity's ancestors evolved over "fifty million years" to eat fat and protein—stating that the pair's natural ratio is 40–60—with carbohydrates near zero.[55] These numbers beg citations that Atkins omitted. Chapter 1 mentioned that the keto, grapefruit, and paleo diets resemble his formulation. Viewed from this vantage point, Perlmutter is the latest to laud fat and excoriate carbohydrates.

Fatty diets' proliferation did not eliminate concerns about saturated fat. Since the 1980s, these worries shifted consumption from animal products rich in saturated fat and cholesterol to plant oils with monounsaturated and polyunsaturated fats.[56] This transition did not reduce fat intake because fast foods and processed items had abundant lipids as well as salt and sucrose. The rest of this chapter examines how fat affected ancient and modern health. The next chapter evaluates carbohydrates as sucrose, honey, and high fructose corn syrup (HFCS).

10.3 OLIVE OIL

10.3.1 Olive Oil versus Most Vegetable Oils

As noted, an example of a domesticated tree that yields fat is the olive. Olive oil is among the few plant lipids—avocado (*Persea americana*) oil is another—derived from fruit that surrounds the seed rather than from the seed. Because each olive has just one seed, it is known as a drupe. The fact that olives are about 80 percent water by mass necessitates oil extraction by crushing the fruit, a mechanical process known as pressing.[57] Pressing preserves the oil's flavor and aroma. In contrast, extraction of seed oils, once done by pressing, is now accomplished chemically. The chemical's removal at extraction's end is also a chemical process, rendering the oil insipid and odorless. Although such characteristics satisfy some consumers, others are willing to pay a premium for olive oil because it is distinctive. The lure of high prices has long tempted entrepreneurs to adulterate this oil.

10.3.2 Origins of Oleiculture

Since the nineteenth century, competing hypotheses have proposed the olive tree's origin in Asia, Africa, or Europe.[58] The Mediterranean basin, touching all three, may be the tree's homeland. Fossilized seeds on Italian islands Sicily and Sardinia and in southeastern Italy's Puglia date between 12,000 and 3000 BCE, though the oldest may predate domestication. Domestication may have occurred around 6000 BCE in the southern Caucasus Mountains between the Black and Caspian Seas, a region that bridges Asia to the east and Europe to the west.[59] By the fourth millennium BCE, olive trees were in southwestern Asia, from where they spread west throughout the Mediterranean.[60] This chronology denies that the tree originated in the Mediterranean. By 3000 BCE, oleiculture was established in Lebanon and on the Greek island of Crete. About 2300 BCE, papyri documented olive trees in Egypt. Around 1754 BCE, the Code of King Hammurabi (1811–1750 BCE) mentioned them in Babylon, a city whose remnants are 94 kilometers (59 miles) southwest of Baghdad, Iraq.[61] Fifteenth-century BCE Hamitic-Semitic peoples plants olive trees in Syria and Turkey.[62] Roman naturalist Pliny the Elder (23–79 CE) praised Syrian olives for their excellence.[63]

10.3.3 Oleiculture in Egypt

In northeasternmost Africa, Egypt arose as an olive producer and consumer. Chapter 4 discussed its history, geography, economy, diets, nutrition, and health. Egyptian graves had olive branches and leaves. Because only the wealthy could afford elaborate burials, these items indicated olives' elite status. Pharaoh Ramses III (1217–1166 BCE) planted olive trees around the Temple of Thebes and offered their oil to the god Ra, confirmation of olives' eminence and association with royalty and divinity.[64] Egypt's aridity confined olive trees, and all farming, to the narrow band of land inundated annually by the Nile River. Consequently, Egypt was not a large olive producer but instead imported oil. In the fourth century BCE, Greek botanist Theophrastus (c. 372–c. 287 BCE) disparaged Egypt's olive oil. Before then—between the twenty-first and fifteenth centuries BCE—Egypt took olive trees south to what are today Sudan, South Sudan, and Ethiopia.

10.3.4 Oleiculture in Greece

Trading throughout the Mediterranean from their base in the Levant—whose geography Chapter 14 describes—sixteen-and-fifteenth-centuries BCE Phoenicians planted Syrian olive trees on the island of Cyprus, which Greeks colonized in antiquity and which is independent today.[65] From Cyprus, oleiculture spread to Greek islands Rhodes and Samos. On mainland Greece, olive cultivation may predate 3500 BCE. "Olive oil entered its golden age with the Greeks, who held the olive tree sacred," wrote Tom Mueller, journalist and author of *Extra Virginity: The Sublime and Scandalous World of Olive Oil* (2012).[66] Law forbade owners from annually pruning over 0.6 meters (2 feet) from a tree.[67] Greek archon (lawgiver) Solon (c. 630–c. 560 BCE) prohibited an owner from cutting down over two trees yearly.[68] Solon encouraged cultivation by allowing farmers to export only olive oil.[69] Greek philosopher Aristotle (384–322 BCE) advocated death for anyone who destroyed a tree.[70]

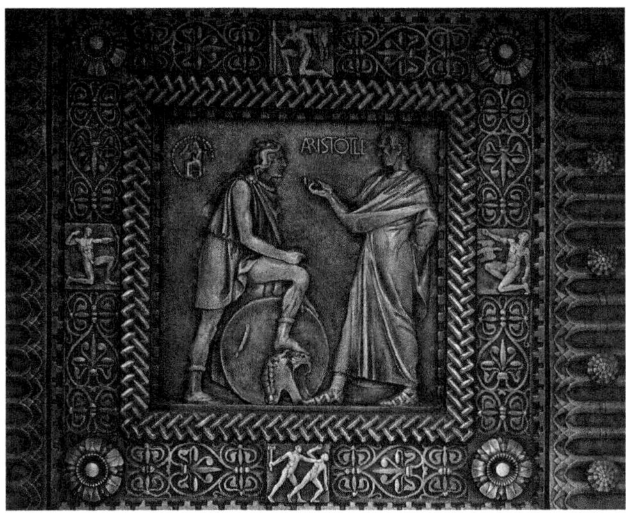

FIGURE 10.1 Aristotle. (Photo courtesy of Library of Congress. https://www.loc.gov/pictures/item/2011631954/.)

10.3.5 Oleiculture in the Roman Empire

By the first millennium BCE, olive oil production and trade were huge enterprises. A press dating around 800 BCE in Palestine—now Palestine and Israel—was large enough to make 500,000 liters (132,086 gallons) of oil annually.[71] Seventh-century BCE Greeks, Phoenicians, or both planted olive trees on Italian islands Sicily and Sardinia, though a previous paragraph mentioned earlier introductions. Whether these plantings spread north into the peninsula is uncertain, though within a century olive trees were as far north as Italy's Po River. Roman agricultural writers Cato the Elder (234–149 BCE), Marcus Terentius Varro (116–27 BCE), and Lucius Junius Moderatus Columella (4–70 CE), Pliny the Elder, and poets Virgil (70–19 BCE) and Horace (65–8 BCE) esteemed olives and gave advice on their culture.[72]

The Romans regarded olive oil as a profitable commodity. Its wealth elevated families into the elite. For example, Emperor Hadrian (76–138 CE) was the scion of Spanish olive magnates.[73] Emperor and Stoic philosopher Marcus Aurelius (121–180) traced his paternal ancestry to Spanish olive tycoons. Emperor Septimius Severus (145–211) descended from prominent Libyan olive planters.

Libya may have acquired olive trees from Egypt to the east. Alternatively, olives may have reached Libya from Tunisia to the west, where the Phoenicians may have introduced them upon founding Carthage—now a suburb of the city Tunis—in the ninth century BCE. A third possibility involves

5386 Crushing Oil from the Olive Nablus Palestine.
Copyrighted 1903 by William H. Rau

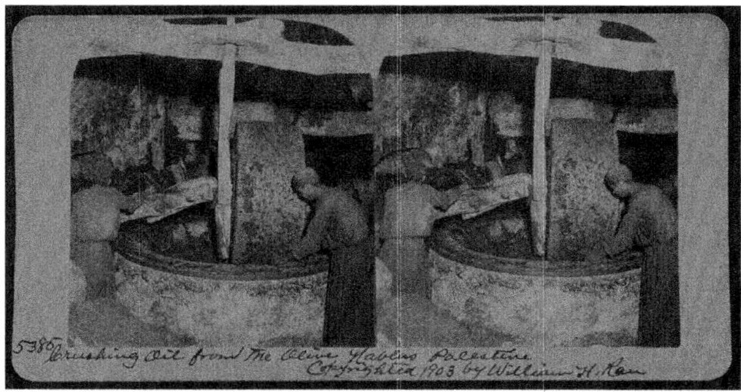

FIGURE 10.2 Olive presses. (Photo courtesy of Library of Congress. https://www.loc.gov/pictures/item/2006679669/.)

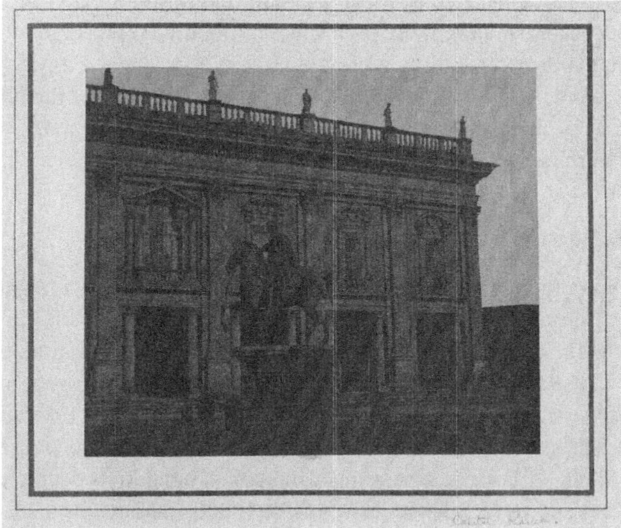

FIGURE 10.3 Marcus Aurelius. (Photo courtesy of Library of Congress. https://www.loc.gov/pictures/item/2019640546/.)

the Greeks, who during the eighth and seventh centuries BCE may have planted olive trees in the region of eastern Libya known in antiquity as Cyrenaica.[74] From Tunisia, olives spread west to what are today Algeria and Morocco. Independent of these developments, the Berbers, early inhabitants of North Africa, may have begun cultivating olives in the fourth century BCE.

Although Spain entered Rome's orbit in the third century BCE because of war with Carthage, interest in olives had begun earlier. Spaniards ate wild ones as early as the fourth millennium BCE. The Phoenicians planted *O. europaea* in what are today Spain and Portugal around the eleventh century BCE. Rome intensified cultivation, especially in the province Hispania Baetica, which lies in southwestern Spain and includes Gibraltar. Spain shipped olive oil to Italy, Britain, and what are now Switzerland, Germany, Belgium, and the Netherlands. Northeast of Baetica, the province Hispania Terraconensis produced olive oil for local consumption. Together Baetica and Terraconensis occupied Mediterranean Spain and so commanded Iberia's best olive lands.

Rome conquered Carthage in the second century BCE, enlarging it into the province of North Africa during the next century, though emperors administered it separate from Egypt, which was annexed in 30 BCE.[75] Rome promoted oleiculture throughout North Africa—which was expected to furnish the empire 3 million liters (792,516.2 gallons) of oil yearly—Egypt, and other Mediterranean territories.[76] Soldiers furthered this objective by planting olive trees in these lands. Olive trees integrated an area into the economy by supplying the oil that Romans prized. The trees symbolized civilization and so concretized Rome's ambition to spread high culture wherever it went. Olive trees also symbolized peace—evident in Genesis—communicating soldiers' desire to diffuse tensions as they occupied territory.[77]

When the empire expanded into northern Europe, however, farmers discovered its unsuitability for olive trees. This disappointment never diminished Rome's enthusiasm for olives and olive oil. Like other Mediterranean peoples, Romans ingested olive oil as their primary fat, consuming as many as 50 liters (13.2 gallons) per person annually.[78] In the second century CE, Emperor Trajan (53–117 CE) required North African farms without olive trees to plant them. His successor Hadrian suspended ten years' taxes for those who grew olives on land that had been abandoned. Although they could not own this land, Hadrian's edict granted them and their descendants a perpetual right to lease it. This law furthered a policy of encouraging agriculturists to occupy and improve uncultivated hectarage, reflecting Roman opinion that land fulfilled its purpose only if productive; otherwise, it was useless, a circumstance deemed wasteful and immoral. In 301, Emperor Diocletian (245–311) attempted to establish maximum prices for commodities.[79] It set three for olive oil, recognizing differences in quality by awarding a premium for virgin, defined as oil from the first pressing.[80] These prices implied that the wealthy had long been able to purchase the finest oil, a possibility that Rome had realized by integrating Mediterranean lands into a single market. Consequently, the best Spanish oil, for example, was never far from buyers in Greece, Turkey, Syria, or Jordan.

10.3.6 Oleiculture in the Middle Ages

Olive cultivation, commerce, and consumption survived the empire's fragmentation in the fourth and fifth centuries. Originating in the High Empire (c. 200 BCE–c. 200 CE), Christianity preserved Rome's knowledge about oleiculture. Reading Roman agricultural texts, monks produced olive oil for their own use, for sale, and for burning during liturgy. By generating light, this last act reminded worshippers that Jesus was "the light of the world."[81] At the same time, Christians grappled with olive oil's pre-Christian uses in gymnasia, theaters, and pagan temples. In these contexts, the oil symbolized lasciviousness and abandon. The church deemphasized this past by claiming that saints worked miracles with olive oil. Religious authorities made it the de facto frying agent by banning meat and animal fat during the year's over 100 fast days including Lent's forty, treated in Chapter 5.

Medieval (c. 500–c. 1500) and Renaissance (c. 1450–c. 1600) Puglia produced a plurality of the world's olive oil. Like oil from Spanish island Mallorca in the Mediterranean Sea, Liguria in northwestern Italy, and Catalonia in northeastern Spain, however, Puglia's harvest occupied the second tier. The best came from Lake Garda in northern Italy, Gaeta and Tuscany in central Italy, and Le Marche on Italy's Adriatic coast. Calabria in southwestern Italy and Andalusia in southern Spain yielded the worst, thought suitable only for making soap.

10.3.7 Defense of Olive Oil

Mueller asserted, first, that olive oil is healthful because it is fat, which does not cause overweight, obesity, heart disease, or cancers, ills he blamed on carbohydrates.[82] Second, olive oil promotes vitality because it is "the crux of the Mediterranean diet."[83] The implication is that it must benefit consumers because it is central to a diet universally praised.

10.3.8 Criticism of Olive Oil's Defense

Taking these issues in order, the attempt to fault carbohydrates rather than fat for the litany of chronic diseases in affluent societies is not novel. Among its proponents are Gary Taubes, American journalist Michael Kevin Pollan (b. 1955), and American physicians William Davis (b. 1957) and David Perlmutter. This chapter includes Davis in this group because his nemesis, wheat, supplies roughly 85 percent of its calories as carbohydrates.[84] This book discusses Davis and Perlmutter's opinions elsewhere and need not comment here. Pollan's *In Defense of Food* (2008) critiqued carbohydrates as responsible for obesity.[85] Mentioned earlier, Taubes condemned carbohydrates—especially the easily digested sugars sucrose and HFCS and starch—in *Good Calories, Bad Calories* (2008) and *Why We Get Fat and What to Do about It* (2011).[86]

In this anti-carbohydrate contingent, Mueller blamed the U.S. Senate Select Committee on Nutrition and Human Needs, the USDA, and the National Institutes of Health (NIH) in the 1970s for excoriating fat as obesity's cause and promoting low-fat foods as the remedy.[87] But because these items have many calories, often as sucrose and other sugars, Americans grew fatter. Between 1980 and 2012, the percentage of obese Americans more than doubled from 14 to 34.[88]

This book acknowledges that surplus energy—whether carbohydrates, fat, protein, alcohol, or their combination—enlarges the body. But Mueller went beyond this arithmetic to target carbohydrates as especially guilty of what has been termed an obesity epidemic. This section refers readers to the next chapter for evidence that sucrose alone is unlikely to have caused rampant obesity. Chapter 12 disagrees that wheat and other grains—noted as carbohydrate rich—cause overweight and obesity but instead amass evidence that inactivity worsens these problems.

Attempts to fault the macronutrient for excessive girth ignore that between roughly 1912 and 2012 U.S. diets diminished from over 56 percent carbohydrates to 47 percent.[89] Moreover, research correlated fat intake—not carbohydrate—and obesity.[90] Troubling are studies that demonstrated body fat enlargement among people who reduced calories but increased fat consumption. These results, despite their health implications, appear not to interest fat's apologists.

Blaming carbohydrates for people's enormity, Mueller ignored the reality that olive oil is among the most caloric foods. One hundred grams have 884 calories compared to 387 and 281 calories in sucrose and HFCS, respectively, per 100 grams.[91] Being pure carbohydrates, sucrose and HFCS are pariahs; yet both have under half olive oil's calories by mass. Despite Mueller's anti-carbohydrate crusade, the arithmetic of calorie counting dictates that olive oil enlarges girth more than pure carbohydrates, all else equal.

Mueller's second claim depends on the existence of a Mediterranean diet, which olive oil undergirds. For this premise to be true, a uniform diet must have existed in lands around the Mediterranean Sea since olives and olive oil became important foods. The previous section found that olive consumption in this region is at least 14,000 years old and that olive oil was produced on a grand scale no later than the first millennium BCE. Muller's argument, therefore, requires the existence of a unitary Mediterranean diet during roughly the last three millennia and probably much longer. In other words, Mueller's Mediterranean diet must hold over a vast duration and diverse peoples. The United Nations Educational, Scientific and Cultural Organization (UNESCO) acknowledges this criterion, stating that "The Mediterranean diet is characterized by a nutritional model that has remained constant over time and space."[92]

But no consensus consensus exists about this diet's elements. Eying antiquity, British classicist Peter David Arthur Garnsey (b. 1938) supplied the simplest list: grains, olives, and grapes (*Vitis vinifera*).[93] To the "Mediterranean triad," he added legumes mentioned in Chapter 8: broad beans (*Vicia faba*), chickpeas (*Cicer arietinum*), peas (*Pisum sativum*), and lentils (*Len culinaris*).[94] These additions were no afterthought, occupying greater geographic breadth than olives and grapes. Chapter 8 examined legumes' health effects in prehistory and history.

British biochemist Richard Hoffman and French epidemiologist Mariette Gerber articulated a similar trio for Phoenicians, Greeks, and Romans: wheat (*Triticum monococcum, T. dicoccon, T. aestivum*, and *T. durum*), grapes, and olives.[95] To these three, the authors add onions (*Allium cepa*), leeks (*Allium ampeloprasum*), lettuce (*Lactuca sativa*), carrots (*Daucus carota ssp. sativus*), asparagus (*Asparagus officinalis*), turnips (*Brassica rapa ssp. rapa*), cabbage (*Brassica oleracea var. capitata*), celery (*Apium graveolens*), artichoke (*Cynara scolymus*), figs (*Ficus carica*), apples

(*Malus domestica*), pears (*Pyrus communis*), cherries (*Prunus cerasus* and *P. avium*), plums (*Prunus domestica*), peaches (*Prunus persica*), apricots (*Prunus armeniaca*), citrons (*Citrus medica*), chestnuts (*C. sativa*), almonds (*Amygdalus communis*), and walnuts (*Juglans regia*) during Roman antiquity (c. 750 BCE–c. 500 CE). This list might have included dates (*Phoenix dactylifera*)—discussed in Chapter 14—which were grown in Roman Asia and North Africa and eaten throughout the empire.

Hoffman and Gerber enlarged this roster for the Middle Ages when Arabs—colonizing several Mediterranean islands, southwestern Asia, North Africa, and parts of Spain—introduced rice, lemon trees (*Citrus limon*), eggplant (*Solanum melongena*), and spices such as saffron (*Crocus sativus*). European contact with the Americas in the late fifteenth century added tomatoes (*Solanum esculentum*) and peppers (*Capsicum annuum*) to the Mediterranean diet.

In 1953, Rockefeller Foundation field director Leland Girard Allbaugh (1896–1991), focusing on Crete, updated this list, writing that "food seemed literally to be 'swimming' in oil."[96] Beyond olive oil, Cretans ate grains, leafy vegetables, fruits, legumes, nuts, and potatoes (*Solanum tuberosum*), the last seldom designated a Mediterranean food. Goat, game, fish, most dairy, eggs, and sucrose were eaten infrequently.[97] The chief grains were wheat, barley (*Hordeum vulgare*), and rice.[98] Emphasizing continuity, Allbaugh stated that Crete's diet changed little over "forty centuries."[99]

In 1999, Artemis Simopoulos, describing her childhood in Greece, highlighted the diversity that fed her family: chicken, goat, mutton, lamb, fish, eggs, olives, pears, figs, plums, pomegranates (*Punica granatum*), and whole-wheat bread.[100] These foods, those in previous paragraphs, and their chronology of adoption indicate the absence of a static Mediterranean diet. Rather than a monolith, the Mediterranean diet—if such language must be employed—changed over time.

It also varied geographically, as the foregoing implied. Even for antiquity, Garnsey emphasized grains as the only universal among the big three.[101] For example, sesame (*Sesamum indicum*) oil was an alternative to olive oil in Roman Asia and Egypt. Among cereals, Hoffman and Gerber's focus on wheat omitted a diversity that included rye (*Secale cereale*), oats (*Avena sativa*), several types of millet (species in Eragrostideae tribe), and barley. Chapter 12 questions wheat's dietary importance during prehistory and much of history. More drought tolerant than wheat (see Chapter 12), barley was especially important in an era of shortages. The danger of crop failure—which meant hunger or starvation—in a region with hot, dry summers led risk-averse farmers to plant barley or millet. Even wheat was diverse because, Chapter 12 notes, the ancients cultivated and ate four species: *Triticum monococcum*, *T. dicoccon*, *T. aestivum*, and *T. durum* plus spelt (*T. spelta*). By contrast, the United States has reduced this quintet to *T. aestivum* for bread and *T. durum* for pasta. Pluralism is also evident in the Roman world's seventy-two types of bread by one count.[102]

Geographic divisions persist. Olive oil consumption is highest in Greece and lowest in Egypt and Turkey.[103] Pork is the principal meat in Spain, southern France, Italy, and the Mediterranean island Malta, whereas beef feeds Croatia, Bosnia, and Albania, lamb sustains Libya, Algeria, Morocco, and Tunisia, and chicken is most popular in Greece, Lebanon, Cyprus, Turkey, and Egypt, though lamb rivals it in Greece.[104] Whole barley and wheat are the chief grains in Libya, Algeria, Morocco, and Tunisia, white flour feeds Croatia, Bosnia, and Albania, and rice rivals wheat in Spain, Italy, southern France, and Malta. Cheese is more popular in Spain, Italy, southern France, Malta, Croatia, Bosnia, and Albania than elsewhere in the Mediterranean. More potatoes are eaten in Spain, southern France, Italy, Malta, Libya, Algeria, Morocco, and Tunisia than elsewhere. Okra (*Abelmoschus esculentus*) is popular only in Greece, Lebanon, Cyprus, Turkey, and Egypt.

Since antiquity, inequalities bifurcated diets between affluent and commoner, a theme evident throughout this book. Chapter 4 described the dietary chasm between ancient Egyptian elites, who feasted on meat, and the poor, who subsisted on plants. Inequality was also manifested throughout the Mediterranean in the reality that commoners might eat an occasional European anchovy (*Engraulis encrasicolus*) but not the sea bream (*Pagrus major* and *Pagellus bogaraveo*), tuna, gray mullet (*Mugil cephalus*), and eels (species in the order Anguilliformes) that the wealthy monopolized.[105] Garnsey noted the "large gulf between the *haute cuisine* of the few and the frugal menus of the mass of the population, rural and urban."[106]

Rather than one diet, therefore, inequalities and numerous food combinations that evolved over centuries characterized the Mediterranean. Sicilian historian and culinary school director Fabrizia Lanza (b. 1961) acknowledged that "it is nearly impossible to find a common link among the various countries that surround the Mediterranean Sea, least of all on culinary grounds."[107]

Complicating this description is insistence that Mediterranean foodways transcend diets by encompassing a way of life. Simopoulos stressed the immediacy of fresh, local produce and the virtue of moderation.[108] Religiosity compels Greeks to fast, even abstaining from olive oil, during Lent and other spartan periods. Lenten fasts lead the devout to lose as many as 4.5 kilograms (10 pounds). Besides austerity, Greeks walk wherever they go and stand during church services. Schools mandate an hour's exercise daily. Elsewhere this book contends that vitality requires exertion.

Hoffman and Gerber likewise considered moderation and activity integral to the "MedDiet" because the word "diet" derives from the Greek *diaita*, meaning "mode of living."[109] These authors and Chapters 1 and 2 stated that outdoor activity enhances health by exposing the body to sunlight, thereby stimulating it to produce vitamin D. Beyond these particulars, Hoffman and Gerber noted the prevalence of siestas, whose healthfulness is unclear, in Spain and Greece. These specifics and those in previous paragraphs undermine belief in a single Mediterranean diet, which olives and olive oil supposedly anchor. Moreover, these particulars do not demonstrate that olive oil maintains or improves vigor.

In championing olive oil, Mueller interpreted evidence in ways that may be challenged. For example, he upheld Puglia as the exemplar of a region where olive oil promoted vitality, writing that "Olive oil has been a staple here [in Puglia] forever."[110] Nineteen pages later, however, he quoted a resident who credited vegetables with Puglia's health: "Pugliesi eat an incredible amount of vegetables—we're like goats."[111] Yet Mueller is silent about vegetables in his preoccupation with olive oil. Chapter 15 avoids this myopia by examining them in ancient Herculaneum.

10.3.9 Olive Oil and Health in Roman Antiquity

Olive oil's importance to ancient Mediterranean peoples suggests their suitability for examining its health effects. Desirable for this investigation is knowledge of how much olive oil they consumed. Such data might seem irretrievable, but in *On Agriculture* (c. 160 BCE), Cato the Elder advised that each slave receive about 6.8 liters (1.8 gallons) yearly.[112] Skeptics might challenge this information given the impossibility of knowing whether readers followed this advice during or after Cato's life. Additionally, the dietary diversity emphasized in the previous section means that Mediterranean peoples consumed different quantities of olive oil, if any. Moreover, his recommendation may reveal nothing about consumption before or after his time.

This section acknowledges these criticisms while arguing that three conditions favor *On Agriculture*'s use as an index of olive oil consumption. First, Rome, like elsewhere in premodern times, was agrarian. The estimate that Rome's farms generally yielded 10 percent surpluses means that agriculture fed farmers plus an extra one-tenth of people: those engaged outside agriculture, namely urbanites.[113] The 90 percent of Romans who lived and worked on farms were within Cato's purview because he specified rations for rural rather than urban laborers.

Second, in targeting farmworkers (slaves), his allowances applied to the masses rather than elites. Such information is invaluable during an era when literate people came from the leisure class and seldom expressed interest in anyone but their peers. In other words, in writing about slaves, Cato revealed information about commoners, whose diets, nutrition, and health are central to this inquiry. The objection that not all nine-tenths of Roman workers were slaves does not weaken this argument because farmworkers, whether slave or free, had to exert themselves to eke out an existence in an era of low yields and rudimentary technology. To put the matter differently, free people and slaves faced the same biological and technological limits to extracting food from the soil. Both toiled under the same conditions.

Third, *On Agriculture* survives. In fact, it is the oldest extant Latin text.[114] At a time of papyri and parchment, documents had to be copied and recopied by hand, an expensive, laborious chore that doomed anything deemed unimportant to oblivion. *On Agriculture*'s persistence over two millennia suggests its value to readers. Varro and Columella quoted it, and Columella praised the manual for teaching "agriculture to speak Latin."[115] Roman author and stylist Aulus Gellius (c. 125–c. 180 CE) admired its vigor and directness.[116] Pliny quoted it sixty-four times in his *Natural History* (c. 77 CE), more than any other source.[117] Such circumstances imply that readers heeded rather than ignored Cato.

His 6.8 liters of olive oil per slave annually is little over half Mueller's 2012 estimate that the average Italian consumed 13 liters (3.4 gallons) per year.[118] Cato's smaller number is unsurprising given ancient agriculture's low yields, mentioned already, and the desire to economize slaves' upkeep. Frugality led Cato to recommend less food for slaves when ill and unable to work.[119] Modern corporations seek the same parsimony even though workers are now free to sell their talents to the highest bidder.

Olive oil does not appear to have improved Roman demography. A woman who reached menopause had to average 4.5–6.5 births just to replace losses from mortality.[120] Youth mortality was so high that three or four times more people died before age ten than reached sixty.[121] Contagion truncated lives, especially in cities. Although epidemics worried authorities, diseases were prevalent even in uneventful times. Ancient life expectancy at birth (e^0) hovered nearer twenty than thirty years.[122] Census data from Roman Egypt, skeletons from North African cemeteries, and the third-century CE legal document Ulpian's life table put e^0 around twenty-two years.[123]

These numbers led Austrian historian Walter Scheidel (b. 1966) to doubt that diets improved during antiquity and to infer poor net nutrition from bone and teeth deformities.[124] Net nutrition is intake minus claims made by work, diseases, and parasites. Intake adequate today might have failed to meet the demands of a precarious existence. Ancient Mediterranean diets were deficient in vitamin A and its precursors, vitamin D, and possibly iron.[125] Iron deficiency is inferred from anemia and is controversial. Because pathogens and parasites deplete iron, diets may contain enough iron by modern reckoning but still not protect against anemia. Such considerations indicate that olive oil cannot be faulted entirely for nutritional shortfalls. On the other hand, its value extending no farther than calories, phytochemicals, and vitamins E and K, olive oil cannot have prevented iron and vitamins A and D deficits. A later section quantifies olive oil's vitamins E and K.

Amid modernity's diverse foods, consumers can do better than olive oil. For example, Chapter 13 recommends the potato as the world's most nourishing food. Readers should favor it over olive oil. If fatty foods are desired, peanuts—Chapter 8 discussed their origin, dispersal, consumption, nutrition, and healthfulness—supply many more nutrients than olive oil. Several nuts in Chapter 9 provide more essential fatty acids than olive oil plus abundant nutrients. These comparisons do not bar it from diets but instead urge consideration of the entire nutrient profile when selecting foods.

10.3.10 Olive Oil and Health in Crete

Besides ancient Rome, post-World War II Crete is a suitable example given Allbaugh's observation, mentioned above, that Cretans ate copious olives and olive oil. The average Cretan consumed 30.5 kilograms (33.4 liters) of olive oil in 1948.[126] Mueller wrote in 2012 that the typical resident of Kritsa, Crete ingested the world's most olive oil at 45.6 kilograms (50 liters) yearly, whereas the mean for all Greeks was 19.2 kilograms (21.1 liters) per person annually.[127] Also in 2012, Hoffman and Gerber stated that the Greek annual average was the world's highest at 15.9 kilograms (17.4 liters) per capita.[128] Italy and Spain ranked second and third in annual intake at 14 kilograms (15.4 liters) and 11.8 kilograms (12.9 liters) per head, respectively. At the bottom of Mediterranean countries were Turkey and Egypt at 0.7 kilograms (700 grams or 767.2 milliliters) and 0.1 kilograms (100 grams or 109.6 milliliters) per person per year, respectively. Tunisian, Moroccan, and French annual averages were not inordinate by Greek standards at 3.4 kilograms (3.7 liters), 2.9 kilograms (3.2 liters), and 1.7 kilograms (1.9 liters) per capita, respectively. These numbers elude easy comparison because they vary markedly. Moreover, Muller on one hand and Hoffman and Gerber on the other disagreed about Greek consumption.

These problems may be skirted by concentrating on Allbaugh, who furnished demographic data. Whereas Mediterranean countries reported mortality between fourteen and eighteen per 1,000 persons in 1948—figures Allbaugh rated "medium high"—Crete totaled from 11.3 to 13.7 before World War II and 10.6 from 1946 to 1948.[129] In the Mediterranean, only Jews and Cypriots approached Cretan mortality, which was 2.5 years lower in countryside than city.[130] In 1948, Crete's modal age at death was forty-eight, eight years later than in 1938. Cretan e^0 in 1948 was roughly fifty-five or fifty-six years. By comparison, U.S. modal age at death in 1948 was fifty-eight years and e^0 was sixty-seven years.

Differences between hinterland and metropolis implied that contagion truncated urban lives. Between 1946 and 1948, pneumonia was Crete's second greatest killer, trailing the natural causes of old age.[131] Tuberculosis killed under 5 percent of Cretans, and, as a group, dysentery, diarrhea, enteritis, and typhoid registered 3 percent of deaths. Reductions in malaria from the use of the insecticide dichlorodiphenyltrichloroethane (DDT) and in influenza likely explained the increase in lifespan between 1938 and 1948.

While malaria and influenza retreated, deaths from heart disease and cancers rose.[132] These chronic diseases may have stemmed from Crete's World War II reliance on imports rather than its traditional foods.[133] Imports did not cease at war's end because in 1953, Allbaugh reported that Crete distributed sucrose, corn, and soybean flour free to its poorest citizens.[134] The ascent of heart disease and cancers implied that sucrose, corn, and soybean flour undermined health. In this context, Chapter 11 critiques sucrose, and Chapter 12 furnishes evidence of corn's shortcomings.

Crete's low death rate by Mediterranean standards raised the possibility that olive oil, as a large component of diets, is healthful, though, as noted, evidence from antiquity is wanting. Crete's favorable mortality may be juxtaposed with its status as part of Greece, Europe's poorest nation in 1948.[135] Because poverty often correlates with morbidity and mortality, as discussed in Chapter 1, Cretans were exceptional in being poor and healthy.

If Cretans in the 1940s and 1950s exemplified vitality and ate much fat, especially olive oil, readers may wish to emulate their diets. To this end, the Cretan model limits fat largely to olive oil. Allbaugh emphasized Crete's paucity of butter and animal fat and near absence of margarine.[136] Moreover, Cretans consumed little sucrose, honey, or other sweeteners, subjects of the next chapter. Crucial is the recognition that Cretan diets necessitated deprivation. One interviewee summarized the island's predicament, stating that "We are hungry most of the time."[137]

Despite hunger, Cretan life mandated strenuous exertions. Allbaugh recorded Cretans' "great amount of daily walking over stony and hilly terrain."[138] This pedestrianism and average of just two cars per 1,000 residents between 1930 and 1940 contrasted with America's automobile addiction, a problem explored in Chapter 12 and elsewhere.[139] Eighty percent of Cretans occupied farms, which they worked without machines.[140] Allbaugh counted only forty tractors on the island.[141] Instead, farmers used little besides a plow, sickle, and hoe. Plowing necessitated continuous walking. The sickle and hoe required enormous hand labor. The sickle—often used while bent near the ground—fatigued workers to a degree unknown and unimaginable in developed nations. Periods of intense labor required daily consumption of 4,500 calories per person.[142]

Emulation of Cretan vitality, therefore, requires more than eating fat. Absent the arduous exertions that Allbaugh documented throughout *Crete: A Case Study of an Underdeveloped Area* (1953), excess fat and calories, as noted, cause overweight and obesity. The Cretan formula requires unremitting toil, self-denial, and hunger. This book doubts that developed countries are ready for such austerity and sacrifice. Among sacrifices, for example, Cretan vigor demanded the automobile's renunciation, a step unthinkable and draconian to the affluent.

Returning to the relationship between health and wealth, a 2009 paper used data from the Great Depression's (1929–1939) early years (1930–1933) to argue that health improves during economic crises.[143] This conclusion contradicts Chapter 1's observation that the wealthiest Americans live almost fifteen years longer than the poorest.[144] To be sure, belief that poverty promotes health resonates in a plutocracy because it justifies the poor's oppression. Yet in 2018, the world's poorest countries by gross domestic product (GDP) per person—the Democratic Republic of the Congo (DRC), Mozambique, Uganda, Tajikistan, and Yemen—ranked near the bottom in e^0.[145] Mozambique was 217th of 228 nations at 54.1 years at birth. Uganda ranked 213th at 54.7 years, and the DRC was 205th at 58.1 years. Of the five poorest nations, only Tajikistan and Yemen ranked above the 200 worst nations in e^0. The richest countries—Qatar, Singapore, Brunei Darussalam, Kuwait, and the United Arab Emirates (UAB)—surpassed the poorest by decades.[146] The second richest, Singapore, ranked third in e^0 at 85.5 years. The other four occupied the top 100 countries while trailing Singapore's e^0 over six years. Aggregate wealth does not guarantee longevity, especially given unequal distribution. In this regard, per person GDP is an inadequate measure because it hides inequalities by averaging wealth across a population.

10.3.11 Olives, Olive Oil, and Health in Egypt

Economics aside, not all Mediterranean peoples exhibited enviable health. In 2018, Egypt ranked 126th in e^0 at 74.4 years, with men dying four years younger than women.[147] Heart disease is the greatest killer at 34 percent of Egyptian deaths according to the World Health Organization (WHO) in Geneva, Switzerland.[148] These data challenge belief that olive oil is "the healthiest fat" and "the best oil for your health," particularly because Egyptians eat numerous olives.[149] If olive oil benefits the body, olives should also confer vitality.[150] That olives do not benefit Egyptians raises doubts about olive oil.

Hoffman and Gerber sidestepped the issue of olive oil by faulting Egyptians for frying foods in ghee (see Chapter 7), which has saturated fat, and for eating too little fish, whose benefits Chapter 5 examined.[151] Despite these authors' concern about ghee, Egyptians' heart disease and modest longevity compared with the rest of the world seem incongruous with their consumption of olives, vegetables, legumes, and little meat.

10.3.12 Olive Oil and Health in Modern Greece

No less troubling is Greece, once the exemplar of Mediterranean vigor. In 1953, Allbaugh gushed at Cretan slenderness, but by 2010 Greece ranked third worst among Organization for Economic Co-operation and Development (OECD) countries in obesity for women and in the middle for men.[152] Half Greek men and one-third women were overweight. Obesity and overweight plagued children in addition to adults. Between roughly 1965 and 2000, increases in meat and dairy intake raised calories from a daily average of 2,900 to 3,700.[153] Parallel to this development, Greeks emulated other developed nations' inactivity. Between 1965 and 2005, the average Cretan gained mass despite cutting daily calories from 2,820 to 2,412. Such circumstances justify this book's emphasis on exertion as essential to health.

10.3.13 Olive Oil and Calories

Although Hoffman and Gerber did not blame olive oil for obesity and overweight, 100 grams of olive oil have 884 calories, as noted. Returning to Table 4.1, olive oil has more calories by mass than the flesh of all six animals: bison, deer, sheep, goat, pig, and cow. Compared to other caloric foods by mass, olive oil has 43.2 percent more calories than walnuts, 47.3 percent more than dry-roasted almonds, 47.8 percent more than dark chocolate, 55.9 percent more than raw peanuts, 56.6 percent more than raw pistachios, 174.5 percent more than egg yolk, and 651.7 percent more than avocado.[154] Among fast foods and similar items, 100 grams of olive oil have more calories than a Burger King Whopper with cheese, two Starbuck's plain bagels, two of its glazed donuts, four Krispy Kreme glazed donuts, or four Dunkin Donuts mocha swirl lattes, each 283.5 grams (10 ounces).[155]

In the context of energy, Chapter 2 listed fat as the densest source at 9.4 calories per gram.[156] That is, no food can surpass 940 calories per 100 grams. This amount functions as a dietary ceiling analogous to the dictum in physics that light speed (299,792 kilometers per second) is the maximum in the universe.[157] Just as no food can exceed 940 calories per 100 grams, nothing can travel faster than light. At 884 calories per 100 grams, olive oil tallies 94 percent of the maximum. Completing the analogy, 94 percent of light speed is around 281,804.5 kilometers per second, an enormous number. This information, coupled with earlier remarks, emphasizes olive oil's status as especially caloric.

Although disconcerting, these numbers may not rule out olive oil, though its abundant calories tread the path toward overindulgence, especially when not offset by strenuous exertions. For example, olive oil's 884 calories in 100 grams supply enough energy for an 83.9-kilogram (185-pound) person to cut grass for over two hours with a push mower or to pedal a bicycle 19.3 kilometers per hour (12 miles/hour) for over one hour.[158] Laxity uses less energy. For example, this individual must stand almost eight hours to metabolize all 884 calories.

Earlier chapters announced this book's determination not to excoriate calories. The issue is less energy than nutrient density. The fact that junk foods are unwholesome is evident to anyone who has consulted their nutrition labels only to find many calories and a long sequence of zeroes beside the various nutrients. The exception is sodium, which is too prevalent in modern diets. Such foods create a strange reality in which consumers eagerly buy products with nonexistent nutrients. In no other sphere of the economy do consumers willingly purchase nothing. They may retort, however, that they have bought something, namely pleasure in the form of deliciousness. Yet this pleasure is transitory, especially when it saps vitality.

10.3.14 Olive Oil's Nutrients

Olive oil transcends junk because Table 10.2 shows that 100 grams have 95.7 percent of the U.S. Food and Drug Administration's (FDA) daily value (DV) for vitamin E and 75.3 percent for vitamin K.[159] Beyond this duo, olive oil has phytochemicals that act as antioxidants and reduce inflammation. Chapter 2 discussed phytochemicals and antioxidants. Olive oil's antioxidants hydroxytyrosol ($C_8H_{10}O_3$), oleuropein ($C_{25}H_{32}O_{13}$), and squalene ($C_{30}H_{50}$) may reduce incidences of colon, breast, ovary, and prostate cancers.[160] Olive oil's anti-inflammatory properties may lessen the risk of atherosclerosis, stroke, and heart attack, and its phytochemicals may protect against Alzheimer's disease.

Olive oil's nutrients invite comparison in Table 10.2 with olives, 100 grams of which supply 105 calories: just 11.9 percent of the calories in the same amount of olive oil.[161] Whereas olive oil lacks fiber, 100 grams of olives furnish 3 grams of it. By mass, olives have only 11.5 percent as much vitamin E as olive oil.[162] Yet 100 grams of olives contain 12 percent DV for copper and 18.4 percent for iron whereas the same amount of olive oil has no copper and 3.1 percent for iron.[163] Whereas 100 grams of olive oil have 75.3 percent DV for vitamin K, as noted, the same quantity of olives has 1.8 percent.

The foregoing shows that olive oil's strengths are vitamins E and K, though other options supply more of both for fewer calories. For example, Table 10.3 indicates that 100 grams of sunflower seeds furnish 35.17 milligrams (234.5 percent) of DV for vitamin E, roughly 2.5 times more than the same amount of olive oil.[164] These seeds' vitamin E is a bargain because by mass they have under two-thirds olive oil's calories. Arithmetic demonstrates that calorie for calorie, sunflower seeds have almost four times more vitamin E than olive oil.

Vitamin K's quantification reinforces this narrative. Table 10.4 reveals that by mass kale, swiss chard, mustard greens, and collard greens all surpass olive oil in vitamin K. For example, 100 grams of kale provide 817 micrograms of the vitamin, 1,021.3 percent DV.[165] By mass, kale has over thirteen times more vitamin K than olive oil.[166] Again appealing to arithmetic, by calorie, kale supplies 242.6 times more vitamin K than olive oil.[167]

TABLE 10.2
Nutrients in Olives and Olive Oil 100 g

Nutrient	Olives	%DV	Olive Oil	%DV
Calories	105	N/A	884	N/A
Protein (g)	0.88	N/A	0	N/A
Fat (g)	9.54	N/A	100	N/A
Carbs (g)	6.06	N/A	0	N/A
Fiber (g)	3	N/A	0	N/A
		Minerals		
Ca (mg)	90	9	1	0.1
Fe (mg)	3.31	18.4	0.56	3.1
Mg (mg)	4	0.01	0	0
P (mg)	3	0.3	0	0
K (mg)	8	0.2	1	0.03
Na (mg)	735	30.6	2	0.08
Zn (mg)	0.22	1.5	0	0
Cu (mg)	0.24	12	0	0
Mn (mg)	0.02	1	0	0
Se (mcg)	0.9	1.3	0	0
		Vitamins		
A (IU)	403	8.1	0	0
B_1 (mg)	<0.01	0.2	0	0
B_2 (mg)	0	0	0	0
B_3 (mg)	0.03	0.2	0	0
B_5 (mg)	0.01	0.1	0	0
B_6 (mg)	0.01	0.5	0	0
B_9 (mcg)	0	0	0	0
B_{12} (mcg)	0	0	0	0
C (mg)	1.1	1.8	0	0
D (IU)	0	0	0	0
E (mg)	1.65	11	14.35	95.7
K (mcg)	1.4	1.8	60.2	75.3

TABLE 10.3
Vitamin E (mg) in Selected Foods (100 g)

Food (100 g)	Vitamin E (mg)	%DV
Sunflower seeds	35.17	234.5
Almonds	25.6	171
Avocado	2.1	14
Spinach	2.1	14
Kiwi	1.5	10
Broccoli	1.5	10
Trout	2.8	19
Shrimp	2.2	15

TABLE 10.4
Vitamin K (mcg) in Selected Foods (100 g)

Food (100 g)	Vitamin K (mcg)	%DV
Kale	817	1,021.3
Mustard greens	593	741.3
Swiss chard	830	1,037.5
Collard greens	407	508.8
Natto	1,103	1,378.8
Spinach	483	603.8
Broccoli	141	176.3
Brussel sprouts	140	175

10.3.15 Olive Oil and High Fat Diets

A diet laden with olive oil, or any caloric item, leaves little room for other foods just as athletes who command extravagant pay reduce the money that may be spent on the rest of the team in sports with a salary cap. An olive oil enthusiast, Simopoulos referenced research that participants who consumed 45 percent of calories from fat lost the same mass and more adipose than those who ingested 26 percent of calories from fat.[168] Total calories were identical for both, but the implication is that diets should lavish rather than limit fat. Simopoulos' results contradicted research, already mentioned, that correlated fat consumption and obesity and that documented body fat enlargement among people who reduced calories but increased fat intake.

Although Simopoulos disavowed "a high-fat diet," her regimen is difficult to characterize otherwise given that the Cleveland Clinic in Cleveland, Ohio, and the Mayo Clinic in Rochester, Minnesota, recommended fat intake between 20 and 35 percent of total calories.[169] The U.S. Department of Health and Human Services (HHS), the National Academy of Sciences, the U.S. Surgeon General's office, the USDA, and Laurence Eyres set 30 percent of calories from fat as the ceiling.[170] As noted, Stanley Boyd Eaton and colleague cautioned against eating over 20 percent of calories from fat. The typical American gets roughly 34 percent of calories from fat, a total almost midway between Spain's 30 percent from fat and Greece's 40 percent.[171] These percentages prompted Hoffman and Gerber to concede that "the traditional MedDiet is not a low fat diet."[172] Yet even these numbers trail Simopoulos' 45 percent.

She counseled dieters to restrict calories to 1,200 or 1,500 per day.[173] With 45 percent coming from olive oil—her favorite—or another fat, weight watchers have only between 660 and 825 calories to spare daily for all other foods. Many combinations of low-calorie items such as celery, lettuce, and kindred vegetables fit these parameters, allowing the consumption of salads with dressing for flavor and fat. Following this rationale, U.S. women consume dressing as their primary fat.[174] The result is a meal with more calories and fat than had they eaten meat or dairy. Consequently, American women double men in obesity, an outcome contrary to belief that fatty diets promote weight loss.[175]

The issues of overweight and obesity aside, Simopoulos' austerity allows only 660–825 calories, as noted, for nutrients besides fat. All cannot receive treatment, though the U.S. Centers for Disease Control and Prevention (CDC) in Atlanta, Georgia, reported in 2016 that many women ingest too little iodine, that over 30 percent of African Americans are deficient in vitamin D, and that more African American and Mexican American women under-consume iron than white women.[176] Vitamin D may be obtained from sunlight, as mentioned elsewhere, and American anthropologist Susan Kent (1952–2003) judged iron deficiency uncommon in the developed world.[177]

This situation leaves iodine—whose content Table 10.5 lists for eight foods—as the test case. Governments worldwide urge adults to ingest 150 to 200 micrograms daily.[178] Pregnant and lactating women should exceed this range. The issue, therefore, is whether 660–825 calories allow intake

TABLE 10.5
Iodine (mcg) in Selected Foods (100 g)

Food (100 g)	Iodine (mcg)	%DV
Seaweed, Nori	1470	980
Cod	256	170.7
Shrimp	100	66.7
Eggs	50	33.3
Tuna, fresh	18	12
Haddock	325	216.7
Cheese	37.5	25
Salmon	14	9.3

of at least 150 micrograms of iodine daily, leaving aside pregnant and lactating women. This exercise is not abstract; in 2017, the WHO judged iodine intake insufficient for 2 billion of the world's 7.6 billion people.[179] Iodine deficiency, Chapter 13 notes, may cause goiter and mental impairment.

Iodine-rich foods include seaweed, seafood, eggs, dairy, lima beans (*Phaseolus lunatus*), and prunes. Plums also have iodine, though less per gram than prunes because of higher water content. Cod, tuna, and shrimp (species in the infraorder Caridea) are good choices among fish and shellfish. For example, 100 grams of cod supply on average 256 micrograms of iodine and 69 calories.[180] That is, 40.4 calories of cod furnish the daily iodine minimum of 150 micrograms, leaving 619.6–784.6 calories for derivation of other nutrients. Simopoulos' recommendations, therefore, permit adequate nutrition from diets with high fat but few total calories.

10.3.16 Olive Oil and Omega 9 Fatty Acids

Olive oil's chief fat, oleic acid ($C_{18}H_{34}O_2$), is an antioxidant and anti-inflammatory agent thought to benefit the immune system, brain, heart, and skin. By volume, olive oil is 55–85 percent oleic acid.[181] Chemists classify it a monounsaturated omega 9 fatty acid. Unlike polyunsaturated omega 3 and omega 6 fatty acids, omega 9s are unessential because the body can manufacture them from other compounds. Unessential does not mean unimportant. Most of the body's cells use more omega 9s than other fatty acids to construct membranes. Readers may recall from Chapter 2 and an earlier section that the brain is about 70 percent fat and so requires many omega 9 fatty acids. Oleic acid and other omega 9s may protect against type 2 diabetes.[182] Research credits them with reducing triglycerides and cholesterol—Chapter 2 defines both—in blood.

10.3.17 Comparisons among Olive, Soybean, and Peanut Oils

Olive oil is not the only fat under scrutiny. Soybean oil receives attention because it totals three-quarters of U.S. vegetable oil consumption and supplies about 20 percent of Americans' calories.[183] In 2008, the average American ingested over 300 more calories daily than in 1985.[184] Ninety-three percent of this increase came from sucrose, HFCS, and fat. This fat was largely soybean oil, which supplied, and continues to furnish, most omega 6 fatty acids in U.S. diets.[185] A 2018 paper ranked soybean oil first among vegetable oils in consumption worldwide between 2009 and 2011, the latest years for which it had data.[186] During this time, soybean oil tallied 30.3 percent of world vegetable oil intake, nearly 12 percent above second-place palm oil's 18.6 percent.

During maturation, soybeans store fat chiefly as triglycerides at over 99 percent of oil by weight after processing.[187] Of the fatty acids in these triglycerides, the omega 6 linoleic acid—whose formula was stated earlier—constitutes 53.2 percent and the omega 3 linolenic acid ($C_{18}H_{30}O_2$) totals 7.8 percent.[188] The ratio of omega 6 to omega 3 in soybean oil, therefore, is 6.8:1, not the 1:1

recommendation mentioned throughout this chapter.[189] Soybean oil is 23.4 percent oleic acid, about one-third olive oil's value.

Compared to soybean oil, olive oil is 10 percent linoleic acid and 0.6 percent linolenic acid, for a 16.7:1 omega 6 to omega 3 ratio.[190] Simopoulos criticized American and European diets for eating fourteen to twenty times more omega 6s than omega 3s.[191] Yet olive oil has a worse omega 6 to omega 3 ratio than soybean oil. Readers may question olive oil's healthfulness given that she implicated fatty-acid imbalance in heart disease, stroke, cancers, obesity, type 2 diabetes, asthma, rheumatoid arthritis, lupus, mental illness, and Alzheimer's disease.[192]

With olive oil in the Mediterranean and soybean oil in the United States, geography broadens by examining peanut oil, which is popular for frying in Africa and East, South, and Southeast Asia and which is 31.4 percent linoleic acid but lacks linolenic acid.[193] This disparity cannot approach a balanced fatty acid ratio. Among peanut oil's fatty acids, half are monounsaturated, 30 percent are polyunsaturated, and the remaining 20 percent are saturated.[194]

Besides fatty acids, 100 grams of olive oil, as mentioned, supply 95.7 percent DV for vitamin E and 75.3 percent for vitamin K. The USDA lists no other vitamins and few minerals for olive oil.[195] By comparison, Table 10.6 indicates that 100 grams of soybean oil have 54.5 percent DV for

TABLE 10.6
Calories and Nutrients in Soybean and Peanut Oils 100 g

Nutrient	Soybean Oil	%DV	Peanut Oil	%DV
Calories	884	N/A	884	N/A
Protein (g)	0	N/A	0	N/A
Fat (g)	100	N/A	100	N/A
Carbs (g)	0	N/A	0	N/A
Fiber (g)	0	N/A	0	N/A
		Minerals		
Ca (mg)	0	0	0	0
Fe (mg)	0.05	0.3	0.03	0.2
Mg (mg)	0	0	0	0
P (mg)	0	0	0	0
K (mg)	0	0	0	0
Na (mg)	0	0	0	0
Zn (mg)	0.01	0.06	0.01	0.06
Cu (mg)	0	0	0	0
Mn (mg)	0	0	0	0
Se (mcg)	0	0	0	0
		Vitamins		
A (IU)	0	0	0	0
B_1 (mg)	0	0	0	0
B_2 (mg)	0	0	0	0
B_3 (mg)	0	0	0	0
B_5 (mg)	0	0	0	0
B_6 (mg)	0	0	0	0
B_9 (mcg)	0	0	0	0
B_{12} (mcg)	0	0	0	0
C (mg)	0	0	0	0
D (IU)	0	0	0	0
E (mg)	8.18	54.5	15.69	104.6
K (mcg)	183.9	229.9	0.7	0.9

vitamin E, 229.9 percent for vitamin K, under 1 percent for iron and zinc, and no other nutrients.[196] One hundred grams of peanut oil exceed vitamin E's DV and provide 0.9 percent of vitamin K's DV, below 1 percent for iron and zinc, and no other nutrients.[197] All three oils have plentiful vitamin E, and olive oil and soybean oil are also rich in vitamin K.

NOTES

1 Lenka Kourimska and Anna Adamkova, "Nutritional and Sensory Qualities of Edible Insects," *NSF Journal* 4 (July 16, 2016): 22, https://www.researchgate.net/publication/305396814_Nutritional_and_sensory_quality_of_edible_insects.
2 Tom Mueller, *Extra Virginity: The Sublime and Scandalous World of Olive Oil* (New York and London: Norton, 2012), 94.
3 George Wolf, "Vitamin A," in *The Cambridge World History of Food*, vol. 1, ed. Kenneth F. Kiple and Kriemhild Conee Ornelas (Cambridge, UK: Cambridge University Press, 2000), 744.
4 Ibid.; David I. Thurnham, "Vitamin A and Carotenoids," in *Essentials of Human Nutrition*, 5th ed., ed. Jim Mann and A. Stewart Truswell (Oxford: Oxford University Press, 2017), 191.
5 Jacqueline L. Dupont, "Essential Fatty Acids," in *The Cambridge World History of Food*, vol. 1, ed. Kenneth F. Kiple and Kriemhild Conee Ornelas (Cambridge, UK: Cambridge University Press, 2000), 876.
6 Mark R. Jenike, "Nutritional Ecology: Diet, Physical Activity and Body Size," in *Hunter-Gatherers: An Interdisciplinary Perspective*, ed. Catherine Panter-Brick, Robert H. Layton, and Peter Rowley-Conwy (Cambridge, UK: Cambridge University Press, 2001), 208–209.
7 Ibid.
8 Artemis P. Simopoulos, "Evolutionary Aspects of the Dietary Omega-6/Omega-3 Fatty Acid Ratio: Medical Implications," in *Evolutionary Thinking in Medicine: From Research to Policy and Practice*, ed. Alexandra Alvergne, Crispin Jenkinson, Charlotte Faurie (Switzerland: Springer, 2016), 119.
9 Mueller, 137.
10 David Perlmutter, *Grain Brain: The Surprising Truth about Wheat, Carbs, and Sugar—Your Brain's Silent Killers*, rev. ed. (New York: Little, Brown Spark, 2018), 35.
11 Ibid.
12 Gary Taubes, *Why We Get Fat and What to Do About It* (New York: Knopf, 2011), 163.
13 Ibid.
14 Blake F. Donaldson, *Strong Medicine* (Garden City, NY: Doubleday, 1962), 33–34.
15 Ibid., 32–33.
16 William Rubel, *Bread: A Global History* (London: Reaktion Books, 2011), 11–12.
17 Helen W. Atwater, "Food for Farm Families," in *U.S. Department of Agriculture Yearbook, 1920* (Washington: GPO, 1921), 476.
18 Ofer Bar-Yosef, "Eat What Is There: Hunting and Gathering in the World of the Neanderthals and Their Neighbors," *International Journal of Osteoarchaeology* 14, nos. 3–4 (May 2004): 333–337.
19 Ibid., 337.
20 Jenike, 208–209.
21 S. Boyd Eaton and Melvin Konner, "Paleolithic Nutrition: A Consideration of Its Nature and Current Implications," in *Nutritional Anthropology: Biocultural Perspectives on Food and Nutrition*, 2nd ed., ed. Darna L. Dufour, Alan H. Goodman, and Gretel H. Pelto (New York and Oxford: Oxford University Press, 2013), 53.
22 Loren Cordain, *The Paleo Diet: Lose Weight and Get Healthy by Eating the Foods You Were Designed to Eat*, rev. ed. (Hoboken, NJ: Wiley, 2011), 11.
23 Perlmutter, 34; Taubes, *Why We Get Fat*, 163.
24 Stanley Ulijaszek, Neil Mann, and Sarah Elton, *Evolving Human Nutrition: Implications for Public Health* (New York: Cambridge University Press, 2012), 50.
25 Laurence Eyres, "Fats and Oils," in *Essentials of Human Nutrition*, 5th ed., ed. Jim Mann and A. Stewart Truswell (Oxford: Oxford University Press, 2017), 292.
26 Kenneth F. Kiple, "The Question of Paleolithic Nutrition and Modern Health: From the End to the Beginning," in *The Cambridge World History of Food*, vol. 2, ed. Kenneth F. Kiple and Kriemhild Conee Ornelas (Cambridge, UK: Cambridge University Press, 2000), 1705.
27 Eyres, 292.

28 "Eggs, Pasture-Raised," *The World's Healthiest Foods*, May 13–19, 2019, accessed May 14, 2019, http://www.whfoods.com/genpage.php?tname=foodspice&dbid=92#nutritionalprofile.
29 Stephanie Green, *Optimum Nutrition* (New York: Alpha Books, 2015), 72.
30 Mike Lean and Emilie Combet, *Barasi's Human Nutrition: A Health Perspective*, 3rd ed. (Boca Raton, FL: CRC Press, 2017), 315; Julian E. Spallholz, L. Mallory Boylan, and Judy A. Driskell, *Nutrition Chemistry and Biology*, 2nd ed. (Boca Raton, FL: CRC Press, 1999), 202.
31 Green, 72.
32 John Cummings and Jim Mann, "Carbohydrates," in *Essentials of Human Nutrition*, 5th ed., ed. Jim Mann and A. Stewart Truswell (Oxford: Oxford University Press, 2017), 33.
33 Louise Eaton and Kara Rogers, eds., *Examining Basic Chemical Molecules* (New York: Britannica, 2018), 221.
34 Darna L. Dufour and Richard L. Bender, "Nutritional Transitions: A View from Anthropology," in *Nutritional Anthropology: Biocultural Perspectives on Food and Nutrition*, 2nd ed., ed. Darna L. Dufour, Alan H. Goodman, and Gretel H. Pelto (New York and Oxford: Oxford University Press, 2013), 372.
35 Lawrence Kaplan, "Legumes in the History of Human Nutrition," in *The World of Soy*, ed. Christine M. Du Bois, Chee-Beng Tan, and Sidney W. Mintz (Urbana and Chicago: University of Illinois Press, 2008), 28.
36 Arnold van Huis, Joost Van Itterbeeck, Harmke Klunder, Esther Mertens, Afton Halloran, Giulia Muir, and Paul Vantomme, *Edible Insects: Future Prospects for Food and Feed Security* (Rome, Italy: Food and Agriculture Organization of the United Nations, 2013), xiv.
37 Ibid., 72.
38 Ibid.; J. N. Kinyuru, G. M. Kenji, S. N. Muhoho, and M. Ayieko, "Nutritional Potential of Longhorn Grasshopper (*Ruspolia differens*) Consumed in Siaya District, Kenya," *Journal of Agriculture, Science and Technology* (November 2009), accessed July 11, 2019, https://www.researchgate.net/publication/268186085_Nutritional_potential_of_longhorn_grasshopper_Ruspolia_differens_consumed_in_Siaya_District_Kenya.
39 S. Boyd Eaton and Stanley B. Eaton III, "Hunter-Gatherers and Human Health," in *The Cambridge Encyclopedia of Hunters and Gatherers*, ed. Richard B. Lee and Richard Daly (Cambridge, UK: Cambridge University Press, 2004), 449.
40 Ibid., 454.
41 "Nuts, Raw, Cashew Nuts," *Nutrition Facts Exposed*, 2019, accessed May 15, 2019, https://www.nutritionvalue.org/Nuts%2C_raw%2C_cashew_nuts_nutritional_value.html.
42 Ibid.
43 Ibid.
44 Catherine J. Nock, Craig M. Hardner, Juan D. Montenagro, Ainnatul A. Ahmad Termizi, Satomi Hayashi, Julia Playford, David Edwards, and Jacqueline Batley, "Wild Origins of Macadamia Domestication Identified through Intraspecific Chloroplast Genome Sequencing," *Frontiers in Plant Science* (March 21, 2019), https://www.frontiersin.org/articles/10.3389/fpls.2019.00334/full.
45 "Cheese, Parmesan, Hard," *USDA FoodData Central*, April 1, 2019, accessed February 12, 2020, https://fdc.nal.usda.gov/fdc-app.html#/food-details/170848/nutrients.
46 Eyres, 296.
47 Ibid., 293.
48 "Oil, Palm," *USDA FoodData Central*, April 1, 2019, accessed February 12, 2020, https://fdc.nal.usda.gov/fdc-app.html#/food-details/171015/nutrients.
49 Eyres, 293.
50 Ancel Keys, *Seven Countries: A Multivariate Analysis of Death and Coronary Heart Disease* (Cambridge, MA and London: Harvard University Press, 1980), 315–320.
51 Eyres, 293.
52 T. Colin Campbell, *Whole: Rethinking the Science of Nutrition* (Dallas, TX: BenBella Books, 2013), 7.
53 Robert C. Atkins, *Dr. Atkins' Diet Revolution: The High Calorie Way to Stay Thin Forever* (New York: David McKay, 1972), 2–3.
54 Ibid., 10. This quote retains the original italics.
55 Ibid., 55, 132.
56 Eyres, 292.
57 Adda Bjarnadottir, "Olives 101: Nutrition Facts and Health Benefits," *Healthline*, May 21, 2019, accessed May 23, 2019, https://www.healthline.com/nutrition/foods/olives; Mueller, 19.

58 Giorgio Bartolini and Raffaella Petruccelli, *Classification, Origin, Diffusion and History of the Olive* (Rome: Food and Agriculture Organization of the United Nations, 2002), 14–15.
59 Ibid., 27.
60 Ibid., v, 28–34.
61 *The Oldest Code of Laws in the World: The Code of Laws Promulgated by Hammurabi, King of Babylon, B.C. 2285–2242*, trans. C. H. W. Johns (Union, NJ: Lawbook Exchange, 2000), 38, 49.
62 Bartolini and Petruccelli, 28–29.
63 Ibid., 28.
64 Ibid., 29.
65 Ibid., 30.
66 Mueller, 35.
67 Bartolini and Petruccelli, 36.
68 Mueller, 37.
69 Sean Francis O'Keefe, "An Overview of Oils and Fats, with a Special Emphasis on Olive Oil," in *The Cambridge World History of Food*, vol. 1, ed. Kenneth F. Kiple and Kriemhild Conee Ornelas (Cambridge, UK: Cambridge University Press, 2000), 377.
70 Mueller, 37.
71 Ibid., 29.
72 John Train, *The Olive Tree of Civilization* (Easthampton, MA and Woodbridge, UK: Antique Collectors' Club, 2004), 44.
73 Mueller, 43.
74 Bartolini and Petruccelli, 33.
75 Robin W. Winks, Crane Brinton, John B. Christopher, and Robert Lee Wolff, *A History of Civilization, vol. 1: Prehistory to 1715*, 7th ed. (Englewood Cliffs, NJ: Prentice Hall, 1988), 69; Nel Yomtov, *Ancient Egypt* (New York: Scholastic, 2013), 90
76 Fabrizia Lanza, *Olive: A Global History* (London: Reaktion Books, 2011), 22.
77 Gen. 8:11 (New American Bible).
78 Mueller, 42–43.
79 Maria Prantl, "Diocletian's Edict on Maximum Prices of 301 AD. A Fragment Found in Aigeira," *historia. scribere* 3 (2011): 360, https://webapp.uibk.ac.at/ojs/index.php/historiascribere/article/viewFile/208/105.
80 Ibid., 372.
81 John 8:12 (New American Bible).
82 Mueller, 137.
83 Ibid., 138.
84 "Wheat Flour, Whole-Grain (Includes Foods for USDA's Food Distribution Program)," *USDA FoodData Central*, April 1, 2019, accessed February 12, 2020, https://fdc.nal.usda.gov/fdc-app.html#/food-details/168893/nutrients.
85 Michael Pollan, *In Defense of Food: An Eater's Manifesto* (New York: Penguin Press, 2008), 58–60.
86 Gary Taubes, *Good Calories, Bad Calories: Challenging the Conventional Wisdom on Diet, Weight Control, and Disease* (New York: Knopf, 2008), 454; Taubes, *Why We Get Fat*, 134, 136.
87 Mueller, 136.
88 Ibid., 137.
89 Vishwanath Sardesai, *Introduction to Clinical Nutrition*, 3rd ed. (Boca Raton, FL: CRC Press, 2012), 49–50.
90 Gillian Pocock, Christopher D. Richards, and David A. Richards, *Human Physiology*, 5th ed. (Oxford: Oxford University Press, 2018), 748.
91 "Olive Oil," *USDA FoodData Central*, April 1, 2019, accessed December 12, 2019, https://fdc.nal.usda.gov/fdc-app.html#/food-details/343873/nutrients; "Sugars, Granulated," *USDA FoodData Central*, April 1, 2019, accessed February 12, 2020, https://fdc.nal.usda.gov/fdc-app.html#/food-details/169655/nutrients; "Syrups, Corn, High-Fructose," *USDA FoodData Central*, April 1, 2019, accessed June 22, 2019, https://fdc.nal.usda.gov/fdc-app.html#/food-details/169659/nutrients.
92 Richard Hoffman and Mariette Gerber, *The Mediterranean Diet: Health and Science* (West Sussex, UK: Wiley-Blackwell, 2012), 6.
93 Peter Garnsey, *Food and Society in Classical Antiquity* (Cambridge, UK: Cambridge University Press, 1999), 13.
94 Ibid., 13, 15.
95 Hoffman and Gerber, 2.

96 Leland G. Allbaugh, *Crete: A Case Study of an Underdeveloped Area* (Princeton, NJ: Princeton University Press, 1953), 100.
97 Ibid., 99–100.
98 Ibid., 106–107.
99 Ibid., 100.
100 Artemis P. Simopoulos and Jo Robinson, *The Omega Diet: The Lifesaving Nutritional Program Based on the Diet of the Island of Crete* (New York: Harper, 1999), xii.
101 Garnsey, 14.
102 Ibid., 9.
103 Hoffman and Gerber, 138.
104 Ibid., 8.
105 Garnsey, 116–117.
106 Ibid., 113.
107 Lanza, 77.
108 Simopoulos and Robinson, xii.
109 Hoffman and Gerber, 1, 12, 14, 16.
110 Mueller, 13.
111 Ibid., 32.
112 Marcus Porcius Cato, *On Agriculture*, trans. William Davis Hooper (Cambridge, MA: Harvard University Press, 1979), 73.
113 Garnsey, 25.
114 "Introduction," in *On Agriculture*, by Marcus Porcius Cato, trans. William Davis Hooper and Harrison Boyd Ash (Cambridge, MA: Harvard University Press, 1967), xiii.
115 K. D. White, *Roman Farming* (Ithaca, NY: Cornell University Press, 1970), 19, 35–36.
116 "Introduction."
117 White, 28.
118 Mueller, 81.
119 Cato, 9.
120 Walter Scheidel, "Demography," in *The Cambridge Economic History of the Greco-Roman World*, ed. Walter Scheidel, Ian Morris, and Richard Saller (Cambridge, UK: Cambridge University Press, 2007), 41.
121 Ibid., 40.
122 Ibid., 38; Garnsey, 59.
123 Scheidel, 39.
124 Ibid., 61.
125 Garnsey, 46–47, 56.
126 Allbaugh, 114; "Useful Number Conversions," *Everything but the Olive*, 1998–2019, accessed May 29, 2019, https://www.oliveoilsource.com/page/useful-number-conversions.
127 Mueller, 81; "Useful Number Conversions."
128 Hoffman and Gerber, 138.
129 Allbaugh, 136.
130 Ibid., 137.
131 Ibid., 139.
132 Ibid.
133 Ibid., 15.
134 Ibid., 101.
135 Ibid., 15.
136 Ibid., 111–112.
137 Ibid., 105.
138 Ibid., 119.
139 Ibid., 196–197.
140 Ibid., 16–17.
141 Ibid., 17.
142 Ibid., 119.
143 Jose A. Tapia Granados and Ana V. Diez Roux, "Life and Death during the Great Depression," *Proceedings of the National Academy of Sciences* 106, no. 41 (October 13, 2009): 17290–17295, https://www.ncbi.nlm.nih.gov/pmc/articles/PMC2765209.

144 Peter Dizikes, "New Study Shows Rich, Poor Have Huge Mortality Gap in U.S." MIT News, April 11, 2016. http://news.mit.edu/2016/study-rich-poor-huge-mortality-gap-us-0411.

145 "The Poorest Countries in the World," *FocusEconomics*, November 19, 2018, accessed May 29, 2019, https://www.focus-economics.com/blog/the-poorest-countries-in-the-world; "The World: Life Expectancy (2018)," *geoba.se*, 2019, accessed May 29, 2019, http://www.geoba.se/population.php?pc=world&type=015&year=2018&st=country&asde=&page=1.

146 John Harrington, "From Bahrain to Qatar: These Are the 25 Richest Countries in the World," *USA Today*, November 28, 2018, accessed May 29, 2019, https://www.usatoday.com/story/money/2018/11/28/richest-countries-world-2018-top-25/38429481; "The World: Life Expectancy (2018)," *geoba.se*, 2019, accessed May 29, 2019, http://www.geoba.se/population.php?pc=world&type=015&year=2018&st=rank&asde=d&page=3.

147 "The World: Life Expectancy (2018);" Hoffman and Gerber, 21.

148 Hoffman and Gerber, 22.

149 Mueller, 138; Hoffman and Gerber, 138; Michael van Straten and Barbara Griggs, *SuperFoods: Nutrient-Dense Foods to Protect Your Health* (London: DK, 2006), 14.

150 Hoffman and Gerber, 22.

151 Ibid.; Egyptians call ghee *samna*.

152 Ibid., 23; Allbaugh, 105.

153 Hoffman and Gerber, 24.

154 "Olive Oil"; "Peanuts, All Types, Raw," *USDA FoodData Central*, April 1, 2019, accessed December 12, 2019, https://fdc.nal.usda.gov/fdc-app.html#/food-details/172430/nutrients; Allan Borushek, *The CalorieKing Calorie, Fat, and Carbohydrate Counter* (Huntington Beach, CA: Family Health Publications, 2019), 99, 130; "Chocolate, Dark, 70–85% Cacao Solids," *USDA FoodData Central*, April 1, 2019, accessed December 12, 2019, https://fdc.nal.usda.gov/fdc-app.html#/food-details/170273/nutrients; "Egg, Yolk, Raw, Fresh," *USDA FoodData Central*, April 1, 2019, accessed December 12, 2019, https://fdc.nal.usda.gov/fdc-app.html#/food-details/172184/nutrients.

155 Blossom Paravattil, "Fast Food Facts: Calories and Fat," *National Center for Health Research*, 2019, accessed May 30, 2019, http://www.center4research.org/fast-food-facts-calories-and-fat.

156 Lean and Combet, 314.

157 Nola Taylor Redd, "How Fast Does Light Travel? The Speed of Light," *Space*, March 7, 2018, accessed December 12, 2019, https://www.space.com/15830-light-speed.html.

158 "Calories Burned in 30 Minutes for People of Three Different Weights," *Harvard Medical School*, July 2004, last modified August 13, 2018, accessed May 30, 2019, https://www.health.harvard.edu/diet-and-weight-loss/calories-burned-in-30-minutes-of-leisure-and-routine-activities.

159 "Olive Oil."

160 Mueller, 104.

161 "Olives, Black," *USDA FoodData Central*, April 1, 2019, accessed January 24, 2020, https://fdc.nal.usda.gov/fdc-app.html#/food-details/343670/nutrients.

162 Ibid.; "Olive Oil."

163 "Olives," *The World's Healthiest Foods*, 2001–2019, accessed June 29, 2019, http://www.whfoods.com/genpage.php?tname=foodspice&dbid=46; "Oil, Olive, Salad or Cooking Nutrition Facts and Calories," *SelfNutritionData*, 2018, accessed June 29, 2019, https://nutritiondata.self.com/facts/fats-and-oils/509/2.

164 "Olive Oil"; "Seeds, Sunflower Seed Kernels, Dried," *USDA FoodData Central*, April 1, 2019, accessed December 12, 2019, https://fdc.nal.usda.gov/fdc-app.html#/food-details/170562/nutrients.

165 Atli Arnarson, "20 Foods That Are High in Vitamin K," *Healthline*, September 6, 2017, accessed June 29, 2019, https://www.healthline.com/nutrition/foods-high-in-vitamin-k.

166 Ibid.; "Olive Oil."

167 Arnarson; "Olive Oil"; Borushek, 159.

168 Simopoulos and Robinson, 17.

169 Ibid; "Fat: What You Need to Know," *Cleveland Clinic*, November 28, 2014, accessed June 1, 2019, https://my.clevelandclinic.org/health/articles/11208-fat-what-you-need-to-know; Katherine Zeratsky, "Nutrition and Healthy Eating," *Mayo Clinic*, May 3, 2019, accessed June 1, 2019, https://www.mayoclinic.org/healthy-lifestyle/nutrition-and-healthy-eating/expert-answers/fat-grams/faq-20058496.

170 "Choose Sensibly," *U.S. Department of Health and Human Services*, accessed June 1, 2019, https://health.gov/dietaryguidelines/dga2000/document/choose.htm; "Improving America's Diet and Health: From Recommendations to Action," *National Academy of Sciences*, 1991, accessed June 2, 2019, https://www.ncbi.nlm.nih.gov/books/NBK235267; Eyres, 294.

171 Hoffman and Gerber, 3.

172 Ibid.
173 Simopoulos and Robinson, 193.
174 Leslie Sue Lieberman, "Obesity," in *The Cambridge World History of Food*, vol. 1, ed. Kenneth F. Kiple and Kriemhild Conee Ornelas (Cambridge, UK: Cambridge University Press, 2000), 1066–1067.
175 Ibid., 1065.
176 "Are We Getting Enough Vitamins and Nutrients?" *CDC*, last modified March 2, 2016, accessed June 1, 2019, https://blogs.cdc.gov/yourhealthyourenvironment/2016/03/02/are-we-getting-enough-vitamins-and-nutrients.
177 Susan Kent, "Iron Deficiency and Anemia of Chronic Disease," in *The Cambridge World History of Food*, vol. 1, ed. Kenneth F. Kiple and Kriemhild Conee Ornelas (Cambridge, UK: Cambridge University Press, 2000), 920.
178 Sheila Skeaff and Christine D. Thomson, "Iodine," in *Essentials of Human Nutrition*, 5th ed., ed. Jim Mann and A. Stewart Truswell (Oxford: Oxford University Press, 2017), 178.
179 Ibid., 173; "Sustainable Development Goals," *UN Press Release*, June 21, 2017, accessed June 1, 2019, https://www.un.org/en/development/desa/population/events/pdf/other/21/21June_FINAL%20PRESS%20RELEASE_WPP17.pdf.
180 Kaitlyn Berkheiser, "9 Healthy Foods That Are Rich in Iodine," *Healthline*, February 2, 2018, accessed June 2, 2019, https://www.healthline.com/nutrition/iodine-rich-foods; "Fish, Cod, Pacific, Raw (May Have Been Previously Frozen)," *USDA FoodData Central*, April 1, 2019, accessed February 12, 2020, https://fdc.nal.usda.gov/fdc-app.html#/food-details/174191/nutrients.
181 Mueller, 92.
182 Ruairi Robertson, "Omega 3-6-9 Fatty Acids: A Complete Overview," *Healthline*, January 15, 2017, accessed May 31, 2019, https://www.healthline.com/nutrition/omega-3-6-9-overview.
183 Pollan, 116–117.
184 Ibid., 122.
185 Ibid., 122, 131.
186 Joe Parcell, Yasutomo Kojima, Alice Roach, and Wayne Cain, "Global Edible Vegetable Oil Market Trends," *Biomedical Journal of Scientific and Technical Research* 2, no. 1 (January 22, 2018): 2284–2285, https://biomedres.us/pdfs/BJSTR.MS.ID.000680.pdf.
187 KeShun Liu, *Soybeans: Chemistry, Technology, and Utilization* (New York: Chapman and Hall, 1997), 27.
188 Ibid., 29.
189 Simopoulos and Robinson, 5.
190 Liu, 29.
191 Simopoulos and Robinson, 5.
192 Ibid., 5–6.
193 Sylvia A. Johnson, *Tomatoes, Potatoes, Corn, and Beans: How the Foods of the Americas Changed Eating around the World* (New York: Atheneum Books, 1997), 57–58; Liu, 29.
194 Jillian Kubala, "Is Peanut Oil Healthy? The Surprising Truth," *Healthline*, November 10, 2017, accessed May 31, 2019, https://www.healthline.com/nutrition/is-peanut-oil-healthy#section2.
195 "Olive Oil."
196 "Vitamin E Fact Sheet for Health Professionals," *NIH Office of Dietary Supplements*, last modified August 17, 2018, accessed May 31, 2019, https://ods.od.nih.gov/factsheets/VitaminE-HealthProfessional; "Soy Bean Oil Amounts Converter," *Convert-to.com Units Converter*, 2019, accessed May 31, 2019, http://convert-to.com/565/soy-bean-oil-nutrition-info-and-amounts-conversion.html; "Soybean Oil Nutrition Facts," *Nutrition-And-You*, 2009–2019, accessed May 31, 2019, https://www.nutrition-and-you.com/soybean-oil.html.
197 "Oil, Peanut, Salad or Cooking," *USDA FoodData Central*, April 1, 2019, accessed February 12, 2020, https://fdc.nal.usda.gov/fdc-app.html#/food-details/171410/nutrients; "Vitamin K Fact Sheet for Health Professionals," *NIH Office of Dietary Supplements*, last modified September 26, 2018, accessed June 1, 2019, https://ods.od.nih.gov/factsheets/VitaminK-HealthProfessional/#h2.

11 Sweeteners
Honey, Sucrose, and High Fructose Corn Syrup

11.1 HONEY

11.1.1 HONEYBEES

Honey's past is rooted in honeybees' (*Apis mellifera*) evolution and dispersal. Related to ants (species in the family Formicidae) and wasps (species in the family Vespidae), bees (species in the clade Anthophila) may have evolved from the latter about 125 million years ago.[1] A more recent genealogy puts their origin roughly 50 million years ago with the evolution of the genus *Electrapis*, whose fossils have been found near northern Europe's Baltic Sea. A third possibility is origin 40 million years ago in South or Southeast Asia. The last two dates parallel primates' colonization of Africa and South America. Although these geographies do not overlap, primates may have eaten honey from an early date. Primatologists have documented its gathering among chimpanzees (*Pan troglodytes*), monkeys, and other primates. Although some 20,000 bee species produce honey, modern humans favor *Apis mellifera*. Of *Apis*' nine species, *A. mellifera* arose perhaps 300,000 years ago in North Africa or Asia.[2] Modern humans originated about 150,000 years ago, noted Chapter 3, and arrived late to the narrative of bees and honey.

Like other bees, *A. mellifera* collects nectar and pollen from flowers. From its proboscis, a honeybee sucks nectar into its honey sac, where enzymes break the sugars into simpler compounds. Regurgitation deposits the liquid into honeycombs, where evaporation yields honey. Sizable quantities require huge aggregates of bees given that one bee produces under 0.6 grams (one-twelfth of a teaspoon) of honey in a lifetime.[3] This sticky, sweet substance has roughly equal portions of glucose and fructose. Both monosaccharides are $C_6H_{12}O_6$ (mentioned in Chapter 2 and the abstract) but have different structures—making them isomers (see Chapter 2)—and metabolic pathways in the body. These sugars are important as energy and in building the disaccharide sucrose ($C_{12}H_{22}O_{11}$), treated later.

The necessity of bees for producing honey restricted it to regions with them. Yet hunter-gatherers did not limit themselves to what honeybees made but instead collected several species' honey. Hunter-gatherers' persistence into modernity allowed anthropologists to identify honey collection and consumption among indigenes, including the Central African Republic's Aka; Kenya's Okiek; southwestern India's Nayaka; Andhra Pradesh, India's Chenchu; the Paliyan on the border between Tamil Nadu and Kerala, India; the Philippines' Batak; and Paraguay's Ache, whose diets Chapter 4 detailed.[4]

Humankind's ingestion of honey from *A. mellifera* focused the sweetener's early prehistory on North Africa, Central, South, and Southeast Asia, Europe, and Central America. Chapter 3 stated that some of the oldest evidence of modern humans comes from North Africa. That North Africa also may have been the honeybee's cradle suggests that the earliest modern peoples may have eaten honey among their first foods.

Valencia, Spain's cave art from roughly 10,000 BCE depicts honey collection, making European consumption at least that old.[5] Five-thousand-year-old Georgian pottery retains honey residues, evincing Eastern Europe's collection and consumption no later than this date.[6] The gathering of wild honey predated *A. mellifera*'s domestication by millennia. British journalist Henry Hobhouse (1924–2016) believed that domestication preceded Egypt's oldest reference to honeybees in 5551 BCE whereas American folklorist and food scholar Lucy M. Long favored a date between 3000 and 2000 BCE.[7]

11.1.2 Honey as Luxury

An early inventor of writing, Egypt memorialized some of honey's oldest recipes. Egyptians mixed the sweetener with wheat (*Triticum monococcum*, *T. dicoccon*, *T. aestivum*, and *T. durum*) flour before baking, an addition that raised bread prices above commoners' means. Honey's inclusion in beer and wine had the same effect. French author Maguelonne Toussaint-Samat (1926–2018) posited that royalty and priests monopolized what Egypt produced, leaving commoners to collect wild honey.[8] American anthropologists Naomi Frances Miller and Wilma Wetterstrom widened the chasm between elites and the masses, asserting the improbability "that lower classes ever saw honey."[9] That is, it highlighted the divide between haves and have nots. As other chapters argue, food sharpens inequalities by demarcating classes or castes.

Beyond Egypt, Greek historian Polybius (c. 208–c. 125 BCE) deemed honey a luxury.[10] That the Greeks imported it from Central Asia must have raised its price. The dynamics of distant trade might have operated in ancient Mesopotamia—now Iraq and parts of Syria, Turkey, and Iran—where only the wealthy consumed honey.[11]

Its prestige was apparent in Rome, where the rich added the sweetener to meat, vegetable, and cheese dishes. Elites sweetened omelets with honey. Roman gourmet Marcus Gavius Apicius (c. 25 BCE–c. 37 CE)—advisor to Emperors Augustus (63 BCE–14 CE) and Tiberius (42 BCE–37 CE)—is thought to have compiled recipes for honey and other foods in a cookbook attributed to him.[12] Because of his status, Apicius, if these recipes' source, memorialized culinary habits of elites rather than underclass.

11.1.3 Apiculture

Honeybees' domestication was intertwined with apiculture (beekeeping), an occupation that yielded a dependable supply. Keeping honeybees, Egypt pioneered their breeding in hopes of increasing honey production. Even so, collection from the wild was the principal method of acquisition into the seventh century BCE. Because gathering exposed humans to bee stings, it required courage and, like hunting, was thought proper for men.[13] By the seventh century Egypt, Persia (today Iran), India, Babylon, and Ur—the last two being ruins in what is now Iraq—collected honey from the wild and produced it in artificial hives. Its importance is evident in Egyptians' belief that the god Ra gave them honey. Hinduists and Buddhists also held honey sacred.

Both religions began in India, where bakers topped flatbreads and dough balls with honey to affix sesame (*Sesamum indicum*) seeds. Indians, Central Asians, and Greeks added it to yogurt. Central Asia, western Asia, Arabia, and Mediterranean lands made pastries—baklava for example—with honey. Arabs and North Africans added it to durum (*Triticum durum*) porridge or gruel, though dates (*Phoenix dactylifera*) were the chief sweetener. Farther east, the Chinese used honey more as seasoning than sweetener as early as 200 BCE, though those who desired sweetness added it to tea (*Camellia sinensis*). Unlike its western neighbors, China deemphasized honey.

Between Egypt and East Asia, Phoenicians, Assyrians, and Arabs collected honey from the wild and produced it in manmade hives. To their east, Central Asians traded it as early as 2000 BCE. In the first millennium BCE, the Persian Empire valued it as food and for income. Merchants pursued honey along the Silk Road—a group of overland routes between Mediterranean Sea and Pacific Ocean—as far east as China. These arteries gave Russia honey beyond the local supply.

Fourth-century BCE Romans began keeping bees.[14] Roman authors Cato the Elder (234–149 BCE), Marcus Terentius Varro (116–27 BCE), Virgil (70–19 BCE), and Pliny the Elder (23–79 CE) esteemed the sweetener and apiculture.[15] Rome's integration of the Mediterranean into a single trade zone encouraged honey commerce. Commercialization predated Rome in Egypt, which imported honey as early as 2500 BCE. Rome's expansion into northern Europe reinforced honey consumption among peoples who had long collected it. Celts, Germans, and Slavs ate honey and fermented it into mead, possibly the oldest alcoholic beverage.[16]

11.1.4 Honey's Early Prevalence

Centuries before Jesus, Europeans made honey the primary sweetener and mead the chief alcoholic drink between Ireland in the west and the Ural Mountains in the east.[17] Christianity and its monasteries preserved interest in, and literature about, honey and mead during the Middle Ages (c. 500–c. 1500 CE). As charity, English and Irish monks distributed the sweetener free to the poor. Medieval Bavaria in southeastern Germany, Bohemia in what is now the Czech Republic, and the Baltic region of what are today Estonia, Latvia, and Lithuania emerged as large honey—paired with milk, meat, fish, and eggs—and mead producers and consumers. The quest for balance led Europeans to flavor savory dishes with honey. Like salt, honey's status as preservative recommended its addition to perishables.

Its popularity stemmed partly from its cheapness relative to sugar through the Middle Ages, a fact that a later section demonstrates. Aiming to increase production, Frankish King Charlemagne (742–814) ordered each farm in the Carolingian Empire—now France, Germany, and part of Italy—to keep bees and pay two-third of honey in taxes.[18] By the fifteenth century, however, honey was in retreat as northern Europeans drank more beer than mead. The continent increased sucrose imports as ties strengthened with Asia—notably India, China, and what is today Indonesia—the source of tea and spices.

In the eighteenth century, industrialization further weakened honey by attracting people to cities, which kept no bees. By 1850, it was more expensive than sucrose, making honey a luxury and sucrose a mass commodity. Even as honey languished in Europe, Britain took honeybees to Australia during the nineteenth century.[19] In recent decades, honey revived as people equated it with nature and sucrose and HFCS with corporations.

Besides these developments, Mesoamerica and South America arose as western-hemisphere centers of honey production and consumption. Beginning around 7000 BCE, a succession of peoples in Mexico and Central America collected wild honey.[20] By roughly 1500 BCE, the Olmec practiced apiculture to augment this supply. Between Mexico and the southernmost Incan outposts in Chile, Amerindians added honey to cornbread, beans (*Phaseolus vulgaris*, *P. lunatus*, *P. acutifolius*, and *P. coccineus*), squashes (*Cucurbita* species), chili peppers (*Capsicum* species), and game and ate honeybees for extra nutrients and calories.

11.1.5 Honey, Nutrition, and Health

The abstract stated that unlike sucrose and HFCS, honey has minerals and vitamins. One hundred grams of raw honey have 1.1–100 percent of the U.S. Food and Drug Administration's (FDA) daily value (DV) for potassium, 1–30 percent for copper, 1–100 percent for manganese, 0.3–13.3 percent for zinc, and 0.5–16 percent for vitamin B_6.[21] No other nutrient equals or exceeds 5 percent DV. Minerals and vitamins vary because bees collect irregular amounts of nectar and pollen from numerous florae.

Honey may be compared with molasses ($C_6H_{12}NNaO_3S$), the most popular U.S. sweetener before the twentieth century.[22] One hundred grams have 20.5 percent of DV for calcium, 26.2 percent for iron, 60.5 percent for magnesium, 41.8 percent for potassium, and 33.5 percent for vitamin B_6.[23] No other nutrient equals or surpasses 5 percent DV. These numbers show that molasses has more calcium, iron, magnesium, and vitamin B_6 than raw honey, for which the amounts of copper, potassium, manganese, and zinc vary too markedly for comparison.

Honey may be evaluated by examining hunter-gatherers. Previous sections indicated that wild collection predated apiculture. Hunter-gatherers' persistence into modernity, as noted, furnishes information about their health. For example, American anthropologists Kim R. Hill (b. 1953) and Ana Magdalena Hurtado quantified Ache honey consumption at roughly 8 percent the daily total of over 2,700 calories per person.[24] That is, each individual averaged above 216 calories from honey daily.

This amount trailed the roughly 78 percent (2,106 calories) from meat but should not be construed to minimize honey's value. Chapter 4 emphasized that the Ache needed many calories. Parasites and pathogens sapped energy and nutrients, and moving camp, hunting, and gathering necessitated almost continuous exertions. Men hunted about seven hours per day.[25] Women gathered plants two hours daily, relocated camp another two hours, and cared for children. On their feet much of the day, Ache traversed difficult terrain. American anthropologist Stephen Le estimated that preagricultural men walked 14.5 kilometers (9 miles) and women covered 9.7 kilometers (6 miles) daily.[26] These guesses need not match Ache nomadism to intimate their lives' arduousness. Honey's calories and nutrients fueled Ache activity, contributing to their vigor.

Besides hunter-gatherers, honey may be evaluated in antiquity. A previous section mentioned honey's restriction to Egyptian elites. Chapter 4 detailed Egypt's geography, history, economy, diets, nutrition, and health. Readers may remember that overeating and idleness contributed to the wealthy's obesity and heart disease. Chapter 4 amassed evidence for atherosclerosis (sometimes rendered arteriosclerosis) and heart attacks among them. By supplying calories, honey must have aggravated these conditions, especially obesity, which worsens chronic diseases.

Considered together, the Ache and Egyptian elites underscore the importance of context, as emphasized throughout this book. Differences in activity put them on divergent trajectories, highlighting that diet and nutrition cannot be isolated from total circumstances. At its essence, food is a biological commodity understood in terms of chemistry and physics, Chapter 2 argued, and is inseparable from the biology of organisms that consume it. Within the realms of science and nature, insects, parasites, and pathogens exact energy and nutrients from their hosts. The chemistry of metabolism, accelerated by exertions, determines how many calories and nutrients are used and how fast. These factors, varying over time and space, caution against overgeneralizations about foods.

Egypt concretized the previous section's description of honey as extravagance rather than mass commodity. To be sure, this rule had exceptions. For example, the poor among Britain's Celts added honey to beer, but Greeks and Romans regarded them as oddities whose behavior proved unsophistication.[27] This deviation from the norm does not weaken the generalization that the rich monopolized honey in antiquity.

Wealthy ancients were taller than the underclass on average, important evidence given this book's emphasis on height as health gauge.[28] Giving the rich energy and some nutrients, honey may have contributed to this disparity, though other foods were likely more important. For example, Chapter 4

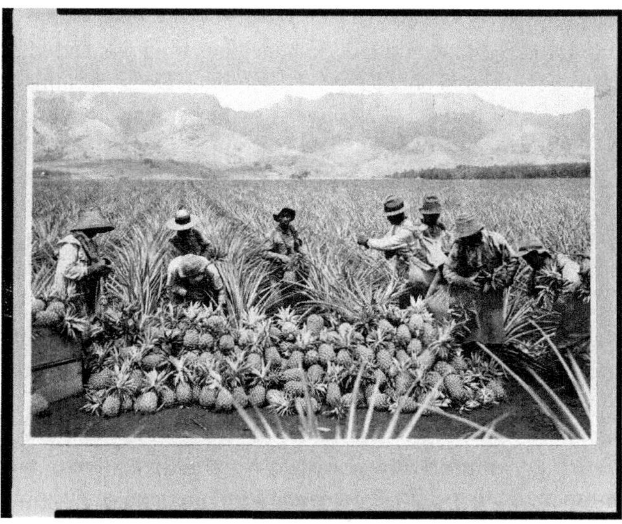

FIGURE 11.1 Pineapples. (Photo courtesy of Library of Congress. https://www.loc.gov/pictures/item/93511081/.)

documented meat's promotion of height. Readers may recall that nineteenth-century Plains Indians ate bison (*Bison bison*), antelopes (species in Bovidae family), elk (*Cervus species*), deer (*Odocoileus* species), wolves (*Canis lupus*), foxes (*Vulpes vulpes*), bears (*Ursus americanus*), beavers (*Castor canadensis*), muskrats (*Ondatra zibethicus*), mink (*Mustela vison*), weasels (*Mustela nivalis*), raccoons (*Procyon lotor*), mutton, lamb, and beef. American anthropologist Joseph M. Prince and American economist Richard Hall Steckel (b. 1944) credited diet with making these indigenes the world's tallest about 1850.[29]

Using Ache and Plains Indians as evidence, this section argues that meat was a larger dietary component and a greater determiner of height than honey among these hunter-gatherers. Egypt, Greece, and Rome typified a pattern whereby the wealthy ate more meat than honey and more meat than the poor. In these instances, too, meat played a larger role than honey in height disparities. This inquiry does not recommend against honey's consumption, though it cautions against extravagant claims about the sweetener's benefits and against overeating.

11.2 SUCROSE

11.2.1 Chemistry

Chapter 2 classified all sugars as carbohydrates and described several sugars, though this section treats only sucrose, the disaccharide meant by casual use of the word "sugar." Chapter 2 introduced, and the abstract reiterated, its formula. As a disaccharide, a sucrose molecule unites one fructose and one glucose molecule. Both fructose and glucose are monosaccharides with the formula ($C_6H_{12}O_6$), Chapter 2 and a previous section stated. The linkage of one fructose and one glucose molecule liberates a water molecule (H_2O) to yield sucrose's $C_{12}H_{22}O_{11}$.

Chapter 3 contrasted animals, which store most surplus energy as fat, with plants, which store excess as carbohydrates, whether starch, sugars, or both. Because of this ability, many plants have some sucrose. For example, 100 grams of mangos (*Mangifera indica*) have 7 grams of sucrose.[30] Sucrose, fructose, and glucose impart sweetness to pineapples (*Ananas comosus*), apricots (*Prunus armeniaca*), dates, figs (*Ficus carica*), and many other dessert fruits. Although less sweet, vegetables and legumes may also have sucrose. For example, despite dissimilar flavors, identical amounts of pineapples and peas have the same quantity of sucrose.[31] Of the global florae, two plants—sugarcane (*Saccharum officinarum*) and sugar beet (*Beta vulgaris ssp. vulgaris*)—feed the world's sucrose addiction.

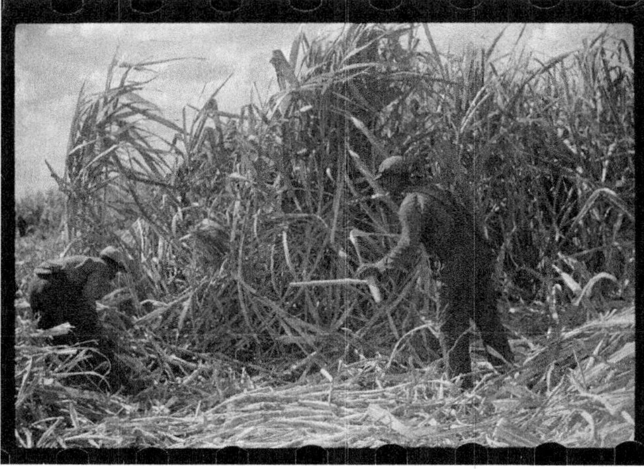

FIGURE 11.2 Sugarcane. (Photo courtesy of Library of Congress. https://www.loc.gov/pictures/item/2017754366/.)

11.2.2 Biology of Craving

Demand for sugars has a biological component because the mouth's roughly 10,000 taste buds—spread among the tongue, palate, cheek, esophagus, and epiglottis—detect sweetness.[32] In response to sucrose and other sugars, taste buds send neurotransmitters to the brain, which increases appetite. A hearty appetite must have benefited humans during all but recent history by enlarging the intake of calories and nutrients. Spurts of gluttony helped people survive the food scarcity that prevailed most of the time. Moreover, the craving for sweetness prodded newborns to nurse in order to ingest mother's milk, rich in the sugar lactose ($C_{12}H_{22}O_{11}$), which Chapters 2 and 7 described.[33] Newborns and infants who gained mass stood better odds of survival upon weaning, when food became scant, than runts. American economist, historian, and 1993 Nobel laureate in economics Robert William Fogel (1926–2013) reported that mortality was higher for underweight than average infants among Trinidad and U.S. slaves.[34] Avoidance of underweight—which Fogel equated with shortness absent data for mass—helped slaves in Trinidad and the American South reach adulthood.

11.2.3 Sugarcane

Of the two sucrose-rich plants, sugarcane is millennia older. A tropical grass in the Poaceae or Gramineae family, it is related to wheat, rye (*Secale cereale*), corn, rice (*Oryza* species), oats (*Avena sativa*), triticale (*Triticosecale rimpaui*), barley (*Hordeum vulgare*), sorghum (*Sorghum bicolor*), the millets (species in Eragrostideae tribe), and other grains. Native to Polynesia, sugarcane supplied energy to prehistoric peoples who chewed stems' interior for the sweet juice.[35] The stem, also termed stalk or culm, is about 16 percent sucrose by mass, with the rest as water and fiber.[36]

The first species to attract humankind is unknown, though *Saccharum robustum* is a candidate because people early used its leaves for roofing huts and erecting fences. Familiarity with it may have led Polynesians to chew stems, though the species' sucrose is minimal. Domestication of *Saccharum officinarum*, richer in the sugar, occurred west of Polynesia on New Guinea about 7000 BCE.[37]

Equatorial latitudes gave the tropical grass long, warm, humid growing seasons absent frost and did not impede movement east and west from these islands. Frost not only damages or kills plants but renders stems unsuitable for juice's extraction by crushing. Warmth's necessity limited the crop's movement to higher latitudes. Most sugarcane is raised between 20 degrees north and 20 degrees south, though its range extends another 15 degrees in both directions.[38]

From New Guinea, *S. officinarum* spread east throughout Melanesia and into Polynesia around 6000 BCE. West and north of New Guinea, the species reached India, where it was "widely used," about two millennia later.[39] Emulating the islanders, Indians chewed stems for sweetness and energy. By 3000 BCE, sugarcane was grown in India, southern China, Southeast Asia including the Philippines, New Guinea, and several other Pacific Islands. Around 500 BCE Bihar, India, pioneered sucrose crystallization by heating the juice to evaporate water.[40] This invention made sucrose a solid rather than the liquid of sugarcane stems, changing how humans consumed it.

11.2.4 Production and Prices

Tropical Asia produced most of the world's crop before Europe encountered the Americas, though before 1500 CE sugarcane and appetite for sweetness had spread west throughout the Old World. Important in this diffusion was Iran's adoption of the grass before 600 CE and Islam's ascent in the seventh century.[41] Arab converts carried the new faith east and west. Encountering sugarcane in Iran, they planted it in Syria, Palestine (today Israel and Palestine), Greek islands Rhodes, Cyprus (now independent), and Crete, Italian island Sicily, many smaller Mediterranean islands, North Africa—today Libya, Tunisia, Algeria, and Morocco—Egypt, and Mediterranean Spain by the eighth century.

With Syria and Palestine in the eastern Mediterranean, many Greek islands, and Sicily all able to produce sucrose in the Middle Ages, Europe, at last, could purchase it. England began importing the sugar in 1319, Denmark in 1374, and Sweden in 1390. University of Toronto food historian Jeffrey M. Pilcher (b. 1965) wrote in 2006 that the disaccharide was "relatively plentiful" in medieval Europe.[42]

Abundance usually means inexpensiveness, but prices suggest scarcity during the Middle Ages, a judgment that University of Toronto geographer Jock H. Galloway confirmed.[43] The mean price for 4.5 kilograms (10 pounds) of sucrose in London, England, Paris, France, and Amsterdam, the Netherlands equaled the value of 9.9 grams (0.35 ounces) of gold between 1350 and 1400.[44] Thereafter prices diminished so that 4.5 kilograms of sucrose were worth 6.9 grams (0.24 ounces) of gold between 1401 and 1450, 5.4 grams (0.19 ounces) between 1451 and 1500, and 2.5 grams (0.09 ounces) between 1501 and 1550. American botanist Beryl Brintnall Simpson (b. 1942) and American botanist and science educator Molly Conner Ogorzaly rated the sweetener dearer in Europe than these numbers indicate, equating 0.5 kilograms (roughly 1 pound) of sucrose to 9.4 grams (0.33 ounces) of gold in 1500.[45]

Honey prices followed these reductions. The mean price for 4.5 kilograms of honey in London, Paris, and Amsterdam fell from being worth 0.9 grams (0.03 ounces) of gold between 1350 and 1400 to 0.6 grams (0.02 ounces) between 1401 and 1450, 0.4 grams (0.014 ounces) between 1451 and 1500, and 0.3 grams (0.011 ounces) between 1501 and 1550.[46] Over these two centuries, sucrose inundated markets, driving down demand and prices for honey.

Toward the end of this period, Europe began importing sucrose from a new source: tropical America, notably the West Indies and Brazil. In 1493 or 1494 Italian-Spanish mariner Christopher Columbus (1451–1506) planted sugarcane on Caribbean island Hispaniola, today Haiti and the Dominican Republic.[47] Around 1500 Spain's rival Portugal began growing the grass in its colony Brazil.[48] Unwilling to let Iberia control New World production, Britain, France, the Netherlands, and Denmark carved out plantations in the Caribbean. Attempts to force indigenes to toil in the fields failed as they succumbed to Old-World diseases. This mortality led planters to enslave Africans to produce sucrose in the Caribbean, South America, and Mexico in the sixteenth century, and in Texas and Louisiana in the eighteenth century. This system's inhumanity defies description.

Slavery's abolition in the nineteenth century did not weaken sucrose output. In the United States, for example, the Thirteenth Amendment—ratified in 1865—retained slavery and involuntary servitude "as punishment for a crime."[49] Plantation owners forced convicts to work the fields (see Chapter 8), and twentieth-century South Florida replicated slave-like conditions on sugar estates. Even before statehood in 1959, Hawaii produced sucrose for export to the mainland, using Chinese, Japanese, Korean, and Filipino laborers.

11.2.5 Consumption, Nutrition, and Health

Sucrose consumption had been "a mere pinch per head" in medieval Europe.[50] Households used it less as a sweetener than as a spice to complement other flavors. They also added just enough to medicines to reduce bitterness. Such parsimony is unsurprising given the high prices already mentioned. Sixteenth-century Europeans averaged 4 grams (one teaspoon) of sucrose per person annually.[51] In the eighteenth century sucrose was dearer than bread.[52] Commoners' poverty throughout history, emphasized throughout this book, precluded sucrose's purchase until it was cheap.

Medieval Europe's sparing use permits evaluation of health before sucrose became ubiquitous. Introduced in Chapter 8, military records between roughly 800 and 1300 showed that northern European men were tall even by nineteenth-century standards.[53] They stood taller than some Plains Indians (see Chapter 4), who as a group were the world's tallest in the nineteenth century. Because nutrition and height correlate, as noted throughout this book, northern Europeans were well nourished without sucrose.

An earlier section deemed honey the chief prehistoric, ancient, and medieval sweetener. Although, as mentioned, Mediterranean lands produced sucrose beginning in the Middle Ages, their inhabitants—consuming grapes (*Vitis vinifera*) and wine—used less than northern Europe, where sucrose began to rival honey in the fifteenth century.[54] An exception was Russia, where temperate sugar beet's arrival only in the nineteenth century allowed tardy sucrose production. Into the 1860s, honey remained an important sweetener there.

Strong demand for sucrose kept prices high, as mentioned, through the eighteenth century as Europeans and North Americans added it to coffee (*Coffea* species) and tea (*Camellia sinensis*).[55] Earlier chapters stated that expensive foods like meat marked status by affirming their consumers as elites. The less affluent wanted to emulate their superiors by eating these items. This dynamic applied to sucrose while it was a luxury. Even as prices declined, it remained a costly source of energy. In 1800, sucrose cost five times more than bread, and tenfold above potatoes, per calorie in England.[56] By then, however, the sweetener—dubbed "white death"—was undermining health.[57] As early as 1598, a Dutch visitor wrote about teeth blackened from too much sucrose.[58]

Less visible were the body's biochemical adjustments to it. Foods rich in fiber, minerals, vitamins, and phytochemicals take time and energy to digest. But without nutrients, sucrose exemplifies empty calories and is too readily absorbed. Adapting to it, the digestive system streamlines operations by suppressing enzymes necessary to assimilate nutrients but superfluous absent them. Consequently, before 1800, the English favored white flour and white bread because their bodies produced too few enzymes to digest whole grains.[59] The next chapter details shortcomings in white flour, white bread, and white rice. Not only devoid of nourishment, therefore, sucrose reinforced preferences for unwholesome foods.

Sucrose prices fell during the nineteenth and twentieth centuries, permitting consumption on a vast scale. About 1810, the average American ate 5.4–5.9 kilograms (12–13 pounds) of sucrose annually, whereas in 1929 his or her consumption reached 49.4 kilograms (109 pounds) according to American anthropologists Gretel H. Pelto and Pertti J. Pelto (b. 1927).[60] Thereafter U.S. per person annual consumption plateaued at roughly 45.4 kilograms (100 pounds), the amount West Palm Beach, Florida's Hippocrates Health Institute (HHI) reported for 2005.[61]

American neuroscientist Stephan J. Guyenet's numbers match HHI's 2005 value, though not the Peltos' statistics around 1810 and 1929.[62] Although Guyenet retrogressed to 1822 rather than 1810, his figure of 2.87 kilograms (6.34 pounds) per American for 1822 requires sucrose intake to have decreased between roughly 1810 and 1822, an unlikelihood given increase afterward. Whereas the Peltos stated that the average American consumed 49.4 kilograms of sucrose in 1929, as noted, Guyenet put intake at 36.47 kilograms (80.41 pounds). Perhaps more important, comparison of the Peltos' numbers and HHI's 2005 figure implies stasis between 1929 and 2005 whereas Guyenet reported increase between 1929 and 2005. Indeed, Graph 11.1 shows that he documented enlargement in sucrose ingestion from 1822 to 2005.

Guyenet's data and HHI's 2005 figure agree with a 2009 paper, which stated that in 1970 sucrose added 400, and in 2005 476, calories to the typical daily American diet.[63] At 3.87 calories per gram,

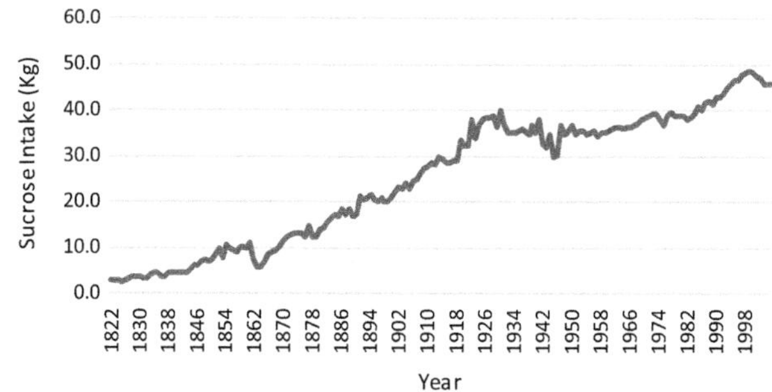

GRAPH 11.1 Annual sucrose intake per average American, 1822–2005. Courtesy of Dietra Cumo.

400 calories of sucrose have a mass of 103.36 grams (3.65 ounces), the amount consumed daily in 1970. This daily intake enlarges to 37.73 kilograms (83.18 pounds) per year, a quantity near Guyenet's 38.48 kilograms (84.83 pounds) in 1970.[64] Repeating these calculations, 476 calories of sucrose yield 44.89 kilograms (98.97 pounds) of the sugar ingested in 2005, a value near Guyenet's 45.74 kilograms (100.84 pounds) and HHI's 45.4 kilograms that year.

England's per person ingestion surged to 50.8 kilograms (112 pounds) in 1960, dipped briefly, and then resumed its ascent.[65] In 2015, American food historian Andrew Francis Smith (b. 1946) estimated per person annual sucrose consumption at 60 kilograms (132 pounds) in the United States, at 45 kilograms (99 pounds) in Mexico, Brazil, Argentina, and Australia, but only at 1.8 kilograms (4 pounds) in China.[66] Worldwide, the average annual per capita sucrose intake is 4.4 kilograms (9.7 pounds). Smith's statistics indicate that U.S. individual consumption rose over 30 percent between 2005 and 2015.

These numbers, though worrisome, do not correlate well with the obesity epidemic, which began after 1970 according to American cardiology William Davis (b. 1957)—introduced in Chapter 1—in the 1970s, late 1970s, or around 1980 according to American journalist and food writer Michael Kevin Pollan (b. 1955), or after 1980, reckoned American science writer Gary Taubes (b. 1956).[67] These dates acknowledge that the nineteenth-century surge in sucrose consumption did not produce obesity despite concern from American cardiologist Robert Coleman Atkins (1930–2003), introduced in Chapter 4, about its "fattening power."[68] Chapter 12 indicates that American men and women retained roughly the same mass for their age and height between 1885 and 1900 and that masses rose with twentieth-century adoption and spread of the automobile.[69] Masses increased after roughly 1920, around the time sucrose consumption reached stasis according to the Peltos. Moreover, Davis, Pollan, and Taubes' timing of this epidemic about or after 1970 came over 150 years after Americans began to eat more sucrose. According to the trio, obesity leapt after sucrose intake had plateaued, again referencing the Peltos.

Research about U.S. and U.K. diets contradicts attempts to blame sucrose, and carbohydrates in general, for obesity. Last chapter previewed the finding that growth in fat intake relative to sucrose and other carbohydrates and to total calories enlarges body fat.[70] Sucrose consumption correlates inversely with obesity but increases in both fat and sucrose predispose people to obesity. Besides diet, studies support this book's argument that inactivity, even if not the sole cause, contributes to obesity.[71] Chapter 12 indicates that the longer people are in an automobile, and the more television they watch, the fatter they grow.

Retaining an international perspective, Americans and Europeans consume similar sucrose quantities yet differ in obesity.[72] In 2017, the Organization for Economic Cooperation and Development (OECD) in Paris, France, reported the worst rate for the United States, where 38.2 percent of Americans were obese.[73] The United Kingdom exhibited Europe's greatest obesity with 26.9 percent of Brits obese. Finland, Germany, Ireland, the Czech Republic, Latvia, and Luxembourg exceeded 20 percent of inhabitants as obese. At the other extreme, under one in ten Italians was obese. Brazil averaged over 50 kilograms (110.2 pounds) of sucrose per person in 2017 but had fewer obese denizens (20.8 percent) than the United States.[74] Cuba had the world's highest intake at 60 kilograms (132.3 pounds) per person in 2015 and the greatest obesity at over 43 percent of the population.[75] These statistics yield no pattern—neither indicting nor exonerating sucrose for obesity—an unsurprising outcome given that numerous factors influence body mass.

Beyond concerns about body fat, the large increase in U.S. sucrose intake between 1810 and 1929 caused no upsurge in chronic diseases. For example, in 1925—with Americans near peak consumption—British physician and professor John William McNee (1887–1984) characterized atherosclerosis as a "rare disease" in the United States, having identified only two cases.[76] In the United States and other affluent nations, heart disease mortality rose only around 1950, peaking about twenty years later.[77] Sucrose is an unlikely villain in these deaths because its 1929 zenith, according to the Peltos, predated the apex of U.S. heart disease deaths by roughly forty years. Chapter 12 notes that during the 1950s, the United States began building interstate highways to buttress the nation's car culture. Chronic diseases, uncommon before the automobile, rose after its adoption and as Americans increased dependence on it.

Even if the links among sucrose, obesity, and chronic diseases are questionable, trends in U.S. stature and longevity suggest that sucrose does not enhance vitality. Military records indicated that American white men's heights grew most rapidly before about 1710.[78] Sucrose consumption must have been minuscule then and would not begin to increase for another century. Seventeenth-century American diets, largely absent sucrose, must have been nourishing to permit marked height gains. Between about 1710 and 1780, stature continued to rise, though more slowly than during the seventeenth century. Nonetheless, by mid-eighteenth century, Americans were as tall as today, reaching modern stature before many Europeans and before sucrose ingestion began to climb.

During the 1790s, U.S. life expectancy at age ten (e^{10}) began to decrease, a trend that continued into the 1840s as shown in Table 11.1.[79]

TABLE 11.1
E^{10} for American White Men 1701–1925

Dates	E^{10}, American White Men (yr)
1701–1725	50.3
1726–1750	55.5
1751–1775	58.8
1776–1800	51.9
1801–1825	52.3
1826–1850	48.9
1851–1875	55.3
1876–1900	N/A
1901–1925	56.9

After roughly 1830, American heights likewise began to decline, shrinking 3 centimeters (1.2 inches) on average during the next twenty years.[80] If the 1790s were the pivot between improvement and degradation, sucrose cannot bear full blame because consumption did not start to rise until about 1810. Yet, once intake was on the ascent, heights began to shorten. Although correlation does not prove causation, sucrose—bereft of nutrients—cannot have benefited Americans who trailed earlier generations in longevity and stature.

Other factors complicate the relationship between sucrose and health in the United States. First, the Americas presented unusual opportunities for demographic expansion. Chapter 6 documented that from earliest contact, Europeans carried Old World diseases to which Amerindians lacked immunities. Their deaths opened the New World to colonization. In the American colonies and early republic, the population of Europeans and their descendants grew from roughly 250,000 in 1700 to over 10 million in the 1820s.[81] Before 1914, the United States surpassed 100 million inhabitants. This growth expanded west as Americans migrated toward the Pacific Ocean after the Revolutionary War (1775–1783). So long as population was sparse, epidemics seldom threatened. But as cities swelled—U.S. urban population more than tripled between 1790 and 1850—pathogens, pests, and parasites multiplied, and mortality rose.[82]

Second, cities grew with the demand for labor in factories, mills, and shops. Open borders and the promise of jobs attracted immigrants such that surplus workers drove down wages. Management amplified this development by hiring women and children, groups it overworked and underpaid.[83] British economist David Ricardo's (1772–1823) "iron law of wages" expressed pay's tendency to sink to subsistence.[84] Bucking this reality, real wages plateaued or rose between 1820 and 1860.[85] Some of this money fueled the increase in sucrose consumption, noted earlier, which may have exacerbated declines in lifespan and stature during these decades when half to three-quarters of incomes fetched food.

Robert Fogel argued that wage gains benefited workers with skills and education rather than laborers, increasing inequalities.[86] Widespread poverty exacerbated squalor. Crowding and the absence of sanitation in slums spread pathogens, pests, parasites, and death. Consequently, commoners' longevity and stature declined. Whatever factors were involved, sucrose consumption increased while health, as measured by e^{10} and height, diminished.

Third, as mentioned, molasses rather than sucrose was the primary sweetener in the United States before roughly 1900. Like sucrose, molasses derives from sugarcane. Sugar beet, grapes, and sorghum yield a similar substance. Unlike sucrose, however, molasses has more than carbohydrates, a previous section quantifying its minerals and vitamins. Obesity and other chronic conditions were minor in the United States while molasses was the principal sweetener, possibly because it is not just empty calories. Chronic diseases worsened in the twentieth century when sucrose surpassed it.

Like HFCS examined in the next section, sucrose adds inconspicuous calories to processed foods and beverages. For example, a McDonald's medium Minute Maid orange juice has 41 grams of sugars and 200 calories, 10 percent of a 2,000-calorie diet.[87] Because the juice lacks fat and has just 3 grams of protein, nearly all calories come from these sugars. Neither McDonald's nor the U.S. Department of Agriculture (USDA) identified orange juice's sugars.[88] The Florida Department of Citrus stated only that the sugars are "naturally occurring."[89] Even without added sucrose, orange juice has this sugar because it, along with fructose and glucose, is a component of oranges (*Citrus sinensis*). American neurologist David Perlmutter (b. 1954), introduced in chapter 1, cautioned against orange juice because of its "hidden sugars."[90] Other examples need not be entertained to demonstrate that sucrose adds calories to foods that need no enhancement.

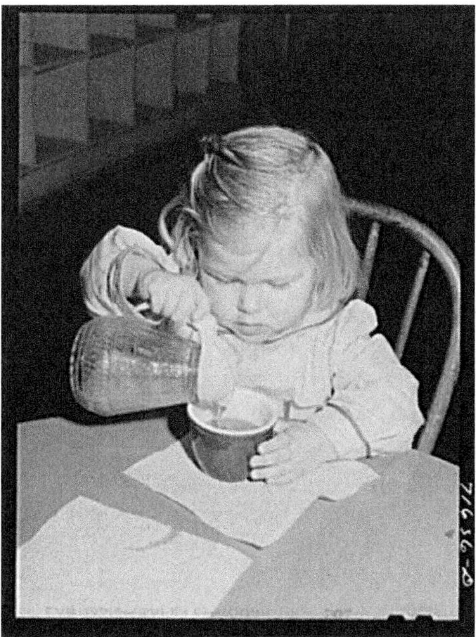

FIGURE 11.3 Orange juice. (Photo courtesy of Library of Congress. https://www.loc.gov/pictures/item/2017817209/.)

An earlier section mentioned the prehistoric practice of chewing sugarcane stems for the juice. The USDA defined this liquid as almost pure sucrose and water, with 100 milliliters (3.4 ounces) supplying 12.9 grams of the sugar.[91] The only nutrient the USDA listed is sodium, which is excessive in many diets.

Yet unprocessed sugarcane juice is more than sucrose, water, and sodium. *The Daily Observer*, a newspaper on Caribbean island Antigua, declared in 2015 that the juice has calcium, magnesium, iron, potassium, manganese, and antioxidants.[92] The anonymous author claimed that the liquid increases protein in the body, aids digestion and kidney function, and fights tooth decay, fevers, infections, and cancers. These assertions lack evidence and may stem from the desire to protect a crop grown on the island since the seventeenth century.

Although sweeping, the newspaper's comments are rooted in eighteenth-century observations that slaves appeared most vigorous at harvest.[93] This perception countered expectations given this labor's strenuousness. Onlookers attributed slaves' vitality to unlimited access to cane juice during harvest, a liberty otherwise unavailable. A mix of molasses and brown sugar, this juice supplied nutrients because molasses, has calcium, iron, magnesium, potassium, manganese, and vitamin B_6. Even brown sugar has these minerals and B_6 because of molasses.

Asserting that carbohydrates cause obesity and chronic diseases, Gary Taubes began the prologue to *Good Calories, Bad Calories* (2008) by quoting English physician Thomas Hawkes Tanner (1824–1871), who wrote in 1869 that wherever sugarcane was grown, blacks and cows (*Bos taurus*) became "remarkably stout" when able to consume copious cane juice.[94] The choice of Tanner as a putatively impartial observer is unfortunate because his equation of Africans and cattle revealed the racism common among white elites, a class that fabricated the absurdity that blacks preferred slavery to freedom.[95]

Tanner's selection is also regrettable because he and Taubes failed to clarify whether the focus was slave or free labor.[96] The context was unclear in 1869 because tropical America had no uniform policy. France outlawed slavery in its Caribbean colonies in 1794, but French emperor Napoleon Bonaparte (1769–1821) nullified the law in 1802.[97] Two years later French colony Saint Domingue—roughly the western one-third of Hispaniola—proclaimed independence as Haiti and abolished slavery. In 1813, Argentina enacted a policy of gradual emancipation. Ten years later Chile ended slavery. Colombia and Peru followed in 1851 and 1854, respectively. But bondage remained legal in Puerto Rico, Cuba, and Brazil at Tanner's death. The issue of slavery versus freedom need not be resolved, however, if slave-like conditions persisted after emancipation. Chapter 8 argued that free labor did not differ markedly from slavery in arduousness wherever greed and ruthlessness prevailed.

Tanner's belief that Africans grew fat during sugarcane harvest conflicts with their "systematic semistarvation" in the British Caribbean.[98] As early as 1688, legislators on Caribbean island Barbados admitted that starvation drove slaves to steal food.[99] Whites retaliated by executing transgressors, for example, hanging a slave on Caribbean island Montserrat in the 1690s for stealing nothing more consequential than two turkeys (*Meleagris gallopavo f. domestica*).[100] Because the youngest and oldest slaves were least able to work, some Caribbean planters starved them to cut expenses.[101]

This system was so brutal that slaves seldom survived four years beyond their arrival in the West Indies.[102] The risk of death was great during the transition to this new environment, a period known as "seasoning."[103] The tropical climate nurtured insects, pathogens, and parasites, problems Europeans worsened by importing killers such as malaria and yellow fever through the slave trade. American historian Richard Slator Dunn (b. 1928) described mortality as "frightfully high," writing that Caribbean slaves "died much faster than they were born."[104] This circumstance encouraged owners to regard Africans as "disposable."[105]

Sugarcane juice's limitations were evident on Barbados. When food was unavailable, this liquid was slaves' lone intake.[106] Although brief, such privation undermined health. Examination of 101 skeletons revealed enamel growth on teeth roots—a condition known as hypercementosis—and enamel hypoplasia (defined in Chapters 1) severe enough to indicate starvation. These defects appeared in infant skeletons, implying that these children starved after weaning when cane juice substituted poorly for mother's milk. Malocclusion (misaligned teeth) confirmed undernourishment. American anthropologists Jerome S. Handler and Robert Spencer Corruccini (b. 1949) concluded from these data that slaves lacked protein, an unsurprising circumstance given its absence in sugarcane juice.[107] Omnipresent hunger and undernutrition emaciated slaves.[108]

Cane juice is blameless for slavery's cruelties, though its nutrients were inadequate. Without lipids, it lacked fat-soluble vitamins A, D, E, and K described in Chapter 2. Besides B_6, the juice had no water-soluble vitamins: the other B vitamins and C, also treated in Chapter 2. Its minerals, though more numerous than vitamins, were also incomplete. Deprivations, nutritional and otherwise, condemned slaves to an early grave.[109]

Slaves throughout the western hemisphere coped with meager diets by eating soil (geophagy).[110] Originating in Africa as the commonest type of pica (consumption of nonfoods) in the tropics, the practice may have helped compensate for diets poor in calcium, manganese, magnesium, iron, potassium, zinc, or their combination.[111] Despite its minerals, cane juice could not avert the behavior because, as noted, the liquid was plentiful only at harvest. Owners and doctors identified gaunt slaves as especially prone to geophagy, which may have caused half of all deaths on some plantations.[112]

Undernutrition was also evident in night blindness, blindness, and other eye afflictions from vitamin A deficiency among slaves.[113] Cane juice could not have remedied these problems because, as stated, it lacked fat-soluble vitamins including A. Rickets' prevalence due to vitamin D dearth, discussed elsewhere, betrayed the juice's absence of this fat-soluble vitamin.[114] Among water-soluble vitamins, B_1's paucity in sugarcane juice caused beriberi, a disease discussed in Chapter 12. By the nineteenth century, the malady was widespread among Cuban slaves.[115]

Barbados and Jamaica were not the only British colonies to ail from sucrose. Canada likewise fell under its spell. In 1583, England established its first Canadian colony at St. John's in what is today the province Newfoundland and Labrador. Additional settlements followed despite opposition from French colonists. Britain's triumph in the Seven Years' War (1756–1763) won it France's Canadian holdings.

Victory opened Canada to widespread British colonization. In the province Ontario, Brits settled what had been the Amerindian village Asukhknosk in 1776, enlarging and renaming it Belleville in 1816. The town grew from roughly 700 settlers in 1829 to over 7,300 in 1871.[116] Belleville's middle and upper classes belonged to the Church of England, known as the Anglican Church, and attended St. Thomas' Anglican Church. Belleville had acquired land for the parish in 1818. Construction finished in 1821 when the church began services and opened its grounds for interment of deceased faithful. Examination of nearly 600 skeletons buried between 1821 and 1874 thus documented middle-and-upper-class health and nutrition.[117]

Chapter 1 indicated that economic, social, and political inequalities created an America in which the richest live almost fifteen years longer than the poorest.[118] Not all gains resulted from the wealthy's medical care, lifestyle, and diet. By itself, affluence appears to benefit its possessors in ways difficult to quantify. If this mechanism operated in the past, St. Thomas' skeletons should demonstrate that parishioners were healthier than the poor.

Yet these skeletons put life expectancy at birth (e^0) at just twenty-one years.[119] Readers may recall from earlier chapters that this number typified rather than exceeded e^0 before roughly 1900. For example, only about one-quarter of Neanderthals and contemporary modern humans reached age forty, and British chemist Walter Bruno Gratzer (b. 1932) asserted that few surpassed twenty during prehistory.[120] Ancient Egyptians lived on average between nineteen and twenty-five years.[121] In the Middle Ages, forty years marked life's end.[122] French anthropologist and paleontologist Henri Victor Vallois (1889–1981) summarized humanity's frailty, lamenting that "few individuals passed forty years, and it is only quite exceptionally that any passed fifty."[123] Indigenous, African, and European skeletons in the Americas revealed that before the twentieth century, few surpassed age forty-five.[124] Between Neanderthal prehistory and 1900, e^0 seldom departed over five years either way of twenty-five years, and half of all children died before puberty.[125]

Moreover, St. Thomas' mortality was highest in life's first year, a pattern Canadian anthropologist Shelley Rae Saunders (1950–2008) and colleagues attributed to undernutrition and diseases.[126] The fact that almost three-fifths of skeletons had enamel hypoplasia confirmed undernutrition.[127] Infant mortality rose over time, reaching 143 deaths per 1,000 births between 1856 and 1875.[128] This trend correlated with Belleville's population expansion. As the town grew crowded, contagion spread more readily, especially because officials were slow to institute public health measures that are basic today. For example, in the mid-1870s, Belleville's drinking water harbored the cholera bacterium *Vibrio cholerae* because sewage polluted the water.[129] Poor hygiene brought typhus from lice (*Pediculus humanus capitis*, *Pediculus humanus corporis*, and *Pthirus pubis*) and fleas (*Pulex irritans*). Inadequate sanitation and hygiene were unsurprising in an era when the Germ Theory of Disease was novel enough to encounter resistance and disbelief.

Although diseases truncated life, Saunders and coauthors, as noted, also implicated diets. Early in Belleville's history, sucrose and white flour were "very important".[130] The next chapter discusses white flour's unwholesomeness. This section notes that these junk foods—mentioned as common among the English—made Belleville's middle and upper classes sicker than mid-nineteenth-century occupants of the Monroe County Alms House in Rochester, New York.[131] Crowding and the poorhouse's dismal sanitation and hygiene implied that diseases killed Rochester's poor as surely as Belleville's affluent. American anthropologist Rosanne L. Higgins and coworkers described the almshouse as less humane than prison around 1850.[132] Harsh conditions deterred the poor from seeking entrance and economized expenses.

These circumstances implied that poorhouse moldy bread and coffee were more nourishing than sucrose, white flour, and the other items on Belleville plates: meat, corn porridge, and fruits and vegetables when available.[133] Saunders and coauthors did not specify how often fruits and vegetables were eaten, but they must have been infrequent given the characterization of early-nineteenth-century Canadian diets as fatty and starchy.[134] Chapter 4 argued that meat caused heart disease among Egypt's inert elites. Saunders and her team did not discuss lifestyle, but comparison between Belleville and Egypt may be apt because both featured affluent people who could evade labor by hiring the poor. The previous chapter examined fat. Chapter 12 documents corn's shortcomings in prehistory and history. Although the poorhouse cannot be lauded for serving deteriorating bread, the impetus to save money must have led officials to favor whole grain over white bread. Because wheat was most expensive, almshouse bread was likely barley, rye, or their combination. The next chapter corroborates the axiom that whole grains are more nutritious than white flour, thereby furthering the argument that Rochester's poor were healthier than Belleville's affluent.

A third line of evidence against sucrose came from England rather than its colonies. Hardship during the first half of the nineteenth century forced commoners to economize. Among the first items to go was sucrose; its per person consumption fell over one-third between 1801 and 1821, Table 11.2 reveals.[135] Gradual decrease followed so that by 1840 the average Brit halved sucrose intake.[136]

TABLE 11.2
Average Annual Sucrose Intake (kg) per Englishman 1801, 1811, 1821, and 1830–1840

Year	Per Englishman Intake (kg)
1801	13.9
1811	13.3
1821	8.7
1830	9
1831	9.1
1832	8.6
1833	8.2
1834	8.3
1835	8.7
1836	7.5
1837	8.3
1838	8.3
1839	7.8
1840	6.9

This decline occurred amid an apparently favorable interlude given increase in heights between roughly 1751 and 1826 as measured by British military records.[137] The first two-thirds of the gain preceded sucrose diminution—eliminating it as a factor—though the decrease may have enhanced health as reflected by stature increase during the first quarter of the nineteenth century.

Besides the trend in heights, Table 11.3 reports that e^0 rose from 35.9 to 39.2 years between 1801 and 1821, the decades of swift reduction in sucrose intake.[138] E^0's expansion in the first two decades of the nineteenth century contrasted with the past's stasis. Between 1541 and 1641, for example, England's e^0 held nearly constant, diminishing from 33.8 to 33.7 years.[139] By 1741, e^0 had slumped to 31.7 years. The next century, however, witnessed improvement to an e^0 of 40.3 years in 1841.

Most of this enlargement happened by 1821, when e^0 registered 39.2 years after twenty years' decrease in sucrose intake, as mentioned. Between roughly 1826 and 1876, e^0 plateaued and military recruits were shorter.[140] This reversal coincided with worsening poverty and widespread hunger during the 1830s and 1840s.[141] Following sucrose's decline, mentioned above, consumption rebounded after 1845.[142] Ingestion of these empty calories correlated with the last thirty years of soldiers' diminishing heights.

TABLE 11.3
E^0 in England 1541, 1641, and 1741–1871 in 5-yr Increments

Year	E^0 (yr)
1541	33.8
1641	33.7
1741	31.7
1746	35.3
1751	36.6
1756	37.3
1761	34.2
1766	35
1771	35.6
1776	38.2
1781	34.7
1786	35.9
1791	37.3
1796	36.8
1801	35.9
1806	38.7
1811	37.6
1816	37.9
1821	39.2
1826	39.9
1831	40.8
1836	40.2
1841	40.3
1846	39.6
1851	39.5
1856	40.4
1861	41.2
1866	40.3
1871	41.3

United Kingdom pharmacologist Paul Clayton and historian Judith D. Rowbotham (b. 1952), both introduced in Chapter 1, argued that British health worsened after 1870 because consumption of fatty, salty meat, canned fruit, and sucrose increased.[143] These authors faulted canned fruit for its sugary syrup. Thereafter the "decline was astonishingly rapid."[144] By 1900, the army rejected half of recruits as underfed, causing authorities to fear that commoners were too feeble to defend the nation.

11.3 HIGH FRUCTOSE CORN SYRUP (HFCS)

11.3.1 Origins

Chapter 12 remarks that corn was an American staple millennia before Columbus encountered it on Hispaniola or Cuba in October or November 1492.[145] Europeans amplified its importance, feeding it to pigs (*Sus scrofa domesticus*) and cattle and distilling it into whiskey in the first centuries after settlement. As hectarage and production increased, scientists sought new uses for the grass. Ethanol (C_2H_5OH) as automobile fuel is a familiar example. In *The Story of Corn* (1992), American author and historian Betty Harper Fussell (b. 1927) mentioned fifty-six additional products from corn.[146]

Among her items were sweeteners, a redundancy in the United States given sucrose extraction from sugarcane grown in Florida, Hawaii, Texas, and Louisiana and from sugar beet cultivated in Michigan, Minnesota, North Dakota, Colorado, Montana, Nebraska, Wyoming, California, Idaho, Oregon, and Washington. Other sources of sweetness come from maple syrup made in Vermont, New York, Maine, Wisconsin, New Hampshire, Maine, Pennsylvania, Ohio, Connecticut, Michigan, and Massachusetts and from honey produced in North Dakota, South Dakota, Florida, Montana, California, and several other states.

With most of its carbohydrates as starch—defined and discussed in Chapter 2—corn was not an obvious raw material for sweetness. Fussell asserted that the Molasses Act of 1733 spurred interest in corn's use as a sweetener.[147] That year Parliament began to tax molasses imported into its colonies from outside them to force its purchase from the British Caribbean. Because this tax raised molasses' price, Americans sought a cheaper alternative.

Beyond colonialism's internal dynamics, attention on corn is best understood as part of a broad search for temperate plants that yielded sucrose in sizable quantities and that might, therefore, free Europe and British North America from dependence on tropical sugarcane. In 1747, German chemist Andreas Marggraf (1709–1782) moved toward this goal by isolating sucrose from the roots of two *Beta* species and in skirret (*Sium sisarum*), a perennial eaten as a famine food.[148] This discovery stimulated research that would culminate in sucrose's extraction from sugar beet.

Demonstration that these plants were sources of sweetness intensified the quest for others during the Napoleonic Wars (1803–1815), when England's navy blockaded France.[149] Unable to import sucrose from the tropics, temperate France wanted its own sweeteners. Napoleon offered 100,000 francs for discovery of a new sweetener. The prize motivated Russian chemist Gottlieb Sigismund Constantin Kirchhoff (1764–1833) in 1811 to derive glucose from potato starch by treating it with hydrochloric acid (HCl).[150]

This method worked on other starchy plants, for example, yielding corn syrup from corn. After the Civil War (1861–1865), American businesses led by New York's Union Sugar Company began experimenting with enzymes and acids to derive the most sweetness from cornstarch at least cost.[151] The goal of potency required more than glucose, which tastes less sweet than fructose or sucrose. Because the sweetest of the three is fructose, chemists aimed to convert cornstarch's glucose into fructose. In 1967, Clinton, Iowa's Clinton Corn Processing Company converted 14 percent of glucose into fructose by treating it with the enzyme xylose isomerase.[152] Although manufacturers may derive HFCS with up to 90 percent fructose, the product is typically 55 percent fructose and 45 percent glucose.[153]

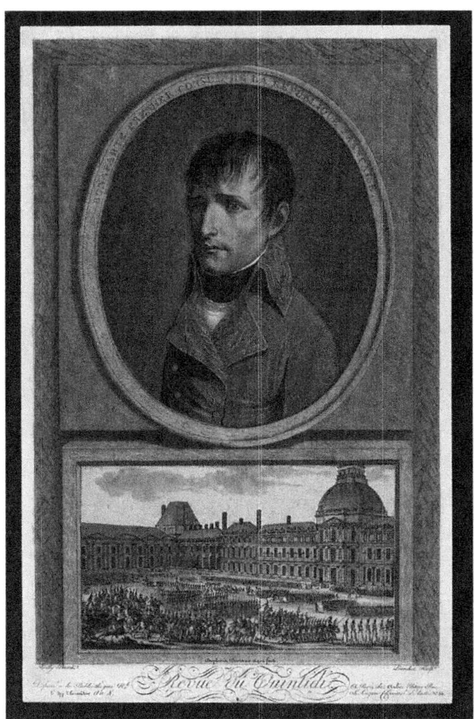

FIGURE 11.4 Napoleon Bonaparte. (Photo courtesy of Library of Congress. https://www.loc.gov/pictures/item/2007685781/.)

Being about half glucose and half fructose, the new product, HFCS, resembled honey in chemical composition. Produced from corn, which the United States raised in abundance, HFCS became a mass commodity able to undercut sucrose prices. Manufacturers favored HFCS—which sweetened beverages, baked goods, ice cream and other frozen desserts, salad dressing, mayonnaise, ketchup, pickles, and innumerable kindred processed items—wherever sweetness and inexpensiveness were the only criteria. Sucrose retained a place in the food industry wherever consumers desired its crystalline appearance. Nonetheless, competition from the new sweetener led candy and chocolate makers, which had relied on sucrose, to invest in HFCS.

11.3.2 Competition between HFCS and Sucrose

An early adopter, Coca-Cola announced in 1974 that Sprite, Mr. Pibb, and Fanta were 25 percent HFCS by mass.[154] Royal Crown Cola and Canada Dry publicized similar figures. By 1983, Pepsi was half, and the next year Coca-Cola was three-quarters, HFCS. The sweetener invisible in beverages, consumers engorged themselves on hidden calories as consumption per American leapt from an average of 1.8 kilograms (4 pounds) in 1974 to 30.4 kilograms (67.1 pounds) in 1987.[155] Per American average intake declined to 18 kilograms (39.8 pounds) in 2017.[156]

11.3.3 Concerns about HFCS as Cause of Overweight and Obesity

HFCS is too new to evaluate its health effects in history, though its relationship to overweight and obesity merits commentary. The increase in consumption between 1974 and 1987 overlapped the obesity epidemic's core years as envisioned by William Davis, Michael Pollan, and Gary Taubes, whose chronologies an earlier section mentioned. Support for their conception of obesity as a phenomenon

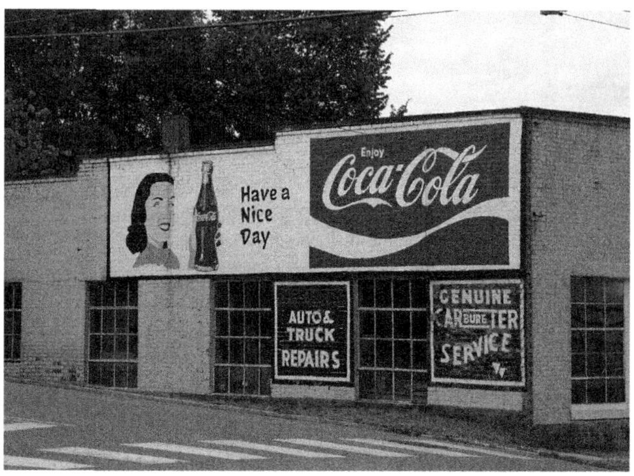

FIGURE 11.5 Coca-Cola sign. (Photo courtesy of Library of Congress. https://www.loc.gov/pictures/item/2017880268/.)

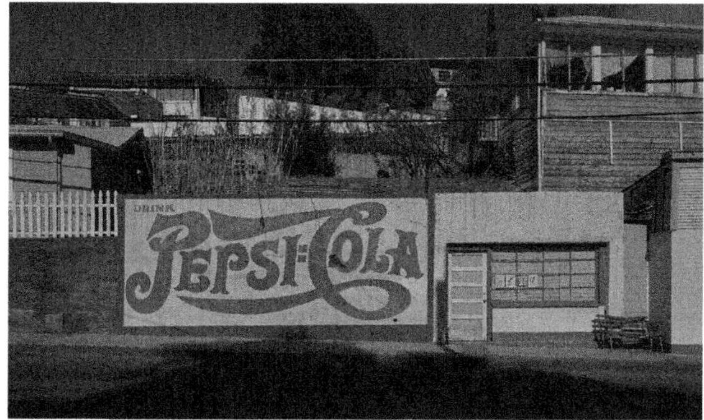

FIGURE 11.6 Pepsi sign. (Photo courtesy of Library of Congress. https://www.loc.gov/pictures/item/2018663397/.)

of roughly the last half century came from the U.S. National Health and Nutrition Examination survey, which recorded an 8 percent increase in the proportion of overweight adults between the mid-1970s and 1991.[157] Although this book argues that the automobile and concomitant inactivity best explain twentieth-century increases in overweight and obesity, the gargantuan rise in HFCS intake benefits only the corporations that market it.

Translation of HFCS consumption into calories concretizes its dangers to developed nations' inert inhabitants. One and eight-tenths kilograms of HFCS per American in 1974 yielded 4.9 grams (0.01 pounds) daily. The USDA counts 2.8 calories in 1 gram of HFCS or 13.7 calories in a day's 4.9 grams.[158] This amount ballooned to 160.3 grams in 1987, adding 448.8 calories to the day's rations. A consumer who ingests an extra 448.8 calories daily without increasing activity will gain 1 kilogram (2.2 pounds) of fat roughly every seventeenth day or 21.5 kilograms (47.3 pounds) in one year.

These calculations justify Davis, Pollan, and Taubes' concerns over expanding waistlines during recent decades. Summarizing this trend, American internist and endocrinologist George A. Bray (b. 1931), American nutritional epidemiologist Samara Joy Nielsen, and American food scientist Barry Michael Popkin (b. 1944) wrote that "The increased use of HFCS in the United States mirrors the rapid increase in obesity."[159]

11.3.4 Concerns about Many Causes of Overweight and Obesity besides HFCS

Although this correlation is obvious, causation is hard to prove. Part of the problem is that Americans have been eating more of many items, not just HFCS, during the past half century. For example, between 1982 and 1994 U.S. aggregate consumption of olive oil leapt from 29 million kilograms (64 million pounds) to 113.3 million kilograms (250 million pounds).[160] Not only is this jump large, but chapter 10 demonstrated that olive oil is among the most caloric foods, with 884 calories compared to 387 and 281 calories in sucrose and HFCS, respectively, per 100 grams.[161] All else equal, calorie counting's arithmetic dictates that olive oil enlarges girth more than pure carbohydrates.

The issue of blame aside, Davis, Pollan, Taubes, Bray, Nielsen, and Popkin are understandably worried about overweight and obesity. But restriction of treatment to the United States does not pinpoint HFCS as a cause of these ills. The previous chapter noted the popularity of salads among dieters. Yet consumers, many of them women, cover low-calorie lettuce (*Lactuca sativa*) and other vegetables with fattening dressing. Consequently, American women are twice as obese as men.[162] American anthropologist Leslie Sue Lieberman criticized this situation while noting salad bars' ubiquity in the United States.[163]

This prevalence does not exonerate HFCS, which American historian of science and technology Deborah Jean Warner identified as a salad dressing ingredient.[164] Even with HFCS, the USDA reports that fat supplies 97.4 percent of ranch dressing's calories.[165] Fat furnishes 68.4 percent of calories in low-calorie blue or Roquefort cheese dressing.[166] Examples need not be multiplied to demonstrate that fat provides most calories in salad dressings. Unfortunately for consumers, and as stated, fat intake better predicts obesity than sucrose consumption.[167] This finding should apply to HFCS, which has fewer calories per gram than sucrose or fat.

11.3.5 HFCS, Overweight, and Obesity in the Netherlands

The Netherlands illuminates these matters. Its 1960s' youth culture rejected Europe's post-World War II austerity. The desire for pleasure and indulgence quadrupled wine consumption and more than doubled soft drink and beer intake between 1965 and 1990.[168] Emulating the United States, the Dutch adopted hamburgers, French fries, and kindred fast foods. Processed and convenience items became popular between and during meals. Previous paragraphs mentioned HFCS's presence in such fare and soft drinks. Wine and beer had it if added after fermentation, though addition beforehand was irrelevant because yeast (*Saccharomyces cerevisiae*) converted it to alcohol.

Alcohol aside, since the 1960s Netherlands' HFCS consumption rose while causing less overweight and obesity than elsewhere in Europe. Data from 1994, in Tables 11.4 and 11.5, ranked Dutch overweight and obesity the continent's lowest.[169] These statistics rated 5 percent of Dutchmen and 10 percent of women between fifty and sixty-four years overweight; 4.2 percent of men and 5 percent of women aged thirty-five to forty-nine were obese. In 2017, 52 percent of Dutchmen and 45 percent of women were overweight.[170] Thirteen percent of men and 15 percent of women were obese.

Dutch nutritionist Fred J. P. H. Brouns (b. 1950) stated in 2018 that his compatriots were too heavy, though the Netherlands compared favorably with the United States.[171] In 2017, the U.S. Centers for Disease Control and Prevention (CDC) in Atlanta, Georgia, classified 40.8 percent of men and 44.7 percent of women between ages forty and fifty-nine obese.[172] Obesity neared 50 percent among Hispanics and African Americans.

HFCS alone has not caused these problems, else the Dutch should approximate Americans because consumption increased among both as the Netherlands mimicked U.S. habits. The two differ in activity given that "the Dutch move a lot," remarked Brouns.[173] They cycle and walk whereas this book emphasizes Americans' automobile addiction. The Dutch average 2.5 kilometers (1.5 miles) daily by bicycle, the most in Europe.[174] By contrast, under one-third of Americans rode a bicycle even once in 2014.[175] The Netherlands demonstrates that health requires activity, a message throughout this book.

TABLE 11.4
Global Overweight (%) in 1980s and 1990s

Population	Age (yr)	Male (%)	Female (%)
US overall	20–74	31	35
US White	20–74	32	34
African American	20–74	31	49
Mexican American	20–74	36	47
US Seminole	Adult	>50	>50
US Pima	Adult	>50	>50
US Zuni	Adult	29–35	55–66
Canada overall	25–64	9	8
Canada Cree, Ojibwa	Adult	45–54	>90
Micronesia	Adult	85	93
Polynesia	Adult	48	79
Melanesia	Adult	31	65
Asia	Adult	12	36
Hawaii, Indigene	Adult	85	52
England	18–84	13	15
Italy	45–64	10	11
Finland	50–59	12	30
Netherlands	50–64	5	10
Australia	25–64	7	9
South Africa	15–84	15	18
Costa Rica	40–45	8	14
El Salvador	40–45	0	2
Guatemala	40–45	0	6
Nicaragua	40–45	3	16
Panama	40–45	2	2
Honduras	40–45	3	6

11.3.6 HFCS, Overweight, and Obesity among Native Peoples

Concentration on Americans and Europeans should not deflect attention from indigenes. By 2000, over half U.S. Seminole and Pima men and women were overweight, indicated Table 11.4.[176] In the American Southwest, nearly two-thirds of Zuni women and roughly one-third of men were overweight. Over 45 percent of Canadian Cree and Ojibwa men and above 90 percent of women were overweight. Eighty-five percent of native Hawaiian men and 52 percent of women were overweight. Roughly half Samoan men and women were obese, noted Table 11.5.[177]

Northwest of Samoa is Micronesia, where 93 percent of women and 85 percent of men were overweight by 2000, stated Table 11.4.[178] Georgetown University's Center for Strategic and International Studies (CSIS) faulted U.S. corporations for inundating the islands with "many processed junk foods."[179] The center decried turkey tails, which Americans eschewed because of their fattiness, but which were sold to Micronesians. Among processed foods, CSIS mentioned ramen noodles and packaged beverages. Although CSIS did not mention corn syrup or HFCS, Maruchan ramen noodles have "corn syrup solids," and corn syrup or HFCS pervades junk foods.[180] The center also implicated inactivity in Micronesian obesity.[181] Another factor is the connection between size and status in traditional Pacific societies.[182] Along similar lines, some islanders find girth attractive. These elements suggest that HFCS alone has not made Micronesians fat. More generally, this book affirms the consensus that overweight and obesity have many causes, not all dietary.

TABLE 11.5
Global Obesity (%) in 1980s and 1990s

Population	Age (yr)	Male (%)	Female (%)
US White	40–49	14.8	16.4
African American	40–49	23.1	33
US Hispanic	40–49	18.5	38.7
US Pima	35–44	64	75
Canada	35–44	12	16
France	16–84	7	8
Sweden	15–44	4.8	3.9
Italy	45–64	9.9	11.1
Netherlands	35–49	4.2	5
United Kingdom	35–49	7.9	8.6
Germany	25–69	16	16
Costa Rica	40–45	5.7	14.4
El Salvador	40–45	0	1.5
Guatemala	40–45	0	5.6
Honduras	40–45	2.8	6
Australia	25–64	8.6	13.3
South Africa	35–44	14.3	15.6
Solomon Islands	35–54	19	43
Samoa	45–54	45	55
India	15–76	6.2	10.7
Thailand	>30	11.1	11.1

NOTES

1 Lucy M. Long, *Honey: A Global History* (London: Reaktion Books, 2017), 15.
2 Ibid.; Maguelonne Toussaint-Samat, *A History of Food*, expanded ed., trans. Anthea Bell (Chichester, UK: Wiley-Blackwell, 2009), 14.
3 Long, 9; Frank Whittemore, "How Many Calories in a Teaspoon of Honey?" *Livestrong*, accessed June 7, 2019, https://www.livestrong.com/article/307017-how-many-calories-in-a-teaspoon-of-honey.
4 Serge Bahuchet, "Aka Pygmies," in *The Cambridge Encyclopedia of Hunters and Gatherers*, ed. Richard B. Lee and Richard Daly (Cambridge, UK: Cambridge University Press, 2004), 191; Corinne A. Kratz, "The Okiek of Kenya," in *The Cambridge Encyclopedia of Hunters and Gatherers*, ed. Richard B. Lee and Richard Daly (Cambridge, UK: Cambridge University Press, 2004), 221; Nurit Bird-David, "Introduction: South Asia," in *The Cambridge Encyclopedia of Hunters and Gatherers*, ed. Richard B. Lee and Richard Daly (Cambridge, UK: Cambridge University Press, 2004), 232; James F. Eder, "The Batak of Palawan Island, the Philippines," in *The Cambridge Encyclopedia of Hunters and Gatherers*, ed. Richard B. Lee and Richard Daly (Cambridge, UK: Cambridge University Press, 2004), 294; Kim Hill and A. Magdalena Hurtado, "The Ache of Paraguay," in *The Cambridge Encyclopedia of Hunters and Gatherers*, ed. Richard B. Lee and Richard Daly (Cambridge, UK: Cambridge University Press, 2004), 93–94.
5 Toussaint-Samat, 15.
6 Long, 17–18.
7 Ibid., 16; Henry Hobhouse, *Seeds of Change: Six Plants That Transformed Mankind* (New York: Shoemaker and Hoard, 2005), 54.
8 Toussaint-Samat, 27.
9 Naomi F. Miller and Wilma Wetterstrom, "The Beginnings of Agriculture: The Ancient near East and North Africa," in *The Cambridge World History of Food*, ed. Kenneth F. Kiple and Kriemhild Conee Ornelas, vol. 2 (Cambridge, UK: Cambridge University Press, 2000), 1135.
10 David Braund, "Food among Greeks of the Black Sea: The Challenging Diet of Olbia," in *A Companion to Food in the Ancient World*, ed. John Wilkins and Robin Nadeau (Malden, MA: Wiley Blackwell, 2015), 297.

11 Karen Rhea Nemet-Nejat, *Daily Life in Ancient Mesopotamia* (Westport, CT and London: Greenwood Press, 1998), 160.
12 Long, 60.
13 Toussaint-Samat, 24.
14 Hobhouse, 55.
15 Long, 24–25.
16 Hobhouse, 55; Long, 79.
17 Hobhouse, 55.
18 Toussaint-Samat, 26.
19 Long, 66–67.
20 Ibid., 62–63.
21 Abdulwahid Ajibola, Joseph P. Chamunorwa, and Kennedy H. Erlwanger, "Nutraceutical Values of Natural Honey and Its Contribution to Health and Wealth," *Nutrition and Metabolism* 9 (June 20, 2012), https://www.ncbi.nlm.nih.gov/pmc/articles/PMC3583289.
22 Andrew F. Smith, *Peanuts: The Illustrious History of the Goober Pea* (Urbana and Chicago: University of Illinois Press, 2002), 72.
23 "Molasses," April 1, 2019, accessed February 13, 2020, https://fdc.nal.usda.gov/fdc-app.html#/food-details/168820/nutrients; "FDA Vitamins and Minerals Chart," *FDA*, April 24, 2019, https://www.accessdata.fda.gov/scripts/interactivenutritionfactslabel/factsheets/vitamin_and_mineral_chart.pdf.
24 Hill and Hurtado, 93.
25 Ibid.
26 Stephen Le, *100 Million Years of Food: What Our Ancestors Ate and Why It Matters Today* (New York: Picador, 2016), 4.
27 Martin Pitts, "'Celtic' Food: Perspectives from Britain," in *A Companion to Food in the Ancient World*, ed. John Wilkins and Robin Nadeau (Malden, MA: Wiley Blackwell, 2015), 329.
28 Peter Garnsey, *Food and Society in Classical Antiquity* (Cambridge, UK: Cambridge University Press, 1999), 52; Bernard Harris, "Height and Nutrition," in *The Cambridge World History of Food*, vol. 2, ed. Kenneth F. Kiple and Kriemhild Conee Ornelas (Cambridge, UK: Cambridge University Press, 2000), 1427.
29 Joseph M. Prince and Richard H. Steckel, *Tallest in the World: Native Americans of the Great Plains in the Nineteenth Century* (Cambridge, MA: National Bureau of Economic Research, 1998), 1.
30 Joanne Marie, "Foods Containing Sucrose," *Livestrong*, accessed May 21, 2019, https://www.livestrong.com/article/142823-foods-containing-sucrose; "Mangos, Raw," *USDA FoodData Central*, accessed June 8, 2020, , https://fdc.nal.usda.gov/fdc-app.html#/food-details/169910/nutrients.
31 Marie.
32 Andrew F. Smith, *Sugar: A Global History* (London: Reaktion Books, 2015), 7.
33 Hattie Ellis, *Sweetness and Light: The Mysterious History of the Honeybee* (New York: Harmony Books, 2004), 36.
34 Robert William Fogel, "Nutrition and the Decline in Mortality Since 1700: Some Preliminary Findings," in *Long-Term Factors in American Economic Growth*, ed. Stanley L. Engerman and Robert E. Gallman (Chicago and London: University of Chicago Press, 1986), 471–472.
35 Hobhouse, 54; J. G. Vaughan and C. Geissler, *The New Oxford Book of Food Plants* (Oxford: Oxford University Press, 1997), 16.
36 J. E. Bowen and D. L. Anderson, "Sugar-Cane Cropping Systems," in *Field Crop Ecosystems*, ed. C. J. Pearson (Amsterdam: Elsevier, 1992), 156; Philippus D. R. van Heerden, Gillian Eggleston, and Robin A. Donaldson, "Ripening and Postharvest Deterioration," in *Sugarcane: Physiology, Biochemistry, and Functional Biology*, ed. Paul H. Moore and Frederik C. Botha (Ames, IA: Wiley Blackwell, 2014), 58–59.
37 Deborah Jean Warner, *Sweet Stuff: An American History of Sweeteners from Sugar to Sucralose* (Washington, DC: Smithsonian Institution Scholarly Press, 2011), 5.
38 Bowen and Anderson, 144; Paul H. Moore, Andrew H. Paterson, and Thomas Tew, "Sugarcane: The Crop, the Plant, and Domestication," in *Sugarcane: Physiology, Biochemistry, and Functional Biology*, ed. Paul H. Moore and Frederik C. Botha (Ames, IA: Wiley Blackwell, 2014), 1.
39 Hobhouse, 54.
40 Bill Laws, *Fifty Plants that Changed the Course of History* (Buffalo, NY and Richmond Hill, Ontario: Firefly Books, 2015), 166.
41 Matthew Parker, *The Sugar Barons: Family, Corruption, Empire, and War in the West Indies* (New York: Walker, 2011), 10.

42 Jeffrey M. Pilcher, *Food in World History* (New York and London: Routledge, 2006), 31.
43 J. H. Galloway, "Sugar," in *The Cambridge World History of Food*, vol. 1, ed. Kenneth F. Kiple and Kriemhild Conee Ornelas (Cambridge, UK: Cambridge University Press, 2000), 443.
44 Hobhouse, 56.
45 Beryl Brintnall Simpson and Molly Conner Ogorzaly, *Economic Botany: Plants in Our World*, 3rd ed. (Boston: Houghton Mifflin, 2001), 188.
46 Hobhouse, 56.
47 Ibid., 54; Warner, 5.
48 Parker, 11.
49 U.S. Const. amend. XIII.
50 Hobhouse, 53.
51 Ibid.; Diane Rellinger, "How to Convert Grams of Sugar into Teaspoons," Michigan State University, January 2, 2013, accessed May 22, 2019, https://www.canr.msu.edu/news/how_to_convert_grams_of_sugars_into_teaspoons
52 Hobhouse, 53.
53 Richard H. Steckel, *Health and Nutrition in the Preindustrial Era: Insights from a Millennium of Average Heights in Northern Europe* (Cambridge, MA: National Bureau of Economic Research, 2001), i, 18.
54 Hobhouse, 55.
55 "Sugarcane," in *The Cambridge World History of Food*, vol. 2, ed. Kenneth F. Kiple and Kriemhild Conee Ornelas (Cambridge, UK: Cambridge University Press, 2000), 1860.
56 Hobhouse, 59.
57 Laws, 166.
58 Pilcher, 31–32.
59 Hobhouse, 59.
60 Gretel H. Pelto and Pertti J. Pelto, "Diet and Delocalization: Dietary Changes since 1750," *Journal of Interdisciplinary History* 14, no. 2 (Autumn 1983): 516.
61 "The Sugar Timeline," *Hippocrates Health Institute*, September 9, 2016, accessed May 26, 2019, https://hippocratesinst.org/the-sugar-timeline.
62 "Sugar Consumption in the U.S. Diet between 1822 and 2005," accessed January 12, 2020, http://onlinestatbook.com/2/case_studies/sugar.html.
63 Rachel K. Johnson, Lawrence J. Appel, Michael Brands, Barbara V. Howard, Michael Lefevre, Robert H. Lustig, Frank Sacks, Lyn M. Steffen, and Judith Wylie-Rosett, "Dietary Sugar Intake and Cardiovascular Health," *Circulation* 120, no. 11 (September 15, 2009), https://www.ahajournals.org/doi/10.1161/CIRCULATIONAHA.109.192627.
64 Ibid.; "Sugar Consumption in the U.S. Diet between 1822 and 2005."
65 Pelto and Pelto, 516; "More Sugar!—The Causes of the Rise in British Sugar Consumption," *Chocolate Class*, March 11, 2019, accessed January 31, 2020, https://chocolateclass.wordpress.com/2019/03/11/more-sugar-the-causes-of-the-rise-in-british-sugar-consumption.
66 Smith, 135.
67 Michael Pollan, *The Omnivore's Dilemma: A Natural History of Four Meals* (New York: Penguin Books, 2016), 102; Michael Pollan, *In Defense of Food: An Eater's Manifesto* (New York: Penguin Books, 2009), 50, 185–186; Gary Taubes, *Good Calories, Bad Calories: Challenging the Conventional Wisdom on Diet, Weight Control, and Disease* (New York: Knopf, 2008), xviii.
68 Robert C. Atkins, *Dr. Atkins' Diet Revolution: The High Calorie Way to Stay Thin Forever* (New York: David McKay, 1972), 264.
69 Milicent L. Hathaway, "Trends in Heights and Weights," *Yearbook of Agriculture, 1959*, ed. Alfred Stefferud (Washington, DC: GPO), 181–185, ps://naldc.nal.usda.gov/download/IND43861419/PDF.
70 Leslie Sue Lieberman, "Obesity," in *The Cambridge World History of Food*, ed. Kenneth F. Kiple and Kriemhild Conee Ornelas, vol. 1 (Cambridge, UK: Cambridge University Press, 2000), 1066.
71 Ibid.
72 Galloway, 437.
73 "Obesity Update 2017," OECD, accessed July 5, 2019, https://www.oecd.org/els/health-systems/Obesity-Update-2017.pdf, 3.
74 Galloway, 437; "Obesity Update 2017," 3.
75 Galloway, 437; J. J. Nieves, "Cuba: An Overweight Country," *Havana Times*, May 6, 2015, accessed July 5, 2019, https://havanatimes.org/features/cuba-an-overweight-country.
76 Mark J. Messina, "Soyfoods: Their Role in Disease Prevention and Treatment," in *Soybeans: Chemistry, Technology, and Utilization*, KeShun Liu (New York: Chapman and Hall, 1997), 442.

77 Jim Mann and Rachael McLean, "Cardiovascular Diseases," in *Essentials of Human Nutrition*, ed. Jim Mann and A. Stewart Truswell, 5th ed. (Oxford: Oxford University Press, 2017), 382.
78 Fogel, 465–466.
79 Ibid., 465.
80 Ibid., 495.
81 Jeremy Atack and Peter Passell, *A New Economic View of American History: From Colonial Times to 1940*, 2nd ed. (New York and London: Norton, 1994), 213.
82 Ibid., 239; Fogel, 502–503.
83 Atack and Passell, 179.
84 John P. McKay, Bennett D. Hill, John Buckler, Clare Haru Crowston, Merry E. Wiesner-Hanks, and Joe Perry, *Understanding Western Society: A Brief History* (Boston and New York: Bedford/St. Martin's, 2012), 622.
85 Fogel, 497.
86 Ibid., 498.
87 "Minute Maid Premium Orange Juice," McDonald's Nutrition Calculator, 2017–2019, accessed May 22, 2019, https://www.mcdonalds.com/us/en-us/about-our-food/nutrition-calculator.html.
88 Ibid.; "Orange Juice, Raw (Includes Foods for USDA's Food Distribution Program)," April 1, 2019, accessed February 13, 2020, https://fdc.nal.usda.gov/fdc-app.html#/food-details/169098/nutrients.
89 "FAQs: 100% OJ and Sugar," Florida Department of Citrus, accessed May 22, 2019, https://www.floridacitrus.org/newsroom/citrus-411/100-juice-and-sugar/faqs-100-oj-and-sugar.
90 David Perlmutter, "The #1 Reason to Avoid Orange Juice," accessed May 22, 2019, https://www.drperlmutter.com/avoid-orange-juice.
91 "Taisun, Sugarcane Juice," April 1, 2019, accessed February 13, 2020, https://fdc.nal.usda.gov/fdc-app.html#/food-details/500321/nutrients.
92 "Ten Health Benefits of Sugarcane Juice," *The Daily Observer*, September 28, 2015, accessed May 22, 2019, https://antiguaobserver.com/ten-health-benefits-of-sugarcane-juice.
93 Kenneth F. Kiple and Virginia H. Kiple, "Deficiency Diseases in the Caribbean," in *Caribbean Slavery in the Atlantic World: A Student Reader*, ed. Verene A. Shepherd and Hilary McD. Beckles (Princeton, NJ: Markus Wiener Publishers, 2000), 790.
94 Taubes, *Good Calories, Bad Calories*, ix.
95 Richard S. Dunn, *Sugar and Slaves: The Rise of the Planter Class in the English West Indies, 1624–1713* (Chapel Hill: University of North Carolina Press, 1972), 246.
96 Thomas Hawkes Tanner, *The Practice of Medicine*, 5th ed. (Philadelphia: Lindsay and Blakiston, 1866), 142–143; Taubes, Good Calories, Bad Calories, ix.
97 Johannes Postma, *The Atlantic Slave Trade* (Westport, CT and London: Greenwood Press, 2003), xx.
98 Dunn, 324.
99 Ibid., 242.
100 Ibid., 244.
101 Ibid., 320.
102 Linda Civitello, *Cuisine and Culture: A History of Food and People*, 3rd ed. (Hoboken, NJ: Wiley, 2011), 134–135.
103 Postma, 31.
104 Dunn, 301.
105 Civitello, 135.
106 Jerome S. Handler and Robert S. Corruccini, "Plantation Slave Life in Barbados: A Physical Anthropological Analysis," *Journal of Interdisciplinary History* 14, no. 1 (Summer 1983): 75.
107 Ibid., 74.
108 Ibid., 79.
109 Dunn, 301–302.
110 Handler and Corruccini, 77; Kiple and Kiple, 789; Margaret J. Weinberger, "Pica," in *The Cambridge World History of Food*, vol. 1, ed. Kenneth F. Kiple and Kriemhild Conee Ornelas (Cambridge, UK: Cambridge University Press, 2000), 969, 971.
111 Weinberger, 969–970.
112 Ibid., 969; Kiple and Kiple, 789.
113 Kiple and Kiple, 789.
114 Ibid., 790.
115 Ibid., 791.

116 Shelley R. Saunders, Ann Herring, Larry Sawchuk, Gerry Boyce, Rob Hoppa, and Susan Klepp, "The Health of the Middle Class: The St. Thomas' Anglican Church Cemetery Project," in *The Backbone of History: Health and Nutrition in the Western Hemisphere* (Cambridge, UK: Cambridge University Press, 2002), 139–140.
117 Ibid., 130.
118 Peter Dizikes, "New Study Shows Rich, Poor Have Huge Mortality Gap in U.S." MIT News, April 11, 2016, accessed February 13, 2020, http://news.mit.edu/2016/study-rich-poor-huge-mortality-gap-us-0411.
119 Saunders, Herring, Sawchuk, Boyce, Hoppa, and Klepp, 146.
120 Sindya N. Bhanoo, "Life Span of Early Man Same as Neanderthals'," *New York Times*, January 10, 2011, accessed January 18, 2019, https://www.nytimes.com/2011/01/11/science/11obneanderthal.html; Walter Gratzer, *Terrors of the Table: The Curious History of Nutrition* (Oxford: Oxford University Press, 2005), 44.
121 Ann E. M. Liljas, "Old Age in Ancient Egypt," March 2, 2015, accessed January 18, 2019, https://blogs.ucl.ac.uk/researchers-in-museums/2015/03/02/old-age-in-ancient-egypt; Roger S. Bagnall and Bruce W. Frier, The Demography of Roman Egypt (Cambridge, UK and New York: Cambridge University Press, 2006), 109.
122 McKay, Hill, Buckler, Crowston, Wiesner-Hanks, and Perry, 212.
123 Henri V. Vallois, "The Social Life of Early Man: The Evidence of Skeletons," in *Social Life of Early Man*, ed. Sherwood L. Washburn (Chicago: Aldine, 1961), 222.
124 Richard H. Steckel and Jerome C. Rose, "Introduction," in *The Backbone of History: Health and Nutrition in the Western Hemisphere*, ed. Richard H. Steckel and Jerome C. Rose (Cambridge, UK: Cambridge University Press, 2002), 6; Richard H. Steckel, Paul W. Sciulli, and Jerome C. Rose, "A Health Index from Skeletal Remains," in *The Backbone of History: Health and Nutrition in the Western Hemisphere*, ed. Richard H. Steckel and Jerome C. Rose (Cambridge, UK: Cambridge University Press, 2002), 72.
125 Edward S. Deevey Jr., "The Human Population," *Scientific American* 203, no. 9 (September 1, 1960), 202.
126 Saunders, Herring, Sawchuk, Boyce, Hoppa, and Klepp, 145.
127 Ibid., 151.
128 Ibid., 146.
129 Ibid., 135.
130 Ibid., 136.
131 Ibid., 148.
132 Rosanne L. Higgins, Michael R. Haines, Lorena Walsh, and Joyce E. Sirianni, "The Poor in the Mid-Nineteenth-Century Northeastern United States," in *The Backbone of History: Health and Nutrition in the Western Hemisphere*, ed. Richard H. Steckel and Jerome C. Rose (Cambridge, UK: Cambridge University Press, 2002), 165.
133 Ibid., 176; Saunders, Herring, Sawchuk, Boyce, Hoppa, and Klepp, 136.
134 Saunders, Herring, Sawchuk, Boyce, Hoppa, and Klepp, 135.
135 John Burnett, *Plenty and Want: A Social History of Diet in England from 1815 to the Present Day* (London: Scolar Press, 1979), 24.
136 Ibid.; Roderick Floud, Kenneth Wachter, and Annabel Gregory, *Height, Health and History: Nutritional Status in the United Kingdom, 1750–1980* (Cambridge, UK: Cambridge University Press, 1990), 301.
137 Floud, Wachter, and Gregory, 136–138.
138 E. A. Wrigley and R. S. Schofield, *The Population History of England, 1541–1871: A Reconstruction* (Cambridge, UK: Cambridge University Press, 1989), 230.
139 Ibid.
140 Floud, Wachter, and Gregory, 136–138; 292.
141 Ibid., 305.
142 Ibid., 301.
143 Paul Clayton and Judith Rowbotham, "How the Mid-Victorians Worked, Ate and Died," *International Journal of Environmental Research and Public Health* 6, no. 3 (March 2009): 1235–1253, https://www.ncbi.nlm.nih.gov/pmc/articles/PMC2672390.
144 Ibid.
145 Paul C. Mangelsdorf, *Corn: Its Origin, Evolution, and Improvement* (Cambridge, MA: Harvard University Press, 1974), 1; Betty Fussell, *The Story of Corn* (New York: Knopf, 1992), 17; Sylvia A. Johnson, *Tomatoes, Potatoes, Corn, and Beans: How the Foods of the Americas Changed Eating around the World* (New York: Atheneum Books, 1997), 7.

146 Fussell, 7–8.
147 Ibid., 269.
148 Martin S. Staum, "Marggraf, Andreas Sigismund," in *Dictionary of Scientific Biography*, vol. 9, ed. Charles Coulston Gillispie (New York: Charles Scribner's Sons, 1981), 105.
149 Fussell, 269.
150 Ibid.; A. N. Shamin and A. I. Volodarsky, "Kirchhof, Konstantin Sigizmundovich," in *Dictionary of Scientific Biography*, vol. 7, ed. Charles Coulston Gillispie (New York: Charles Scribner's Sons, 1981), 378.
151 Fussell, 269–270.
152 Ibid., 273.
153 Ibid., 274; Gary Taubes, *The Case against Sugar* (New York: Knopf, 2016), 25.
154 Warner, 141.
155 Ibid., 142.
156 "Per Capita Consumption of High Fructose Corn Syrup in the United States from 2000 to 2017 (in Pounds)," *Statista*, 2019, accessed June 12, 2019, https://www.statista.com/statistics/328893/per-capita-consumption-of-high-fructose-corn-syrup-in-the-us.
157 Lieberman, 1064.
158 "Syrups, Corn, High-Fructose," *USDA FoodData Central*, April 1, 2019, accessed June 12, 2019, https://fdc.nal.usda.gov/fdc-app.html#/food-details/169659/nutrients.
159 George A. Bray, Samara Joy Nielsen, and Barry M. Popkin, "Consumption of High-Fructose Corn Syrup in Beverages May Play a Role in the Epidemic of Obesity," *American Journal of Clinical Nutrition* 79, no. 4 (April 2004): 537, https://academic.oup.com/ajcn/article/79/4/537/4690128.
160 Fabrizia Lanza, *Olive: A Global History* (London: Reaktion Books, 2011), 82.
161 "Olive Oil," *USDA FoodData Central*, April 1, 2019, accessed December 12, 2019, https://fdc.nal.usda.gov/fdc-app.html#/food-details/343873/nutrients; "Sugars, Granulated," *USDA FoodData Central*, April 1, 2019, accessed February 13, 2020, https://fdc.nal.usda.gov/fdc-app.html#/food-details/169655/nutrients; "Syrups, Corn, High-Fructose," *USDA FoodData Central*, April 1, 2019, accessed June 22, 2019, https://fdc.nal.usda.gov/fdc-app.html#/food-details/169659/nutrients.
162 Lieberman, 1065.
163 Ibid., 1066.
164 Warner, 140.
165 "Salad Dressing, Ranch Dressing, Regular," *USDA FoodData Central*, April 1, 2019, accessed February 13, 2020, https://fdc.nal.usda.gov/fdc-app.html#/food-details/173592/nutrients.
166 "Salad Dressing, Blue or Roquefort Cheese, Low Calorie," *USDA FoodData Central*, April 1, 2019, accessed February 13, 2020, https://fdc.nal.usda.gov/fdc-app.html#/food-details/169876/nutrients.
167 Lieberman, 1066.
168 Anneke H. van Otterloo, "The Low Countries," in *The Cambridge World History of Food*, vol. 2, ed. Kenneth F. Kiple and Kriemhild Conee Ornelas (Cambridge, UK: Cambridge University Press, 2000), 1238.
169 Lieberman, 1063–1064.
170 "1 in 5 Obese Adults Satisfied with Body Weight," *Centraal Bureau voor de Statistiek*, September 25, 2018, accessed June 16, 2019, https://www.cbs.nl/en-gb/news/2018/37/1-in-5-obese-adults-satisfied-with-body-weight.
171 Ibid.
172 Craig M. Hales, Margaret D. Carroll, Cheryl D. Fryar, and Cynthia L. Ogden, "Prevalence of Obesity among Adults and Youth: United States, 2015–2016," *NCHS Data Brief*, U.S. Department of Health and Human Services, October 2017, accessed February 13, 2020, https://www.cdc.gov/nchs/data/databriefs/db288.pdf, 2.
173 Conor Dillon, "Obese? Not Us! Why the Netherlands Is Becoming the Skinniest EU Country," *Deutsche Welle*, September 6, 2015, accessed June 16, 2019, https://www.dw.com/en/obese-not-us-why-the-netherlands-is-becoming-the-skinniest-eu-country/a-18503808.
174 Ibid.
175 Joe Lindsey, "One in Three Americans Rides a Bike," *Bicycling magazine*, March 3, 2015, accessed June 16, 2019, https://www.bicycling.com/news/a20010688/cycling-advocacy-1.
176 Lieberman, 1063.
177 Ibid., 1064.
178 Ibid., 1063.

179 Elise Green, "Exporting Obesity: Micronesia as a Microcosm," Center for Strategic and International Studies, 2019, accessed June 13, 2019, https://www.csis.org/npfp/exporting-obesity-micronesia-microcosm.

180 "Maruchan Ramen Noodles, Creamy Pesto," *Fooducate*, 2010–2019, accessed June 13, 2019, https://www.fooducate.com/product/Maruchan%20Ramen%20Noodles%20Creamy%20Pesto/A2175722-E10A-11DF-A102-FEFD45A4D471.

181 Green.

182 Nancy Davis Lewis, "The Pacific Islands," in *The Cambridge World History of Food*, vol. 2, ed. Kenneth F. Kiple and Kriemhild Conee Ornelas (Cambridge, UK: Cambridge University Press, 2000), 1359.

12 Grains

12.1 TERMINOLOGY

The word "grain" derives from the Latin *granum*, meaning "seed." This etymology reveals few specifics because innumerable plants produce seeds: packages of embryos and nutrients to hasten germination. Terminology reflects this inexactitude given that agronomists apply "grain" to seeds not just of cereals but of edible legumes, designated "grain legumes," remarked Chapter 8.[1] Complicating matters is British English's archaic tendency to call cereal grains "corn" even though American English reserves the word for the Mesoamerican grass *Zea mays*, known as maize. This book follows convention by confining "corn" to maize and "grain" to cereals.

12.2 EVOLUTION OF GYMNOSPERMS

The first plants to produce seeds—gymnosperms—may have occupied the genera *Elkinsia* and *Archaeosperma*, specimens of which originated before 360 million years ago and resembled bushes.[2] Grains did not arise from them, however, but from grasses that originated 70–55 million years ago and dispersed widely between 9 and 4 million years ago.[3] Self- or wind-pollinated, they need neither bees nor other animals to reproduce. Grasses tolerate low carbon dioxide concentrations and efficiently photosynthesize. Although they colonized many latitudes, temperate grasses catalyzed agriculture in the parts of Asia that specialized in seed plants.

12.3 WHEAT

12.3.1 Wheat and Barley in Southwestern Asia

The shift toward farming appears to have begun in southwestern Asia, where rainfall was greater 14,000 years ago than today.[4] Rain supported vegetation, including wheat (*Triticum monococcum, T. dicoccon, T. aestivum,* and *T. durum*) and barley's (*Hordeum vulgare*) precursors. Emphasizing this area's shape and agricultural importance, historians call it the Fertile Crescent. Its easternmost protrusion begins at the northern end of the Persian Gulf, moving northwest along the Tigris and Euphrates Rivers, then southwest along the eastern shore of the Mediterranean Sea, and south along the Nile River through Upper Egypt. In tracing this path, the Fertile Crescent passed through what are today southeastern Turkey, Iraq, Syria, Lebanon, Jordan, Israel, and northern Egypt.

These nations tend to be labeled the Middle East. This book avoids such language as imprecise because the Middle East does not appear to be the middle of any easily defined location. Because Syria, Lebanon, Israel, and Egypt border the Mediterranean Sea, they are better described as Mediterranean countries. Alternatively, given that Syria, Lebanon, Jordan, and Israel are in westernmost Asia, they might be identified as part of western Asia, or more precisely southwestern Asia, rather than of a nebulous Middle East. Of Egypt, only the Sinai Peninsula is in Asia, challenging the claim that the nation is part of the East, if East means Asia. Egypt is rightfully an African country even though Lower Egypt—defined in Chapter 4—has ancient ties to the Mediterranean.

Fertile Crescent hunter-gatherers, known as Natufians, ate grass seeds among other edibles. When rainfall diminished and temperatures cooled during the Younger Dryas (10,800–9500 BCE), plants became less plentiful.[5] The Natufians compensated for this dearth by planting seeds to grow food rather than simply relying on what nature provided. This behavior deepened the association between plants and people, making Natufians participants in floral evolution. In shaping plants, they derived the earliest varieties of barley and wheat. Of the two, wheat is more widespread today, though this circumstance was untrue from agriculture's origin to the Middle Ages (c. 500–c. 1500 CE).[6] Better tolerating cold, drought, and excessive moisture, barley was the safer option. Moreover, people favored it for making beer, which may have contributed to the early enthusiasm for grain farming.[7]

12.3.2 Wheat's Dispersal

From southwestern Asia, wheat descended south into Egypt about 5000 BCE.[8] From there, it moved west through North Africa, today Libya, Tunisia, Algeria, and Morocco. Mediterranean lands proved suitable for *Triticum durum*, which is today made into pasta and noodles, though ancients use it for bread, porridge, and gruel. In southwestern Asia, Egypt, and North Africa, durum is still made into bread and is popular in couscous and bulgar. Another route took wheat west into Mediterranean Europe, Greece, acquiring the grain around 6000 BCE.[9] Movement west and north spread it from Scandinavia to Britain between 4000 and 2000 BCE. Independent of these developments, archeology put it in Mehrgarh, Pakistan, about 4000 BCE. In the next millennium, the grass spread along Pakistan and India's Indus River.

Although many Americans associate wheat with bread, it was not the grain's primary use 12,000 years ago. The species most widely grown today and most often made into bread, *Triticum aestivum*, arose about 7000 BCE.[10] The first cultivated *Triticum* species appear to have been emmer (*Triticum dicoccon*), einkorn (*Triticum monococcum*), and possibly spelt (*Triticum spelta*). Spelt must have been an early cultivar if *T. aestivum* evolved from it. Adding water or milk to these grains yielded gruel or porridge depending on the proportion of liquid and solid. Despite its suitability for bread, *T. aestivum* was a latecomer; people initially used emmer for this purpose. Unaware of yeast (*Saccharomyces cerevisiae*), southwestern Asians made flatbread before 3000 BCE. The Egyptians, Mesopotamians (people in what are today Iraq and parts of neighboring countries), or both harnessed yeast to leaven bread around 1000 BCE. Besides these developments, bread fed early farmers in what is today Pakistan. A pariah in some circles, gluten—a complex of over one hundred proteins in wheat, barley, rye (*Secale cereale*), and triticale (*Triticosecale rimpaui*)—makes dough sticky and elastic, helping it cohere and rise during baking. These properties equip gluten for breadmaking.

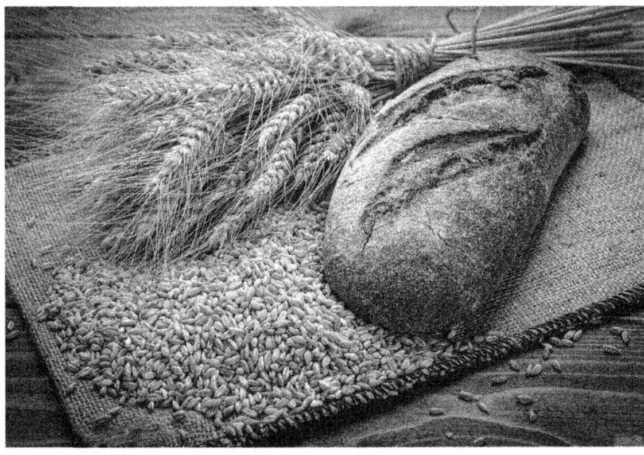

FIGURE 12.1 Whole-wheat bread. (Photo from Shutterstock.)

Europe's expansion after roughly 1500 CE carried wheat and preference for bread worldwide. Sixteenth-century Spain planted the grain in Mexico, Argentina, Chile, and California.[11] In 1620, the Pilgrims brought wheat to Massachusetts. During the next two decades, New York, New Jersey, and Delaware planted varieties from Sweden and the Netherlands. By 1892, Americans grew over 470 varieties. Important were soft red and soft white winter wheats; their yields surpassed those of hard varieties and their kernels were easier to process into flour. In 2017, CGIAR—once known as the Consultative Group for International Agriculture Research—in Montpellier, France, estimated world hectarage at 215 million and the number of consumers at 2.5 billion.[12]

12.3.3 *Wheat Belly* and *Grain Brain*

Perhaps, no food has suffered such intense recent criticism as wheat and grains in general. Chapters 1 and 3 remarked that American cardiologist William R. Davis (b. 1957) launched the first salvo in 2011, publishing *Wheat Belly*. Emmaus, Pennsylvania's Rodale Publishing Company, capitalized on strong sales the next year by releasing a new edition titled *Lose the Wheat, Lose the Weight*!

Davis' attack has two parts. The first claimed that into the 1960s, Americans were trim but thereafter grew fat.[13] The second blamed obesity on genetically altered wheat varieties, which have gliadins, proteins in gluten that Davis blamed for overstimulating appetite.[14] He conjectured that they bind to brain receptors, creating pleasure by diminishing pain, slowing breathing, and calming agitation. Clinicians designate this area opiate receptors because opium and its derivatives act on it. But if gliadins stimulate appetite by acting on opiate receptors, as Davis supposed, readers may wonder why opium, attaching to the same receptors, dulls appetite. Moreover, gliadins are not unnatural as Davis claimed because wheat always had them. If gliadins overstimulate appetite now, this effect must have existed since southwestern Asians began to eat wheat's prehistoric precursors. If gliadins act as Davis posited, people should not have been slender into the 1960s, as he claimed, because wheat must have caused them to overeat whenever and wherever food was abundant. Admittedly, food's scarcity during all but recent times must have prevented all but elites from overeating regardless of what stimulated the appetite.

In attempting to sketch obesity's chronology, Davis plowed into trouble at the outset, writing that old family photos demonstrated "how *thin* everyone looks."[15] This claim preceded assertions that are an odd mix of specificity and vagueness. The photos, he stipulated, should date from the grandparents or parents' generation. A range of two generations is imprecise. Later paragraphs indicated time by mentioning the 1950s and 1960s and "40 or 50 years ago."[16] Forty or fifty years' retrogression from the 2011 copyright yields 1961 or 1971. Davis must have had in mind, therefore, sometime between the 1950s and 1970s.

If his chronology is hazy, the specifics he pinned to it are precise, provided the reader lets him entertain notions of likelihood: between the 1950s and 1970s women "probably" were size four, men had 81.3 centimeter (thirty-two inch) waists, no man exceeded this norm by 25.4 or more centimeters (ten or more inches), and no teen was 90.7 kilograms (200 pounds).[17] Such specificity should have been, but was not, cited.

All cannot receive treatment, but for the sake of illustration consider the proposition that between the 1950s and 1970s women wore size four clothes. Davis did not specify geography, implying worldwide uniformity. If he is right and if evidence exists, it should be possible to track global sales of women's clothing during these decades such that size four apparel outsold all other sizes. Yet Davis supplied no evidence of any kind, making his assertion akin to the declaration, for example, that between the 1950s and 1970s dragonflies (species in the infraorder Anisoptera) were larger or smaller, faster or slower, or more or less numerous than today. Neither pronouncement furnishes any reason for belief. Both are so peculiar that, without evidence, disbelief is more reasonable than affirmation.

Even if family photos merit treatment as evidence of a sort, I have not intruded into others' lives by asking to view ancestral photos, though my experience falsifies Davis' generalization. My mother was obese, as was her mother. My maternal grandfather was smaller than both, but nonetheless had a protruding belly. These comments intend no disparagement. After my mother's early death and her husband's passing, my maternal grandmother suppressed her grief to do everything in her power to parent me. Her memory is never far from my thoughts. My father and his mother were svelte, and my paternal grandfather was neither fat nor thin but resembled the sturdy peasants from whom he descended. My lineage demonstrates that everyone was not slender once upon a time, contrary to *Wheat Belly*.

Moreover, belief in universal slenderness contradicts wealthy Egyptians' corpulence, discussed in Chapter 4. Greek physician Hippocrates (460–377 BCE) observed that the obese died younger than lean individuals.[18] In the second century CE, Greek anatomist and author Galen (130–210 CE), physician to Roman emperor Marcus Aurelius (121–180 CE), warned his wealthy patients against obesity, criticizing people too fat to walk without perspiring.[19] Roman frescos featured women with ample physiques.

In the sixth century CE, Pope Gregory I (c. 540–604), known as Gregory the Great, listed seven deadly sins: gluttony, sloth, and lust among them. Although modern people associate the third with sex, Gregory meant to encompass all physical excesses, including overeating. The seven deadly sins thus twice condemned gluttony. Warnings against intemperance indicated that not everyone was gaunt and underfed. People who ate much and did little were fat enough to alarm religious authorities. Eating well and inert, for example, medieval monks had triple the obesity of commoners.[20]

Flemish artist Peter Paul Rubens (1577–1640), Dutch artist Rembrandt Harmenszoon van Rijn (1606–1669), and French painters Edgar Degas (1834–1917), Pierre Auguste Renoir (1841–1919), and Henri Matisse (1869–1954) depicted fleshy nudes. German composer Johann Sebastian Bach (1685–1750), American scientist, inventor, and statesman Benjamin Franklin (1706–1790), and English historian Edward Gibbon (1737–1794) were rotund. Twenty-seventh U.S. President William Howard Taft (1857–1930) weighed 160.6 kilograms (354 pounds) at his 1909 inauguration.[21]

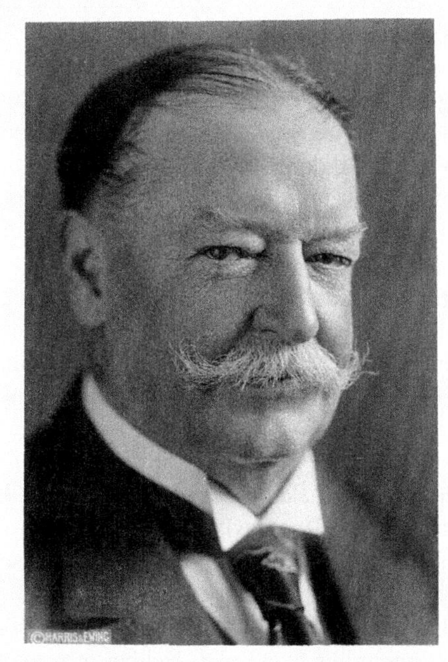

FIGURE 12.2 William Howard Taft. (Photo courtesy of Library of Congress. https://www.loc.gov/pictures/item/2017669059/.)

Yet Davis supposed that humans were uniformly lean before roughly 1970. This idea is untenable for a species that has long displayed diverse phenotypes. Treating him gently, his belief may be rephrased as the proposition that into the 1960s Americans were thinner and lighter on average than afterward. Assessment of this statement requires surveying the past to determine whether leanness and lightness held sway until after 1970. Absent inspection of innumerable photos, the claim of smallness can be investigated by substituting mass for size. Measurements from several sources show that American men and women retained roughly the same mass for their age and height between 1885 and 1900.[22] Absent earlier numbers, late-nineteenth century stasis intimates that changes must have occurred in the twentieth century.

12.3.4 Motorization Rather than Wheat as Cause of Obesity

Data reveal that Americans gained weight during that century, but not just after roughly 1970 as Davis asserted. Increases occurred in two phases: between the two world wars and after World War II.[23] The wars less reshaped physiques than stifled demand. During World War I, for example, government discouraged indulgence.[24] Americans were to buy war bonds with spare income. War's end opened the floodgates of consumerism, the target of which was the automobile.

A nineteenth-century invention, the horseless carriage was initially designed and priced for the affluent. Earlier chapters drew attention to inequalities and the tendency of economic systems and foodways to sharpen them. This thinking defined the automobile until the twentieth century, when American automaker Henry Ford (1863–1947) reconceptualized it as a mass commodity. Achievement of this aim required him to cut prices. Whereas the average car cost $1,600 in 1901, Ford introduced the Model N in 1906 for $600.[25] Two years later, he unveiled the Model T, cutting the price from $850 that year to $490 in 1914, $325 in 1916, and $310 in 1921. Low prices changed transportation as American automakers produced 1.9 million cars in 1920 and nearly 4.5 million in 1929.[26] The United States had 8.1 million registered vehicles in 1920 (1 car per every third household) and 23.1 million in 1929 (1 car for every 1.3 households). Prioritizing the automobile, Americans that decade skimped on groceries and clothes to afford it.[27]

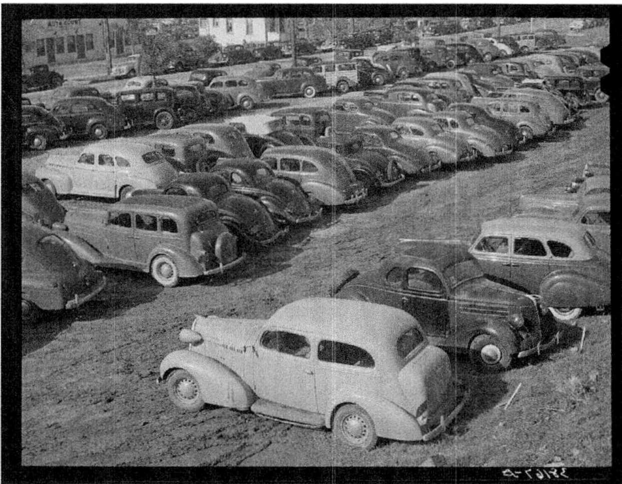

FIGURE 12.3 Automobiles. (Photo courtesy of Library of Congress. https://www.loc.gov/pictures/item/2017788354/.)

Many authors have detailed how the automobile changed the United States and the world. Our objective is to reiterate earlier chapters' remarks that it opened a chasm between those who lived without and with it. United Kingdom (UK) pharmacologist Paul Clayton and historian Judith D. Rowbotham (b. 1952)—both introduced in Chapter 1—stated that before the automobile, people walked wherever they went.[28] During the 1920s, as noted, Americans bought cars, permitting movement without exertion. This idleness corresponded to mass increases between World Wars I and II.

New York City typified motorization's effects on the physique. Like other cities, cars enabled the Big Apple to grow as Americans settled its suburbs. Retaining its position as the largest U.S. metropolis, New York City more than doubled from 4 to 9.4 million inhabitants between 1900 and

1930.[29] Entering it in 1934, German pediatrician Hilde Bruch (1904–1984) encountered overweight and obese children at schools, in hospitals, on streets, and on the subway.[30] The last, opening in 1904, presaged mass motorization by allowing movement without toil. Although Bruch concentrated on under and overeating as disorders, dependence on the automobile and consequent weight gain are pathologies in their own right.

World War II reestablished World War I's austerity. Demand for materiel led U.S. factories to transition from consumer goods to armaments. Although Americans earned generous wartime wages, they had little to buy because rationing constricted purchasing. As was true of World War I's end, peace in 1945 unleashed consumerism. Between 1946 and 1955, U.S. annual automobile production rose from 2 million to 8 million.[31] In 1956, Congress extended the automobile's range with the Interstate Highway Act, which allocated $26 billion to lay over 64,370 kilometers (40,000 miles) of highways.

Businesses conformed to the postwar landscape. McDonald's took the lead among fast food restaurants in locating along highways to attract weary travelers. Rather than require from drivers and passengers the minimal exertions of parking, exiting a car, and walking into a restaurant, McDonald's and its imitators established drive-through windows. Drivers needed only approach a window, order food, inch forward to collect a purchase, and exit the parking lot to consume a meal without taking a stride. Today, countless businesses offer drive-through services, enabling Americans to slouch toward death. This postwar renewal and expansion of America's commitment to motorization corresponds to the second increase in mass. This pattern corroborates earlier chapters in implicating the automobile and consequent inactivity in obesity and related chronic maladies. Davis was wrong to heap all the blame on wheat.

If diets must be faulted, wheat and other grains are unlikely villains. Paralleling the automobile's twentieth century ascent, U.S. consumption of bread and other grain products declined from 308.4 kilograms (680 pounds) per person annually in 1910 to 204.1 kilograms (450 pounds) in 1970.[32] During these years, daily vegetable oil ingestion more than doubled from 20 to 50 grams per American. These data correlate fat rather than grains with mass increase. Chapter 10 examined fat's health effects.

None of the foregoing challenges Davis' assertions that Americans have grown fatter since the 1970s and that waistlines continue to expand. Given what has been called an obesity epidemic, critics are safe to fault wheat or another convenient scapegoat. Courage or rashness is necessary to challenge the automobile, which has become the centerpiece of American life.

Whichever quality is involved, statistics collected between 1985 and 2007 showed that the more miles Americans drove, the fatter they became.[33] "When you are sitting in a car, you are doing nothing, so your body is burning the least amount of energy possible," remarked American computer scientist, statistician, and data analyst Sheldon Howard Jacobson. "And if you are eating food in your car, it becomes even worse." Journalists marvel at families with four or five cars to enable parents and adolescents to work and socialize.[34] Youths who begin driving around age fifteen absorb America's culture of ease, comfort, and inertness, growing into adulthood without having exerted themselves.

In this context, Davis correctly targeted the 1970s, but not because of wheat. During the 1973 oil crisis, U.S. gasoline prices sextupled, prompting U.S. Secretary of State Henry Alfred Kissinger (b. 1923) to describe the shock as "the most devastating blow to economic development in this decade."[35] Gas stations limited purchases, and angry drivers fought each other with fists and guns. Theft's prevalence led automakers to design cars with locking gas caps.[36] Truckers parked their rigs across interstate highways to halt traffic. Their brazenness arose from the conviction that as Americans, they were entitled to inexpensive fuel. Such actions concretized an umbilical attachment to the automobile and the indolence it permits. Clayton and Rowbotham lamented in 2009 that "Our levels of physical activity...are at an historical low."[37] Contrasting past exertions with today's torpor, they concluded that "because they [mid-nineteenth-century Britons] were so much more physically active than we are today, overweight and obesity hardly existed at the working class level."

12.3.5 Contrast between Inactivity and Activity

Focusing on seventeenth-century Maryland and nineteenth-century Illinois, American anthropologist Clark Spencer Larsen (b. 1952) reached the same conclusion: Survival amid rustic conditions and rudimentary technologies compelled labor too strenuous to permit overweight and obesity.[38] Contrasting these rigors with today's lassitude, he asserted that "One of the most profound lifestyle changes to occur in recent memory is the growing sedentism of late twentieth-century Americans, resulting in unprecedented levels of obesity."[39] No imagination is necessary to identify the automobile as lethargy's enabler.

These conclusions jibe with a 2015 finding that 88 percent of Americans owned at least one automobile.[40] Although large, this percentage underreported the reality that 95 percent of U.S. households owned at least one car.[41] By comparison, 85 percent of Germans owned at least one automobile; yet 23.6 percent of Germans were obese in 2017 compared with 38.2 of Americans.[42] The difference may stem from activity. Eighty percent of Germans owned a bicycle, regarding it as transportation rather than a toy. By contrast, only 53 percent of Americans had one, 85 percent of whom commuted by car.[43]

12.3.6 Diminution in Wheat Intake

Davis also rightly singled out the 1970s because in 1972 American cardiologist Robert Coleman Atkins (1930–2003), introduced in Chapter 4, published *Dr. Atkins' Diet Revolution: The High Calorie Way to Stay Thin Forever*. In the context of American inertness, the book advocated the non sequitur that caloric foods produced slenderness.[44] Since publication of *Dr. Atkins' Diet Revolution*, per American annual wheat consumption has fallen 6.8–9 kilograms (15–20 pounds).[45] If wheat causes obesity, then fatness should have declined with reduced intake. Instead, as Davis emphasized, Americans have enlarged. Given this trend, it seems strange to blame overweight and obesity on a food whose consumption is diminishing. Rather than confront inactivity and gluttony, Davis faulted wheat even though per Italian wheat consumption more than doubled that in the United States, and Table 11.5 reported only 9.9 percent of Italian men aged forty-five to sixty-four and 11.1 percent of women obese.[46]

Attempts to ignore facts and excoriate wheat and other grains contradict the reality that their consumption, as implied, has declined since roughly 1800.[47] For example, Chapter 7 stated that eighteenth-century pensioners in Gevaudan, France, ate the equivalent of slightly over fourteen slices of rye-barley bread daily. Using averages, Chapter 7 calculated that bread totaled 703.5 grams of the day's 724.1 grams of food, or 97.2 percent of Gevaudan diets by mass. Although not wheat, rye and barley also have gluten and therefore should cause the problems attributed to wheat. If grains cause obesity, Gevaudans should have been massive. Instead, British historian Olwen H. Hufton (b. 1938), quoted in Chapter 9, described them as "puniest."[48] French scholar R. J. Bernard indicated in Chapters 7 and 9 that they were poor and hungry and so seldom ate enough.[49]

This example suggests that obesity results more from how much is eaten than from what is consumed. If wheat and kindred grains caused obesity, fatness should have peaked around 1800 and decreased thereafter. Instead, it increased during the twentieth century as grains retreated. If diet is obesity's sole factor, the culprit should be foods whose intake increased in the twentieth century: fats, sucrose ($C_{12}H_{22}O_{11}$), high-fructose corn syrup, eggs, meat, fruits, and vegetables.[50]

Vegetables are a catchall whose nutrition and healthfulness are examined in Chapter 15. Dearth of calories makes them unlikely to increase body fat. Not all fruits, however, have this virtue. Dried fruits such as dates (*Phoenix dactylifera*), figs (*Ficus carica*), prunes, and raisins are caloric. Ample fat gives 100 grams of avocado (*Persea americana*) 160 calories.[51] Even more potent, 100 grams of coconut (*Cocos nucifera*) furnish 354 calories.[52] Chapter 4 noted that meat has many calories. One hundred grams of hen's egg have 155 calories.[53] At 9.4 calories per grams, Chapter 2 noted, 100 grams of fat have 940 calories. One hundred grams of olive oil, for example, have 884 calories.[54]

These 100 grams do not total 940 calories because olive oil is not pure fat, having sodium and vitamins E and K. Minerals and vitamins, discussed in Chapter 2, lack calories. One hundred grams of sucrose supply 387 calories.[55] Tables in earlier chapters list calories, fat, and carbohydrates in various foods. Meat, eggs, lard and oils, sugars, and some fruits are caloric and have increased in consumption, but Davis omitted them in chastising wheat.

12.3.7 Broad Criticisms That Grains Undermine Health

Despite Davis' weak assertions, American neurologist David Perlmutter (b. 1954), introduced in Chapter 1, expressed "love" for *Wheat Belly*.[56] He enlarged Davis' critique by implicating all gluten-containing grains in dementia, writing that "Modern grains are silently destroying your brain."[57] Fundamental to his criticisms is belief that grains, having many carbohydrates, are unnatural given the supposition, challenged in Chapter 10, that ancestral diets were 75 percent fat and only 5 percent carbohydrates.[58]

Perlmutter's position depends on the premise that people eat lots of bread, breakfast cereals, pastries, and related products and that these items harm the body. Yet the claim that these foods are unhealthy contradicts his admission of a "dramatic reduction" in deaths from heart disease, stroke, and some cancers between 2000 and 2014.[59] Sickness and death should increase rather than diminish amid consumption of harmful foods. As mortality from heart disease and cancers declined, as Perlmutter conceded, people must succumb to other conditions. Despite life's implacable limits, he appears to inhabit a counterfactual universe where humans can exist in a utopia free from all maladies. Such naivete ignores life's finitude. Despite fervent wishes otherwise, death spares no one.

12.3.8 Gluten as Straw Man

At the microlevel—Chapter 2 distinguished between macrolevel and microlevel explanations—and as previous paragraphs noted, the attack against wheat targets gluten, mentioned earlier as a group of over one hundred proteins in several grains. Celiac disease sufferers cannot ingest it without harming the small intestine, though critics go beyond this fact to assert that everyone should eschew gluten in the belief that it irritates the digestive system irrespective of celiac disease. These detractors believe that the immune system retaliates by inflaming the digestive tract's cells. This information convinced 63 percent of Americans that reducing or eliminating gluten may enhance health.[60]

The rationale against gluten, however, requires that if something injures a subset of people, it must distress many others. Such reasoning is faulty because what troubles some may not affect others. For example, the Centers for Disease Control and Prevention (CDC) in Atlanta, Georgia, reported that influenza killed roughly 80,000 Americans in late 2017 and early 2018.[61] But this mortality does not necessitate that it will kill me. The danger exists but is unknown. Such uncertainty might lead people to think me irrational should I refuse to leave home or admit anyone for fear of influenza, particularly because I receive an annual flu vaccine. In this context, readers might question the logic that everybody should fear gluten irrespective of its risks.

Manufacturers leverage fear—a primal emotion that tends to overwhelm the capacity for deliberation—by offering gluten-free products whose ingredients include "tapioca, corn, rice flour, potato starch, and xanthan gum."[62] Chapter 13 defines tapioca as cassava starch, which lacks micronutrients.[63] Later sections discuss corn and rice's health effects in prehistory and history. Chapter 13 amasses evidence that the potato (*Solanum tuberosum*) is the world's most nourishing food. Like tapioca, however, potato starch is just carbohydrates without additional nutrients.[64] Fermented from sucrose, mentioned earlier and discussed in Chapters 2 and 11, xanthan gum lacks nutrients and may impair breathing and digestion.[65]

Moreover, gluten-free items tend to have little fiber, iron, or vitamins B_2 (riboflavin) and B_3. Lack of fiber promotes rapid digestion, during which the pancreas produces the hormone insulin to tell cells to absorb the sugar glucose ($C_6H_{12}O_6$) in carbohydrates. Insulin signals the liver to store excess glucose and to release it when needed. In these ways, insulin regulates glucose in blood. But the hormone surges when digestion is fast in fiber's absence. These overloads weaken cells' response to insulin, causing diabetes. Boston's Celiac Center at Beth Israel Deaconess Medical Center discouraged people from wasting money on gluten-free items absent medical necessity.[66]

Rejection of Davis and Perlmutter's assertions, and the fears they heighten, leads this chapter to caution against a priori biases against grains. Preconceptions, ahistoricism, and speculation should be alien to empirical fields like the natural sciences and medicine. This section concludes that no evidence condemns all grains because of gluten or fear of overstimulating the appetite. The rest of this chapter examines grains' consumption worldwide and their prehistoric and historic health effects.

12.3.9 The Obesity Epidemic as Context

Although *Wheat Belly* has flaws, Davis rightly worries about obesity. Physicians and scientists express alarm that an "obesity epidemic" assails humanity.[67] In February 2018, the World Health Organization (WHO) in Geneva, Switzerland, announced that the number of obese children and adults had tripled worldwide since 1975.[68] Chapter 1 defined overweight and obesity as statistical designations, and Tables 11.4 and 11.5 listed global percentages of overweight and obesity by ethnicity. Being a type of excessive massiveness, obesity indicates abnormal fatness. Because muscle is denser than fat, American nutritionist and chef Monica Reinagel conceded that lean bodybuilders may satisfy obesity's statistical definition.[69] But they are a tiny subset of the population. Almost all obese individuals are overfat.

The issue is whether wheat and other grains worsen obesity. A previous section correlated mass increases with greater motorization and consequent inactivity. At their core, overweight and obesity result from surfeit left after subtracting metabolism. Because inertness minimizes metabolism and is the norm in developed countries and increasingly in developing nations, calorie restriction is necessary to guard against mass gain. This arithmetic rejects American science writer Gary Taubes's (b. 1956) belief that hormones, not overconsumption, cause overweight and obesity.[70] The issue therefore is the number of calories in grains and other foods. If grains are fattening, as critics contend, they must provide inordinate energy.

12.3.10 Calories and Nutrients in Grains

Our foci are corn, rice, and wheat, which the abstract introduced as humanity's principal foods. This book follows convention in using 100 grams as the standard for foods and does not depart here, though the U.S. Food and Drug Administration (FDA) designates 45 grams of grain a serving.[71] The U.S. Department of Agriculture (USDA) favors an even smaller amount, 28 grams, as a serving. One hundred grams of corn (as cornmeal) have 362.2 calories. The same amount of brown rice has 367 calories. Depending on type, 100 grams of whole wheat have between 327 and 342 calories. Despite Davis' animus, wheat has fewer calories by weight than rice or corn. Of the grains that the Whole Grains Council catalogs, 100 grams of oats (*Avena sativa*) have most calories at 389 and sorghum (*Sorghum bicolor*) least at 329.

Of course, people do not eat pure grain seeds, whose tough outer coat—known as the husk, hull, or chaff—is indigestible, but rather preparations like bread or noodles. The USDA tabulates between 141.1 and 142.2 calories in two slices of whole wheat bread.[72] By comparison, two slices of whole rye bread have 130 calories.[73] Belief that toast has fewer calories than the same amount of untoasted bread is false. Bread may have ingredients such as oats, corn, millet (species in Eragrostideae tribe), or potatoes, but if leavened, wheat or rye is a constituent. Chapter 7 stated that eighteenth-century France's poor extended bread with barley, a practice common where it was grown. Bread variants include bagels, muffins, buns, baguettes, rolls, and ciabattas. Consumers also eat wheat in noodles or pasta. Table 12.1 compares calories in bread and kindred items.[74]

TABLE 12.1
Calories in Bread and Similar Products 100 g

Food	Calories
Bread, whole wheat	252
Bread, white	266
Bread, rye	259
Bread, oat	262
Bread, barley	268
Bread, potato	266
Pasta, unenriched	371
Pasta, gluten free	179
Pasta, whole grain	362
Pasta, chickpea	333
Pasta, lentil	350
Pasta, black bean	376

Recalling that 100 grams of whole grain surpass 300 calories irrespective of type, comparisons may be made with foods in earlier tables. For example, calories in fruits appear in Table 1.1, in vegetables, fruits, and fungi in Table 2.1, in fruits, eggs, nuts, and peanuts (*Arachis hypogaea*) in Table 2.2, in meat in Table 4.1, in seafood in Tables 5.1 through 5.4, in poultry and eggs in Table 6.1, in legumes including peanuts in Tables 8.1 and 8.3, in nuts in Tables 9.1, 9.3, and 9.4, and in vegetable oils in Tables 10.2 and 10.6.

These comparisons imply no criticisms because eggs, legumes, and nuts have many nutrients in addition to calories, as Chapters 6, 8, and 9 and their accompanying tables emphasized. Other chapters indicate that low-calorie foods such as vegetables, some fruits, and potatoes are nourishing. Chapter 13 argues that potatoes are the world's most nutritious food. Dieters may count calories, but no less important is the endeavor to make calories count by selecting foods with ample nutrients per calorie just as shoppers aim to buy products that deliver value on the dollar.

None of the foregoing denies grains' nutrients, shown in Table 12.2.[75] Among whole cornmeal, rice, and wheat, the last has the most protein, calcium, phosphorus, potassium, zinc, copper, manganese, and vitamin B_9 (folate, folic acid, or pteroylmonoglutamic acid).[76] Among wheats, Table 12.3[77] indicates that durum has the most calcium, magnesium, phosphorus, zinc, copper, selenium, and vitamins B_2, B_3, B_6 (pyridoxine), and B_9 by mass. Wheat ranges from 0 micrograms of selenium for hard white to 89.4 for durum and from 4.38 milligrams of vitamin B_3 for hard white to 6.74 for durum per 100 grams.

The same amount of rice has 23.3 micrograms of selenium and 6.5 milligrams of B_3, and corn has 15.6 micrograms of selenium and 3.6 milligrams of B_3. Corn and wheat have similar amounts of iron and magnesium though corn's phytic acid binds to iron, calcium, magnesium, and zinc, hindering their absorption from corn and all foods eaten with it. Corn is not alone in this defect because some legumes and nuts also have phytic acid. For this reason, Chapters 4, 5, and 6 indicated that the body better absorbs these nutrients from animal products. Rice has the least iron and the most vitamins B_1 (thiamine or thiamin), B_5 (pantothenic acid), and B_6. Corn has the most vitamin B_2. The Whole Grains Council calculated that corn has over ten times the carotenoids (vitamin A precursors) in other grains.[78] Yellow kernels have more carotenoids than white. Corn, rice, and wheat lack vitamins C and D. Grains are not the best sources of fat-soluble vitamins, whose functions where discussed in Chapter 2.

TABLE 12.2
Nutrients in Selected Grains 100 g

Nutrient	Cornmeal	%DV	Brown Rice	%DV	Rye	%DV	Oats	%DV
Calories	362.2	N/A	366.7	N/A	337.8	N/A	388.9	N/A
Protein (g)	8.1	N/A	7.5	N/A	10.3	N/A	16.9	N/A
Fat (g)	3.6	N/A	3.2	N/A	1.6	N/A	6.9	N/A
Carbs (g)	76.9	N/A	69.6	N/A	75.9	N/A	66.3	N/A
Fiber (g)	7.3	N/A	3.6	N/A	15.1	N/A	10.7	N/A
Minerals								
Ca (mg)	6.67	0.67	8.89	0.89	24.44	2.44	53.33	5.33
Fe (mg)	3.44	19.1	1.29	7.2	2.62	14.6	4.71	26.2
Mg (mg)	126.67	31.7	115.56	28.9	111.11	27.8	177.78	44.4
P (mg)	240	24	311.11	31.11	331.11	33.11	522.22	52.22
K (mg)	286.67	8.2	248.89	7.1	511.11	14.6	428.89	12.3
Na (mg)	35.56	1.5	4.44	0.2	2.22	0.1	2.22	0.1
Zn (mg)	1.82	12.1	2.13	14.2	2.64	17.6	3.98	26.5
Cu (mg)	0.2	10	0.29	14.5	0.38	19	0.62	31
Mn (mg)	0.49	24.5	3.73	186.5	2.58	129	4.91	245.5
Se (mcg)	15.56	22.2	23.33	33.3	14	20	28.9	41.3
Vitamins								
A (IU)	214	4.3	0	0	11	0.2	0	0
B_1 (mg)	0.38	25.3	0.53	35.3	0.31	20.7	0.76	50.7
B_2 (mg)	0.2	11.8	0.09	5.3	0.24	14.1	0.13	7.6
B_3 (mg)	3.62	18.1	6.49	32.5	4.27	21.4	0.96	4.8
B_5 (mg)	0.42	4.2	1.49	14.9	1.47	14.7	1.36	13.6
B_9 (mcg)	24.44	6.1	22.22	5.6	37.78	9.5	55.56	13.9
B_{12} (mcg)	0	0	0	0	0	0	0	0
C (mg)	0	0	0	0	0	0	0	0
D (IU)	0	0	0	0	0	0	0	0
E (mg)	0.42	2.8	0.6	4	0.85	5.7	0.42	2.8
K (mcg)	0.3	0.4	0.6	0.8	5.9	7.4	2	2.5

12.3.11 Wheat around the World

An earlier section referenced CGIAR's 2017 estimate that 2.5 billion people worldwide eat wheat. Although this chapter rejects Davis and Perlmutter's alarmism, American agricultural chemist Donald Kasarda conceded that some people may have difficulty digesting wheat, displaying "gluten sensitivity."[79] He is uncertain, however, that gluten is at fault. Readers may recall that Davis blamed scientists for deriving unnatural wheats since the 1960s, but Kasarda and others documented no changes in wheat proteins because of scientific manipulation.[80] If wheat is unhealthful now, if its proteins are the problem, and if they have not changed over time, then wheat was never wholesome. Under these circumstances, prehistory and history should reveal instances of illness among wheat eaters.

The search for past wheat consumers is less easy than might be imagined. An earlier section implied that wheat was unknown in North and South America before the sixteenth century. It cannot therefore have harmed pre-Columbian peoples. Chapters 3, 4, and 5 indicated that high latitudes have long, harsh winters and short growing seasons. Humans responded to these limitations by favoring animal products. In this context, Chapter 7 documented dairy's importance in northern

TABLE 12.3
Nutrients in Wheat by Type 100 g

Nutrient	Hard White	%DV	Hard Red Spring	%DV	Hard Red Winter	%DV	Durum	%DV
Calories	342	N/A	329	N/A	327	N/A	339	N/A
Protein (g)	11.31	N/A	15.4	N/A	12.61	N/A	13.68	N/A
Fat (g)	1.71	N/A	1.92	N/A	1.54	N/A	2.47	N/A
Carbs (g)	75.9	N/A	68.03	N/A	71.18	N/A	71.13	N/A
Fiber (g)	12.2	N/A	12.2	N/A	12.2	N/A	3.9	N/A
Minerals								
Ca (mg)	32	3.2	25	2.5	29	2.9	34	3.4
Fe (mg)	4.56	25.33	3.6	20	3.19	17.7	3.52	19.6
Mg (mg)	93	23.3	124	31	126	31.5	144	36
P (mg)	355	35.5	332	33.2	288	28.8	508	50.8
K (mg)	432	12.3	340	9.7	363	10.4	431	12.3
Na (mg)	2	0.08	2	0.08	2	0.08	2	0.08
Zn (mg)	3.33	22.2	2.78	18.5	2.65	17.7	4.16	27.7
Cu (mg)	0.36	18	0.41	20.5	0.43	21.5	0.55	27.5
Mn (mg)	3.82	191	4.06	203	4	200	3.01	150.5
Se (mcg)	0	0	70.7	101	70.7	101	89.4	127.7
Vitamins								
A (IU)	9	0.2	9	0.2	9	0.2	0	0
B_1 (mg)	0.39	26	0.5	33.3	0.38	25.3	0.42	28
B_2 (mg)	0.11	6.5	0.11	6.5	0.12	7.1	0.12	7.1
B_3 (mg)	4.38	21.9	5.71	28.6	5.46	27.3	6.74	33.7
B_5 (mg)	0.96	9.6	0.94	9.4	0.96	9.6	0.94	9.4
B_6 (mg)	0.37	18.5	0.34	17	0.3	15	0.42	21
B_9 (mcg)	38	9.5	43	10.8	38	9.5	43	10.8
B_{12} (mcg)	0	0	0	0	0	0	0	0
C (mg)	0	0	0	0	0	0	0	0
D (IU)	0	0	0	0	0	0	0	0
E (mg)	1.01	6.7	1.01	6.7	1.01	6.7	N/A	N/A
K (mcg)	1.9	2.4	1.9	2.4	1.9	2.4	N/A	N/A

Europe. At the other extreme, the tropics, Chapter 13 observes, situated root and tuber agriculture. Wheat has been absent or unimportant in these areas.

A later section remarks that West Africa grew rice (*Oryza glaberrima*). Elsewhere in Africa, sorghum, millet, and, after 1500, corn were the chief grains. Rice (*Oryza sativa*) was the staple in South, Southeast, and much of East Asia. Rice dominated south of China's Yangtze River, and wheat had to compete with millet and corn north of the river. Northern India and Pakistan have long grown wheat, but even in these areas, people often ate rice and the poor subsisted on millet bread.[81] In southwestern Asia, Iranians and Arabs preferred rice to wheat.[82] The masses ate millet or wheat bread. Turks ate wheat and rice.[83] Between the Tigris and Euphrates Rivers—in ancient Mesopotamia—barley bread was the staple.[84] Ancient Rome's granary, Egypt—whose diets were detailed in Chapter 4—produced millet, sorghum, barley, and wheat. Egyptians favored *T. dicoccon*, or less often barley, for bread.[85] Even then, bread was a component of diets that featured lettuce (*Lactuca sativa*), turnips (*Brassica rapa* ssp. *rapa*), cabbage (*Brassica oleracea var. capitata*), beets (*Beta vulgaris*), radishes (*Raphanus raphanistrum* ssp. *sativus*), broad beans (*Vicia faba*), peas (*Pisum sativum*), lentils (*Lens culinaris*), chickpeas (*Cicer arietinum*), garlic (*Allium sativum*), onions (*Allium cepa*), leeks (*Allium ampeloprasum*), cucumbers (*Cucumis sativus*), papyrus (*Cyperus papyrus*) roots, watermelons (*Citrullus lanatus*), figs, dates, grapes (*Vitis vinifera*) and raisins, and plums (*Prunus domestica*). In the seventh century CE, Arabs further broadened food choices by bringing rice from India. Wheat never monopolized Egypt's palate. Only in Syria, Jordan, and Lebanon was preference for wheat longstanding.[86]

Even where grown, wheat was too expensive for the masses, who ate barley, millet, buckwheat (*Fagopyrum esculentum*), or chestnut porridge or gruel.[87] Bread eaters consumed what was available: combinations of at least two grains, known as maslin. Shortages led bakers to augment bread with bark, soil, legumes such as peas and vetch (*Vicia* species), chestnuts (*Castanea* species), beechnuts (*Fagus sylvatica*), and weeds.[88] Even nobles ate maslin, though wheat formed the mixture's majority whereas commoners' maslin had little if any of the grain.

Wheat's premodern scarcity may surprise Christians who assume that Jesus and his apostles ate wheat bread, thereby making it the norm. Religion aside, dearth suggests a solution to the complaint of indigestibility. From the past's perspective, wheat is a novelty for most societies. Not having evolved from a lineage of wheat eaters, some modern people may have trouble digesting it. Rather than gluten sensitivity, therefore, some humans' digestive tract may treat wheat as alien irrespective of gluten. The link between novelty and indigestibility may explain food allergies. For example, a 2011 study documented peanut allergy among those of African descent, an unsurprising result given peanuts' South American origin Chapter 8 mentioned.[89] An ocean away, Africans were not exposed to them until after 1500.

Wheat's dearth or absence may not have undermined health. The grain lacks essential amino acids lysine and isoleucine.[90] Chapter 2 noted the necessity of ingesting such amino acids because of the body's inability to make them from other compounds. Fortunately, populations dependent on wheat often consumed dairy—discussed in Chapter 7—a source of complete proteins. Another shortcoming was wheat's inadequate zinc where grown on soils deficient in the mineral, as happened in southwestern Asia and North Africa. Even adequate soils did not solve the problem because the grass' phytic acid binds with zinc, inhibiting absorption. Chapter 1 mentioned zinc's importance in growth.[91] For this reason, wheat consumers without another dietary source of the mineral did not reach full stature.[92] Consequently, southwestern Asia's farmers were shorter than their hunter-gatherer predecessors, a development detailed in Chapter 14.[93]

12.3.12 Milling

Even if wheat harms consumers because it is foreign to their digestive system and because of insufficient amino acids and zinc, milling rather than gluten causes most problems. Humans have processed kernels to increase digestibility and palatability, an operation known as milling and performed by abrading kernels with stones throughout prehistory and most of history. The earliest millstones date to roughly 18,000 BCE, though people must have removed the husk with some abrasive when they began eating grains at least 22,500 years ago.[94] Millstones usually crushed seeds, mixing rather than separating their components: husk, bran, embryo (known as germ), and endosperm. Retention of all parts conserved nutrients.

By stopping short of pulverization, breadmakers could sift grain to separate endosperm from other components. Retention of only endosperm yielded white flour. This extra step increased labor and wasted grain because sifting discarded half the harvest. Labor and losses made white flour scarce and expensive. For this reason, only the affluent ate white bread, which served to differentiate elites from commoners. Although the masses wanted to emulate their superiors by consuming white bread, from a nutritional perspective they were fortunate to eat coarse, whole grains.

Enthusiasm for white flour did not corrupt everyone. In the first half of the nineteenth century, American minister Sylvester Graham (1794–1851) decried it as unnatural because God, having created the entire kernel, intended people to eat it whole.[95] Milling was therefore sinful, and sinfulness could produce nothing but illness. Instead of white flour, Graham promoted whole-wheat wafers known as Graham crackers.

Graham's argument could not retard technology. In 1832, Swiss inventor Jakob Sulzberger revolutionized milling by building the first roller mill, which used steel rather than stone to strip away all but the starchy endosperm, yielding white flour.[96] By the 1870s, flour makers in many countries, including the United States and United Kingdom (U.K.), replaced millstones with roller mills. Churning out flour faster than was previously possible, these mills made white bread plentiful and inexpensive. Consumers liked the price, ease of chewing, and texture. In the 1880s, however, U.S. and U.K. physicians reported increases in indigestion, heart disease, and diabetes.[97]

This development spurred a search for the cause. Doctors who sounded the alarm in the 1880s suspected white flour but lacked evidence to make their case. Among its most charismatic opponents, American bodybuilder and vegetarian Bernarr Adolphus Macfadden (1868–1955) in the 1920s labeled white flour the "staff of death."[98] He asserted that dogs that fed only it died as quickly as if they ate nothing. This warning was not hyperbole. Vermin had long raided whole grains in storage, but they avoided white flour.[99] Mice perished from eating it. In the 1920s, while Macfadden condemned white flour, American chemist Benjamin Ricardo Jacobs (1879–1963) quantified its near absence of iron and vitamins B_1, B_2, B_3, and B_9 and linked it to pellagra and beriberi, discussed in Chapter 2 and later sections.

These shortfalls raised consternation only in 1940, when Congress reinstituted conscription while war engulfed Europe and Asia. Half the first 1 million conscripts were too undernourished for induction.[100] Military and civilian leaders blamed unenriched white flour, and in 1942, the U.S. Army announced that it would feed troops only bread and pasta made from fortified flour. Such flour could still be white, but in 1943, Congress required manufacturers to add iron and vitamins B_1, B_2, B_5, and B_6.[101] Calcium was optional, but breadmakers could not label their products "fortified" without it.

No panacea, fortification failed to ennoble white bread, which African American author James Arthur Baldwin (1924–1987) denounced as "blasphemous and tasteless foam rubber."[102] This language underscored white bread's inherent unnaturalness, a critique that expressed unease with modernity's artificiality. White flour's unhealthfulness and blandness suggest that critics have wrongly attacked gluten rather than milling.

12.4 RICE

12.4.1 Rice in Asia

Like barley and wheat in parts of southwestern Asia, *O. sativa* fed South, East, and Southeast Asia. Farmers may have begun cultivating it along China's Yangtze River between 8000 and 6000 BCE.[103] As early as 7000 BCE, people were raising it on the border between China and India. Rice husks in Koldihwa, India, date between 6570 and 4530 BCE, though kernels from this site are more recent.[104] Chinese geneticist Te-Tzu Chang (1927–2006) believed that what are today India's Uttar Pradesh and Bihar provinces began growing and eating rice between 2000 and 1500 BCE.[105] Progress south was slow, with Andhra Pradesh and Tamil Nadu provinces acquiring it only about 300 BCE. From India, it reached western Asia around 1000 BCE and Sri Lanka before 543 BCE.[106] From China, rice migrated to Korea before 1030 BCE and to Japan around 1000 BCE. Independent acquisitions occurred in Vietnam between 4000 and 2000 BCE, in Thailand around 3500 BCE, in the Philippines—home to the International Rice Research Institute (IRRI)—about 1400 BCE, and in Indonesia by 500 CE. From an early date, people grew and ate two subspecies of *O. sativa*. *O. sativa* ssp. *japonica* has shorter seeds (grains or kernels) than *O. sativa ssp. indica*. Each may have been domesticated independent of the other.

Like wheat, humans removed the husk from the time they began eating rice. Rice processing has multiple steps depending on the product desired. Ten-thousand-year-old stones in what is today Shangshan, China, supply the earliest evidence of milling.[107] Husk's removal yields brown rice, a whole grain with intact layers of bran, germ, and endosperm. As with other grains, retention of these components provides greatest nourishment. Table 12.2 shows that brown rice by mass is 69.6 percent carbohydrates, 3.2 percent fat, and 7.5 percent protein. Chang ranked the quality of brown rice's amino acids behind only oats among grains.[108] For example, rice has more of the amino acid lysine than wheat, corn, or sorghum. These considerations did not impress Clark Spencer Larsen, who judged rice "remarkably deficient in protein, even in its brown or unmilled form."[109] Table 12.2 indicates that 100 grams—roughly half a serving—have sizable amounts of manganese, selenium, phosphorus, magnesium, and vitamins B_3 and B_6.

Brown rice, however, is less popular than white, whose milling removes bran and embryo, halving iron and B vitamins.[110] Table 12.4 shows that the product, being mostly starch, is 79.34 percent carbohydrates, 0.58 percent fat, and 6.61 percent protein by mass.[111] One hundred grams have 55 percent the FDA's daily value (DV) for manganese, 21.6 percent for selenium, 10.8 percent for phosphorus, and 13.4 percent for vitamin B_5. White rice lacks vitamins A, B_{12}, C, D, and K. If rinsed before cooking, rice loses most or all water-soluble vitamins: B complex and C.

The United States counteracts some of these deficiencies by requiring manufacturers to fortify white rice with iron and vitamins B_1 and B_3. Soaking, steaming, and drying kernels before milling, a method known as parboiling, lessens shortfalls by allowing nutrients—in Table 12.5—to

TABLE 12.4
Nutrients in White Rice 100 g

Nutrient	White Rice	%DV
Calories	360	N/A
Protein (g)	6.61	N/A
Fat (g)	0.58	N/A
Carbs (g)	79.34	N/A
Fiber (g)	0.4	N/A
	Minerals	
Ca (mg)	9	0.9
Fe (mg)	0.8	4.4
Mg (mg)	35	8.8
P (mg)	108	10.8
K (mg)	86	2.5
Na (mg)	1	0.04
Zn (mg)	1.16	7.7
Cu (mg)	0.11	5.5
Mn (mg)	1.1	55
Se (mcg)	15.1	21.6
	Vitamins	
A (IU)	0	0
B_1 (mg)	0.07	4.7
B_2 (mg)	0.05	2.9
B_3 (mg)	1.6	8
B_5 (mg)	1.34	13.4
B_6 (mg)	0.15	7.5
B_9 (mcg)	9	2.3
B_{12} (mcg)	0	0
C (mg)	0	0
D (IU)	0	0
E (mg)	0.11	0.7
K (mcg)	0	0

TABLE 12.5
Nutrients in Parboiled Rice 100 g

Nutrient	Parboiled Rice	%DV
Calories	374	N/A
Protein (g)	7.51	N/A
Fat (g)	1.03	N/A
Carbs (g)	80.89	N/A
Fiber (g)	1.8	N/A
	Minerals	
Ca (mg)	71	7.1
Fe (mg)	0.74	4.1
Mg (mg)	27	6.8
P (mg)	153	15.3
K (mg)	174	5
Na (mg)	2	0.08
Zn (mg)	1.02	6.8
Cu (mg)	0.28	14
Mn (mg)	1.04	52
Se (mcg)	19.9	28.4
	Vitamins	
A (IU)	0	0
B_1 (mg)	0.22	14.7
B_2 (mg)	0.05	2.9
B_3 (mg)	5.05	25.3
B_5 (mg)	0.67	6.7
B_6 (mg)	0.45	22.5
B_9 (mcg)	8	2
B_{12} (mcg)	0	0
C (mg)	0	0
D (IU)	0	0
E (mg)	0.03	0.2
K (mcg)	0.1	0.1

penetrate the endosperm and so may be thought natural enrichment of white rice.[112] Parboiled rice is 80.9 percent carbohydrates, 1 percent fat, and 7.5 percent protein by mass. One hundred grams have 25.3 percent DV for vitamin B_3, 22.5 percent for B_6, 14.7 percent for B_1, 6.7 percent of B_5, 52 percent for manganese, 28.4 percent for selenium, 15.3 percent for phosphorus, 14 percent for copper, 6.8 percent for magnesium and zinc, 7.1 percent for calcium, 5 percent for potassium, and 4.1 percent for iron. Parboiled rice lacks vitamins, A, B_{12}, C, and D. Chapter 2 discussed these nutrients and others.

Raising and eating roughly 95 percent of the world's rice, Asians' dependence on it invites comparisons with potatoes in Ireland before the mid-nineteenth century and cassava (*Manihot esculenta*) in parts of Africa today.[113] Because rice yields more calories and protein per hectare than many other grains, Asia long had denser populations than rye, oat, barley, and wheat-eating Europe and the cornfed Americas. Rice supplies roughly 60 percent of calories in Southeast Asia, whereas the percentage is around 35 in East and South Asia. Indigenes in Myanmar, Laos, Thailand, and Vietnam eat the grain thrice daily.[114] The poor in Bangladesh, India, Nepal, Pakistan, Sri Lanka, and parts of West Africa consume about one-fifth of the world's harvest, preferring parboiled rice. At roughly 130–180 kilograms (287–397 pounds) per person annually and 55–80 percent of daily calories, consumption is highest in Bangladesh, Cambodia, Indonesia, Laos, Myanmar, Thailand, and Vietnam.[115]

12.4.2 Rice in Africa and the Americas

West Africans domesticated a different species, *O. glaberrima*—known as African, black, or red rice—in the Niger River valley.[116] American geographer Judith Ann Carney (b. 1946) and independent scholar Richard Nicholas Rosomoff referenced 3000 BCE as the probable beginning of cultivation, though domestication must have come later.[117] American plant breeder C. Wayne Smith favored domestication around 1500 BCE along the Niger and a possible second taming about 500 years later near Guinea's coast.[118] Chang offered a later estimate for the Guinean domestication at 1000–1200 CE.[119] *O. glaberrima* has a nuttier flavor and more nutrients, requires less labor, and tolerates insects, weeds, and poor soils better than *O. sativa*. Lower yields, however, have made *O. glaberrima* a minor crop since the nineteenth century CE. From the Niger valley, African rice spread west to Senegal between 1700 and 800 BCE. The species migrated north by the sixteenth century CE to Morocco and west to the Cape Verde Islands. Today, *O. glaberrima* is absent outside West Africa.[120]

O. sativa may have reached Africa as early as 1000 BCE, when traders are thought to have brought it to Madagascar in the Indian Ocean south of the equator.[121] Persians from what is today Iran may have given Egypt Asian rice by 300 BCE.[122] From the Indian Ocean, Arabs brought it to East Africa between the sixth and eleventh centuries CE. In the eighth century, they carried rice throughout North Africa and into Spain. Another opinion, however, put *O. sativa* in Africa only after 1500.[123] Although Asian rice usually yields more than its African counterpart, Africa's weeds and insects reduced *O. sativa*'s yields. Weed control required inundation and extra labor, delaying *O. sativa*'s progress. Crossing from Madagascar to Mozambique, this species reached what are today the Democratic Republic of the Congo and the Republic of the Congo only in the nineteenth century.

The slave trade opened a market for rice in the sixteenth century, as Portuguese captains provisioned ships with it, assigning African women the traditional job of preparing it for crew and slaves. Uncooked grains must have remained viable in the Americas, bringing rice agriculture and cuisine to the Caribbean islands and Mexico in the 1520s, Brazil and Uruguay about 1570, the Gulf of Mexico by 1579, Virginia in 1609, and South Carolina around 1685.[124] Early accounts assigned South Carolina's first planting to *O. glaberrima,* though if Madagascar was the source, *O. sativa* was a possibility given its early introduction into the island. Carney and Rosomoff argued from primary sources that *O. glaberrima* was the first rice in South Carolina, though Smith believed that North America had only *O. sativa*.[125]

After 1680, South Carolina imported slaves from the Caribbean and Africa to grow rice.[126] In the eighteenth century, expertise was obtained by purchasing slaves from West Africa's rice-growing areas. Their knowledge and exertions expanded rice agriculture south from coastal South Carolina through Georgia and northern Florida and north to North Carolina's Cape Fear River.[127] Planters exported rice to Europe, where it could be eaten, fermented into alcohol, or processed into paper. Catholics ate it with fish during Lent—whose dietary restrictions were discussed in Chapter 5—and on other meatless days throughout the year. For this reason, Catholic Portugal and Spain were large buyers. Britain imported colonial America's rice, selling it on the continent and in India. Rice concentrated wealth among a plantocracy that shaped regional, national, and transatlantic policies.

In the Caribbean, Mexico, Brazil, South Carolina, and Georgia, slaves ate variants of rice and legumes. Chapter 8 stated that the cowpea (*Vigna unguiculata*), also known as black-eyed pea, had been a West African staple since roughly 3000 BCE.[128] The Portuguese introduced beans (*Phaseolus vulgaris*) into West Africa in the sixteenth century, adding another legume. Slaves employed these possibilities in the Americas. Those in the West Indies ate black *Phaseolus* beans and rice, whereas

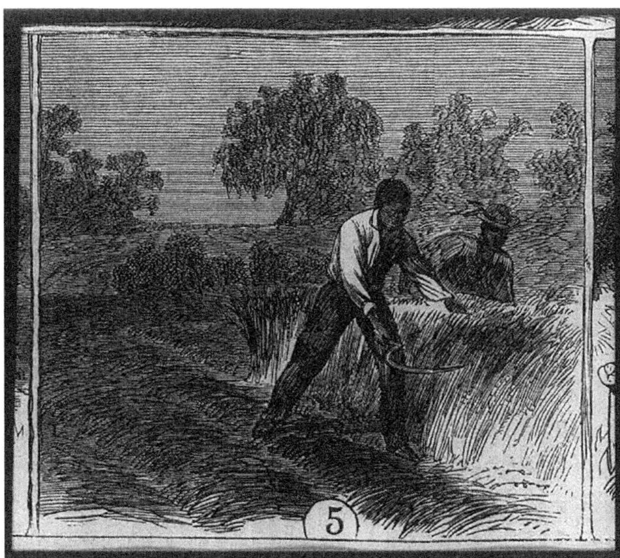

FIGURE 12.4 North Carolina rice plantation. (Photo courtesy of Library of Congress. https://www.loc.gov/pictures/item/2007677025/.)

New Orleans, Louisiana, specialized in red kidney beans and rice. South Carolinian and Georgian slaves paired cowpeas and rice. On the Sea Islands off the coast of South Carolina, Georgia, and Florida, the preferred cowpea was the sea island red pea.

Whole grain rice and legumes complement each other. Although rice has lysine, as noted, the amount is small. Legumes such as beans surmount this disadvantage by furnishing enough of the amino acid.[129] Beans lack the essential amino acid methionine, which rice supplies. White or parboiled rice lacks fiber, which legumes provide. Beans, peas, cowpeas, lentils, and other legumes contribute potassium, iron, manganese, magnesium, and vitamin B_9. More nourishing, beans are also more expensive than rice throughout much of the world, causing the poor to skimp on them while eating more rice and reducing nutrients in the process, noted Chapter 8.[130] Improvements might include supplanting white rice with brown to increase fiber and nutrients. Inclusion of tomatoes (*Solanum esculentum*) or peppers (*Capsicum annuum*) adds vitamin C. A side of carrots (*Daucus carota ssp. sativus*) or spinach (*Spinacia oleracea*) boosts vitamins A (as beta carotene) and C. Chapter 8 discussed legumes' healthfulness.

12.4.3 Rice, Milling, and Deficiency Diseases

Chapter 2 mentioned that since the nineteenth century, physicians and scientists have associated rice with beriberi, a potentially fatal disease. Medical practitioners categorize it by type and list symptoms that include vomiting, diarrhea, insomnia, apathy, disorientation, hallucinations, memory loss, muscle weakness and soreness, atrophy, anorexia, ataxia, neuritis, difficulty breathing, swelling that begins in the feet and ascends to the face, double vision, involuntary eye movements, weak or paralyzed eye muscles, and heart failure. American internist and anthropologist Frederick L. Dunn (1928–2014) suspected that the disease predated agriculture.[131] Beriberi's origins may never be pinpointed because it leaves no traces in bones or teeth and so cannot be detected among prehistoric peoples who left little beyond their skeletons. The association with rice is misleading in the sense that whole grains do not cause the disease. Chapter 2 identified the cause as insufficient vitamin B_1. This book notes that whole grains, legumes, nuts, yeast, meat, fish, and some dairy products have adequate

B_1, other B vitamins, and additional vitamins, minerals, protein, and phytochemicals. Pork and eggs provide the most B_1, though milk is not rich in it.

Chinese texts mentioned a disease like beriberi in the first millennium BCE, though neither rice nor processing was likely the villain because milling probably removed no bran, which along with the husk has B_1.[132] In other words, ancient Chinese ate whole grain rice. Whatever this malady's cause, brown rice prevents beriberi because bran is intact. Problems emerged after roughly 1870 upon introduction of steam mills into East and Southeast Asia. Milling, now powerful enough to remove all layers of bran, produced a polished kernel deficient in B_1 and many more nutrients. An earlier paragraph and Tables 12.2 and 12.4 detailed the nutritional chasm between brown and white rice. Especially vulnerable were the poor, prisoners, soldiers, sailors, the mentally ill in asylums, and anyone else who subsisted on polished rice. The disease was absent, however, from much of India, where rice was parboiled. Readers may recall from an earlier section and Table 12.5 that parboiling retains nutrients otherwise lost during milling. Only in India's Andhra Pradesh, where parboiled rice was unpopular, did beriberi arise.[133] Besides polished rice eaters, the malady afflicted Thais who ate rotting raw fish and twentieth century Canada's Newfoundland and Labrador fishers who subsisted on white flour during winters.

Beyond beriberi, polished rice imperiled vision due to vitamin A deficiency, a problem rice's inadequate protein compounded.[134] Identifying 1,400 Japanese children who ate white rice and had dry, inflamed corneas and mucus membranes of the eyes and eyelids (xerophthalmia), researchers in 1904 connected vision problems to polished rice.[135] This insight focused attention on undernutrition among Indonesia, India, Bangladesh, the Philippines, Afghanistan, Nepal, Sri Lanka, Haiti, Nigeria, Ghana, and Brazil's poor who ate white rice and suffered partial or total blindness. To be fair, rice was not alone in undermining vision. People who subsisted on corn, white flour, cassava, or beans had the same troubles.

Scientists in Japan, Europe, and the United States pinpointed undernutrition as the culprit. In 1929, British biochemist Frederick Gowland Hopkins (1861–1947) shared the Nobel Prize in physiology or medicine for identifying "the growth-stimulating vitamins."[136] As a practical matter, the honor awarded him priority for discovering vitamin A, though several others contributed to this achievement. Notably, in 1912, American nutritionist Elmer Verner McCollum (1879–1967) named vitamin A and announced its solubility in fat.[137]

Vitamins' twentieth-century identification has not eliminated deficiency diseases, which result more from poverty than inadequate knowledge. A 1992 estimate counted 750,000 Bangladeshi preschoolers with xerophthalmia because of insufficient vitamin A.[138] Another 45,000 Bangladeshi schoolchildren were partially blind and 12,000 lacked sight because polished rice furnished no carotenoids. Additionally, xerophthalmia afflicted roughly 3 million children below age 5 in eastern and southern Africa.[139] Worldwide, xerophthalmia bedeviled over 40 million infants in 2017.[140]

12.5 CORN

12.5.1 Origins and Dispersal

Like prehistoric peoples in the eastern hemisphere, American hunter-gatherers ate wild seeds. Although several proto grains were domesticated, none rivalled corn over the long term. Mexicans in the Tehuacan Valley began cultivating the grass between 8000 and 5000 BCE.[141] Fossilized cobs from New Mexico suggest that people in the American Southwest were growing corn around 4500 BCE.[142] This northern migration took corn into Canada during pre-Columbian times, movement that required Amerindians to transform a tropical grass into a temperate plant through selection of hardy lines. From southern Mexico, corn also trekked south into Panama about 4900 BCE, Ecuador around 4000 BCE, and Peru by roughly 3000 BCE.[143] At its full extent, corn spanned the Americas from roughly 50 degrees north to 50 degrees south.[144]

CORN
THE FOOD OF THE NATION
SERVE SOME WAY
EVERY MEAL
APPETIZING
NOURISHING
ECONOMICAL
CORN
MEAL
GRITS
HOMINY
UNITED STATES FOOD ADMINISTRATION

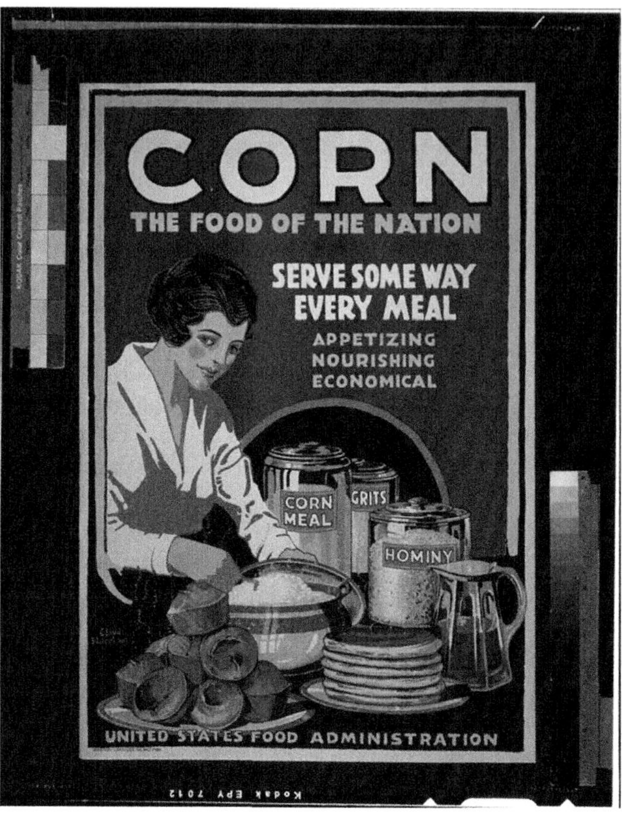

FIGURE 12.5 Corn. (Photo courtesy of Library of Congress. https://www.loc.gov/pictures/item/2002711987/.)

12.5.2 Corn in Amerindian Diets

Before the fifteenth century CE, corn was a staple from Chile to Canada. Mayan, Aztec, and, to a lesser extent, Incan civilizations depended on it. The grain fed Mesoamerica, South America, and the Caribbean. Hopi weddings treated guests to finely ground corn combined with squash (*Cucurbita* species), sunflower (*Helianthus annuus*), or watermelon seed oil, whereas everyday life called for corn dumplings, pancakes, and grits. In contrast to squashes and sunflower, watermelon was an African rather than an American indigene; it reached the western hemisphere only in the sixteenth century. Hopi *piki* looked and tasted like unsweetened cornflakes. Whether as taco, burrito, tamale, empanada, torta, or another item, corn is basic to Mexican cuisine. Summarizing its importance, Hopi chief Don Talayesva remarked in 1942 that "Corn is life."[145]

As succotash—the "most universal Indian dish, found almost everywhere"—corn and *Phaseolus* beans fed Native Americans and might have been part of the 1621 Thanksgiving.[146] Great Plains' Hidatsa baked cornbread known as *naktsi*.[147] The Seneca and Cherokee added berries, beans, apples (*Malus domestica*), chestnuts (*Castanea dentata*), venison, or their combination to cornbread. Mesoamericans ate tortillas, beans, and squash seeds, which American anthropologist Ellen Messer (b. 1948) described a "nutritious and balanced diet."[148] A previous section and Chapter 8 discussed the benefits of combining beans or another legume with a whole grain. Depending on preferences, corn, beans, and squashes were consumed with leafy vegetables, chili peppers (*Capsicum annuum*) or chili sauce, meat, sucrose, or a mix of ingredients.

Hominy, whose preparation leveraged an intuitive understanding of chemistry, fed Mesoamerica. Its production necessitated immersing corn kernels in alkaline water. Such liquid, having a pH over 7—the number signifying neutrality—may be obtained by dissolving ashes in water. Another option is calcium hydroxide [$Ca(OH)_2$], known as limewater, whose pH is also above 7. Numbers over 7 signify bases, whereas those below 7 are acids. The greater the pH, the more caustic the solution. Alkaline water is caustic enough to loosen the husk, whose removal increases digestibility of nutrients and calories. For example, the solution separates vitamin B_3 from indigestible hemicellulose, permitting the vitamin's absorption. Greater availability of B_3 and amino acid tryptophan protects against pellagra. Husk's removal eases grinding the rest of the kernel and forming dough. Lacking gluten, the dough does not leaven and is not hominy: the remains of kernels after alkaline water treatment, a process known as nixtamalization. Nixtamalization removes some bran, raising the issue of whether hominy is a whole grain. The USDA categorized nixtamalized corn as whole grain, specifying tortillas made from it as such but omitting reference to hominy.[149] Boston, Massachusetts' Whole Grains Council likewise withheld judgment about hominy.

Today, the average Mexican, Guatemalan, and Honduran consumes nearly 100 kilograms (220 pounds) of corn yearly, most of it as tortillas.[150] The grass supplies up to 70 percent of their calories, though it has not eliminated deprivation.[151] Mexican anthropologist Arturo Warman (1937–2003) described hunger and undernutrition as typical for poor peasants in Mexico, Central America, and many more parts of the world.[152]

12.5.3 Corn and Amerindian Health

Economists and other anthropologists provided prehistorical and historical depth to this reality by uncovering evidence of diseases and brief lives in skeletons of Amerindians who subsisted on corn. Chapters 1 and 3 documented life's worldwide brevity during all but recent times. In the western hemisphere, diseases such as anemia worsened, heights diminished, teeth decayed, and infant mortality increased wherever people made corn their staple.[153] For example, women shrunk 4 centimeters (1.6 inches) on average and men shortened 2 centimeters (0.8 inches) during the transition from hunting, gathering, and fishing to corn growing on Georgia's coast.[154] That women shrank more than men suggests that men monopolized animal protein, leaving corn for women.

Stunting is unsurprising because corn lacks essential amino acids lysine, tryptophan, and isoleucine.[155] As with zinc discussed earlier, Chapter 1 indicated that humans cannot reach full stature without consuming complete proteins. Beans' inclusion with corn restored adequate essential amino acid balance, but beans and squashes did not return health to preagricultural levels.[156] Among pre-Columbian peoples, corn and anemia plagued southeastern North America's Mississippian civilization between 1100 and 1300 CE, the American Southwest, and the Maya in Mexico's Chichen Itza. For example, fourteen of twenty-one Mayan skulls from children aged 6–12 years displayed porotic hyperostosis, which Chapter 1 described as evidence of anemia.[157] Researchers have not documented the disease among precontact Americans who subsisted on potatoes, sweet potatoes (*Ipomoea batatas*), cassava, or yams (*Dioscorea trifida*), all subjects of the next chapter.

Confirmation of corn's limitations came from Amerindians along the Midwest's Ohio and Illinois rivers. Initially hunter-gatherers, they relied increasingly on corn by roughly 1150 CE. These corn consumers suffered 50 percent more enamel hypoplasia—defined in Chapter 1—than their predecessors, three times more bone deformities from diseases, and four times more anemia.[158] Osteoarthritis became more prevalent, implying that raising corn was more arduous than hunting, gathering, and fishing. Life expectancy at birth (e^0) fell from 26 years before corn was the staple to nineteen afterward.

Yet Warman's "botanical bastard" cannot shoulder all the blame for misery. Globally, the transition from hunting and gathering to farming and livestock raising stunted growth, shortened lives, and exacerbated diseases—Chapter 3's critics charged—as people reduced dietary diversity and crowded settlements, in the process polluting their environment and hastening proliferation of rodents, insects, parasites, and pathogens.[159] Warfare intensified as combatants fought over farmland and pasture.[160] These factors operated among Mississippians, Southwestern peoples, and the Maya.[161]

For example, anthropologists suspect that yaws or syphilis—similar diseases though only syphilis can be venereal—may have caused anemia among Maya.[162] Yaws may be eliminated from consideration if it arose only in Africa because Africa and the Americas had no contact before the sixteenth century. Moreover, Amerindians in the Southeast, Southwest, and Mexico ate more than corn. Dietary diversity, even if less than for hunter-gatherers, implies that iron and B vitamins may have been adequate and that other factors may have caused anemia. The interplay among nutrition, pathogens, parasites, and insects demonstrates that not every instance of anemia signified dietary distress.

12.5.4 Corn, Caribbean Slaves, and Health

In October 1492, Italian-Spanish mariner Christopher Columbus (1451–1506) observed corn on Caribbean island Hispaniola, now Haiti and the Dominican Republic.[163] This encounter opened the Americas to Europeans, Africans, and others. Preferring wheat bread, Spaniards avoided corn, whereas necessity drove seventeenth-century English colonists to imitate Native Americans by growing and eating it. Africans' acquaintance with corn may have begun aboard slave ships—where it was a common ration before 1800—and continued on plantations.[164]

For example, slaves ate corn throughout the Caribbean. Planting okra (*Abelmoschus esculentus*)—whose origins are disputed—on the islands, slaves combined it with corn to make *coo-coo*. Others added the grass to stews, making *fungee*. On Barbados, slaves ate corn, sorghum, vegetables, and sugarcane (*Saccharum officinarum*) juice, the last examined in Chapter 11. When food was scarce, slaves relied on cane juice for short durations. Besides these items, American anthropologists Jerome S. Handler and Robert Spencer Corruccini (b. 1949) mentioned "root crops."[165] Literally understood, this language should eliminate yams and potatoes, which Chapter 13 classifies as tubers. In contrast, sweet potatoes and cassava, being enlarged roots, satisfy Handler and Corruccini's terminology. Columbus mentioned them in the Caribbean in 1492, unsurprising evidence for their presence on the islands because both originated in tropical America.[166] Everyday use of the expression "root crop" includes tubers, of which yam species *D. trifida* fed Caribbean indigenes. Chapter 13 indicates, however, that potatoes need coolness and so cannot have thrived in tropical lowlands. Beyond these foods, slaves sometimes had rum and molasses, though meat, eggs, and dairy were uncommon. Infrequent salted fish supplied complete protein. Wild plants supplemented this fare.

These victuals, including corn and sorghum, were nourishing enough that slaves born on Caribbean islands Cuba and Trinidad were taller than West African arrivals.[167] Statistics between 1751 and 1800 showed that Trinidad's slaves were better nourished than London's poorest adults and children.[168] Moreover, data collected between 1810 and 1863 revealed that on the American South's tobacco, rice, and cotton plantations, slaves who ate corn stood taller than those who did not.[169]

Nonetheless, Caribbean slaves' nutrition was unenviable. Comparisons with West Africans exaggerated slaves' vitality given poor diets in West Africa and appalling conditions aboard slave ships. Data collected between 1813 and 1815 contextualized Trinidadian slaves' health, indicating that they were shorter than 99 percent of British laborers.[170] Slave children suffered the severe protein deficiency disease kwashiorkor, which a later paragraph links to corn consumption. Chapter 8 acknowledged the difficulties of comparing slaves and free people.

Hunger and possibly nutritional deficiencies drove slave children and adults to eat soil, a practice known as geophagy. Nutritional shortfalls were acute when cane juice was the lone edible, stated Chapter 11. Deprivation emaciated slaves. Examination of 101 skeletons revealed abnormal growths on teeth roots, known as hypercementosis, which Handler and Corruccini attributed to undernutrition.[171] Hypoplasia was severe in teeth from skeletons aged about 3 or 4 years, implying starvation after weaning. Malocclusion (misaligned teeth) confirmed undernourishment's magnitude.

12.5.5 Corn in Europe

Corn entered Europe upon Columbus' 1493 return to Spain.[172] Within 25 years, farmers grew the grass throughout the Mediterranean, where Spain, Portugal, and Italy were early adopters. In 1622, famine prompted Leonardo Scincia da Sermoneta, duke of Italian city Tossignano, to give residents free corn porridge, known as polenta, to prevent starvation.[173] The city commemorates the day with an annual festival that serves participants polenta with sausage and tomatoes. To the east, Romania planted corn around 1600.[174] By the eighteenth century, much of central Europe, including Hungary, grew it. As it penetrated the region, corn extended into eastern France, where rye bread was a staple and potatoes were emerging as the poor's sustenance; Chapters 7 and 13 discuss these developments. In Mediterranean and central Europe, corn attracted smallholders because of minimal labor requirements. Where wheat or rye was scant, bakers extended bread with corn.

Northern Europeans, however, were unenthusiastic. In 1597, English barber-surgeon and botanist John Gerard (1545–1612) wrote that corn was "a more convenient food for swine than for man," a prejudice that persisted during the seventeenth century.[175] He rated the grass less nourishing than wheat, rye, barley, and oats.[176] Despite this hostility, about 1550 corn had become a world crop that fed people and livestock, especially pigs.

12.5.6 Corn, China, and Population Increase

Like potatoes in Europe and cassava and sweet potatoes in tropical Africa and Asia—foods discussed in Chapter 13—corn entered China when population threatened to exceed the land's capacity to feed it. Adopting the grain in 1516 from Portugal, farmers grew it in Manchuria, the Yangtze River delta, Yunnan and Szechwan's mountains, and southwestern China.[177] By 1550, what are today Vietnam, Laos, and Cambodia had corn. During the next century, it migrated west to Thailand, south to Indonesia, and east to the Philippines.[178] After roughly 1700, China's population rose as corn, potatoes, and sweet potatoes yielded more calories per hectare than rice. Chapter 13 emphasizes that potatoes supplied more nutrients per unit land than any alternative. Today, corn trails only rice and wheat as a source of calories in China, where it supplements bread and noodles and sustains the poor.[179] Additionally, corn feeds some 18 million in Indonesia, where the equatorial location permits three crops yearly.[180] Popular sequences are rice followed by two plantings of corn and rice followed by corn and then either soybeans (*Glycine max*) or cassava.

12.5.7 Corn in Africa

Portugal was also active in East Africa, introducing corn in the sixteenth century.[181] As noted, that century captains provisioned slave ships with it. Returning to West Africa, crews planted leftovers, though the gold coast—today Ghana—acquired the grass from the Caribbean in the seventeenth century. By 1800, it penetrated the interior as far as Lake Chad in what are today Niger, Nigeria, Chad, and Cameroon. Independent of the slave trade, Arabs carried corn to North Africa. By 1900, the grain fed laborers including miners. During the twentieth century, extension agents encouraged farmers throughout Africa to plant corn.

Africans ground corn, cooking it in water to make mush, known as *kpekple* in Ghana, as *bidia* in the Democratic Republic of the Congo (DRC), as *sadza* in Zimbabwe, as *posho* or *ugali* throughout East Africa, and as *putu* in South Africa. Corn was popular in stews with meat, insects, fish, vegetables, or a combination of ingredients. Among the world's largest corn consumers, Kenyans, Malawians, Zambians, and Zimbabweans rival Mexicans, Guatemalans, and Hondurans, already mentioned, in averaging almost 100 kilograms annually.[182]

Tables 12.2 through 12.5 listed nutrients among corn, rice, and wheat. About 10 percent protein by mass, corn is deficient in lysine, isoleucine, and tryptophan, as mentioned.[183] Mexicans and Central Americans improve nutrition by eating corn with chili peppers, tomatoes, and vegetables, which add vitamin C and increase carotenoids. Africans and Asians consume corn with peanuts and leafy vegetables. Chapter 8 reported that peanuts supply fatty acids, protein, vitamins B_1, B_2, B_3, B_5, B_6, and E, magnesium, phosphorus, potassium, zinc, iron, copper, manganese, selenium, and choline, which is classified as neither vitamin nor mineral. Leafy vegetables have vitamins C and K, carotenoids, iron, calcium, and antioxidants.

12.5.8 Corn and Pellagra

Dietary diversity yields more nutrients than corn alone. Overreliance on it causes pellagra, which French author Maguelonne Toussaint-Samat (1926–2018) blamed on its "very low vitamin content."[184] Chapters 1 and 2 noted that the disease results primarily from insufficient vitamin B_3, which the body cannot absorb from unnixtamalized corn. Symptoms, mentioned in Chapter 1, arose in the 1730s in Spain, where perhaps 20 percent of the population ailed into the early twentieth century, and in Italy, where they persisted until the 1930s.[185] In the nineteenth century, French physician Jean-Baptiste Victor Theophile Roussel (1816–1903) suspected corn the villain. At his urging, French officials encouraged addition of wheat and meat to diets. By the early twentieth century, pellagra had diminished in France. Decades earlier, the disease spread throughout Egypt, South Africa, Austria, Russia, and the Ottoman Empire: today Turkey, Hungary, Greece, Albania, Bosnia and Herzegovina, Bulgaria, Croatia, Kosovo, North Macedonia, Montenegro, Romania, Serbia, Slovenia, Syria, Iraq, Israel, Egypt, Libya, Tunisia, Algeria, and parts of Ukraine and Arabia.

By 1910, pellagra reached "epidemic proportions" in the American South.[186] In 1914, U.S. Public Health Service (PHS) physician and epidemiologist Joseph Goldberger (1874–1929) determined that corn was part of the larger problems of poverty and narrow diets because the poor could not afford the breadth of foods that promoted vitality. Here, as this book emphasizes, food exacerbated inequalities. Hoping to counteract uniform diets, Goldberger advocated consumption of meat, dairy, and eggs, particularly the yolk. Disastrous in many ways, the Great Depression (1929–1939) reduced pellagra. As markets for cotton vanished, farmers instead planted vegetables for their own use, improving health in the process. Although it receded from many nations, pellagra lingers in South Africa, Lesotho, Tanzania, Egypt, and India.

12.5.9 Corn and Kwashiorkor

Another disease associated with corn is kwashiorkor, which Jamaican physician Cicely Delphine Williams (1893–1992) named in 1933.[187] She noted the condition in Ghanaian children who ate little but corn. Investigators thereafter found kwashiorkor in Central America and Brazil's corn consumers. Symptoms included edema, especially in the feet, ankles, and belly, where swelling was conspicuous. Victims suffered fatigue, weakness, diarrhea, sores on mucus membranes, fatty liver, peeling skin on legs and forearms, and irritability. Fatal when untreated, kwashiorkor retards growth and impairs the immune system. In 1952, the World Health Organization (WHO) blamed insufficient protein intake as the cause and noted kwashiorkor's ubiquity among tropical and subtropical poor. Corn is not the lone culprit because the condition also afflicts cassava, rice, millet, and sorghum eaters.

NOTES

1 Vincent E. Rubatzky and Mas Yamaguchi, *World Vegetables: Principles, Production, and Nutritive Values*, 2nd ed. (New York: Chapman and Hall, 1997), 474.
2 Stanley A. Rice, *Encyclopedia of Evolution* (New York: Facts on File, 2007), 182.
3 Elizabeth A. Kellogg, "Evolutionary History of the Grasses," *Plant Physiology*, March 2001, accessed March 4, 2020, http://www.plantphysiol.org/content/125/3/1198#ref-21; Bonnie F. Jacobs, John D. Kingston, and Louis L. Jacobs, "The Origin of Grass-Dominated Ecosystems," *Annals of the Missouri Botanical Garden* 86, no. 2 (Spring 1999): 590.
4 Naomi F. Miller and Wilma Wetterstrom, "The Beginnings of Agriculture: The Ancient Near East and North Africa," in *The Cambridge World History of Food*, vol. 2, ed. Kenneth F. Kiple and Kriemhild Conee Ornelas (Cambridge, UK: Cambridge University Press, 2000), 1123–1124; Joy McCorriston, "Wheat," in *The Cambridge World History of Food*, vol. 1, ed. Kenneth F. Kiple and Kriemhild Conee Ornelas (Cambridge, UK: Cambridge University Press, 2000), 162.

5 David R. Harris, "Origins and Spread of Agriculture," in *The Cultural History of Plants*, ed. Ghillean Prance and Mark Nesbitt (New York and London: Routledge, 2005), 15.
6 Mark Nesbitt, "Grains," in *The Cultural History of Plants*, ed. Ghillean Prance and Mark Nesbitt (New York and London: Routledge, 2005), 49.
7 Phillip A. Cantrell II, "Beer and Ale," in *The Cambridge World History of Food*, vol. 1, ed. Kenneth F. Kiple and Kriemhild Conee Ornelas (Cambridge, UK: Cambridge University Press, 2000), 619–620; Joy McCorriston, "Barley," in *The Cambridge World History of Food*, vol. 1, ed. Kenneth F. Kiple and Kriemhild Conee Ornelas (Cambridge, UK: Cambridge University Press, 2000), 81–82.
8 McCorriston, "Wheat," 170.
9 J. G. Vaughan and C. Geissler, *The New Oxford Book of Food Plants: A Guide to the Fruit, Vegetables, Herbs and Spices of the World* (Oxford: Oxford University Press, 1997), xv.
10 Linda Civitello, *Cuisine and Culture: A History of Food and People*, 3rd ed. (Hoboken, NJ: Wiley, 2011), 7.
11 McCorriston, "Wheat," 170.
12 "Wheat in the World," CGIAR, 2017, accessed April 25, 2019, https://wheat.org/wheat-in-the-world.
13 William Davis, *Wheat Belly: Lose the Wheat, Lose the Weight, and Find Your Path Back to Health* (Emmaus, PA: Rodale, 2011), ix–x.
14 Fred J. P. H. Brouns, Vincent J. van Buul, and Peter R. Shewry. "Does Wheat Make Us Fat and Sick?" *Journal of Cereal Science* 58, no. 2 (September 2013): 209–215, https://www.sciencedirect.com/science/article/pii/S0733521013000969#!.
15 This quote retains the original's italics. Davis, ix.
16 Ibid.
17 Ibid.
18 D. Haslam, "Weight Management in Obesity—Past and Present," *International Journal of Clinical Practice* 70, no. 3 (February 26, 2016): 206–217, https://www.ncbi.nlm.nih.gov/pmc/articles/PMC4832440.
19 Peter Garnsey, *Food and Society in Classical Antiquity* (Cambridge, UK: Cambridge University Press, 1999), 115; Haslam.
20 Jennifer Viegas, "Fat Jolly Monks Had Painful Secrets," ABC, July 26, 2004, accessed March 28, 2019, http://www.abc.net.au/science/news/health/HealthRepublish_1161819.htm.
21 Gina Kolata, "In Struggle with Weight, Taft Used a Modern Diet," *New York Times*, October 14, 2013, accessed March 29, 2019, https://www.nytimes.com/2013/10/15/health/in-struggle-with-weight-william-howard-taft-used-a-modern-diet.html.
22 Milicent L. Hathaway, "Trends in Heights and Weights," *Yearbook of Agriculture, 1959*, ed. Alfred Stefferud, 181–185 (Washington, DC: GPO, 1959), ps://naldc.nal.usda.gov/download/IND43861419/PDF.
23 John Komlos and Marek Brabec, "The Evolution of BMI Values of US Adults: 1882–1986," *Vox*, August 31, 2010, accessed March 18, 2019, https://voxeu.org/article/100-years-us-obesity.
24 Nancy A. Hewitt and Steven F. Lawson, *Exploring American Histories: A Brief Survey with Sources* (Boston and New York: Bedford/St. Martin's, 2013), 638–639.
25 Christopher Cumo, *Science and Technology in 20th Century American Life* (Westport, CT and London: Greenwood Press, 2007), 21–22.
26 Jeremy Atack and Peter Passell, *A New Economic View of American History: From Colonial Times to 1940*, 2nd ed. (New York and London: Norton, 1994) 578.
27 Diane Bailey, *How the Automobile Changed History* (Minneapolis, MN: Abdo Publishing, 2016), 54.
28 Paul Clayton and Judith Rowbotham, "How the Mid-Victorians Worked, Ate and Died," *International Journal of Environmental Research and Public Health* 6, no. 3 (March 2009): 1235–1253, https://www.ncbi.nlm.nih.gov/pmc/articles/PMC2672390.
29 Gary B. Nash, Julie Roy Jeffrey, John R. Howe, Peter J. Frederick, Allen F. Davis, and Allan M. Winkler, *The American People: Creating a Nation and a Society*, vol 2, since 1865, 2nd ed. (New York: HarperCollins *Publishers*, 1990), 788.
30 Gary Taubes, *Why We Get Fat and What to Do about It* (New York: Knopf, 2011), 3.
31 Nash, Jeffrey, Howe, Frederick, Davis, and Winkler, 923.
32 Gretel H. Pelto and Pertti J. Pelto, "Diet and Delocalization: Dietary Changes since 1750," *Journal of Interdisciplinary History* 14, no. 2 (Autumn 1983): 517.
33 Phil Ciciora, "Study: Surge in Obesity Correlates with Increased Automobile Usage," Illinois News Bureau, May 11, 2011, accessed April 2, 2019, https://news.illinois.edu/view/6367/205328.
34 Ralph Vartabedian, "One-Car Family? That's So 1959," *Los Angeles Times*, February 14, 2007, accessed April 1, 2019, https://www.latimes.com/archives/la-xpm-2007-feb-14-hy-wheels14-story.html.

35 Albert Marrin, *Black Gold: The Story of Oil in Our Lives* (New York: Knopf, 2012), 101; Bradley L. Bowman, "Middle East, Relations with (Except Israel)," in *Postwar America: An Encyclopedia of Social, Political, Cultural, and Economic History*, vol. 3, ed. James Ciment (Armonk, NY: Sharpe Reference, 2007), 859.
36 Wil Mara, *Inside the Oil Industry* (Minneapolis, MN: ABDO, 2017), 58.
37 Clayton and Rowbotham.
38 Clark Spencer Larsen, *Skeletons in Our Closet: Revealing Our Past through Bioarchaeology* (Princeton, NJ and Oxford, UK: Princeton University Press, 2000), 222–223.
39 Ibid, 222.
40 Tanvi Misra, "Global Car, Motorcycle, and Bike Ownership, in 1 Infographic," *City Lab*, April 17, 2015, accessed April 17, 2019, https://www.citylab.com/transportation/2015/04/global-car-motorcycle-and-bike-ownership-in-1-infographic/390777.
41 Robin Chase, "Does Everyone in America Own a Car?" U.S. Department of State, March 2010, accessed April 17, 2019, https://static.america.gov/uploads/sites/8/2016/04/You-Asked-Series_Does-Everyone-in-America-Own-a-Car_English_Lo-Res_508.pdf.
42 Misra; "Study Finds Nearly Quarter of German Population Obese," *Xinhua*, May 19, 2017, accessed April 17, 2019, http://www.xinhuanet.com//english/2017-05/19/c_136296081.htm.
43 Ibid.; Chase.
44 Robert C. Atkins, *Dr. Atkins' Diet Revolution: The High Calorie Way to Stay Thin Forever* (New York: David McKay, 1972), 2–3, 10, 134.
45 Ibid., 59.
46 Stephen Yafa, *Grain of Truth: The Real Case for and against Wheat and Gluten* (New York: Avery, 2015), 28.
47 H. J. Teutenberg, "The General Relationship between Diet and Industrialization," in *European Diet from Pre-Industrial to Modern Times*, ed. Elborg Forster and Robert Forster (New York: Torchbooks, 1975), 68; Pelto and Pelto, 520.
48 Olwen Hufton, "Social Conflict and the Grain Supply in Eighteenth-Century France," *Journal of Interdisciplinary History* 14, no. 2 (Autumn 1983): 308.
49 R. J. Bernard, "Peasant Diet in Eighteenth-Century Gevaudan," in *European Diet from Pre-Industrial to Modern Times*, ed. Elborg Forster and Robert Forster (New York: Torchbooks, 1975), 35, 42.
50 Teutenberg, 67–68.
51 "Avocados, Raw, All Commercial Varieties," *USDA FoodData Central*, April 1, 2019, accessed February 14, 2020, https://fdc.nal.usda.gov/fdc-app.html#/food-details/171705/nutrients.
52 "Nuts, Coconut Meat, Raw," *USDA FoodData Central*, April 1, 2019, accessed February 14, 2020, https://fdc.nal.usda.gov/fdc-app.html#/food-details/170169/nutrients.
53 "Egg, Whole, Cooked, Hard-Boiled," *USDA FoodData Central*, April 1, 2019, accessed February 14, 2020, https://fdc.nal.usda.gov/fdc-app.html#/food-details/173424/nutrients.
54 "Oil, Olive, Salad or Cooking," *USDA FoodData Central*, April 1, 2019, accessed February 14, 2020, https://fdc.nal.usda.gov/fdc-app.html#/food-details/171413/nutrients.
55 "Sugars, Granulated," *USDA FoodData Central*, April 1, 201p, accessed February 14, 2020, https://fdc.nal.usda.gov/fdc-app.html#/food-details/169655/nutrients.
56 David Perlmutter, *Grain Brain: The Surprising Truth about Wheat, Carbs, and Sugar—Your Brain's Silent Killers*, rev. ed. (New York: Little, Brown Spark, 2018), 43.
57 Ibid., 12.
58 Ibid., 35.
59 Ibid., 5.
60 Robert Shmerling, "Ditch the Gluten, Improve Your Health?" *Harvard Medical School*, May 2015, last modified April 12, 2017, accessed April 18, 2019, https://www.health.harvard.edu/staying-healthy/ditch-the-gluten-improve-your-health.
61 Lena H. Sun, "Flu Broke Records for Deaths, Illnesses in 2017–2018, New CDC Numbers Show," *Washington Post*, September 27, 2018, accessed April 18, 2019, https://www.washingtonpost.com/national/health-science/last-years-flu-broke-records-for-deaths-and-illnesses-new-cdc-numbers-show/2018/09/26/97cb43fc-c0ed-11e8-90c9-23f963eea204_story.html?noredirect=on&utm_term=.7b7839dfdccc.
62 Yafa, 49.
63 "Tapioca Starch," *USDA FoodData Central*, April 1, 2019, accessed February 14, 2020, https://fdc.nal.usda.gov/fdc-app.html#/food-details/483350/nutrients.
64 "Potato Starch," April 1, 2019, accessed February 14, 2020, https://fdc.nal.usda.gov/fdc-app.html#/food-details/359697/nutrients.

65 Caroline Pullen, "Xanthan Gum—Is This Food Additive Healthy or Harmful?" *Healthline*, May 27, 2017, accessed April 18, 2019, https://www.healthline.com/nutrition/xanthan-gum.

66 Holly Strawbridge, "Going Gluten-Free Just Because? Here's What You Need to Know," *Harvard Medical School*, February 20, 2013, last modified January 18, 2018, accessed April 18, 2019, https://www.health.harvard.edu/blog/going-gluten-free-just-because-heres-what-you-need-to-know-201302205916.

67 Nia Mitchell, Vicki Catenacci, Holly R. Wyatt, and James O. Hill, "Obesity: Overview of an Epidemic," *Psychiatric Clinics of North America* 34, no. 4 (December 2011): 717–732, https://www.ncbi.nlm.nih.gov/pmc/articles/PMC3228640.

68 "Obesity and Overweight," World Health Organization, February 16, 2018, accessed April 13, 2019, https://www.who.int/news-room/fact-sheets/detail/obesity-and-overweight.

69 Monica Reinagel, "Can You Be Overweight and Still Be Healthy?" *Scientific American*, July 31, 2013, accessed April 13, 2019, https://www.scientificamerican.com/article/can-you-be-overweight-still-be-healthy.

70 Taubes, 8–9.

71 "GrainsCompared2017_SR28," Whole Grains Council, accessed April 14, 2019, https://wholegrainscouncil.org/whole-grains-101/health-studies-health-benefits/compare-nutrients-various-grains.

72 "Bread, Whole-Wheat, Commercially Prepared," *USDA FoodData Central*, accessed April 14, 2019, https://fdc.nal.usda.gov/fdc-app.html#/food-details/172688/nutrients; "Bread, Whole-Wheat, Commercially Prepared," *USDA FoodData Central*, accessed April 14, 2019, https://fdc.nal.usda.gov/fdc-app.html#/food-details/335240/nutrients.

73 "Bread, Rye," *USDA FoodData Central*, accessed April 14, 2019, https://fdc.nal.usda.gov/fdc-app.html#/food-details/172684/nutrients.

74 "Pasta, Penne, Black Bean," *Nutritionix Grocery Database*, last modified March 9, 2017, accessed January 25, 2020, https://www.nutritionix.com/i/livegfree/pasta-penne-black-bean/58733743192bd626082dd409; "Pasta, Dry, Unenriched," *USDA FoodData Central*, April 1, 2019, accessed January 24, 2020, https://fdc.nal.usda.gov/fdc-app.html#/food-details/168927/nutrients; "Bread, Whole Wheat," *USDA FoodData Central*, April 1, 2019; accessed January 25, 2020, https://fdc.nal.usda.gov/fdc-app.html#/food-details/339612/nutrients; "Bread, White," *USDA FoodData Central*, April 1, 2019, accessed January 25, 2020, https://fdc.nal.usda.gov/fdc-app.html#/food-details/339504/nutrients; "Bread, Rye," *USDA FoodData Central*, April 1, 2019, accessed January 25, 2020, https://fdc.nal.usda.gov/fdc-app.html#/food-details/339660/nutrients; "Pasta, Gluten Free," *USDA FoodData Central*, April 1, 2019, accessed January 25, 2020, https://fdc.nal.usda.gov/fdc-app.html#/food-details/340356/nutrients; "Pasta, Whole Grain, 51% Whole Wheat, Remaining Unenriched Semolina, Dry," *USDA FoodData Central*, April 1, 2019, accessed January 25, 2020, https://fdc.nal.usda.gov/fdc-app.html#/food-details/168915/nutrients; "Bread, Oat Bran," *USDA FoodData Central*, April 1, 2019, accessed January 25, 2020, https://fdc.nal.usda.gov/fdc-app.html#/food-details/339677/nutrients; "Bread, Barley," *USDA FoodData Central*, April 1, 2019, accessed January 25, 2020, https://fdc.nal.usda.gov/fdc-app.html#/food-details/339697/nutrients; "Bread, Potato," *USDA FoodData Central*, April 1, 2019, accessed January 25, 2020, https://fdc.nal.usda.gov/fdc-app.html#/food-details/339547/nutrients; "Chickpea Pasta," *Fat Secret*, 2019, accessed April 14, 2019, https://www.fatsecret.com/calories-nutrition/banza/chickpea-pasta; "Red Lentil Pasta-Pasta, MyFitnessPal, 2020, accessed January 25, 2020, https://www.myfitnesspal.com/food/calories/red-lentil-pasta-pasta-568563489.

75 "GrainsCompared2017_SR28;" "Cornmeal, Whole-Grain, Yellow," *USDA FoodData Central*, April 1, 2019, accessed January 25, 2020, https://fdc.nal.usda.gov/fdc-app.html#/food-details/169697/nutrients; "Rice, Brown, Long-Grain, Raw (Includes Foods for USDA's Food Distribution Program)," *USDA FoodData Central*, April 1, 2019, accessed January 25, 2020, https://fdc.nal.usda.gov/fdc-app.html#/food-details/169703/nutrients; "Rye Grain," *USDA FoodData Central*, April 1, 2019, accessed January 25, 2020, https://fdc.nal.usda.gov/fdc-app.html#/food-details/168884/nutrients; "Oats, Raw," *USDA FoodData Central*, April 1, 2019, accessed January 25, 2020, https://fdc.nal.usda.gov/fdc-app.html#/food-details/340734/nutrients.

76 "GrainsCompared2017_SR28."

77 "Wheat, Hard White," *USDA FoodData Central*, April 1, 2019, accessed January 25, 2020, https://fdc.nal.usda.gov/fdc-app.html#/food-details/169719/nutrients; "Wheat, Hard Red Spring," *USDA FoodData Central*, April 1, 2019, accessed January 25, 2020, https://fdc.nal.usda.gov/fdc-app.html#/food-details/168889/nutrients; "Wheat, Hard Red Winter," *USDA FoodData Central*, April 1, 2019, accessed January 25, 2020, https://fdc.nal.usda.gov/fdc-app.html#/food-details/168890/nutrients; "Wheat, Durum," *USDA FoodData Central*, April 1, 2019, accessed January 25, 2020, https://fdc.nal.usda.gov/fdc-app.html#/food-details/169721/nutrients; "Semolina, Unenriched," *USDA FoodData Central*, April 1, 2019, accessed January 25, 2020, https://fdc.nal.usda.gov/fdc-app.html#/food-details/168933/nutrients.

78 "Corn—October Grain of the Month," Whole Grains Council, accessed April 12, 2019, https://wholegrainscouncil.org/whole-grains-101/easy-ways-enjoy-whole-grains/grain-month-calendar/corn-%E2%80%93-october-grain-month.
79 Yafa, 99.
80 Ibid.; Brouns, van Buul, and Shewry; Peter R. Shewry and Sandra Hey, "Do "Ancient" Wheat Species Differ from Modern Bread Wheat in Their Contents of Bioactive Components?" *Journal of Cereal Science* 65 (September 2015): 236–243, https://www.sciencedirect.com/science/article/pii/S073352101530045X.
81 Delphine Roger, "The Middle East and South Asia," in *The Cambridge World History of Food*, vol. 2, ed. Kenneth F. Kiple and Kriemhild Conee Ornelas (Cambridge, UK: Cambridge University Press, 2000), 1149.
82 Ibid., 1145.
83 Ibid., 1147.
84 Ibid., 1141.
85 Miller and Wetterstrom, 1133; William Rubel, *Bread: A Global History* (London: Reaktion Books, 2011), 28.
86 Roger, 1146.
87 Maguelonne Toussaint-Samat, *A History of Food*, expanded ed., trans. Anthea Bell (Chichester, UK: Wiley-Blackwell, 2009), 125, 129–131.
88 Ibid., 129, 132.
89 Rajesh Kumar, Hui-Ju Tsai, Xiumei Hong, Xin Liu, Guoying Wang, Colleen Pearson, Katherin Ortiz, Melanie Fu, Jacqueline A. Pongracic, Howard Bauchner, and Xiobin Wang, "Race, Ancestry, and Development of Food-Allergen Sensitization in Early Childhood," *Pediatrics* 128, no. 4 (October 2011): 821–829, https://www.ncbi.nlm.nih.gov/pmc/articles/PMC3182844.
90 Clark Spencer Larsen, "Dietary Reconstruction and Nutritional Assessment of Past Peoples: The Bioanthropological Record," in *The Cambridge World History of Food*, vol. 1, ed. Kenneth F. Kiple and Kriemhild Conee Ornelas (Cambridge, UK: Cambridge University Press, 2000), 15.
91 Alan H. Goodman and Debra L. Martin, "Reconstructing Health Profiles from Skeletal Remains," in *The Backbone of History: Health and Nutrition in the Western Hemisphere*, ed. Richard H. Steckel and Jerome C. Rose (Cambridge, UK: Cambridge University Press, 2002), 20.
92 Larsen, "Dietary Reconstruction and Nutritional Assessment of Past Peoples," 15.
93 J. Lawrence Angel, "Health as a Crucial Factor in the Changes from Hunting to Developed Farming in the Eastern Mediterranean," in *Paleopathology at the Origins of Agriculture*, ed. Mark Nathan Cohen and George J. Armelagos (Orlando, FL: Academic Press, 1984), 62; Patricia Smith, Ofer Bar-Yosef, and Andrew Sillen, "Archaeological and Skeletal Evidence for Dietary Change during the Late Pleistocene/Early Holocene in the Levant," in *Paleopathology at the Origins of Agriculture*, ed. Mark Nathan Cohen and George J. Armelagos (Orlando, FL: Academic Press, 1984), 112.
94 Rubel, 11–12.
95 Yafa, 38–39.
96 "What's Lacking?" *Einkorn.com*, 2015, accessed April 19, 2019, https://www.einkorn.com/whats-lacking.
97 Yafa, 84.
98 Ibid., 42.
99 Ibid.; James F. Fixx, *The Complete Book of Running* (New York: Random House, 1977), 172.
100 Yafa, 85.
101 Ibid., 87.
102 James Baldwin, "From The Fire Next Time," in *The Norton Anthology of American Literature*, 2nd ed., Nina Baym, Francis Murphy, Ronald Gottesman, Hershel Parker, Laurence B. Holland, William H. Pritchard, and David Kalstone (New York and London: Norton, 1986), 2384.
103 Te-Tzu Chang, "Rice," in *The Cambridge World History of Food*, vol. 1, ed. Kenneth F. Kiple and Kriemhild Conee Ornelas (Cambridge, UK: Cambridge University Press, 2000), 135; Nesbitt, 56.
104 Chang, 134.
105 Ibid.
106 Ibid., 139.
107 Sarah Zhang, "Rice Was First Grown at Least 9,400 Years Ago," *The Atlantic*, May 29, 2017, accessed April 3, 2019, https://www.theatlantic.com/science/archive/2017/05/rice-domestication/528288.
108 Chang, 144.
109 Larsen, "Dietary Reconstruction and Nutritional Assessment of Past Peoples," 15.

110 Chang, 144.
111 "Rice, White, Medium Grain, Raw, Unenriched," *USDA FoodData Central*, April 1, 2019, accessed January 25, 2020, https://fdc.nal.usda.gov/fdc-app.html#/food-details/169760/nutrients; "Rice Flour, White, Unenriched," *USDA FoodData Central*, April 1, 2019, accessed January 25, 2020, https://fdc.nal.usda.gov/fdc-app.html#/food-details/169714/nutrients.
112 "Rice, White, Long-Grain, Parboiled, Unenriched, Dry," *USDA FoodData Central*, April 1, 2019, accessed January 25, 2020, https://fdc.nal.usda.gov/fdc-app.html#/food-details/169758/nutrients.
113 Chang, 132.
114 Ibid., 144.
115 Ibid., 132.
116 Nesbitt, 56.
117 Judith A. Carney and Richard Nicholas Rosomoff, *In the Shadow of Slavery: Africa's Botanical Legacy in the Atlantic World* (Berkeley: University of California Press, 2009), 22.
118 C. Wayne Smith, *Crop Production: Evolution, History, and Technology* (New York: Wiley, 1995), 224.
119 Chang, 135.
120 Smith, 223.
121 Chang, 139.
122 Meredith Sayles Hughes, *Glorious Grasses: The Grains* (Minneapolis, MN: Lerner Publications, 1999), 34.
123 Nesbitt, 56.
124 Smith, 228, 232; Henry C. Dethloff, *A History of the American Rice Industry, 1685–1985* (College Station: Texas A & M University Press, 1988), 4.
125 Carney and Rosomoff, 150–151; Smith, 233.
126 Jill Dubisch, "Low Country Fevers: Cultural Adaptations to Malaria in Antebellum South Carolina," *Social Science and Medicine* 21, no. 6 (February 1985): 643.
127 Bill Laws, *Fifty Plants that Changed the Course of History* (Buffalo, NY and Richmond Hill, Ontario: Firefly Books, 2015), 145.
128 Vaughan and Geissler, 48.
129 Jimmy Louie, "Breads and Cereals," in *Essentials of Human Nutrition*, 5th ed., ed. Jim Mann and A. Stewart Truswell (Oxford, UK: Oxford University Press, 2017), 274; Bernard Venn, "Legumes," in *Essentials of Human Nutrition*, 5th ed., ed. Jim Mann and A. Stewart Truswell (Oxford, UK: Oxford University Press, 2017), 277.
130 Sarah Zielinski, "Man Cannot Live on Rice and Beans Alone (But Many Do)," *NPR*, May 3, 2012, accessed June 23, 2019, https://www.npr.org/sections/thesalt/2012/05/03/151932410/man-cannot-live-on-rice-and-beans-alone-but-many-do.
131 Frederick L. Dunn, "Beriberi," in *The Cambridge World History of Food*, vol. 1, ed. Kenneth F. Kiple and Kriemhild Conee Ornelas (Cambridge, UK: Cambridge University Press, 2000), 914.
132 Ibid., 915.
133 Ibid., 916.
134 Larsen, "Dietary Reconstruction and Nutritional Assessment of Past Peoples," 15.
135 Elmer Verner McCollum, *A History of Nutrition: The Sequence of Ideas in Nutrition Investigations* (Boston: Houghton Mifflin, 1957), 230.
136 "Sir Frederick Hopkins," The Nobel Prize Organisation, 2019, accessed May 17, 2019, https://www.nobelprize.org/prizes/medicine/1929/hopkins/facts.
137 George Wolf, "Vitamin A," in *The Cambridge World History of Food*, vol. 1, ed. Kenneth F. Kiple and Kriemhild Conee Ornelas (Cambridge, UK: Cambridge University Press, 2000), 744; David I. Thurnham, "Vitamin A and Carotenoids," in *Essentials of Human Nutrition*, 5th ed., ed. Jim Mann and A. Stewart Truswell (Oxford: Oxford University Press, 2017), 191.
138 Jennifer A. Woolfe, *Sweet Potato: An Untapped Food Resource* (Cambridge, UK: Cambridge University Press, 1992), 147.
139 George Thottappilly, "Introductory Remarks," in *The Sweetpotato*, ed. Gad Loebenstein and George Thottappilly (Dordrecht: Springer, 2009), 5.
140 Thurnham, 199.
141 Ellen Messer, "Maize," in *The Cambridge World History of Food*, ed. Kenneth F. Kiple and Kriemhild Conee Ornelas (Cambridge, UK: Cambridge University Press, 2000), 100.
142 *The Illustrated Encyclopedia of Fruits, Vegetables, and Herbs* (New York: Chartwell Books, 2017), 228.
143 Messer, 100.
144 Ibid., 98.

145 Betty Fussell, *The Story of Corn* (New York: Knopf, 1992), 167.
146 Waverley Root and Richard de Rochemont, *Eating in America: A History* (Hopewell, NJ: Ecco Press, 1995), 34; Aimee Tucker, "Succotash," *Yankee* magazine, July 28, 2015, accessed April 1, 2019, https://newengland.com/yankee-magazine/food/succotash-recipe-with-a-history.
147 Fussell, 186.
148 Messer, 103.
149 "Corn—October Grain of the Month."
150 Messer, 99.
151 Ibid., 108.
152 Arturo Warman, *Corn and Capitalism: How a Botanical Bastard Grew to Global Dominance*, trans. Nancy L. Westrate (Chapel Hill and London: University of North Carolina Press, 2003): 215.
153 Richard H. Steckel, Jerome C. Rose, Clark Spencer Larsen, and Phillip L. Walker. "Skeletal Health in the Western Hemisphere from 4000 BC to the Present." *Evolutionary Anthropology* 11, no. 4 (August 13, 2002): 149–150.
154 Larsen, "Dietary Reconstruction and Nutritional Assessment of Past Peoples," 21.
155 Ibid., 15.
156 Ibid.; Steckel, Rose, Larsen, and Walker, 149–150.
157 Susan Kent, "Iron Deficiency and Anemia of Chronic Diseases," in *The Cambridge World History of Food*, vol.1, ed. Kenneth F. Kiple and Kriemhild Conee Ornelas (Cambridge, UK: Cambridge University Press, 2000), 923–924.
158 Jared Diamond, "The Worst Mistake in the History of the Human Race," *Discover*, May 1, 1999, accessed July 21, 2019, http://discovermagazine.com/1987/may/02-the-worst-mistake-in-the-history-of-the-human-race.
159 Clark Spencer Larsen, *Our Origins: Discovering Physical Anthropology* (New York and London: Norton, 2017), 393, 406–411.
160 Ibid., 392–393, 396–397.
161 Kent, 923–924.
162 Ibid.
163 Walton C. Galinat, "Maize: Gift from America's First Peoples," in *Chilis to Chocolate: Food the Americas Gave the World*, ed. Nelson Foster and Linda S. Cordell (Tucson and London: University of Arizona Press, 1992), 47.
164 Messer, 105–106.
165 Jerome S. Handler and Robert S. Corruccini, "Plantation Slave Life in Barbados: A Physical Anthropological Analysis," *Journal of Interdisciplinary History* 14, no. 1 (Summer 1983): 75.
166 Sylvia A. Johnson, *Tomatoes, Potatoes, Corn, and Beans: How the Foods of the Americas Changed Eating around the World* (New York: Atheneum Books, 1997), 110.
167 Kenneth F. Kiple and Virginia H. Kiple, "Deficiency Diseases in the Caribbean," in *Caribbean Slavery in the Atlantic World: A Student Reader*, ed. Verena A. Shepherd and Hilary McD. Beckles (Princeton, NJ: Markus Wiener Publishers, 2000), 786.
168 Ibid., 473–474.
169 Robert W. Fogel, Stanley L. Engerman, Roderick Floud, Gerald Friedman, Robert A. Margo, Kenneth Sokoloff, Richard H. Steckel, T. James Trussell, Georgia Villaflor, and Kenneth W. Wachter, "Secular Changes in American and British Stature and Nutrition," *Journal of Interdisciplinary History* 14, no. 2 (Autumn 1983): 469–470.
170 Robert William Fogel, "Nutrition and the Decline in Mortality Since 1700: Some Preliminary Findings," in *Long-Term Factors in American Economic Growth*, ed. Stanley L. Engerman and Robert E. Gallman (Chicago and London: University of Chicago Press, 1986), 471.
171 Handler and Corruccini, 72.
172 Jean-Louis Flandrin, "Introduction: The Early Modern Period," in *Food: A Culinary History from Antiquity to the Present*, Jean-Louis Flandrin and Massimo Montanari, trans. Clarissa Botsford, Arthur Goldhammer, Charles Lambert, Frances M. Lopez-Morillas, and Sylvia Stevens (New York: Columbia University Press, 1999), 355.
173 Hughes, 55.
174 Warman, 108.
175 Messer, 105.
176 Warman, 101.
177 Cynthia Clampitt, *Midwest Maize: How Corn Shaped the U.S. Heartland* (Urbana: University of Illinois Press, 2015), 9; Warman, 42–44.

178 Messer, 106.
179 Ibid.
180 Ibid., 106–107.
181 Ibid., 105–106.
182 Ibid., 99.
183 Ibid., 108.
184 Toussaint-Samat, 157.
185 Messer, 109.
186 Ibid.
187 J. D. L. Hansen, "Protein-Energy Malnutrition," in *The Cambridge World History of Food*, vol. 1, ed. Kenneth F. Kiple and Kriemhild Conee Ornelas (Cambridge, UK: Cambridge University Press, 2000), 980.

13 Roots and Tubers

13.1 DEFINITIONS

The simplest definition of plants bifurcates them into aboveground (shoot) and underground (root) portions. Recognition that plants were more than shoots enlarged the food supply among humanity's predecessors. Division of plants into shoot and root risks equating all subterranean components as roots, the structures that anchor plants in the ground. From soil, roots absorb water and minerals, both discussed in Chapter 2. A root crop is often a swollen taproot. Examples are carrot (*Daucus carota ssp. sativus*), radish (*Raphanus raphanistrum ssp. sativus*), rutabaga (*Brassica napobrassica*), and turnip (*Brassica rapa ssp. rapa*), are considered vegetables, and are excluded from this chapter. In contrast to roots, which grow downward, plants have stems, which grow upward. The subterranean part of a stem is a bulb, corm, rhizome, stolon, or tuber depending on its structure. A tuber may be visualized as an enlarged, short, underground stem. This chapter examines the tubers potato (*Solanum tuberosum*) and yam (*Dioscorea species*), and the roots cassava (*Manihot esculenta*) and sweet potato (*Ipomoea batatas*). Like root crops, tubers are vegetables. Potatoes, yams, sweet potatoes, and cassava's status as world staples mandates treatment separate from Chapter 15's consideration of vegetables.

Swollen roots and tubers—which store water and nutrients upon which plants draw during lean times—are evolutionary innovations to environments with uneven rainfall. This function leads scientists to classify both as underground storage organs (USOs). USOs may have minerals, vitamins, proteins, and carbohydrates. Tubers tend to have more starch and therefore more calories than roots. For example, 100 grams of potato have seventy-seven calories, whereas the same amount of carrot has forty-one calories.[1] Neither has inordinate energy because water is the main constituent, potatoes being 79.3 percent and carrots 88.3 percent. For few calories, potatoes supply ample vitamins B_6 (pyridoxine) and C, potassium, magnesium, fiber, and phytochemicals that complement vitamin C's role as antioxidant. Carrots have vitamin A precursor β-carotene, vitamins B_6, B_7 (biotin), and K, potassium, fiber, and antioxidants. Although consumers seldom conceive tubers as protein sources, potatoes have all essential amino acids. Chapter 2 discussed these nutrients and others. Later sections quantify potato, sweet potato, cassava, and yams' nutrients.

The previous paragraphs cautioned against the colloquial equation of tubers and roots. A tuber such as potato yields many potatoes per plant, whereas a root like as carrot, enlarging its taproot, produces just one edible per plant. Sweet potato, however, thickens several roots and so produces many edibles per plant. In this way, it resembles tubers more than taproot crops such as carrot, beet, radish, and turnip, all mentioned earlier. Moreover, a tuber can regenerate into a new plant. For example, a single potato produces several buds, known as eyes. It may be cut into sections, each with at least one eye. When these sections are planted, each germinates into a new plant. Crops that develop from the taproot cannot produce new plants if the edible part is planted. Not a taproot, the sweet potato may be propagated from parts of a root or vine. Tubers' capacity for regeneration must have recommended them to prehistoric peoples for cultivation. Domestication of potato, sweet potato, cassava, and at least one yam species occurred in South America, Mesoamerica, the Caribbean Islands, or their combination, whereas Africa and Asia domesticated other yams. Potato, sweet potato, cassava, and yam became world crops during the global plant exchanges that followed Italian Spanish mariner Christopher Columbus' (1451–1506) voyages.

13.2 DIETARY DISSONANCE

Europeans' New World incursion created dietary dissonance. Heirs to southwestern Asia's seed agriculture, they had long eaten wheat (*Triticum monococcum, Triticum dicoccon, Triticum aestivum,* and *Triticum durum*), oats (*Avena sativa*), rye (*Secale cereale*), barley (*Hordeum vulgare*), peas (*Pisum sativum*), cabbage (*Brassica oleracea var. capitata*), and other plants propagated by seeds. These crops yielded their edible portions above ground, leading Europeans to treat such circumstances as natural. Even taproot crops such as carrots and turnips germinated from seeds. Cassava, sweet potato, yam, and potato being propagated from buds, however, tropical America deviated from this pattern. Suspicious of novelties, Europeans adopted potatoes slowly, as discussed later.[2] Additionally, temperate Europe lacked the tropical conditions best for cassava, sweet potatoes, and yams. Originating in cool Andean highlands, potatoes were suited to northern Europe's climate. But their homeland, being in the tropics, had uniform daylengths absent in Europe. Consequently, the initial attempts to grow them in Europe failed because its long summer days stimulated plants to yield abundant foliage at tubers' expense. Being toxic, foliage was worthless as food and feed. In these ways, the European encounter with American tubers and roots underscored earlier chapters' emphasis on geography's role in shaping diets.

13.3 ROOTS

13.3.1 Sweet Potato

Derided as "poor man's food," "poor man's crop," and 'women's work,' sweet potatoes resemble yams, but their differences—discussed later—include separate prehistories and histories.[3] The root's origins are uncertain. A candidate is the region between the Yucatan Peninsula in the west and Colombia and Venezuela as far east as the Orinoco River. The isthmus that connects North

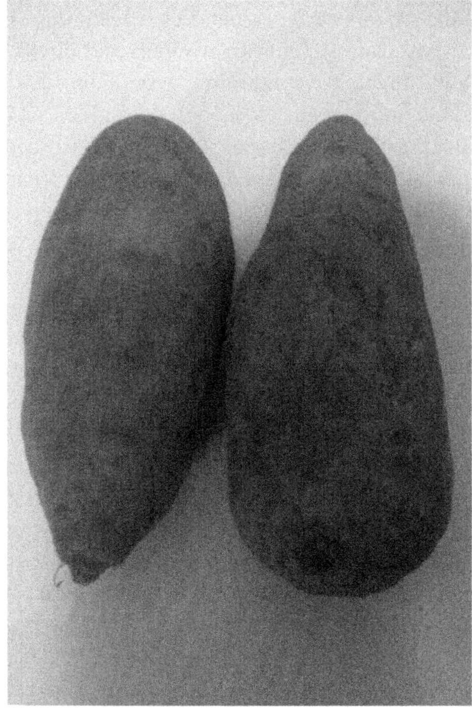

FIGURE 13.1 Sweet potatoes. (Photo from author.)

and South America, and is designated Central America, has the greatest diversity of sweet potato varieties and so might be home to the earliest cultivation.[4] In Central America, Panama has emerged as sweet potatoes' probable birthplace. Another hypothesis gives this distinction to the Caribbean because the wild relative *Ipomoea tiliacea* is a native. Alternatively, the wild relative *Ipomoea trifida*, indigenous to Mexico, makes it the possible ancestral homeland.

These locations disclosed *Ipomoea batatas*' tropical origins. Although cultivated in the subtropics and in temperate locales with warm, long growing seasons, plant and roots cease growth below 15 degrees Celsius (59 degrees Fahrenheit).[5] Injury or death occurs below 10 degrees Celsius (50 degrees Fahrenheit). Frost is always lethal. The plant is perennial, though cold intolerance makes it an annual above 23.5 degrees latitude. Moreover, temperate areas' long summer days favor growth of vines over roots, diminishing yields. Lands above 40 degrees latitude do not support sweet potatoes.[6]

13.3.2 Origins and Early Dispersal

The earliest evidence of sweet potato comes from Peru about 8000 BCE, but the root may have been domesticated only later given that the next oldest leftover dates around 2000 BCE.[7] Botanical remains may not pinpoint chronology because preservation is rare, especially in the tropics. Even if sweet potato was not domesticated as early as 8000 BCE, debris from Peru demonstrates consumption. If the root was domesticated later, consumption ten millennia ago would have been of wild precursors. The Inca ate sweet potatoes in addition to potatoes and corn (*Zea mays*). To the north, the root and grass fed the Maya. Although Europeans spread potatoes, tomatoes (*Solanum esculentum*), corn, peanuts (*Arachis hypogaea*), beans (*Phaseolus vulgaris, P. lunatus, P. acutifolius,* and *P. coccineus*), and other edibles worldwide, they played a secondary role in sweet potato diffusion.

Several Pacific islands, including New Zealand, grew sweet potatoes before Columbus' voyages and acquired them from South American natives, Polynesians, ocean currents, birds, or a combination of natural processes. South of the equator, Tongans and Samoans were eating sweet potatoes by 1000 BCE.[8] Western Polynesia's Lapita may have aided this early dispersal. Northeast of these islands, the Marquesas had the root by 300 CE. To the west, sweet potatoes reached Micronesia around 50 CE. East of Micronesia, the Cook Islands had sweet potatoes about 1000. New Zealanders were eating the root by 1300. Between the fifteenth and eighteenth centuries, it spread to Hawaii, Easter Island, and New Guinea. British archeologist Jack Golson (b. 1926) challenged this chronology for New Guinea, arguing that people began clearing forest around 800 CE for sweet potato farming.[9]

13.3.3 Sweet Potatoes, New Guinea, and Health

In New Guinea's Wantoat Valley, sweet potatoes were the primary food and almost the only domesticated plant.[10] The valley typified the mountains, where the root supplied up to 90 percent of calories.[11] Alone among New Guinean crops, sweet potatoes yield food above 1,200 meters (1,312.3 yards or 3,937 feet).[12] International Potato Center researcher Jennifer Woolfe judged them the "staff of life of the highland Papuan."[13] New Guineans tend to harvest part of a root, taking care not to damage the plant so that it continues to produce.[14] New Guinea is well positioned for this practice because vines and roots, being perennials in the tropics as noted, supply edibles year-round. Sweet potatoes may have reached the island only around 1700, but once established, they reconfigured the economy. They were favored over traditional crops such as taro (*Colocasia esculenta*) because they required less labor, better tolerated pests and pathogens, and yielded more calories and nutrients on infertile soils.

New Guineans fed them to pigs (*Sus scrofa domesticus*), symbols of wealth and prestige more than meat. Eating leaves, vines, and roots, pigs welcomed this arrangement, particularly because they preferred sweet potatoes over the taro they had previously consumed. Desire to maximize status through pig herds incentivized sweet potato monoculture over the diversity of plants that had once sustained the island. Undernutrition diminished birthrate and increased infant mortality.

Women suffered inadequate nutrition and excessive workloads. Pregnancies did not spare them the brunt of farm labor. British anthropologist John Reader (b. 1937) estimated that pregnant New Guinean women who ate little besides sweet potatoes got only 40 percent of necessary calories, 74 percent of protein, and 62 percent of iron.[15] Newborns were underweight, and 20 percent died before age 5. Many survivors did not reach full stature and suffered cognitive impairment. Faulting the "dietary inadequacies of the sweet potato," Reader also condemned an economic system that funneled food to pigs and overburdened women, even when pregnant.[16] His analysis implied that sweet potatoes permitted moderate activity but not strenuous exertions.

These criticisms do not justify sweet potatoes' abandonment. In a global economy, New Guinea imports food from Australia and other nations. As meat, white bread, sucrose ($C_{12}H_{22}O_{11}$)—discussed in Chapters 2 and 11—processed foods, and other Western commodities displaced sweet potatoes, New Guineans became obese and suffered heart disease and type 2 diabetes.[17] These maladies indicate that sweet potatoes better nourished them than imports.

13.3.4 Europe's Encounter with Sweet Potatoes

Columbus sampled sweet potatoes in 1492 on Hispaniola and Cuba, comparing their flavor with roasted chestnuts (*Castanea sativa*) and their size with radishes.[18] Another Spaniard compared them with marzipan, a dessert with almonds (*Amygdalus communis*) and sucrose.[19] A third likened their sweetness to jam. Hispaniola's Tainos called sweet potatoes *batatas*, a word the Spanish mispronounced *patatas*.

Spain's encounter with the Andean potato in the 1530s, treated later, confused the situation. The Inca called potatoes *papas*. Superficial similarities between sweet potatoes and potatoes and between *patatas* and *papas* led Spaniards and other Europeans to conflate both as "potatoes." Recognition of differences rendered the tropical root as sweet because it was less starchy than the Andean tuber, which became the white potato to differentiate it from the sweet potato. Some sweet potatoes being white, this language may perpetuate confusion.

13.3.5 Sweet Potatoes' Post-Columbian Dispersal

Columbus returned to Spain in 1493 with sweet potatoes.[20] About 1600 Portugal introduced them to West Africa, mainland Southeast Asia, and Indonesia.[21] Mali and Senegal's Bambara combined them with peanuts, tomatoes, okra (*Abelmoschus esculentus*), and chicken (*Gallus gallus domesticus*) in the stew *mafe*. Later incursions brought the root to India, China, and Japan, though China's acquisition remains controversial. Woolfe asserted that Spain carried sweet potatoes to the Philippines in 1521.[22] Alternatively, Filipinos might have acquired the root later from New Guinea. During World War II, it saved them from undernutrition and starvation when little else was available.[23] In addition to roots, Southeast Asians eat young leaves, petioles, and stem tips, all of which have β-carotene, vitamin C, and protein.

One story avers that a Chinese businessman brought the root from the Philippines to China in 1594, but this year may be too late given probable references to it in Yunnan Province as early as 1563.[24] Its value was well enough known that the rice crop's failure in 1594 led Fukien Province's governor Chin Hsueh-tseng to urge cultivation to prevent famine.[25] Thereafter, Fukien residents designated sweet potatoes the "*Dioscorea* of Governor Chin," an error that confuses them with yams and that persists today. Farmers in southeastern China's Guangdong Province grew sweet potatoes on hills unsuitable for rice (*Oryza sativa*). Although yams were an option, these smallholders preferred sweet potatoes, which produced more food per hectare, and quicker, than yams. High yields made the root a staple as potatoes were in northern Europe. Easy cultivation recommended sweet potatoes in southern China, where the subtropical climate suited them. Besides these areas, the root spread to high latitudes and by 2012 was grown in the northernmost province of Heilongjiang.[26] To the west and south, Inner Mongolia also cultivates sweet potatoes. The root yields in China's sandy loams, where moisture and nutrients are inadequate for many crops. By 2017, China produced almost two-thirds of the world's sweet potatoes.[27]

13.3.6 Sweet Potatoes, Okinawa, and Health

Tradition credited Japanese official Noguni Sokan in 1605 or 1615 with planting sweet potatoes from China on Okinawa Island, where the warm climate accommodated them.[28] Okinawa's vulnerability to typhoons that flattened rice plants led farmers to plant sweet potatoes because their subterranean edibles were safe from storms. Another advantage was roots' resistance to insects that plagued rice and other crops. American internist Bradley J. Willcox and coauthors stated that sweet potatoes' nutrients and calories increased the island's population from 120,000 to 200,000 in "the first decades of the 1600s."[29] A 2016 estimate put Okinawan sweet potato consumption at 70 percent of daily calories.[30]

American physician and holistic-medicine advocate Andrew Thomas Weil (b. 1942) attributed Okinawans' longevity to diet, activity, and sociability.[31] Dubbed "the land of the immortals," Okinawa has thirty-four centenarians per 100,000 inhabitants compared to under ten in the United States.[32] Heart disease, stroke, and cancers are uncommon on the island, a phenomenon Willcox and colleagues ascribed to a plant diet, including sweet potatoes and yams.[33] They lauded both for having phytochemicals—discussed in Chapter 2—like carotenoids (vitamin A precursors), saponins, and flavonoids.

13.3.7 Sweet Potatoes North of Okinawa

North of Okinawa, Japan's four main islands from south to north are Kyushu, Shikoku, Honshu, and Hokkaido. Movement north increased distance from the equator, cooled the climate, shortened growing seasons, and hindered sweet potato agriculture. At 36.2 degrees latitude north, Japan's main islands are at the fringe of the crop's range. Sweet potatoes' absence from the northern islands left Japan vulnerable to the 1732 Kyoho Famine. That year cold rains damaged wheat and barley on Kyushu, Shikoku, and Honshu.[34] Moisture and decaying organic matter increased numbers of insects, which ate wheat, barley, and rice, causing grain shortages. Twenty percent of northern Kyushu's residents may have starved, focusing attention on sweet potatoes as a solution to food insecurity.[35] Perishable, roots could not be grown in the south for shipment north when famine threatened. Northern islands would need their own supply. In 1735, Confucian scholar Konyo Aoki (1698–1769) derived the first sweet potato variety that matured quickly enough for the north's short growing seasons.[36] He sent seed sweet potatoes, known as slips, and cultivation instructions to farmers near Tokyo, ensuring that the capital had enough food to avert future famines.

Like the potato in Europe, sweet potatoes entered Japan when population strained the land's capacity to feed it. When the root entered Okinawa in the early seventeenth century, commoners ate rice, fish, soybeans (*Glycine max*), radishes, kelp (species in the order Laminariales), buckwheat (*Fagopyrum esculentum*), and burdock (*Arctium* species) roots. This diet supplied complete protein, carbohydrates, omega 3 fatty acids, minerals calcium, iron, iodine, phosphorus, potassium, selenium, manganese, magnesium, copper, zinc, vitamins A, B_1 (thiamine or thiamin), B_2, B_3, B_6, B_9 (folate, folic acid, or pteroylmonoglutamic acid), B_{12} (cobalamin), C, D, K, fiber, and phytochemicals.

13.3.8 Divergent Opinions about Sweet Potatoes' Nutriment

Table 13.1 shows that sweet potatoes duplicated many of these nutrients, mostly in meager quantities, while adding vitamins B_5 (pantothenic acid) and E and choline, which nutritionists classify as neither vitamin nor mineral. American olericulturists Vincent E. Rubatzky and Mas Yamaguchi judged sweet potatoes, being 1.5–2.5 percent protein by mass, inadequate in it.[37] Amounts of zinc, selenium, calcium, iron, phosphorus, sodium, and vitamins B_2 (riboflavin), B_3 (niacin or nicotinic acid),

TABLE 13.1
Nutrients in Sweet Potatoes 100 g

Nutrient	Sweet Potato	%DV
Calories	86	N/A
Protein (g)	1.6	N/A
Fat (g)	0.05	N/A
Carbs (g)	20	N/A
Fiber (g)	3	N/A
	Minerals	
Ca (mg)	30	3
Fe (mg)	0.61	3.4
Mg (mg)	25	6.3
P (mg)	47	4.7
K (mg)	337	9.6
Na (mg)	55	2.3
Zn (mg)	0.3	2
Cu (mg)	0.15	7.5
Mn (mg)	0.26	13
Se (mcg)	0.6	0.9
	Vitamins	
A (IU)	14,187	283.7
B_1 (mg)	0.08	5.3
B_2 (mg)	0.06	3.5
B_3 (mg)	0.56	2.8
B_5 (mg)	0.8	8
B_6 (mg)	0.21	10.5
B_9 (mcg)	11	2.8
B_{12} (mcg)	0	0
C (mg)	2.4	4
D (IU)	0	0
E (mg)	0.26	1.7
K (mcg)	1.8	2.3

B_9, B_{12}, C, D, E, and K fall below 5 percent of U.S. Food and Drug Administration (FDA) daily value (DV) per 100 grams of root.[38] The body converts sweet potatoes' α- and β-carotene—in orange and yellow flesh but not white—into vitamin A, a nutrient that fish furnish in traditional Okinawan diets. One hundred grams of orange sweet potato nearly triple the DV of vitamin A equivalents and supply 11.3 percent of manganese and 16.2 percent of vitamin B_6.[39] Besides these nutrients, purple sweet potatoes have anthocyanins: flavonoids that may slow cancer cell growth, sharpen vision, memory, and cognition, and protect against heart disease and pleurisy.[40] Non-Western medicine uses anthocyanins to treat liver problems and high blood pressure.

Sweet potatoes' modest nutriment contrasts with *The Illustrated Encyclopedia of Fruits, Vegetables, and Herbs'* (2017) belief that they "are a highly nutritious food."[41] American nutritionist Stephanie Pedersen touted their "outrageously high nutrient content."[42] American food writer Kelly Pfeiffer listed sweet potatoes, but not potatoes, among "ten superfoods."[43] American economist, historian, and 1993 Nobel laureate in economics Robert William Fogel (1926–2013) and American economist and historian Stanley Lewis Engerman (b. 1936) judged sweet potatoes superior to the potato, praising their vitamins A and C and calcium.[44]

Table 13.1 indicates that sweet potatoes are rich in vitamin A but have only 4 percent DV for vitamin C and 3 percent for calcium per 100 grams. A later section estimates 100 grams of potatoes at roughly 26.7 percent of DV for vitamin C, more than sextupling that in the same quantity of sweet potatoes. Beyond these data, this chapter cautions against undue exuberance for sweet potatoes. It argues that potatoes, not sweet potatoes, are the world's most nourishing food.

13.3.9 Sweet Potatoes, Japan, and Large Populations

Seventeenth-century Japan's burgeoning population needed energy besides nutrients, but sweet potatoes have fewer calories per 100 grams than buckwheat, most fish, soybeans, and rice.[45] The root enhanced Japanese diets by providing more nutrients and calories per hectare than rice, soybeans, buckwheat, radishes, and burdock roots. Inadequate seventeenth-century data complicate comparisons, though Japan's 2014 sweet potato harvest was 23.3 metric tons per hectare.[46] By contrast, that year, Japan averaged 6.7 metric tons of rice per hectare.[47] In 2016, Japan's soybeans yielded 3.1–5.9 metric tons per hectare.[48] Like potatoes in temperate regions, sweet potatoes fed more people per unit land than seed crops.

Sweet potatoes thrived in Japan's volcanic soils, providing an alternative to other vegetables, rice, soybeans, and buckwheat. Dense plantings created leaf canopies that minimized weeds, thereby reducing labor. Although less marketable than rice, sweet potatoes aided subsistence. World War II heightened dependence on them. In August 1945, the United States dropped atomic bombs on Hiroshima and Nagasaki, Japan, irradiating people, livestock, and crops. Their edibles underground, sweet potatoes were among the few safe options. Japanese survived postwar shortages by eating the roots, leaves, and vines with rice, a dish known as *suiton*.[49]

Sweet potatoes remain in Japanese cuisine. Street vendors roast roots to produce the snack *yakiimo*. Urbanites visit shops to sample sweet potato pastries, ice cream, and custards. Students eat *daigaku imo*—university potatoes in English—fried strips that resemble French fries and are topped with sesame (*Sesamum indicum*) seeds and syrup. Japan's expensive restaurants in Kawagoe serve seven courses, all from the root. Patrons choose among sweet potato noodles, sauces, soups, tempura, and desserts. Popular is *suwito poteto*: sweet potato, butter, cream, brandy, cinnamon (*Cinnamomum verum*), vanilla (*Vanilla planifolia*), and nutmeg (*Myristica fragrans*). Connoisseurs favor roots with dry textures and mild sweetness. Humbler is the sweet potato–rice fusion *imo gohan*.

13.3.10 Sweet Potatoes in North America

The root predated Europeans' arrival in North America. In 1540, Spanish conquistador Hernando de Soto (c. 1500–1542) witnessed sweet potato cultivation and consumption from Louisiana in the west to Georgia in the east.[50] Eliminating Europeans as the conduit, sweet potatoes' route from South America to the American Southeast is unknown.

Separate from these developments, Columbus returned to Spain in 1493 with sweet potatoes among several foods, as noted. England appears not to have learned about them until 1564 or 1604, an unsurprising circumstance given that its northern latitude discouraged cultivation.[51] Despite this tardiness, the English brought sweet potatoes to Virginia between roughly 1610 and 1648.[52] Their expansion throughout the American South owed less to Europeans than to Amerindians and African slaves. Earlier was mentioned Portugal's introduction of the crop into West Africa, the source of slaves. Africans came to the Americas knowing how to grow sweet potatoes, yams, rice (*Oryza glaberrima*), okra, cowpeas (*Vigna unguiculate*), and other crops. They shaped southern agriculture and cuisine.

Sweet potatoes sustained slaves, who had only their off hours for subsistence given the requirement that they grow exports like rice, tobacco (*Nicotiana tabacum*), sucrose, and cotton (*Gossypium hirsutum* and *Gossypium barbadense*). Their tendency to call sweet potatoes yams perpetuated confusion about the two. With little land for their own use, slaves grew the root near their cabins and cooking pots. From Virginia, the sweet potato moved south before or during the eighteenth century into the Carolinas, where it became a staple of antebellum agriculture and diets. Whereas roots

TABLE 13.2
US Sweet Potato Consumption

Year	Per American average intake (kg)
1920	13.6
1930	11
1935	11
1939	11
1970	2.45
1975	2.45
1980	2
1985	2.45
1990	2
1995	1.91
2000	1.91
2005	2.04
2006	2.13

nourished slaves, vines and leaves fed swine and cattle (*Bos taurus*). Residues were dug into soils as organic matter.

By 1840 poor whites in Rankin County, Mississippi ate sweet potatoes as entrée and dessert, drank sweet potato coffee, and fed foliage to animals or stuffed it into mattresses.[53] The root, which Union soldiers did not stop to dig or destroy, helped southerners avert starvation during and after the Civil War (1861–1865).[54] Autumn's harvest yielded food and local sweet potato festivals that reinforced southern pride, tradition, and rural values.

Born a slave, agricultural chemist George Washington Carver (1864–1943)—discussed in Chapter 8—devoted his career to expanding uses for southern crops. His work yielded 118 sweet potato derivatives, including shoe polish, glue, rubber, bleach, dyes, and alcohol.[55] Urging southerners to plant sweet potatoes rather than exhaust land through cotton monoculture, he named them among "the greatest gifts God has ever given us."[56]

By 1909, New Jersey, Delaware, Maryland, and Virginia were large producers. Table 13.2 shows that around 1920, Americans ate on average 13.6 kilograms (30 pounds) of sweet potatoes yearly.[57] During the Great Depression (1929–1939), poor southerners who subsisted on sweet potatoes were healthier than those who relied on corn, whose limitations were detailed in Chapter 12. During the depression, per American consumption hovered around 11 kilograms (25 pounds) annually.[58] By 1980, per American yearly consumption had fallen to 2 kilograms (4.5 pounds), an amount that fluctuated little during the next quarter century.

Three factors caused this diminution. First, post–World War II prosperity led Americans to prefer meat and dairy over sweet potatoes and other humble fare.[59] Americans who ate the root during periods of privation—for example the Great Depression—discarded it in affluence. Second, agribusiness favors crops suitable for mechanization such as potatoes, which tolerate rough treatment, over those that demand hand labor, such as sweet potatoes. Third, the desire to reduce immigration challenges sweet potato growers to hire enough migrant farmworkers, increasing the temptation to plant potatoes wherever the climate is cool enough for them.

13.3.11 Sweet Potatoes as World Food

By 2012, sweet potatoes fed over one hundred countries.[60] People throughout tropical Asia and Africa depend on the root. It sustains rural poor, including those with soils too thin and infertile for other crops. High water content, however, makes roots perishable, a disadvantage that favors cassava, which a later section notes can be stored underground up to 3 years. Among roots and tubers, only cassava supplies more calories worldwide than sweet potatoes.[61]

13.3.12 Cassava

Known as manioc, manioca, mandioca, Brazilian arrowroot, or yucca, cassava—from the Arawak *kasabi*—may have been domesticated as early as 7000 BCE.[62] Although later paragraphs document its drawbacks, cassava likely attracted early notice as a potential crop because, as the abstract mentioned, it tolerates drought and infertile and acidic soils. Additionally, its underground edibles are safe from locusts (*Schistocerca gregaria*), wild pigs (*Sus scrofa*), baboons (*Papio* species), and porcupines (*Erethizon dorsatum*). Compared with sweet potatoes, yams, taro, and potatoes, cassava yields the most calories by mass, benefitting the hungry.[63] Among tropical crops, only banana (*Musa × paradisiaca*) yields more food per hectare.[64]

13.3.13 Origins and Early Uses

Cassava's wild progenitor may have originated in Mexico, Belize, Costa Rica, El Salvador, Guatemala, Honduras, Nicaragua, Panama, or lands near South America's Amazon River. Vegetative propagation made cassava easy to grow, a feature that may have led Amerindians to domesticate it before seed crops such as corn (*Zea mays*), beans, and squashes (*Cucurbita* species), known as the three sisters. By roughly 6600 BCE, cassava farming had spread throughout Mexico, the Gulf of Mexico, and Caribbean island Cuba. About 3000 BCE the Tapi-Guarani grew the root in Colombia and Venezuela.[65] During the next few millennia, it spread south from Colombia and Venezuela to Peru and Paraguay, southeast through Brazil, and southeast from Cuba to Caribbean island Hispaniola, today Haiti and the Dominican Republic.

The Maya grew cassava as their principal root in southern Mexico, Guatemala, Belize, Honduras, and El Salvador, as did Mexico's Aztecs. By growing the least bitter varieties—designated sweet—the Maya minimized ingestion of toxic hydrocyanic acid (HCN), which forms salts with metals in Figure 2.9's Periodic Table group 1—the alkali metals—such as sodium or potassium, producing poisons known as cyanides, sodium cyanide (NaCN) and potassium cyanide (KCN) being examples. Cyanide causes dizziness, stomach pain and swelling, and vomiting. Youths, whose lightness concentrates cyanide per kilogram of body mass, are most vulnerable to cyanide toxicity. Cultivating bitter types, Aztecs removed most toxins by soaking roots in water several days or grating and drying them.

13.3.14 Europe's Encounter with Cassava

Africans, Asians, and Europeans were oceans away from these developments and knew nothing about the Americas until Columbus' voyages. In the Caribbean, he described "bread which tasted exactly as if it were made of chestnuts."[66] Because the native Tainos made cassava bread, Columbus must have been the first European to eat it. He praised it and other new foods to entice Spain's monarchs to fund later voyages, though Spaniards and Portuguese thought cassava insipid compared with wheat, rye, or barley bread and were wary of anything masquerading as bread that did not leaven. Cassava's toxicity was evident as early as 1494, when Italian historian Peter Martyr d'Anghieri (1457–1526) warned against "venomous roots."[67]

13.3.15 Cassava in the Old World Tropics

Suspicion did not prevent Portugal from provisioning slave ships with cassava and introducing it into what are today Cameroon, Gabon, the Republic of the Congo, and Angola in the sixteenth century, though it was not popular everywhere.[68] Liberia, Ghana, and Benin preferred yams, corn, millet (species in the tribe Eragrostideae), rice (*O. glaberrima*), sweet potatoes, beans, and peanuts as late as 1800. Production and consumption rose—especially in Nigeria—after roughly 1910, when ex-slaves returned from Brazil and the Caribbean with expertise in cassava agriculture. The root became indispensable as growing populations and hunger necessitated a reliable food supply. By 1950, the Republic of the Congo and the Democratic Republic of the Congo's (DRC) consumption averaged about 1 kilogram (2.2 pounds) per person—enough to give each individual over 1,000 calories from cassava alone—daily.[69]

Portugal brought the root to the Indian Ocean's Reunion Island in 1736.[70] Thereafter, it spread to Madagascar, Zanzibar, and India while Spain planted it in parts of Southeast Asia including the Philippines. By 1800, people from Sri Lanka to the Philippines—a distance over 4,500 kilometers (2,796 miles)—grew and ate cassava.[71] Around 1850, Thailand adopted it.[72] By 1900, tropical farmers worldwide depended on it wherever other crops languished. By the 1980s, Indonesia produced and consumed over one-quarter of Asia's cassava.[73]

Feeding roughly 1 billion people in 2009, the root has become a staple in eighty developing countries, many of them tropical.[74] As a source of energy, it ranks third in the tropics, trailing only rice (*Oryza sativa*) and corn and fourth worldwide after rice, corn, and sugarcane (*Saccharum officinarum*).[75] Cassava yields more metric tons in the tropics than all crops except corn. In southern China, it ranks fifth in metric tonnage behind rice, sweet potato, sugarcane, and corn. Unable to meet domestic demand, China imports the root from Vietnam and Thailand. Brazil grows most American cassava. Other producers are Colombia, Cuba, Haiti, Paraguay, Peru, and Venezuela. Residents in Madagascar, Ghana, Nigeria, Liberia, the Republic of the Congo, Uganda, Tanzania, and Mozambique get about one-sixth of calories from cassava.[76] After roughly 1980 consumption rose in Ghana and Nigeria and decreased in the Republic of the Congo, Tanzania, and Uganda. Between 1989 and 2009, Africa tripled the root's harvest.[77]Nigeria's International Institute of Tropical Agriculture (IITA) in Ibadan projects additional growth in consumption and production.

Nearly half Africa's peoples subsist on cassava. Some eat it thrice daily. In 1982, 90 percent of survey respondents in the DRC's Nord-Ubangi and Sud-Ubangi provinces ate cassava gruel, known as *fufu*, daily.[78] Cassava entered diets there 6 weeks after birth as liquid from a mixture of it and corn.[79] Because Africans eat most of the harvest, under 10 percent goes to livestock or industry. In Nigeria, the world's largest producer, the poor double the cassava consumption of the rich in cities and triple it in the countryside.[80] In 2014, the root supplied roughly 200 calories daily for 50 million Nigerians.[81]

Rwandans pair cassava with beans.[82] Liberians make *gari foto* from it, onion (*Allium cepa*), tomato, and eggs and combine the root, vegetables, and meat or fish. In Asia, Thais fry fish, shrimp (species in infraorder Caridea), or squid (species in the superorder Decapodiformes) in a coating of cassava starch. In Kerala, India, the root and fish are popular together. As in Columbus' time, cassava bread—"inexpensive but not nutritious"—is eaten throughout the Caribbean Islands.[83] Puerto Ricans make *chili de yucca* from cassava and beans. Guatemalans eat cassava souffle. Peruvians consume the root, cheese, and chili peppers (*Capsicum annuum*). Columbians fry cassava strips as Americans do French fries.

13.3.16 Cassava's Inadequacies

Despite cassava's prevalence, Venezuelan nutritionists Benito Infante and Omar Garcia acknowledged its inadequate "protein, fats, minerals, and vitamins."[84] Table 13.3 shows that 100 grams of cassava have 160 calories, 98 percent being carbohydrates, and the rest protein and fat.[85] Several essential amino acids are absent or minute. These 100 grams furnish 34.3 percent of DV for vitamin C—ascorbic acid—19 percent for manganese, and small quantities of most vitamins, minerals, protein, fat, and fiber. Vitamins B_{12} and D are absent. Processing or cooking destroys nutrients. Cassava's tapioca starch and *gari* flour provide little besides carbohydrates, a criticism *The Cambridge World History of Food* (2000) enlarged to the entire root.[86] A 1984 publication documented protein and

TABLE 13.3
Nutrients in Cassava 100 g

Nutrient	Cassava	%DV
Calories	160	N/A
Protein (g)	1.36	N/A
Fat (g)	0.28	N/A
Carbs (g)	38.06	N/A
Fiber (g)	1.8	N/A
	Minerals	
Ca (mg)	16	1.6
Fe (mg)	0.27	1.5
Mg (mg)	21	5.3
P (mg)	27	2.7
K (mg)	271	7.7
Na (mg)	14	0.6
Zn (mg)	0.34	2.3
Cu (mg)	0.1	5
Mn (mg)	0.38	19
Se (mcg)	0.7	1
	Vitamins	
A (IU)	13	0.3
B_1 (mg)	0.09	6
B_2 (mg)	0.05	2.9
B_3 (mg)	0.85	4.3
B_5 (mg)	0.11	1.1
B_6 (mg)	0.09	4.5
B_9 (mcg)	27	6.8
B_{12} (mcg)	0	0
C (mg)	20.6	34.3
D (IU)	0	0
E (mg)	0.19	1.3
K (mcg)	1.9	2.4

vitamin A deficiencies, anemia, and goiter among Indonesia's cassava eaters.[87] Later paragraphs examine the link between cassava and goiter and describe other dangers.

Despite these shortcomings, American nutritionist Stephanie Pedersen praised cassava for reducing risk of stroke. Her citations concern vitamin C without reference to cassava, though because 100 grams of root have 34.3 percent DV for the vitamin—as Table 13.3 mentioned—Pedersen must infer stroke protection for cassava.[88] She asserted that its polyphenols, flavonoids, and saponins—all phytochemicals—"help prevent cancer and shrink tumors."[89] This language appears to go beyond the consensus that diet and nutrition may lessen the risk of some cancers by endowing cassava with anticancer properties.

Sweeping pronouncements seldom advance the study of diet, nutrition, and health. For example, an Internet post asserted that cassava treats cancers because, supposedly being fungal diseases, they are somehow vulnerable to plant therapies.[90] This contention assumed that sinister physicians conceal cancers' true nature from patients to profit from unnecessary surgeries, chemotherapy, and radiation. A 2018 review of PubMed (http://www.ncbi.nlm.nih.gov/pubmed), however, listed no peer-reviewed publications about cassava as cancer preventor or cure.[91]

As noted, processing is necessary to minimize toxins. Even meticulous efforts cannot remove all cyanide. The body uses essential amino acids methionine and cystine to detoxify the remainder. Both being essential for growth, a 2008 paper implicated their metabolism for detoxification in stunting children.[92] Moreover, a by-product of cyanide detoxification is the anion thiocyanate (SCN^-), which hinders the thyroid gland's storage and use of the mineral iodine and which is known as a goitrogen. Without iodine, the thyroid—in a condition known as hypothyroidism—cannot manufacture the hormones thyroxine and triiodothyronine necessary to regulate cells' production of proteins, including enzymes that help control metabolism. The thyroid also makes the hormone calcitonin to regulate calcium in the blood. The gland is part of a cascade that begins with the hypothalamus, a region in the brain central to emotions, sleep, appetite, thirst, and libido. The hypothalamus regulates the thyroid by signaling the pituitary gland to secrete thyroid-stimulating hormone (TSH). The pituitary calibrates TSH by sensing the amounts of thyroxine and triiodothyronine in blood.

Iodine deficiency swells the thyroid in a disease known as goiter, which Chapter 9 mentioned among poor French peasants. Goiter, which threatens wherever cassava is a staple, may cause coughing or hoarseness. Severe enlargement may imperil swallowing and breathing. The danger is acute in developing nations because poverty forces consumption of inexpensive foods such as cassava and because soils often have little iodine for roots' uptake. Soil deficiencies are prevalent because, as noted, the developing world overlaps with the tropics, where soils are often poor and thin because

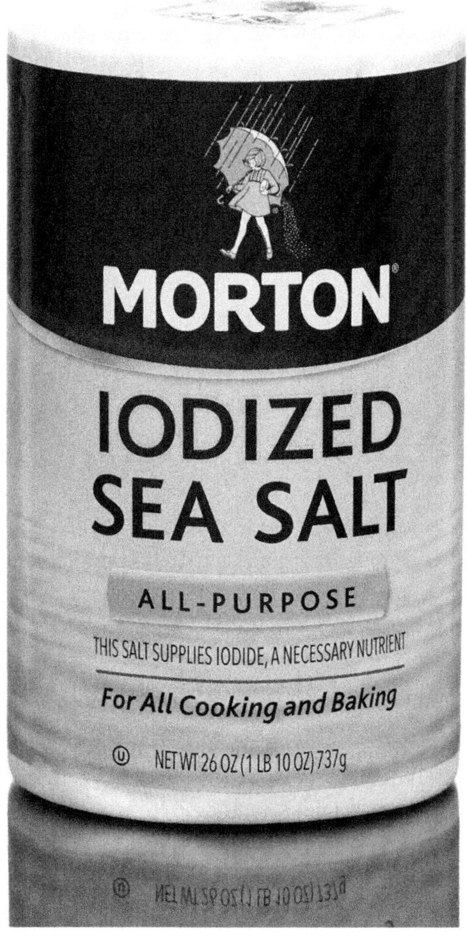

FIGURE 13.2 Iodized salt. (Photo from Shutterstock.)

profuse plants—especially trees—deprive land of nutrients by locking them in roots and foliage. Cassava eaters risk goiter not only by consuming thiocyanate but also by ingesting too little iodine from the root and other crops grown on poor soils. Poverty, geography, climate, soils, agriculture, diet, and nutrition thus interact to perpetuate goiter.

Goiter's frequency rises with increasing cassava consumption.[93] Women with hypothyroidism birth newborns with the same problem.[94] Vulnerable to stunting and brain damage when mothers are iodine deficient, newborns suffer cassava's worst hazards.[95] The World Health Organization (WHO) in Geneva, Switzerland, labeled iodine deficiency, which cassava exacerbates, the greatest cause of global cognitive impairment.[96]

Cyanide poses the greatest dangers when famine threatens from drought. Tolerating aridity better than other crops, cassava may be the only edible to survive, leaving people little else to eat. Yet aridity lowers cassava's water content, concentrating cyanide in roots and other tissues. Insufficient food from poor harvests and cyanide from potent cassava combine to damage the brain, partially paralyzing victims. The disease, known as konzo, usually cripples the legs. Konzo may also impair speech and vision.

In 2005, for example, drought, undernutrition, and toxic cassava increased konzo's incidence in Mozambique.[97] Additionally, famines and warfare dislocate populations. Refugees seldom have time to process cassava, ingesting excessive cyanide. The DRC, where civil war raged between 1994 and 2003 and konzo paralyzed thousands, concretized this reality.

The IITA and United Nations Food and Agriculture Organization (FAO) in Rome, Italy, prioritized derivation of low-cyanide cassava varieties. This effort confronts scientists with the problem of trying to quantify how much cyanide must be ingested to impair health. Even small amounts appear to harm the thyroid. As noted, the gland requires iodine, whose deficiency cassava exacerbates. The connections among the root, cyanide, iodine, and the thyroid are evident in Ghana, where cassava harvests tripled between 1961 and 1999, where iodine is often deficient, and where undernutrition and diseases diminish productivity and cost the economy some $22 million annually.[98] Climate change may intensify aridity in lands prone to droughts, pushing farmers to plant more cassava and thereby exacerbate its ills. Governments in developing countries do little besides recommend consumption of iodized salt and only thoroughly processed cassava. Undernutrition, goiter, cognitive impairment, and konzo require this book to urge cassava's avoidance.

13.4 TUBERS

13.4.1 Potato

From cassava and sweet potatoes' tropical lowlands, ascent into South America's Andes Mountains provided the cool environs where arose the potato. In the tropics, these highlands had ample sunlight for photosynthesis. Harvesting nature required Amerindians to wander the terrain for wild tubers and other edibles. Cultivation may have begun as an attempt to concentrate time and effort by confining plants to a small area efficiently harvested. Tubers must have attracted attention because they yielded more food per hectare than plants targeted for seeds. Despite thin, poor soils due to insufficient organic matter and oxygen deprivation at high altitudes, Andes' indigenes terraced hillsides, irrigated them with water from distant rivers, and developed over 3,000 potato varieties.[99] Insensitive to this diversity, European designation of the potato as white ignores colors that include yellow, orange, pink, purple, red, brown, and black.

13.4.2 Potatoes and Large Populations in Precontact South America

Possibly domesticated as early as cassava in what is today Peru, the potato was among the region's many edible tubers and roots.[100] Initially small and bitter, it might have remained an unpromising candidate for world staple had Amerindians near Lake Titicaca on the border between Peru and

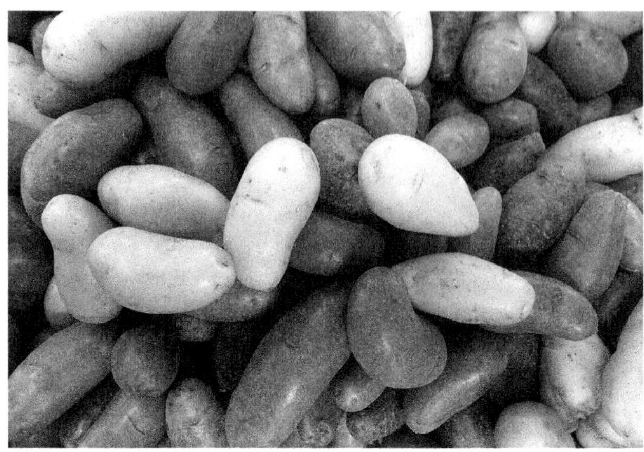

FIGURE 13.3 Potatoes in assorted colors. (Photo from Shutterstock.)

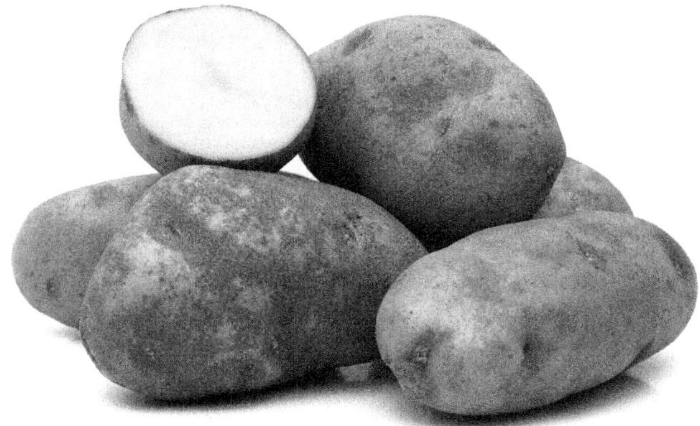

FIGURE 13.4 Russet potatoes. (Photo from Shutterstock.)

Bolivia not selected varieties for size and flavor around 6000 BCE.[101] Peru's Moche civilization (c. 1–c. 800 CE) elevated the potato into a symbol, emblazing pottery with its image.[102] Some pots were shaped like potatoes while displaying human bodies, possibly symbolizing people's dependence on them. A 2018 study identified potato starch in every vessel excavated from Wasi Huachuma, Peru, suggesting the tuber's ubiquity.[103] Arid Pacific coast settlements ate potatoes from the Andes. Bolivia's Tiwanaku Empire (c. 550–c. 1000) used raised beds to trap the sun's heat for potato germination and growth. Ample harvests supported 100,000 residents.[104] Exports throughout Bolivia, Peru, and Ecuador fed another 400,000.[105] The potato sustained the Inca Empire (c. 1400–1533 CE), which grew by 1500 into the largest pre-Columbian polity. At its apex, the empire united Peru and much of Ecuador, Bolivia, and Chile. Its 10 million inhabitants ate potatoes.[106] Later paragraphs detail the connections among potatoes—which supply many nutrients and calories per hectare—population, stature, disease, and longevity.

The Inca rotated potatoes with quinoa (*Chenopodium quinoa*) and canihua (*Chenopodium pallidicaule*), fertilizing fields with llama (*Lama glama*) and alpaca (*Vicugna pacos*) dung, guano (seabird or bat urine), or decaying fish. Following earlier practices, they terraced hillsides, dug irrigation canals, and drained wetlands. Commoners ate *chuno*, a dry, light food prepared since the first millennium BCE that the Spanish likened to bread.[107] At low elevations, corn complemented potatoes or, with sweet potatoes, displaced them where temperatures and humidity were high, but because the grass will not grow above 2,500 meters (2,734 yards or 8,202.1 feet), potatoes were indispensable.[108]

Adding potatoes to soup and stew, Inca ate them with corn, beans, peppers (*C. annuum*), quinoa, guinea pig (*Cavia porcellus*), or their combination. Other Incan foods included tomato, peanut, cashew (*Anacardium occidentale*), squashes, cucumber (*Cucumis sativus*), chili peppers, gourd (*Lagenaria siceraria*), avocado (*Persea americana*), oca (*Oxalis tuberosa*), ulluco (*Ullucus tuberosus*), mashua (*Tropaeolum tuberosum*), maca (*Lepidium meyenii*), carob (*Ceratonia siliqua*), sour cherry (*Prunus cerasus*), pineapple (*Ananas comosus*), elderberry (*Sambucus nigra*), and meat from llama, alpaca, and guinea pig. Game included duck (*Anas platyrhynchos* and *Cairina moschata*) and deer (*Odocoileus* species). The Pacific coast yielded fish. As in ancient Egypt, discussed in Chapter 4, and other stratified societies, only the wealthy regularly ate meat. Commoners ate potatoes, corn, sweet potatoes, and other vegetarian fare. The Inca dried the surplus, especially potatoes, corn, and quinoa, for consumption in lean times. During the precontact period, potatoes were unknown in North America and the Caribbean. Maya and Aztecs, for example, developed civilizations independent of the tuber.

The Inca benefited by eating potatoes whole, a practice that aligned with American nutritionist Thomas Colin Campbell's (b. 1934) opinion that whole foods supply the most nourishment.[109] Law forbade removal of skin (peel), an act that was thought to pain the tuber.[110] Over time, this belief, pervading Incan religion and mores, became unassailable. Skin's retention, a later section indicates, yields maximum nutrients.

13.4.3 Europe's Encounter with the Potato

Its rise to world crop began after Spanish conquistador Francisco Pizarro (c. 1475–1541) conquered the Inca in 1533.[111] Four years later, soldiers discovered Amerindians working in a potato field.[112] Curious, the Spaniards sampled the tuber, whose flavor they esteemed. More interested in gold than Peruvian crops, however, the Spanish neglected it. Even when they turned to agriculture, they focused on transplanting grains and other Old-World florae and raising cattle, pigs, and sheep (*Ovis aries*) rather than on exploiting indigenous plants. Like many Europeans, Spaniards favored bread and meat and wanted to enjoy familiar foods in the Americas.

Stories recount multiple versions of potatoes' entrance into Europe, though the likeliest carrier was Spain. An early participant in the slave trade, it provisioned ships with them. Leftovers might have been planted in sixteenth-century Spain, *The Cambridge World History of Food* (2000) giving 1539 as the year of introduction.[113] Alternatively, Spaniards might have brought potatoes to the Atlantic Ocean's Canary Islands in 1567.[114] From this spot west of Morocco, the Spanish might have introduced them into the motherland. The earliest record of potatoes in Europe dated to 1573, when a hospital in Seville, Spain, served them to patients.[115] Readers may hope that it added them to the menu because they are nourishing. No less plausible, however, is the surmise that inexpensiveness justified inclusion.

13.4.4 Recognition of Potatoes' Nutriment

Sixteenth-century Europe needed the potato. Chapter 7 indicated that between 1500 and 1800, food prices rose faster than wages as burgeoning populations challenged the land's capacity to feed them. The result was premodern Europeans "on the fringe of starvation."[116]

The tuber, yielding more calories per hectare than any plant according to American plant pathologist Gail Lynn Schumann (b. 1951), held potential for feeding the masses.[117] With dense nutrients, potatoes supplied more protein per unit land than any crop but cabbage and broad beans (*Vicia faba*)—also termed fava or faba beans—though the quality of potatoes' protein, as a later paragraph indicates, is superior. American scholars Kenneth Franklin Kiple (1939–2016), Kriemhild Conee Ornelas, and Susan Campbell Bartoletti (b. 1958) esteemed the plant for providing the most nourishment per hectare.[118] British botanist Helen Sanderson in 2005 lauded it as "particularly nutritious."[119] Potatoes' value was evident to English physician Tobias Venner (1577–1660), who wrote in 1622 that they "wonderfully comfort, nourish and strengthen the bodie."[120]

The claim that potatoes require fertile soils is untrue, though like other crops, yields improve with additions of manure or fertilizers.[121] Having evolved in poor rather than fecund ground, the tuber benefitted Europe by producing food in marginal areas, leaving the best for cash crops.[122] Perhaps because farmers consigned it to infertile lands, they fertilized them after 1840, when guano became available from Peru's Chinchas Islands.[123] Peru thereby doubled as source of potatoes and fertilizer.

Table 13.4 shows that calories and nutrients vary by type.[124] Classifying varieties by skin or flesh color, 100 grams each of golden and purple potatoes have 76.3 calories, whereas the same amount of red potatoes has 89 calories.[125] Golden potatoes supply the most fiber and protein, purple varieties provide the most vitamin C and vitamin A precursors β-carotene and lutein, and red tubers have the most potassium and vitamin B_6. With one serving of potatoes being 148 grams, stated the Idaho Potato Commission in Eagle, Idaho, a serving of purple tubers has 770 milligrams of vitamin C, over twelve times the DV according to Pedersen.[126]

This amount, nine times her value by mass for golden potatoes and over forty times her figure for redskins, overshot American anthropologist Ellen Messer's (b. 1948) estimate of 16 milligrams in 100 grams of potatoes by a factor of almost thirty-three.[127] Messer's number, not Pedersen's, approximated potatoes' vitamin C content reported by Potatoes USA in Denver, Colorado, and the Idaho

TABLE 13.4
Nutrients in Potatoes by Type 100 g

Nutrient	Gold Potato	%DV	Purple Potato	%DV	Red Potato	%DV
Calories	76.3	N/A	76.3	N/A	89	N/A
Protein (g)	3.5	N/A	2.3	N/A	2.3	N/A
Fat (g)	0	N/A	0.14	N/A	0.14	N/A
Carbs (g)	17.57	N/A	16.04	N/A	16.04	N/A
Fiber	2.3	N/A	1.2	N/A	1.7	N/A
			Minerals			
Ca (mg)	14	1.4	10	1	10	1
Fe (mg)	1.2	6.7	1.2	6.7	1.2	6.7
Mg (mg)	28.3	7.1	28.3	7.1	28.3	7.1
P (mg)	72.25	7.2	72.25	7.2	72.25	7.2
K (mg)	358.38	10.2	294.8	8.4	545.09	15.6
Na (mg)	0	0	5.88	0.2	5.88	0.2
Zn (mg)	0.2	1.3	0.33	2.2	0.33	2.2
Cu (mg)	0.05	2.5	0.13	6.5	0.13	6.5
Mn (mg)	0.17	8.5	0.17	8.5	0.17	8.5
Se (mcg)	NA	NA	0.49	0.7	0.49	0.7
			Vitamins			
A (IU)	0	0	52	1	7	0.1
B_1 (mg)	0.06	4	0.06	4	0.06	4
B_2 (mg)	0.02	1.2	0.03	1.6	0.03	1.6
B_3 (mg)	1.7	8.5	1.7	8.5	1.7	8.5
B_5 (mg)	0.35	3.5	0.35	3.5	0.35	3.5
B_6 (mg)	0.14	7	0.13	6.5	0.13	6.5
B_9 (mcg)	27.2	6.8	27.2	6.8	27.2	6.8
B_{12} (mcg)	0	0	0	0	0	0
C (mg)	57.8	96.3	520.2	867	12.7	21.2
D (IU)	0	0	0	0	0	0
E (mg)	N/A	N/A	0	0	0	0
K (mcg)	2.9	3.6	2.9	3.6	2.9	3.6

Potato Commission.[128] Messer's value yields 26.7 percent of DV for vitamin C in 100 grams.[129] Skin, having around 30 percent of the vitamin, should be eaten.[130]

Besides minerals, vitamins, and phytochemicals, potato protein ranks first among plants and second to egg whites in its balance of essential amino acids.[131] Especially valuable is skin, which has more fiber, protein, and vitamin B_9 than flesh by mass. Having at least 40 percent fiber, the peel also has vitamins B_2, B_6, and C and other antioxidants. Research credits peel with reducing cholesterol and the sugar glucose ($C_6H_{12}O_6$)—discussed in Chapters 2 and 11—in blood, protecting against insulin surges.[132] These findings recommend against peeling potatoes or eating processed foods such as fries and tater tots. The potato should be eaten whole and never mashed unless peel is retained. Summarizing its value, Reader in 1988 esteemed it "the best all-round package of nutrition known to mankind."[133] American historian and biographer Milton Meltzer (1915–2009) agreed, writing in 1992 that "the potato is the most perfect natural source of nutrition so far discovered."[134]

13.4.5 Potatoes Combated Scurvy

Potatoes' plentiful vitamin C may surprise readers who connect it with citrus fruits. Chapter 2 noted European use of lemon (*Citrus limon*), orange (*Citrus sinensis* and *Citrus aurantium*), and lime (*Citrus aurantiifolia*) aboard ships to prevent scurvy. English captain James Cook (1728–1779) banished it by giving his men pineapple, cabbage (*Brassica oleracea var. capitata*) and other leafy vegetables, yams (*Dioscorea* species), and coconuts (*Cocos nucifera*).[135] But these fruits were absent from U.S. ship *Empress of China*, which in 1784 left New York City for China in the most ambitious American voyage to that date. At sea for 14 months, the crew had no fresh fruit until they gathered oranges at the Cape Verde Islands west of Senegal. Instead, their diet featured pork, beef, bread, and potatoes. Only the last had vitamin C, protecting against scurvy. The medical officer reported no instances of it. Between 1831 and 1836, Britain's *Her Majesty's Ship (H. M. S.) Beagle* circumnavigated Earth. Aboard it, British naturalist Charles Robert Darwin (1809–1882) wrote that the crew ate potatoes collected on Chile's Chiloe Island.[136] Again, the tuber banished scurvy.

Potatoes' value against scurvy led London's Royal Society—England's national scientific society—in 1662 to urge their nationwide planting and consumption.[137] Authors repeated this recommendation through the eighteenth century. The tuber's prevalence, especially in Ireland into the nineteenth century boosted vitamin C intake some fifty times above what was necessary to thwart scurvy. Summarizing these developments, British biochemist Richard Elwyn Hughes (1928–2015) praised potatoes as "the prime protector against scurvy."[138]

13.4.6 Barriers to Potatoes' Adoption

Despite the potato's benefits, impediments slowed adoption. As noted, Europeans favored wheat, rye, peas, and other seed crops. To be sure, the tuber was not unique in yielding food underground given Europe's cultivation of carrots, turnips, and other roots, but it came from a land unknown to almost all Europeans and from heathens, though this circumstance did not delay corn and beans' acceptance. Because carrots and kindred crops were planted from seeds, the Andean preference for planting potato buds rather than seeds discomforted Spaniards.[139]

Clergymen emphasized that the bible would have mentioned the tuber had it been important.[140] This rationale implies that biblical writers knew about the potato and chose to omit it, an impossibility given ignorance of the western hemisphere. Detractors labeled potatoes "Devil's apples" and "forbidden fruit of Eden."[141] Catholics sought to purge seed potatoes (budding sections) of paganism by sprinkling them with holy water before planting.[142] Protestant disdain for Catholic Ireland made the tuber "Ireland's lazy root."[143] Because the potato was lumpy, some Europeans feared it might cause leprosy, among early modernity's most frightful diseases.[144] This supposed danger led seventeenth century Burgundy, France, to outlaw the tuber. Critics who associated potatoes and syphilis with the Americas blamed them for the disease. Syphilis turned attention to sex, with some claiming that potatoes stimulated the libido and others that they caused sterility. Moreover, botanists understood that the potato was a nightshade, belonging to the Solanaceae family. Its members, including the potato plant, contain toxins. Its foliage cannot feed people or livestock.

Geography was another obstacle. As noted, potatoes originated at elevations with a cool climate despite tropical latitude. In Europe, the north had a climate closest to this requirement. But in the tropics, daylength was roughly 12 hours year-round. Having evolved in this environment, potatoes were unsuited to northern Europe's fluctuations in daylength by virtue of its distance from the equator. This disjunction prevented plants from forming tubers until autumn, when daylength approached 12 hours. For this reason, Swiss physician and botanist Casper Bauhin (1560–1624) wrote in 1620 that potatoes were not harvested until November.[145] Only in the eighteenth century did botanists derive varieties suitable for high latitudes, triggering the tuber's expansion and emergence as a staple.

Even the mismatch between potatoes and daylength did not obscure their value. During the Thirty Years' War (1618–1648), armies pillaged central and northern Europe.[146] As they had in previous conflicts, soldiers took grain from barns, leaving peasants nothing. Potatoes temporarily ended confiscation because soldiers would not take time to unearth them. Under these circumstances, the tuber not only improved diets but also became essential to national security. Prussian king Frederick William I (1688–1740) ordered peasants to plant potatoes.[147] Son Frederick II (1712–1786)—who is known as Frederick the Great and whose interest in the tuber was "almost an obsession"—distributed free seed potatoes to enlarge cultivation and consumption.[148] Eastern Europe and Scandinavia emulated Prussia, now part of Germany. In 1778 and 1779, soldiers adjusted to the potato, digging it wherever they halted during the War of the Bavarian Succession (the "potato war").[149]

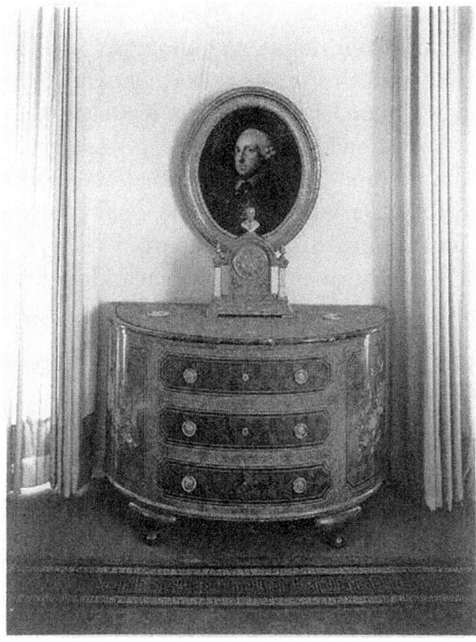

FIGURE 13.5 Frederick the Great. (Photo courtesy of Library of Congress. https://www.loc.gov/pictures/item/2005692976/.)

13.4.7 Potatoes Enlarged Populations and Improved Health

Eighteenth-century enthusiasm for potatoes doubled Europe's food supply by century's end, enlarging populations.[150] The tuber reached Sweden in 1658—the year Swedish physician and naturalist Olaus Rudbeck (1630–1702) mentioned it—though production increased only in the nineteenth century, when the harvest leapt thirteenfold between 1800 and 1850.[151] Population rose as mortality fell, especially among infants. Between 1810 and 1812, Sweden averaged thirty deaths per 1,000 inhabitants. Forty years later, mortality had declined by one-third. Plentiful and inexpensive, the potato nourished Sweden's masses, who had subsisted on oats, rye, and barley. By the mid-nineteenth century, Sweden became a grain exporter because potatoes supplanted it in diets, freeing it for long-distance trade. American economists Lars G. Sandberg and Richard Hall Steckel (b. 1944) summarized the potato's benefits in Sweden, where it "became an essentially new, and very cheap, source of calories, minerals, and vitamins."[152]

Elsewhere in Scandinavia, Finland's population grew after potatoes' arrival, which Chapter 7 mentioned as a poorly documented event. As noted, Sweden acquired them in 1658. To the east, tradition credited Czar Peter I (1672–1725)—known as Peter the Great—with introducing potatoes into Russia in 1697.[153] This date is too late because Russian religious conservatives denounced them as nonbiblical in 1667, implying cultivation and consumption by then.[154] Between the two nations, Finland probably received potatoes about 1660 as they moved east from Sweden.

The conventional account holds that Russian peasants resisted potatoes even after Czarina Catherine II (1729–1796)—known as Catherine the Great—required cultivation in 1765.[155] Czar Nicholas I (1796–1855), frustrated with noncompliance, enforced Catherine's mandate in 1850. This gradualism does not square with population growth after 1650. Between 1600 and 1650, Table 13.5 shows that Russia's population remained 7 million.[156] Its 12 million in 1700 grew to 16 million in 1750, 38 million in 1800, 56 million in 1850, and 97 million in 1900. That is, gains came soon after potatoes' arrival no later than 1667.

Inexpensiveness enabled the tuber to feed the masses. After roughly 1750, the Industrial Revolution cemented the relationship between potatoes and poverty. By paying a pittance, factories forced workers to subsist on the cheapest items, potatoes first among them.[157] By the mid-eighteenth century, therefore, the tuber sustained inequalities in countryside and city.

By then, potatoes yielded five times more food per hectare than wheat in the United Provinces (now the Netherlands), increasing population after 1750.[158] Another estimate put potato yields over tenfold greater than wheat and almost ten times above rye.[159] Growth was sluggish wherever the Dutch clung to grains. In eighteenth- and nineteenth-century German states—Germany became a nation in 1871—the potato "saved many people from starvation because of its high content in starch and vitamin C."[160]

Moving to German state Bavaria in 1785, British-American physicist and inventor Benjamin Thompson (1753–1814)—a forerunner of thermodynamics—encouraged the tuber's cultivation and consumption and established soup kitchens to serve the poor potatoes.[161] He "introduced the potato into Central Europe," wrote American physicist Sanborn Conner Brown (1913–1981).[162] A self-taught nutritionist, Thompson—named Count Rumford in 1793—ranked it among the best foods.[163]

TABLE 13.5
Russia's Population from Lucassen

Year	Population (Millions)
1500	5
1550	5.5
1600	7
1650	7
1700	12
1750	16
1800	38
1850	56
1900	97

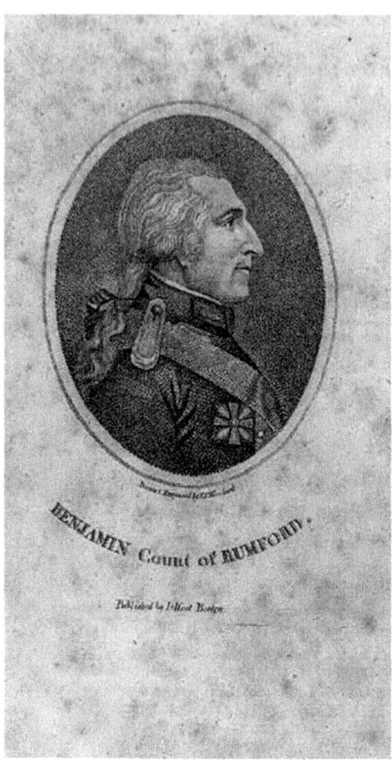

FIGURE 13.6 Benjamin Thompson. (Photo courtesy of Library of Congress. https://www.loc.gov/pictures/item/2005679822/.)

Germans boiled it with apples (*Malus domestica*) and bacon to make *Himmel und Erde* (Heaven and Earth) and shaped it into pancakes with butter and applesauce.[164] European and North American Jews likewise made potato pancakes, known as *latke*. After 1900, Germany's potato consumption declined, and undernutrition and infectious diseases like typhus recurred.[165]

The tuber doubled England and Wales from 9 to 18 million inhabitants between 1801 and 1850.[166] Beneficiaries included Gloucester County Gaol inmates, whose Thursday and Sunday rations featured 0.45 kilograms (1 pound) of potatoes in the early nineteenth century.[167] When officials eliminated them in July 1822, 118 of 850 prisoners exhibited scurvy by February 1823. That April, it afflicted 448 inmates. The sick received oranges, and potatoes were reinstated in 1824. Scurvy vanished. In 1842, a Parliamentary committee recommended potatoes for all English prisoners.[168] Scurvy disappeared from jails nationwide. These improvements led critics to fear that the poor might commit infractions solely to enjoy potatoes and other prison luxuries.

West of England and Wales, Ireland—which other chapters mentioned as dependent on the tuber—adopted it between 1587 and 1602.[169] As in Britain, potatoes protected the Irish from scurvy, sustaining "exceptionally healthy, vigorous (and desperately poor)" farmworkers.[170] Population was about 1.4 million in 1600, 2 million in 1700, and 5 million a century later.[171] Of the 8.5 million Irish in 1845, 4–6 million clung to tiny plots of land and were destitute.[172] Of them, over 3.3 million ate nothing but potatoes and so were vulnerable to shortages.[173] Milton Meltzer estimated that 90 percent of Irish ate little but potatoes, which replaced their past reliance on meat, dairy, and oats, by the nineteenth century.[174] When available, buttermilk—discussed in Chapter 7—and salt supplemented the tuber.

In 1845, the mold *Phytophthora infestans* ruined the crop. Having arisen at elevations with few pests and pathogens, the potato was vulnerable to destruction.[175] Chapters 1 and 3 detailed the ensuing famine. This section emphasizes that suffering and starvation were not due to deficiencies in potatoes' nutriment. Chapter 2 noted that on famine's eve, Irish men ate up to 9.5 kilograms (21 pounds) of potatoes daily, though from 4.5 to 6.5 kilograms (10 to 14 pounds) might have been the norm.[176]

American botanist Beryl Brintnall Simpson (b. 1942) and American botanist and science educator Molly Conner Ogorzaly undercut these numbers, supposing that daily consumption averaged 0.5 kilograms (1.1 pounds) per person.[177] Intake was low, they believed, because the Irish also ingested bread, mutton, butter, sucrose, beer, and tea. This claim of diversity contradicted their reference to "potato monoculture" and their remark that "By the 1840s not only was Ireland fond of potatoes; its population was completely dependent on them."[178] Moreover, had the Irish eaten several foods, absence of one—potatoes—should not have caused catastrophe. When available, milk and vegetables like cabbage and turnips supplemented the tuber but never rivaled it.[179]

Subsisting on the potato, the Irish demonstrated its healthfulness. Travelers unexperienced with it assumed that the tuber was harmful given the above prejudices. Visiting Ireland, they were prepared to criticize it, yet finding the Irish energetic and tall, they acknowledged its virtues.[180] It invigorated men and women for arduous labor.[181] Women were spry and fertile.[182] Eating potatoes, the Irish enjoyed better nutrition than English bread and pork consumers.[183]

Ireland adopted potatoes even in Ulster—a province that is today split between the Republic of Ireland and Northern Ireland—where Scots rather than Irish occupied land. These farmers retained their historic allegiance to oats until 1720, when 2 years' poor harvests convinced them to plant potatoes.[184] Their success convinced the Scottish Highlands to begin growing potatoes around 1730.[185]

Before the 1750s, Torbel, Switzerland, relied on grains, but not even hardy rye grew above 1,100 meters (1,203 yards or 3,608.9 feet).[186] Potatoes provided harvests above 1,500 meters (1,640.4 yards or 4,921.3 feet). Better nourished than in the past, women recovered fertility soon after weaning a child. More infants weaned on softened potatoes and cow, sheep, or goat's milk survived than on substitutes. This phenomenon paralleled Caribbean island Trinidad, where slaves fed potato soup beginning around age 3 had lower mortality and grew more rapidly than on another diet.[187] In American colony Georgia, German immigrant and Lutheran minister John Martin Bolzius (1703–1765) in 1734 praised potatoes as especially nourishing, fortifying slaves for strenuous exertions.[188] The tuber's nutrients and calories strengthened the immune system, reducing respiratory infections.[189] Like Finland, Sweden, Ireland, England, Wales, Scotland, the Netherlands, Russia, Germany, and elsewhere in northern latitudes, Torbel's population swelled as birthrate increased and mortality fell. By the 1880s, Swiss textile workers ate potatoes at breakfast and lunch.[190]

13.4.8 Potatoes Reduced Famines and Mortality

Populations rose faster where the potato became a staple than where grains remained entrenched.[191] It reduced famines' incidence and severity and diminished deaths from undernutrition and attendant diseases.[192] Potatoes produced the surplus labor that fueled the Industrial Revolution and the masses that emigrated to North America; gave Britain, France, Germany, and Russia vast armies that precipitated World War I's horrors; and made Europe a colonial power.[193] These developments prompted German economist Friedrich Engels (1820–1895) in 1884 to judge the tuber humanity's greatest innovation since iron's discovery.[194]

Throughout Europe, mortality began to decline after roughly 1725.[195] This section emphasizes that potatoes became widespread in the eighteenth century and so aided this diminution. They helped fuel what American internist and Rockefeller Foundation president John Hilton Knowles (1926–1979) termed a "second agricultural revolution" that century, causing a "massive increase in available food."[196] Nutritional improvements, which the potato augmented, accounted for half the declining mortality, he estimated.

Potatoes were especially important east of central Europe's Elbe River, where rye was the chief grain. Farmers valued its tolerance of drought, cold, and infertile soils. As the only grain that matured during central, eastern, and northern Europe's short, rainy summers, rye was indispensable to farmers there, though it was vulnerable to the fungus *Claviceps purpurea*.[197] Fungi do not kill rye, but those who eat infested kernels suffer the disease ergotism, which causes nausea, vomiting, hallucinations, convulsions, gangrene, unconsciousness, and death in the worst cases. These

TABLE 13.6
Nutrients in Potatoes and Rye 100 Calories

Nutrient	Potato	%DV	Rye	%DV
Protein (g)	2.66	N/A	2.75	N/A
Fat (g)	0.12	N/A	0.37	N/A
Carbs (g)	22.71	N/A	21.48	N/A
Fiber (g)	2.73	N/A	2.24	N/A
		Minerals		
Ca (mg)	15.58	1.6	3.64	0.4
Fe (mg)	1.05	5.8	0.25	1.4
Mg (mg)	29.87	7.5	8.96	2.2
P (mg)	74.03	7.4	36.41	3.6
K (mg)	551.95	15.8	62.75	1.8
Na (mg)	7.79	0.3	0.56	0.02
Zn (mg)	0.39	2.6	0.37	2.5
Cu (mg)	0.14	7.1	0.06	0.03
Mn (mg)	0.2	10	0.33	16.3
Se (mcg)	0.52	0.7	4.93	7
		Vitamins		
A (IU)	2.6	0.05	0	0
B_1 (mg)	0.11	7	0.09	6.2
B_2 (mg)	0.04	2.4	0.03	1.5
B_3 (mg)	1.38	6.9	0.22	1.1
B_5 (mg)	0.38	3.8	0.19	1.9
B_6 (mg)	0.39	19.4	0.07	3.3
B_9 (mcg)	19.48	4.9	6.44	1.6
B_{12} (mcg)	0	0	0	0
C (mg)	25.58	42.6	0	0
D (IU)	0	0	0	0
E (mg)	0.01	0.09	0.23	0.02
K (mcg)	2.6	3.3	1.65	2.1

symptoms alarmed observers, who suspected witchcraft centuries ago. Where people ate potatoes rather than rye bread, however, ergotism vanished.

Moreover, potatoes yielded roughly four times more calories than rye per hectare.[198] Benefits extended to nutrients, with the mean among golden, purple, and red tubers surpassing rye by mass in iron, potassium, and vitamins B_3, B_9, and C.[199] By calorie, potatoes trump rye in the above plus fiber, carbohydrates, calcium, zinc, sodium, magnesium, phosphorus, copper, and vitamins A (as carotenoids), B_1, B_2, B_5 (pantothenic acid), B_6, and K. By calorie, rye has more fat, protein, manganese, selenium, and vitamin E. Table 13.6 compares U.S. Department of Agriculture (USDA) nutrient summaries for potatoes and rye per 100 calories.

13.4.9 Potatoes Nourished Europe as Had No Previous Food

An earlier paragraph stated that the tuber became widespread in eighteenth century Europe. Table 13.7 indicates that whereas population on the continent, including Russia, fell from 85 million in 1600 to 81.6 million in 1650, it increased to 93.4 million in 1700, 110.2 million in 1750, 160.7 million in 1800, and 233 million in 1850.[200] These numbers, moving from contraction to expansion, show that the potato fed Europe as had no previous food.

TABLE 13.7
Population in Europe and Russia from Lucassen

Year	Population (Millions)
1500	66.6
1550	75.7
1600	85
1650	81.6
1700	93.4
1750	110.2
1800	160.7
1850	233

TABLE 13.8
Population in Europe and World from Civitello

Year	Europe (Millions)	World (Millions)
1650	103	545
1750	144	728
1800	192	906
1850	274	1171
1900	423	1,608
1950	593	2,454
2008	736	6,678

Doubters might identify corn, sweet potatoes, beans, cassava, and peanuts as other viands that became available after roughly 1500. But sweet potatoes and cassava were tropical foods that stored poorly once harvested and were not staples in Europe. Even had they been widespread, earlier sections detailed their nutritional shortcomings. Chapter 12 discussed corn's inadequacies. A world crop by 1550, it did not reverse Europe's population decrease from 1600 to 1650. Peanuts were another tropical food, discussed in Chapter 8, largely neglected in Europe. Even today, Europeans are not avid peanut consumers. For example, they seldom eat peanut butter.[201] Chapter 8 discussed beans' healthfulness. Other than potatoes, they may have helped swell Europe's population.

These additional foods—if not European staples—nonetheless increased global populations, shown in Table 13.8.[202] Comparing European and world growth, this table indicates that the magnitude of increase was similar for both.

Another potato gauge is stature. Beginning in the 1810s, Swedish military statistics document that recruits' heights increased roughly 2.5 centimeters (1 inch) each generation, which demographers estimate at 25 years.[203] By the 1850s, Swedes were as tall or taller than Americans, an achievement Sandberg and Steckel credited to potatoes.[204] Data from 1815 indicate that Irishmen were taller than their English counterparts, a difference Irish historian and economist Cormac O Grada (b. 1945) attributed to the potato.[205] But Englishmen also ate potatoes, complicating comparisons. University of Chicago historian William Hardy McNeill (1917–2016), however, asserted that English laborers, eating bread as well as potatoes, depended less on them than the Irish.[206] French military records indicate that mean height increased nearly 1.3 centimeters (0.5 inches) where potatoes were grown in the seventeenth and eighteenth centuries.[207] Although grain was often traded, potatoes seldom entered the market, suggesting that they were eaten where cultivated and so must explain tallness. In contrast, Chapters 7 and 9 indicated that the shortest French conscripts came from areas dependent on chestnuts or on rye and barley bread and small amounts of cheese, butter, or both. This book correlates tallness with nutrition, though diet is not the lone factor. In this instance, however, little changed besides tuber's adoption.

France's enthusiasm for potatoes owed much to pharmacist Antoine-Augustin Parmentier (1737–1813). While in the French army during the Seven Years' War (1756–1763), he was captured and jailed in Prussia.[208] There rations were little besides potatoes, which he credited with his survival and vitality upon release at war's end. Laboring to make the tuber a national staple, Parmentier won renown and admiration from French nobles, King Louis XVI (1754–1793), and Queen Marie Antoinette (1755–1793). After roughly 1770, potato production increased, France harvesting 21 million hectoliters (554.8 million gallons) of tubers in 1815 and 117 million hectoliters (3.1 billion gallons) in 1840.[209] In his memory, the French eat potato and leek (*Allium ampeloprasum*) soup—*potage Parmentier*—and mashed potatoes, meat, and white wine sauce in potato skins, known as *hachis Parmentier*.[210] France pioneered sliced potatoes, cheese, butter, cream, and breadcrumbs, known as au gratin potatoes, and possibly French fries. Although Belgium may have originated fries, Americans credit France because statesman, scientist, and philosopher Thomas Jefferson (1743–1826) encountered them there while minister between 1785 and 1789.[211] Popularizing the connection between fries and France, he served them at White House dinners as third U.S. president between 1801 and 1809.

Canadian economist Nathan Nunn (b. 1974) and Chinese American economist Nancy Qian concluded that "Because potatoes contain nearly all important vitamins and nutrients, they support life better than any other crop."[212] This judgment reinforces the opinions cited earlier. Potatoes' nutriment, coupled with evidence referenced throughout this chapter, leads this book to recommend them as the world's most nourishing food and as the cornerstone of a varied diet.

13.4.10 Yams

As noted, many people confuse yams and sweet potatoes even though they are different types of angiosperms (flowering plants). For example, African American authors Richard Nathaniel Wright (1908–1960) and Ralph Waldo Ellison (1914–1994) called sweet potatoes yams, an error the USDA

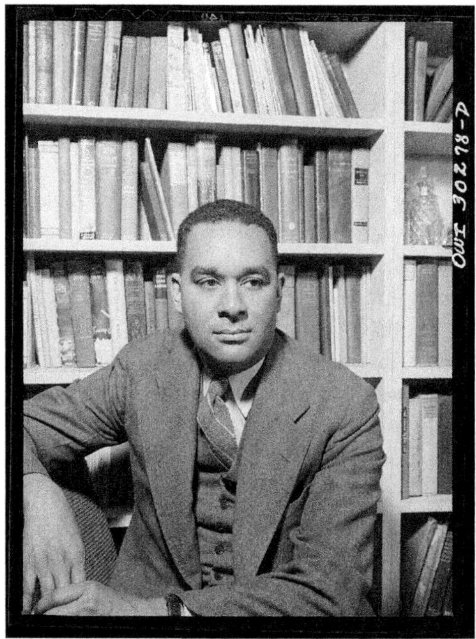

FIGURE 13.7 Richard Wright. (Photo courtesy of Library of Congress. https://www.loc.gov/pictures/item/2017855735/.)

abetted by permitting retailers to brand Puerto Rican sweet potatoes as yams.[213] Sweet potatoes are eudicots, whereas yams are monocotyledons (monocots). These clades evolved separately during roughly the past 130 million years ago.[214] Despite superficial similarities to sweet potatoes, yams are more related to onion, leek, shallot (*Allium ascalonicum*), garlic (*Allium sativum*), and chives (*Allium schoenoprasum*), all monocots. Despite dissimilar appearances, yams are more related to wheat, rye, barley, oats, corn, and other grains because—again—all are monocots than to sweet potatoes.

Even without this confusion, yams have a complex prehistory and history. As mentioned, they are in the genus *Dioscorea*, over 500 species of which inhabit African, Asian, Australian, North American, and South American tropics and subtropics.[215] These continents' peoples ate yams—dubbed "the potatoes of the tropics" because they are staples—millennia before domestication during prehistory.[216] Into the twentieth century wild yams fed India, Southeast Asia, Australia and other Pacific islands, South America, the Caribbean, and Mesoamerica. Plentiful harvests likely delayed domestication because yams fed many people without the effort of cultivation. Of *Dioscorea*'s over 500 species, humans have eaten fifty to one hundred.[217]

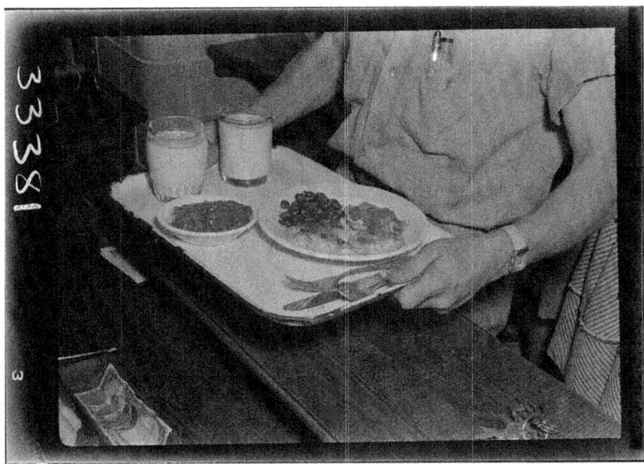

FIGURE 13.8 Candied yams. (Photo courtesy of Library of Congress. https://www.loc.gov/pictures/item/2017858433/.)

Despite yams' diversity, only four species are widely grown. *Dioscorea alata* and *Dioscorea esculenta* originated in Southeast Asia, whereas *Dioscorea rotundata* and *Dioscorea cayenensis* arose in West Africa. Less important was the American species *Dioscorea trifida*, which ceded ground to sweet potatoes and cassava throughout the tropics. Of the major species, *D. rotundata* is grown on the most hectarage worldwide today.[218] Africans make it into dough known as *fufu*. *D. alata* ranks second in area and is the most widespread species with cultivation in Africa, Asia, the Pacific islands, and the Caribbean. *D. esculenta* is seldom grown or eaten outside Southeast Asia. *D. cayenensis* needs the tropics' long, warm growing seasons and languishes in temperate locations. More adaptable, *D. trifida* tolerates the tropics, subtropics, and warm temperate lands. Its tubers, resembling sweet potato roots, exacerbate confusion between yams and sweet potatoes.

Yams evolved at savanna margins with rainy and dry seasons. The tubers hold calories and nutrients to hasten germination at rains' onset. Vines grow during the rains, accumulating energy and nutrients through photosynthesis, a chemical process outlined in Chapter 2. Upon rains' cessation, leaves and vines channel calories and nutrients underground to form tubers, which wait out the dry season. Upon rains' resumption, the cycle repeats. The crucial fact is that yams develop tubers only at the end of each cycle. Premature harvest yields nothing. Those dependent on yams needed patience not to waste time and effort by digging the ground too soon. West Africans, Australian aborigines, and the Andamanese on India's Andaman and Nicobar Islands constructed rituals and festivals to ensure harvest at the proper times.[219]

Yam precursors spread worldwide throughout the tropics by Cretaceous Period's end 65 million years ago.[220] Such dispersal occasioned independent domestications in Southeast Asia, southern China, West Africa, the Caribbean Islands, South America, and possibly Mesoamerica by 3000 BCE.[221] Although northern Australia's indigenes ate wild yams, they appear to have managed rather than domesticated plants.

13.4.11 Yams' Domestication and Dispersal

Domestication may have begun in West Africa, where hunter-gatherers ate wild yams some 60,000 years ago.[222] Between 45,000 and 15,000 years ago, they devised stone and wooden hoes and picks to dig tubers. This work must have been difficult because yams produce edibles deeper underground than potatoes, sweet potatoes, or cassava. Where yams were in forests, people had to penetrate nearby tree roots without metal spades to access tubers. Around 9000 BCE, hunter-gatherers responded to shrinking habitats amid climate change by selecting large yams to maximize food supply. About 3000 BCE, West Africans domesticated *D. rotundata* and *D. cayenensis*. Their farming concentrated in what are today Cote d'Ivoire, Ghana, Togo, Benin, Nigeria, and Cameroon, an area known as the yam belt. Slaves from this region thus knew how to grow yams. Earlier was mentioned their familiarity with sweet potatoes. With this knowledge, they created tuber and root agriculture in the American South, whereas indigenous traditions in tropical America centered on *D. trifida*, sweet potatoes, and cassava and predated the slave trade. Mesoamerican yam consumption and cultivation predated the Maya. In Southeast Asia, the other Old World yam center, *D. esculenta* arose in what are today Vietnam, Laos, and Cambodia. To their west, Thais began eating wild yams between 10,000 and 7000 BCE.[223]

Around 7000 BCE, New Guineans began clearing land for yams.[224] Indonesians were growing them by 5000 BCE. Yam farming spread to Melanesia roughly 3,000 years later. China, acquiring yams before 2000 BCE, may have designated them medicine first and food and pig feed second.[225] In the second millennium BCE, Micronesia adopted yams. The tuber reached eastern Polynesia around 1500 BCE, spreading west through its islands during the first millennium CE. One hypothesis holds that fishers harvested wild yams on island coasts, observing that discards germinated. This discovery led them to plant yams, beginning the process of domestication. In southwesternmost Polynesia, New Zealand began growing yams around 400, though consumption of wild tubers probably preceded cultivation. Yams reached India before 600.[226] Throughout Southeast Asia and Oceania, they joined banana, plantain (*Musa × paradisiaca*), breadfruit (*Artocarpus altilis*), and taro as a staple.[227] Separate from these developments, the Indian Ocean's Madagascar began cultivating yams between the eleventh and fifteenth centuries.[228] They were absent from the Mediterranean—including Egypt—and Arabia.

Reaching India in 1498, the Portuguese learned that Indians and Malaysians provisioned ships with yams. This practice had begun centuries earlier, allowing long voyages across the Indian and Pacific Oceans because yams' vitamin C prevented scurvy.[229] Portugal did likewise. Led by Iberia, Europeans opened their own continent, Africa, Asia, Oceania (including Australia), and the Americas to crop and livestock exchanges.

The western hemisphere's sweet potatoes, cassava, and cacao (*Theobroma cacao*) competed with yams in tropical Africa and Asia. Cassava's inexpensiveness and durability, discussed earlier, made it popular. An earlier section noted its ubiquity in African diets. Despite competition, yams continued to feed Nigeria, Cote d'Ivoire, Benin, Ghana, Togo, Zaire, Ethiopia, Chad, the Central African Republic, New Guinea, Brazil, Haiti, Jamaica, and Japan. Their expensiveness relative to sweet potatoes and cassava in Africa, Asia, Australia, New Guinea and several other equatorial Pacific islands, South America, and the Caribbean indicates strong demand. High prices in West Africa reflect low yields and perishability. In 2016, West African yam production totaled just two-fifths the cassava harvest.[230]

13.4.12 Yams' Nutriment

On average, West Africa's 150 million yam eaters derive over 200 calories daily from the tuber.[231] Among the region's foods, yams supply fewer calories by mass than corn, cassava, or sorghum (*Sorghum bicolor*) and more than sweet potatoes. Carbohydrates furnish most calories. By mass, yams have more calcium than cassava and corn; more iron than cassava; more magnesium than sorghum; more phosphorus than sweet potatoes and cassava; more potassium than corn, cassava, sweet potatoes, and sorghum; more zinc than sorghum; more copper than cassava, sweet potatoes, and sorghum; more manganese than cassava, sweet potatoes, and sorghum; more selenium than sweet potatoes and sorghum; more carotenoids than cassava and sorghum; and more vitamin B_1 than cassava and sweet potatoes; B_5 than corn and sorghum; B_6 than cassava, sweet potatoes, and sorghum; B_9 than corn, sweet potatoes, and sorghum; C than corn, sweet potatoes, and sorghum; E than cassava, sweet potatoes, and sorghum; and K than cassava, corn, sweet potatoes, and sorghum.[232] Table 13.9 shows that 100 grams of yams provide 23.3 percent DV for potassium, 20 percent for manganese, 9 percent for copper, 5.5 percent for potassium, 5.3 percent for magnesium, 28.5 percent

TABLE 13.9
Nutrients in Yams 100 g

Nutrient	Yams	%DV
Calories	118	N/A
Protein (g)	1.53	N/A
Fat (g)	0.17	N/A
Carbs (g)	27.88	N/A
Fiber (g)	4.1	N/A
	Minerals	
Ca (mg)	17	1.7
Fe (mg)	0.54	3
Mg (mg)	21	5.3
P (mg)	55	5.5
K (mg)	816	23.3
Na (mg)	9	0.4
Zn (mg)	0.24	1.6
Cu (mg)	0.18	9
Mn (mg)	0.4	20
Se (mcg)	0.7	1
	Vitamins	
A (IU)	138	2.8
B_1 (mg)	0.11	7.3
B_2 (mg)	0.03	1.7
B_3 (mg)	0.55	2.8
B_5 (mg)	0.31	3.1
B_6 (mg)	0.29	14.5
B_9 (mcg)	23	5.8
B_{12} (mcg)	0	0
C (mg)	17.1	28.5
D (IU)	0	0
E (mg)	0.35	2.3
K (mcg)	2.3	2.9

for vitamin C, 14.5 percent for vitamin B_6, 7.3 percent for B_1, and 5.8 percent for B_9. No other nutrient equals or exceeds 5 percent.

13.4.13 Yams, Yap Island, and Australia

Yams' nutrients and calories increased population on Yap Island—where the tuber occupied 80 percent of arable land—in the North Pacific Ocean's western Caroline Islands.[233] Islanders recounted overcrowding so severe that people had to live on rafts in mangrove swamps.[234] Such stories may be exaggerations, though Yap was crowded when Spaniards attempted to settle it in 1731. Yams alone did not nourish Yapese, who also ate taro, breadfruit, banana, sweet potato, and coconut. As in other places where Europeans encountered indigenes, Old World diseases killed Yapese because they lacked immunity. Yams, sweet potatoes, and other foods deserve no blame for this mortality.

Health data came from Australia's aborigines. In 1982, ten participated in a dietary experiment.[235] All had imitated Europeans, consuming fatty meats, white flour, rice, potatoes, onions, sucrose, sugary beverages, and alcohol and becoming overweight and diabetic. This book absolves the potato from these problems because an earlier section detailed its contributions to nutrition and vitality. Dissatisfied with their predicament, the ten resumed hunting and gathering for 7 weeks, eating only wild produce: seafood, game, yams, figs (*Ficus* species), and honey. By experiment's end, they lost 8.1 kilograms (17.9 pounds) on average, blood pressure and triglycerides declined, and diabetes' symptoms diminished or disappeared. This outcome implies that yams benefited these indigenes, but wild foods and activity also must have invigorated them.

NOTES

1 "Potatoes, Flesh and Skin, Raw," *USDA FoodData Central*, April 1, 2019, accessed February 15, 2020, https://fdc.nal.usda.gov/fdc-app.html#/food-details/170026/nutrients; "Carrots, Raw," *USDA FoodData Central*, April 1, 2019, accessed February 15, 2020, https://fdc.nal.usda.gov/fdc-app.html#/food-details/170393/nutrients.
2 Alan Davidson, "Europeans' Wary Encounter with Tomatoes, Potatoes, and Other New World Foods," in *Chilies to Chocolate: Food the Americas Gave the World*, ed. Nelson Foster and Linda S. Cordell (Tucson and London: University of Arizona Press, 1992), 4–5.
3 Woolfe, 118; George Thottappilly, "Introductory Remarks," in *The Sweetpotato*, ed. Gad Loebenstein and George Thottappilly (Dordrecht: Springer, 2009), 4; Gad Loebenstein, "Origin, Distribution and Economic Importance," in *The Sweetpotato*, ed. Gad Loebenstein and George Thottappilly (Dordrecht: Springer, 2009), 10.
4 Geographers designate this isthmus part of North America, though it is sometimes labeled Central America.
5 Vincent E. Rubatzky and Mas Yamaguchi, *World Vegetables: Principles, Production, and Nutritive Values*, 2d ed. (New York: Chapman and Hall, 1997), 137.
6 Ibid., 132.
7 Patricia J. O'Brien, "Sweet Potatoes and Yams," in *The Cambridge World History of Food*, vol. 1, ed. Kenneth F. Kiple and Kriemhild Conee Ornelas (Cambridge, UK: Cambridge University Press, 2000), 208.
8 Ibid., 210.
9 Jack Golson, "The Making of the New Guinea Highlands," in *The Melanesian Environment*, ed. John H. Winslow (Canberra: Australian National University Press, 1977), 45–46.
10 O'Brien, 211.
11 Woolfe, 541.
12 Ibid., 539.
13 Ibid., 119.
14 Rubatzky and Yamaguchi, 138.
15 John Reader, *Man on Earth* (Austin: University of Texas Press, 1988), 50.
16 Ibid.
17 Woolfe, 548.

18 Hughes and Hughes, 30, 32; Woolfe, 16.

19 Sylvia A. Johnson, *Tomatoes, Potatoes, Corn, and Beans: How the Foods of the Americas Changed Eating around the World* (New York: Atheneum Books, 1997), 71.

20 J. G. Vaughan and C. Geissler, *The New Oxford Book of Food Plants* (Oxford: Oxford University Press, 1997), 192.

21 O'Brien, 209.

22 Woolfe, 16.

23 Ibid., 118.

24 Ping-ti Ho, "The Introduction of American Food Plants into China," *American Anthropologist* 57, no. 2 (April 1955), https://anthrosource.onlinelibrary.wiley.com/doi/pdf/10.1525/aa.1955.57.2.02a00020, 193–194.

25 Frederick J. Simoons, *Food in China: A Cultural and Historical Inquiry* (Boca Raton, FL: CRC Press, 1991), 102.

26 Li and Mu, 156.

27 "China: Sweet Potatoes, Production Quantity (Tons)," *Fact Fish*, 2011–2018, accessed April 23, 2019, http://www.factfish.com/statistic-country/china/sweet%20potatoes%2C%20production%20quantity.

28 Woolfe, 16; Hughes and Hughes, 54.

29 Bradley J. Willcox, D. Craig Willcox, and Makoto Suzuki, *The Okinawa Program: How the World's Longest-Lived People Achieve Everlasting Health—And How You Can Too* (New York: Three Rivers Press, 2001), 160.

30 Janae Wise, "Okinawan Diet: How Much Sweet Potatoes Do Okinawans Really Eat? (Part 2)," *The Okinawan Diet*, 2016, accessed March 28, 2019, http://bring-joy.com/2016/07/31/okinawan-diet-sweet-potatoes.

31 Andrew Weil, "Foreword," in *The Okinawa Program: How the World's Longest-Lived People Achieve Everlasting Health—And How You Can Too*, Bradley J. Willcox, D. Craig Willcox, and Makoto Suzuki (New York: Three Rivers Press, 2001), x.

32 Marina Pitofsky, "What Countries Have the Longest Life Expectancies?" *USA Today*, July 27, 2018, last modified August 5, 2018, accessed April 6, 2019, https://www.usatoday.com/story/news/2018/07/27/life-expectancies-2018-japan-switzerland-spain/848675002; Willcox, Willcox, and Suzuki, 5.

33 Willcox, Willcox, and Suzuki, 69, 160–161.

34 Arne Kalland and Jon Pedersen, "Famine and Population in Fukuoka Domain during the Tokugawa Period," *Journal of Japanese Studies* 10, no. 1 (Winter 1984): 40.

35 Alan Macfarlane, "The Three Major Famines of Japanese History," 2002, accessed March 29, 2019, http://www.alanmacfarlane.com/savage/A-JAPFAM.PDF; Hughes and Hughes, 34.

36 Hughes and Hughes, 34; S. J. Pajonas, "How Sweet Potatoes Saved Japan," April 12, 2016, accessed March 29, 2019, https://www.spajonas.com/2016/04/12/how-sweet-potatoes-saved-japan.

37 Rubatzky and Yamaguchi, 143.

38 "Yam Facts and Figures."

39 Ibid., 5.

40 Li and Mu, 148; Mary Ann Lila, "Anthocyanins and Human Health: An In Vitro Investigative Approach," *Journal of Biomedicine and Biotechnology* 2004, no. 5 (December 1, 2004): 306–313, https://www.ncbi.nlm.nih.gov/pmc/articles/PMC1082894.

41 *The Illustrated Encyclopedia of Fruits, Vegetables, and Herbs* (New York: Chartwell Books, 2017), 154.

42 Pedersen, 37.

43 Kelly Pfeiffer, *Superfood Weeknight Meals: Healthy, Delicious Dinners Ready in 30 Minutes or Less* (Beverly, MA: Quarto Publishing Group, 2017), 10.

44 Robert William Fogel and Stanley L. Engerman, *Time on the Cross: The Economics of American Negro Slavery* (New York and London: Norton, 1995), 113.

45 Pedersen, 35; "100 G, Buckwheat," Fat Secret, 2019, accessed March 30, 2019, https://www.fatsecret.com/calories-nutrition/usda/buckwheat?portionid=62419&portionamount=100.000; "100 G, Grilled Fish," Fat Secret, 2019, accessed March 30, 2019, https://www.fatsecret.com/calories-nutrition/generic/fish-grilled?portionid=479257&portionamount=100.000; "Rice, White, Long-Grain, Regular, Unenriched, Cooked without Salt," USDA FoodData Central, April 1, 2019, accessed February 15, 2020, https://fdc.nal.usda.gov/fdc-app.html#/food-details/169757/nutrients; "100 G, Cooked Soybeans (Fat Not Added in Cooking)," Fat Secret, 2019, accessed March 30, 2019, https://www.fatsecret.com/calories-nutrition/generic/soybeans-cooked-fat-not-added-in-cooking?portionid=51887&portionamount=100.000.

46 Sakio Tsutsui, Yoshihiko Shiga, and Tetsuo Mikami, "Japanese Sweetpotatoes: Production, Cultivars, and Possible Ancestry," *Notulae Botanicae Horti Agrobotanici Cluj-Napoca* 44, no. 1 (June 2016), https://www.notulaebotanicae.ro/index.php/nbha/article/view/10400/7869, 2.

47 "Japan, Basic Statistics," CGIAR, Ricepedia: The Online Authority on Rice, accessed March 30, 2019, http://ricepedia.org/japan.
48 Yohei Kawasaki, Yu Tanaka, Keisuke Katsura, Larry C. Purcell, and Tatsuhiko Shiraiwa, "Yield and Dry Matter Productivity of Japanese and U.S. Soybean Cultivars," *Plant Production Science* 19, no. 2 (2016), https://www.tandfonline.com/doi/full/10.1080/1343943X.2015.1133235, 257.
49 Hughes and Hughes, 35.
50 April McGreger, *Sweet Potatoes* (Chapel Hill: University of North Carolina Press, 2014), 3.
51 "Sweet Potato," in *The Cambridge World History of Food*, vol. 2, ed. Kenneth F. Kiple and Kriemhild Conee Ornelas (Cambridge, UK: Cambridge University Press, 2000), 1863.
52 O'Brien, 209.
53 McGreger, 1–2.
54 Ibid., 7.
55 Hughes and Hughes, 43.
56 McGreger, 3.
57 E. A. Estes, "Marketing Sweetpotatoes in the United States: A Serious Challenge for Small-to-Moderate Volume Growers," in *The Sweetpotato*, ed. Gad Loebenstein and George Thottappilly (Dordrecht: Springer, 2009), 270.
58 T. P. Smith, S. Stoddard, M. Shankle, and J. Schultheis, "Sweetpotato Production in the United States," in *The Sweetpotato*, ed. Gad Loebenstein and George Thottappilly (Dordrecht: Springer, 2009), 291.
59 McGreger, 9.
60 Li and Mu, 148.
61 Ibid., 151.
62 Antonio C. Allem, "The Origins and Taxonomy of Cassava," in *Cassava: Biology, Production and Utilization*, ed. R. J. Hillocks, J. M. Thresh, and A. C. Bellotti (Wallingford, UK and New York: CABI Publishing, 2002), 8.
63 Peng-Gao Li and Tai-Hua Mu, "Sweet Potato: Health Benefits, Production and Utilization in China," in *Potatoes: Production, Consumption and Health Benefits*, ed. Claudio Caprara (New York: Nova Science Publishers, 2012), 151.
64 Jennifer A. Wolfe, *Sweet Potato: An Untapped Food Resource* (Cambridge, UK: Cambridge University Press, 1992), 4.
65 Meredith Sayles Hughes and Tom Hughes, *Buried Treasure: Roots and Tubers* (Minneapolis, MN: Lerner Publications, 1998), 44.
66 Tori Avey, "Christopher Columbus—Foods of the New World," Tori's Kitchen, October 8, 2012, accessed March 20, 2019, https://toriavey.com/history-kitchen/what-christopher-columbus-discovered-foods-of-the-new-world.
67 Mary Karasch, "Manioc," in *The Cambridge World History of Food*, vol. 1, ed. Kenneth F. Kiple and Kriemhild Conee Ornelas (Cambridge, UK: Cambridge University Press, 2000), 183.
68 Ibid, 183–184.
69 Ibid., 184.
70 Rory J. Hillocks, "Cassava in Africa," in *Cassava: Biology, Production and Utilization*, ed. R. J. Hillocks, J. M. Thresh, and A.C. Bellotti (Wallingford, UK and New York: CABI Publishing 2002), 41.
71 Karasch, 185.
72 I. C. Onwueme, "Cassava in Asia and the Pacific," in *Cassava: Biology, Production and Utilization*, ed. R. J. Hillocks, J. M. Thresh, and A.C. Bellotti (Wallingford, UK and New York: CABI Publishing 2002), 58.
73 Karasch, 185.
74 "Cassava's Link to Iodine Deficiency Requires Further Study," *Modern Ghana*, January 17, 2009, accessed March 22, 2019, https://www.modernghana.com/news/198981/cassavas-link-to-iodine-deficiency-requires-further-study.html.
75 A. T. Ciarfella, L. J. Sivoli, and E. E. Perez, "Food Products Developed Using Cassava Roots and Its Derivatives: A Review," in *Cassava: Production, Nutritional Properties and Health Effects*, ed. Francis P. Molinari (New York: Nova Publishers, 2014), 165; "Preface," in *Cassava: Production, Nutritional Properties and Health Effects*, ed. Francis P. Molinari (New York: Nova Publishers, 2014), vii.
76 Hughes and Hughes, 48.
77 Ibid.
78 P. Hennart, P. Bourdoux, R. Lagasse, C. Thilly, G. Putzeys, P. Courtois, H. L. Vis, Y. Yunga, P. Seghers, and F. Delange, "Epidemiology of Goitre and Malnutrition and Dietary Supplies of Iodine, Thiocyanate, and Proteins in Bas Zaire, Kivu, and Ubangi," in *Nutritional Factors Involved in the Goitrogenic Action*

of Cassava, ed. F. Delange, F. B. Iteke, and A. M. Ermans (Ottawa: International Development Research Centre, 1982), 31.

79 J. Vanderpas, M. Vanderpas-Rivera, P. Bourdoux, M. Dramaix, R. Lagasse, P. Seghers, F. Delange, A. M. Ermans, and C. Thilly, "Breast Feeding, Thiocyanate Metabolism, and Thyroid Function in Young Infants in Severe Endemic Goitre," in *Nutritional Factors Involved in the Goitrogenic Action of Cassava*, ed. F. Delange, F. B. Iteke, and A. M. Ermans (Ottawa: International Development Research Centre, 1982), 61.

80 A. O. Akinpelu, L. E. F. Amamgbo, A. O. Olojede, and A. S. Oyekale, "Health Implications of Cassava Production and Consumption," *Journal of Agriculture and Social Research* 11, no. 1 (2011): 118–119, https://www.ajol.info/index.php/jasr/article/view/73684/64364.

81 "Preface," in *Cassava*, vii.

82 Hughes and Hughes, 54.

83 Ciarfella, Sivoli, and Perez, 168.

84 Benito Infante and Omar Garcia, "Cassava Bread (Casabe) in Venezuela: Some Nutritional Considerations," in *Cassava: Production, Nutritional Properties and Health Effects*, ed. Francis P. Molinari (New York: Nova Publishers, 2014), 115.

85 "Cassava, Raw," *USDA FoodData Central*, April 1, 2019, accessed January 25, 2020, https://fdc.nal.usda.gov/fdc-app.html#/food-details/169985/nutrients; "Yam Facts and Figures," accessed April 4, 2019, 5–6, https://www.integratedbreeding.net/attachment/1376/Yam%20Brief.pdf.

86 "Manioc," in *The Cambridge World History of Food*, ed. Kenneth F. Kiple and Kriemhild Conee Ornelas, vol. 2 (Cambridge, UK: Cambridge University Press, 2000), 1810.

87 John A. Dixon, "Consumption," in *The Cassava Economy of Java*, ed. Walter P. Falcon, William O. Jones, Scott R. Pearson, John A. Dixon, Gerald C. Nelson, Frederick C. Roche, and Laurian J. Unnevehr (Stanford, CA: Stanford University Press, 1984), 65.

88 Stephanie Pedersen, *Roots: The Complete Guide to the Underground Superfood* (New York: Sterling 2017), 13.

89 Ibid.

90 Joseph Mason, "Cassava Root: Beats Cancer Instead of Chemo and Radiation! Plus It Doesn't Kill You!" October 16, 2017, https://www.linkedin.com/pulse/cassava-root-beats-cancer-instead-chemo-radiation-plus-%E9%BE%99%E7%9A%84%E5%BB%BA%E9%80%A0%E8%80%85-.

91 Graca Justo, Eloy Macchiute de Oliveira, and Claudia Jurberg, "Functional Foods and Cancer on Pinterest and PubMed: Myths and Science," *Future Science OA* 4, no. 9 (August 9, 2018), https://www.ncbi.nlm.nih.gov/pmc/articles/PMC6225095.

92 Dulce Nhassico, Humberto Muquingue, Julie Cliff, Arnaldo Cumbana, and J. Howard Bradbury, "Rising African Cassava Production, Diseases Due to High Cyanide Intake and Control Measures," *Journal of the Science of Food and Agriculture* 88 (2008), https://biology-assets.anu.edu.au/hosted_sites/CCDN/papers/PAPCYREV.pdf, 2043.

93 C. Abuye, U. Kelbessa, and S. Wolde-Gebriel, "Health Effects of Cassava Consumption in South Ethiopia," *East African Medical Journal* 75, no. 3 (February 28, 1998), http://europepmc.org/article/med/9640816, 166.

94 F. Delange, C. Thilly, P. Bourdoux, P. Hennart, P. Courtois, and A. M. Ermans, "Influence of Dietary Goitrogens during Pregnancy in Humans on Thyroid Function of the Newborn," in *Nutritional Factors Involved in the Goitrogenic Action of Cassava*, ed. F. Delange, F. B. Iteke, and A. M. Ermans (Ottawa: International Development Research Centre, 1982), 50.

95 "Cassava's Link to Iodine Deficiency Requires Further Study."

96 "Micronutrient Deficiencies," World Health Organization, accessed January 1, 2020, https://www.who.int/nutrition/topics/idd/en.

97 "Cassava's Link to Iodine Deficiency Requires Further Study."

98 Ibid.

99 *The Illustrated Encyclopedia of Fruits, Vegetables, and Herbs*, 32.

100 "White Potato," in *The Cambridge World History of Food*, vol. 2, ed. Kenneth F. Kiple and Kriemhild Conee Ornelas (Cambridge, UK: Cambridge University Press, 2000), 1878; Linda Civitello, *Cuisine and Culture: A History of Food and People*, 3d ed. (Hoboken, NJ: Wiley, 2011), 97.

101 John Reader, *Potato: A History of the Propitious Esculent* (New Haven, CT and London: Yale University Press, 2008), 26.

102 Ibid., 52.

103 Kristina Killgrove, "Potatoes Were Not Just a Symbol of the Elite in Ancient Peru, Archaeologists Find," *Forbes*, November 2, 2018, accessed March 26, 2019, https://www.forbes.com/sites/kristinakillgrove/2018/11/02/potatoes-were-not-just-a-symbol-of-the-elite-in-ancient-peru-archaeologists-find/#4c16f90d1877.

104 Reader, *Potato*, 53.
105 "International Year of the Potato," FAO, 2008, accessed March 10, 2020, http://www.fao.org/potato-2008/en/potato/origins.html.
106 Reader, *Potato*, 56–57.
107 Ibid., *Potato*, 38; Johnson, 67.
108 Reader, *Potato*, 57.
109 T. Colin Campbell, *Whole: Rethinking the Science of Nutrition* (Dallas, TX: BenBella Books, 2013), 7.
110 Civitello, 96.
111 John P. McKay, Bennett D. Hill, John Buckler, Clare Haru Crowston, Merry E. Wiesner-Hanks, and Joe Perry, *Understanding Western Society: A Brief History* (Boston and New York: Beford/St. Martin's, 2012), 433.
112 Reader, *Potato*, 68.
113 "White Potato," 1879.
114 Reader, *Potato*, 90–91.
115 Ibid., 88; Hughes and Hughes, 14–15.
116 Waverly Root and Richard de Rochemont, *Eating in America: A History* (Hopewell, NJ: Ecco Press, 1995), 16.
117 Gail L. Schumann and Cleora J. D'Arcy, *Hungry Planet: Stories of Plant Diseases* (St. Paul, MN: American Phytopathological Society, 2012), 6.
118 The Editors, "Introduction," in *The Cambridge World History of Food*, vol. 1, ed. Kenneth F. Kiple and Kriemhild Conee Ornelas (Cambridge, UK: Cambridge University Press, 2000), 3; Susan Campbell Bartoletti, *Black Potatoes: The Story of the Great Irish Famine, 1845–1850* (Boston: Houghton Mifflin, 2001), 20.
119 Helen Sanderson, "Roots and Tubers," in *The Cultural History of Plants*, ed. Ghillean Prance and Mark Nesbitt (New York and London: Routledge, 2005), 64.
120 Reader, *Potato*, 78.
121 Russ Parsons, *How to Pick a Peach: The Search for Flavor from Farm to Table* (Boston and New York: Houghton Mifflin, 2007), 339.
122 Joseph R. O'Neill, *The Irish Potato Famine* (Edina, MN: ABDO Publishing, 2009), 12.
123 Charles C. Mann, "How the Potato Changed the World," *Smithsonian Magazine*, November 2011, accessed February 27, 2020, https://www.smithsonianmag.com/history/how-the-potato-changed-the-world-108470605.
124 Pedersen, 22; "Yukon Gold Potatoes," USDA FoodData Central, April 1, 2019, accessed January 25, 2020, https://fdc.nal.usda.gov/fdc-app.html#/food-details/715214/nutrients; "Yukon Gold Potatoes," USDA FoodData Central, April 1, 2019, accessed January 25, 2020, https://fdc.nal.usda.gov/fdc-app.html#/food-details/472938/nutrients; "Brookshire's, Yukon Gold Potatoes," USDA FoodData Central, April 1, 2019, accessed January 25, 2020, https://fdc.nal.usda.gov/fdc-app.html#/food-details/450096/nutrients; Rachael Link, "Antioxidant-Loaded Purple Potatoes: The Healthy, Versatile Carb," Dr. Axe, August 29, 2019, accessed January 25, 2020, https://draxe.com/nutrition/purple-potatoes; "Potatoes, Red, Flesh and Skin, Raw," Self Nutrition Data, 2018; accessed January 25, 2020, https://nutritiondata.self.com/facts/vegetables-and-vegetable-products/2549/2.
125 Pedersen, 22.
126 Ibid; "A Size Guide to America's Favorite Potato," Idaho Potato Commission, accessed March 27, 2019, https://idahopotato.com/uploads/media/IPC-carton-count-size-guide.pdf; Anitra C. Carr and Balz Frei, "Toward a New Recommended Dietary Allowance for Vitamin C Based on Antioxidant and Health Effects in Humans," *The American Journal of Clinical Nutrition* 69, no. 6 (June 1, 1999): 1086.
127 Pedersen, 22; Ellen Messer, "Potatoes (White)," in *The Cambridge World History of Food*, vol. 1, ed. Kenneth F. Kiple and Kriemhild Conee Ornelas (Cambridge, UK: Cambridge University Press, 2000), 196.
128 "Nutrition Facts," Potatoes USA, accessed October 14, 2019, https://www.potatogoodness.com/wp-content/uploads/2019/04/Potatoes-nutritional-label-2019-ENGLISH-1.jpg; "Potatoes Goodness Unearthed," Idaho Potato Commission, 2012, accessed October 14, 2019, https://idahopotato.com/uploads/media/PPNHandbook_Final.pdf, 2.
129 "FDA Vitamins and Minerals Chart," *FDA*, accessed October 14, 2019, https://www.accessdata.fda.gov/scripts/interactivenutritionfactslabel/factsheets/vitamin_and_mineral_chart.pdf.
130 Sandi Busch, "Does the Skin of a Potato Really Have All the Vitamins?" SF Gate, November 27, 2018, accessed October 14, 2019, https://healthyeating.sfgate.com/skin-potato-really-vitamins-5378.html.
131 Reader, *Man on Earth*, 174.

132 K. H. Sabeena Farvin, A. Surendraraj, and Charlotte Jacobsen, "Composition and Health Benefits of Potato Peel," in *Potatoes: Production, Consumption and Health Benefits*, ed. Claudio Caprara (New York: Nova Science Publishers, 2012), 210–211.
133 Reader, *Man on Earth*, 173.
134 Milton Meltzer, *The Amazing Potato: A Story in Which the Incas, Conquistadors, Marie Antoinette, Thomas Jefferson, Wars, Famines, Immigrants, and French Fries All Play a Part* (New York: HarperCollins*Publishers*, 1992), 43.
135 Kenneth J. Carpenter, *The History of Scurvy and Vitamin C* (Cambridge, UK: Cambridge University Press, 1986), 76–77.
136 Jean Beagle Ristaino and Donald H. Pfister, "'What a Painfully Interesting Subject': Charles Darwin's Studies of Potato Late Blight," *BioScience* 66, no. 12 (December 2016): 1035–1045, https://academic.oup.com/bioscience/article/66/12/1035/2646818.
137 R. E. Hughes, "Scurvy," in *The Cambridge World History of Food*, vol. 1, ed. Kenneth F. Kiple and Kriemhild Conee Ornelas, (Cambridge, UK: Cambridge University Press, 2000), 991.
138 Ibid.
139 Davidson, 4–5.
140 "White Potato," 1879.
141 Messer, 192.
142 Bill Laws, *Fifty Plants that Changed the Course of History* (Buffalo, NY and Richmond Hill, Ontario: Firefly Books, 2015), 182.
143 John Burnett, *Plenty and Want: A Social History of Diet in England from 1815 to the Present Day* (London: Scolar Press, 1979), 36.
144 "White Potato," 1879.
145 Tomas O'Riordan, "The Introduction of the Potato into Ireland," *History Ireland: Ireland's History Magazine*, 2019, accessed March 27, 2019, https://www.historyireland.com/early-modern-history-1500-1700/the-introduction-of-the-potato-into-ireland.
146 William H. McNeill, "How the Potato Changed the World's History," *Social Research* 66, no. 1 (Spring 1999): 72.
147 Johnson, 75–76.
148 Tim Blanning, *Frederick the Great: King of Prussia* (New York: Random House, 2016), 446; Reader, *Potato*, 119.
149 Messer, 191.
150 Mann.
151 Redcliffe N. Salaman, *The History and Social Influence of the Potato*, rev. ed. (Cambridge, UK: Cambridge University Press, 1985), 599; Andrew Griffin, "Eva Ekblad: The Woman Who Brought Potatoes, Flour and Alcohol to the People," Independent, July 10, 2017, accessed January 4, 2020, https://www.independent.co.uk/news/science/eva-ekblad-potato-flour-alcohol-potatoes-google-doodle-swedish-scientist-starch-a7832911.html; Lars G. Sandberg and Richard H. Steckel, "Soldier, Soldier, What Made You Grow So Tall?: A Study of Height, Health and Nutrition in Sweden, 1720–1881," *Economy and History* 23, no. 2 (1980): 100.
152 Ibid.
153 "The Potato Sector," *PotatoPro*, accessed January 4, 2020, https://www.potatopro.com/russian-federation/potato-statistics.
154 Salaman, 116.
155 Johnson, 77.
156 Leo Lucassen, "Total Population Europe, 1500–1900 (Millions)," Research Gate, accessed March 27, 2019, https://www.researchgate.net/figure/2-Total-population-Europe-1500-1900-millions_tbl35_47723061.
157 Meltzer, 38.
158 Gretel H. Pelto and Pertti J. Pelto, "Diet and Delocalization: Dietary Changes Since 1750," *Journal of Interdisciplinary History* 14, no. 2 (Autumn 1983): 512.
159 Blanning, 446.
160 H. J. Teutenberg, "The General Relationship between Diet and Industrialization," in *European Diet from Pre-Industrial to Modern Times*, ed. Elborg Forster and Robert Forster (New York: Torchbooks, 1975), 70.
161 Hughes and Hughes, 16; Herman Erlichson, "Mechanics and Thermodynamics," in *History of Modern Science and Mathematics*, vol. 3, ed. Brian S. Baigrie (New York: Charles Scribner's Sons, 2002), 171–172; "Thompson, Benjamin," in *World Book's Biographical Encyclopedia of Scientists*, vol. 7 (Chicago: World Book, 2003), 139.

162 Sanborn C. Brown, "Thompson, Benjamin (Count Rumford)," in *Dictionary of Scientific Biography*, vol. 13, ed. Charles Coulston Gillispie (New York: Charles Scribner's Sons, 1981), 351.
163 Ibid., 350–351; Hughes and Hughes, 16.
164 Johnson, 82.
165 Teutenberg, 71–73.
166 "History of the Potato," Klondike Brands, 2019, accessed March 27, 2019, http://www.klondikebrands.com/potato-history.
167 J. C. Drummond and Anne Wilbraham, *The Englishman's Food: A History of Five Centuries of English Diet*, rev. ed. (London: Pimlico, 1991), 366–367.
168 Ibid., 368–369.
169 Henry Hobhouse, *Seeds of Change: Six Plants that Transformed Mankind* (New York: Shoemaker and Hoard, 2005), 238; William H. McNeill, "The Introduction of the Potato into Ireland," *Journal of Modern History* 21, no. 3 (September 1949): 221.
170 R. E. Hughes, 991; McNeill, "How the Potato Changed the World's History," 75.
171 Meltzer, 43; Cormac O Grada, "The Population of Ireland, 1700–1900: A Survey," *Annales de Demographie Historique* (1979): 283, https://www.persee.fr/doc/adh_0066-2062_1979_num_1979_1_1425.
172 O'Neill, 26, 35; James S. Donnelly, Jr., *The Great Irish Potato Famine* (Gloucestershire: Sutton Publishing, 2001), 4.
173 O'Neill, 26–27.
174 Meltzer, 43.
175 Parsons, 340, 342.
176 Reader, 156; Shelley Barber, ed. *The Prendergast Letters: Correspondence from Famine-Era Ireland, 1840–1850* (Amherst and Boston: University of Massachusetts Press, 2006), 193; John Percival, *The Great Famine: Ireland's Potato Famine, 1845–51* (New York: Viewer Books, 1995), 36.
177 Beryl Brintnall Simpson and Molly Conner Ogorzaly, *Economic Botany: Plants in Our World*, 3d ed. (Boston: Houghton Mifflin, 2001), 181.
178 Ibid.
179 Johnson, 79.
180 Arthur Young, *Tours in Ireland: 1776–1779*, ed. A. W. Hutton, vol. 2 (London: George Bell and Sons, 1892), 43–45.
181 Messer, 192.
182 Percival, 36.
183 Burnett, 36–37.
184 McNeill, "How the Potato Changed the World's History," 75.
185 Ibid., 77.
186 Reader, 94.
187 Robert William Fogel, "Nutrition and the Decline in Mortality Since 1700: Some Preliminary Findings," in *Long-Term Factors in American Economic Growth*, ed. Stanley L. Engerman and Robert E. Gallman (Chicago and London: University of Chicago Press, 1986), 472.
188 Marcie Cohen Ferris, *The Edible South: The Power of Food and the Making of an American Region* (Chapel Hill: University of North Carolina Press, 2014), 14.
189 Reader, 94.
190 Teutenberg, 83.
191 Nathan Nunn and Nancy Qian, "The Potato's Contribution to Population and Urbanization: Evidence from a Historical Experiment," *Quarterly Journal of Economics* 126, no. 2 (May 2011): 597, https://academic.oup.com/qje/article/126/2/593/1868756.
192 Johnson, 78.
193 McNeill, "How the Potato Changed the World's History," 81–82.
194 Jack Staub, *The Illustrated Book of Edible Plants* (Layton, UT: Gibbs Smith, 2017), 147.
195 Robert William Fogel, *The Escape from Hunger and Premature Death, 1700–2100: Europe, America, and the Third World* (Cambridge, UK: Cambridge University Press, 2004), 5.
196 John H. Knowles, "The Responsibility of the Individual," *Daedalus* 106, no. 1 (Winter 1977): 57.
197 The Editors, 3; Hansjorg Kuster, "Rye," in *The Cambridge World History of Food*, vol. 1, ed. Kenneth F. Kiple and Kriemhild Conee Ornelas (Cambridge, UK: Cambridge University Press, 2000), 151.
198 The Editors, 3.
199 Pedersen, 22; "Potatoes, Flesh and Skin, Raw;" "Rye Flour, Light," USDA FoodData Central, April 1, 2019, accessed October 15, 2019, https://fdc.nal.usda.gov/fdc-app.html#/food-details/168887/nutrients.
200 Lucassen.

201 Alison Spiegel, "You Won't Believe How Hard It Is to Find Peanut Butter in These Countries," *Huffington Post*, April 9, 2014, accessed March 31, 2019, https://www.huffpost.com/entry/peanut-butter_n_5105203.
202 Civitello, 138.
203 Sandberg and Steckel, 100; Donn Devine, "How Long Is a Generation?" Ancestry, 2006–2019, accessed April 23, 2019, http://www.ancestry.ca/learn/learningcenters/default.aspx?section=lib_generation.
204 Sandberg and Steckel, 100–101.
205 Cormac O Grada, *Ireland before and after the Famine: Explorations in Economic History, 1800–1925* (Manchester and New York: Manchester University Press, 1988), 18.
206 McNeill, "How the Potato Changed the World's History," 77.
207 Nunn and Qian, 598.
208 Johnson, 76–77.
209 McNeill, "How the Potato Changed the World's History," 68.
210 Johnson, 83.
211 Ibid.; Hughes and Hughes, 26–27.
212 Nunn and Qian, 599.
213 McGreger, 4, 8.
214 Frederick B. Essig, *Plant Life: A Brief History* (Oxford: Oxford University Press, 2015), 224.
215 Rubatzky and Yamaguchi, 162.
216 Ibid., 178. This language could also be applied to sweet potatoes and cassava.
217 Jack R. Harlan, *Crops and Man*, 2nd ed. (Madison, WI: American Society of Agronomy, Crop Science Society of America, 1992), 130.
218 "Yam Facts and Figures," 1.
219 Harlan, 24.
220 D. G. Coursey, *Yams: An Account of the Nature, Origins, Cultivation and Utilisation of the Useful Members of the Dioscoreaceae* (London: Longmans, 1967), 6.
221 Rubatzky and Yamaguchi, 162.
222 O'Brien, 214.
223 Ibid., 213.
224 Ibid.
225 Ibid.; Coursey, 13.
226 Coursey, 14.
227 Chapter 14 discusses banana and plantain nomenclature.
228 O'Brien, 214.
229 Vaughan and Geissler, 192.
230 "Yam Facts and Figures," 2.
231 Ibid., 4.
232 Ibid., 5–6.
233 Reader, *Man on Earth*, 17.
234 Ibid., 20.
235 Michael Pollan, *In Defense of Food: An Eater's Manifesto* (New York: Penguin Press, 2008), 85–87.

14 Fruits

14.1 DEFINITION AND SEED DISPERSAL

Chapter 9 mentioned that a fruit is a flower's fertilized ovary, which develops to hold seeds. This definition encompasses edibles that popular opinion denies as fruits, including corn (*Zea mays*) kernels, cucumbers (*Cucumis sativus*), peppers (*Capsicum* species), eggplants (*Solanum melongena*), squashes (*Cucurbita* species), almonds (*Amygdalus communis*), pecans (*Carya illinoinensis*), okra (*Abelmoschus esculentus*), legumes (species in the family Fabaceae or Leguminosae) and other pods—though pod's removal eliminates the seeds as fruits—tomatoes (*Solanum esculentum*) and olives (*Olea europaea*).[1] The public discounts these items in the conviction that only sweet, juicy, or pulpy produce not eaten as an entrée qualifies. Desserts such as apples (*Malus domestica*), bananas (*Musa x paradisiaca*), or sweet oranges (*Citrus sinensis*) come to mind as archetypal fruits in the United States, though there is no worldwide standard of what is appropriate for dessert or whether a meal must include it.

A fruit's color, aroma, flavor, or their combination attracts animals to eat it. This occurrence may seem strange because animals flee predators rather than submit to consumption. In this instance, however, comparison between plants and animals is unhelpful because plants' rootedness precludes the mobility evident in animals. More fruitful is recognition that plants, like all life, seek to pass their genes to the next generation.

Every spring my sour cherry trees (*Prunus cerasus*) pollinate, producing fruit that ripens in June. If all cherries fell from the trees, the germinating seedlings would occupy a tiny area. In competition for sunlight, water, and nutrients, each would crowd out its neighbors so that none would survive to maturity and so would fail to perpetuate themselves. But they avoid this fate. Whatever cherries I do not pick lure birds to devour them. They fly away, swallowing each fruit and defecating the pit distant from the trees. Dung fertilizes the soil, aiding germination and growth of seedlings that, no longer facing crowding and competition, grow to maturity if nothing kills them beforehand. In other words, fruit aids seed dispersal, giving seedlings the best prospect for success in a hostile world.

14.2 FRUITS AND PRIMATE EVOLUTION

Among animals drawn to fruits were humanity's forebearers.[2] American nutritionist and exercise physiologist Loren Cordain (b. 1950) stated that fruits were part of "humanity's original way of life."[3] British ecologist Stanley Jan Ulijaszek (b. 1954), Australian nutritional chemist Neil Mann, and British anatomist Sarah Elton traced frugivory (fruit eating) to the first primates.[4] Readers may recall that Chapter 3 dated primate origins no earlier than about 65 million years ago. Fruits were not the lone food, but they were important as sources of fiber, minerals, vitamins, protein, and energy in the form of sugars, especially the monosaccharides glucose and fructose.[5] Chapter 2 noted that both have the formula $C_6H_{12}O_6$ and that glucose is photosynthesis' primary product. Domestic fruits tend to have more sucrose ($C_{12}H_{22}O_{11}$), a disaccharide, than their wild counterparts. Other fruit sugars include sorbitol ($C_6H_{14}O_6$).[6] Sugars made fruits tasty and easy to digest. Through experimentation, primates learned to equate sweetness with edibility and bitterness with toxicity.

Fruit sugars introduced early primates to the alcohol ethanol (C_2H_5OH) through fermentation. Humanity's enthusiasm for ethanol as beer, wine, spirits, and kindred products may derive from primates' exposure to it by eating fruit that had begun to ferment. Dates (*Phoenix dactylifera*) may have been the first fruit that prehistoric peoples converted into wine.[7] Wine from grapes (*Vitis vinifera*) emerged as a beverage throughout the Mediterranean, separating this region from northern

Europe, which relied on beer and—Chapter 11 noted—developed a preference for sucrose in the Middle Ages.[8] Wine or another alcohol diluted with water was a safe beverage because ethanol killed pathogens that contaminated water.

Among nutrients, fruits tend to have vitamin C (ascorbic acid), which Chapter 2 mentioned as water soluble. This characteristic requires the body to consume vitamin C regularly to offset excretion in urine. Humankind's lineage lost the ability to manufacture this vitamin around 60 million years ago, implying that our ancestors had such ample access to fruits, vegetables, and other vitamin C sources that natural selection no longer favored individuals that made the nutrient.[9]

The issue is whether this plentitude was periodic or continuous. The need for regular ascorbic acid intake indicates that humanity's ancestors ingested it often, but this requirement does not prove frequent fruit consumption if other foods could be substituted for the vitamin. American cardiac surgeon Steven R. Gundry averred that fruit was available only seasonally until globalism permitted purchase even when unavailable locally.[10] American neurologist David Perlmutter (b. 1954)—introduced in Chapter 1—agreed, writing that as late as 1900, fruit was eaten only in season.[11]

Seasonality required consumption of vitamin C substitutes when fruit was unobtainable. American anthropologist Stephen Le specified insects in lieu of fruit for vitamin C.[12] This claim is inaccurate because insects tend to be poor sources of it, though many species have B vitamins, E, fiber, minerals, protein, fat, and carbohydrates.[13] Their elimination as vitamin C candidates and fruit unavailability year-round narrows the possibilities to leaves given Ulijanszek, Mann, and Elton's description of primates as frugivores, insectivores, folivores (leaf eaters), or their combination.[14] Because our primate forebearers lived near the equator, only tropical leaves qualify as potential vitamin C sources. A 2010 paper identified leaves of six wild tropical plants as rich in this vitamin.[15] This number does not exhaust the possibilities but suffices to demonstrate that our ancestors could have ingested vitamin C year-round without eating fruit.

The foregoing does not diminish fruits' importance to our predecessors. Avid fruit consumption between roughly 60 and 30 million years ago caused them to evolve flat molars suitable for soft or hard fruits rather than ridged molars ideal for grinding insect exoskeletons.[16] To be sure, our ancestors ate insects, which supplied complete proteins absent in fruits. Leaves too remained in prehuman diets. Like us, our precursors were omnivores and eclectic feeders who targeted many foods. Chapter 3 detailed primate diets' evolution.

Moreover, fruit consumption may have hastened primate brain growth. Chapter 4 discussed anthropologists' belief that meat fueled encephalization during roughly the past 2 million years. This expansion augmented the brain that frugivory had enlarged millions of years earlier. Notable in this regard, frugivorous primates have larger brains than folivores.[17] Ulijaszek, Mann, and Elton believed that enlargement resulted from frugivores' need to map mentally their surroundings to know where and when fruits of various trees ripened.

Cognitive cartography took primates to distant locations when fruit was sparse, developing the nomadism that defined hunter-gatherers.[18] Coverage of long distances in search of fruits may have hastened evolution of bipedalism, an efficient locomotion. Humanity's colonization of every continent—though no one permanently inhabits Antarctica—contrasts with most primates' confinement to the tropics and may have stemmed from the quest for ripe fruit. Chapter 3 described humans' worldwide dispersion.

14.3 FRUITS' CRITICS

Fruits' importance to our evolution has not prevented criticism. Le cited anecdotes of people, notably American businessman Steven Paul Jobs (1955–2011) and American actor Christopher Ashton Kutcher (b. 1978), who sickened from excessive fruit intake.[19] Le implicated fruits' fructose in insulin resistance, pancreatic cancer, abnormal uric acid concentration, gout, metabolic disturbances, and heart disease. He cautioned that birds, bears, and people who eat primarily fruit lose weight, though dieters might welcome this prospect.[20] In contrast, Gundry faulted fruit consumption for overweight among gorillas (*Gorilla gorilla* and *Gorilla beringei*), chimpanzees (*Pan troglodytes*), bonobos (*Pan paniscus*), orangutans (*Pongo pygmaeus, Pongo abelii, Pongo tapanuliensis,* and *Pongo hooijeri*), and us.[21] Beyond this critique, he blamed year-round fruit availability for human illnesses.

As the most strident critic, Gundry equated fruits with Wrigley Company candy Skittles, both being "the same poisonous stuff."[22] He did not specify the worst, though in hopes of finding an example to test, this paragraph notes that Newark, Delaware's Produce Marketing Association listed bananas as the most eaten fruit in the United States in 2018.[23] Because Gundry allowed consumption of green bananas, this paragraph omits them in an effort to accommodate his predilections.[24]

Instead, it references apples, the second most eaten fruit in 2018.[25] Comparison between Skittles and apples in Table 14.1 demonstrates the falsity of equating the two.[26] With only 12.8 percent as many calories by mass, apples furnish more fiber, protein, calcium, iron, zinc, magnesium, phosphorus, potassium, vitamins A, B_1 (thiamin or thiamine), B_2 (riboflavin), B_3 (nacin or nicotinic acid), B_5 (pantothenic acid), B_6 (pyridoxine), B_9 (folate, folic acid, or pteroylmonoglutamic acid), and K, less sodium, and fewer sugars. Calorie for calorie, apples have more of every nutrient—except sodium, B_{12} (cobalamin), and D—than Skittles. Neither apples nor skittles have B_{12} and D.

TABLE 14.1
Nutrients in Skittles and Apples 100 g

Nutrient	Skittles	%DV	Apples	%DV
Calories	405	N/A	52	N/A
Protein (g)	0.19	N/A	0.26	N/A
Fat (g)	4.37	N/A	0.17	N/A
Carbs (g)	90.78	N/A	13.81	N/A
Fiber (g)	0	N/A	2.4	N/A
		Minerals		
Ca (mg)	0	0	6	0.6
Fe (mg)	0	0	0.12	0.7
Mg (mg)	1	0.3	5	1.3
P (mg)	1	0.1	11	1.1
K (mg)	12	0.3	107	3.1
Na (mg)	15	0.6	1	0.04
Zn (mg)	0.02	0.1	0.04	0.3
Cu (mg)	0.04	2	0.03	1.5
Mn (mg)	0.06	3	0.04	2
Se (mcg)	1	1.4	0	0
		Vitamins		
A (IU)	0	0	54	1.1
B_1 (mg)	0	0	0.02	1.3
B_2 (mg)	0.02	1.2	0.03	1.8
B_3 (mg)	0.01	0.05	0.09	0.5
B_5 (mg)	0.01	0.1	0.06	0.6
B_6 (mg)	<0.01	0.2	0.04	2
B_9 (mcg)	0	0	3	0.8
B_{12} (mcg)	0	0	0	0
C (mg)	66.8	111	4.6	7.7
D (IU)	0	0	0	0
E (mg)	0.2	1.3	0.18	1.2
K (mcg)	1.1	1.4	2.2	2.8

14.4 FRUITS' AMBIGUOUSNESS

Critics demonstrate that fruits enjoy no universal acclaim. Their equivocal status may be an evolutionary outcome. An earlier paragraph mentioned that plants use fruit to recruit animals to disperse seeds. This tactic would fail if animals so relished it that they camped by plants to eat all they could stomach. Plants can accomplish the aim of seed dispersal only if they prompt animals to leave after sampling fruit. Tannins, discussed in Chapter 9, and phenols accomplish this goal by imparting bitterness to fruit such that the taste is not pure sweetness.

Fruits' ambiguities, evident in the juxtaposition of sweetness and astringency and of wholesomeness and harmfulness, were apparent in antiquity (c. 3000 BCE–c. 500 CE). Genesis stated that the Hebrew god Yahweh put the first people in a garden for the man to tend.[27] Such language indicated that humans were no longer hunter-gatherers but instead horticulturists. Indeed, the author mentioned nothing about hunting and gathering, as though people had always produced rather than acquired food. If the author meant to convey a time after the hunter-gatherer phase, however, then frugivory was not among Cordain's "original way of life" from the Hebrew literary perspective. On the other hand, if the author supposed that the first people were gardeners, then frugivory met Cordain's condition of earliest subsistence within the Hebrew tradition.

The garden had many trees that yielded edibles.[28] The writer did not specify them until the woman, answering the serpent, identified them as fruits.[29] Even this designation was too imprecise for the exegetes who over the centuries specified several candidates as the forbidden fruit. Most fruits in the garden must have been nourishing, and the author implied that the first people were healthy, the text mentioning neither illness nor death. Yet Yahweh warned against consumption of fruit from a single tree.[30] Upon eating it, the woman and man lost their innocence and incurred Yahweh's anger.[31] He expelled them from the garden, made them mortal, decreased the land's bounty, required them

Blossoms and fruit—Refreshing Tardiff oranges on the tree, Florida.
COPYRIGHT 1906 BY C. L. WASSON.

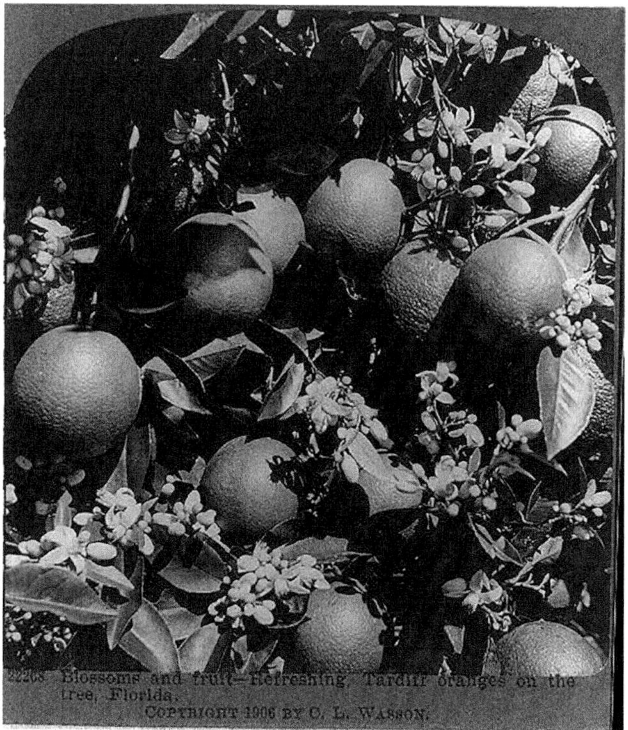

FIGURE 14.1 Oranges. (Photo courtesy of Library of Congress. https://www.loc.gov/pictures/item/2008680464/.)

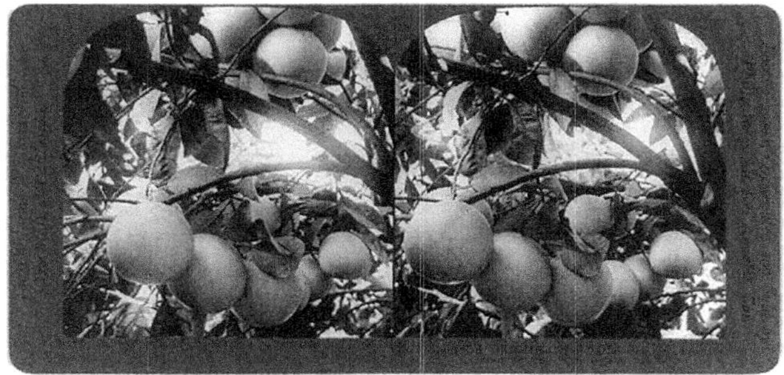

FIGURE 14.2 Grapefruits. (Photo courtesy of Library of Congress. https://www.loc.gov/pictures/item/89712141/.)

to toil for food, and increased the woman's suffering during childbirth.[32] In this story, a single fruit opened Pandora's box.

Such misgivings have not stopped people from eating fruits, which today are consumed in greater breadth than any other type of food.[33] Although American nutritionist Thomas Colin Campbell (b. 1934) urged consumption of whole foods as the best nourishment, as Chapter 13 mentioned, citrus (*Citrus* species) and apples tend to be imbibed as juice rather than eaten.[34] Juices are popular at breakfast, though fiber's absence prevents them from satiating hunger. Additionally, grapefruit (*Citrus paradisi*) juice may concentrate medicines—for example, some statins, antianxiety drugs, antihistamines, and hypertension drugs—in the blood and should be avoided without a physician's approval.[35]

14.5 NUTRIENTS

As noted, many fruits have vitamin C. Chapter 2 discussed its prevention and treatment of scurvy, its antioxidant properties, and its role in helping the body absorb iron. Besides these functions, the body uses vitamin C to synthesize neurotransmitter norepinephrine. Ascorbic acid may improve memory and cognition.[36] Although drying increases fruits' storage, it reduces or eliminates the vitamin.[37] Fruits may have additional nutrients, including potassium, carotenoids (vitamin A precursors), and vitamin B_9, though—as with any food—macro- and micronutrients depend on many factors.

Fruits' nutritional breadth is evident from the fact that 100 grams of grapes have just 3 milligrams of vitamin C, whereas the same amount of guava (*Psidium guajava*) has 230 milligrams of it.[38] Besides ascorbic acid, Table 14.2 lists fruits with the least and most vitamin B_9, potassium, sodium, protein, fat, sugars, β-carotene, and fiber.[39]

Such variance does not characterize protein, of which fruits have little, requiring ingestion of nuts, insects, meat, fish, poultry, eggs, dairy, legumes, or kindred items.[40] Fruits also tend to be deficient in calcium, iron, and zinc. Sodium's dearth recommends fruits to consumers whose diets include too much of the salt sodium chloride (NaCl). Beyond nutrients, fruits contain phytochemicals, discussed in Chapter 2, classified as flavonoids and limonoids. Fruit salicylates may reduce pain and retard pathogen growth.

Contrary to critics mentioned earlier, most scientists and medical authorities advise daily fruit consumption to reduce the risk of heart disease, stroke, and "probably cancer."[41] The connection between fruits and disease prevention is not airtight because fruit intake increases with income. Previous chapters acknowledged that wealth tends to confer health and longevity irrespective of other variables. Affluence as much as diet and nutrition may explain fruit eaters' vitality.

Anticipating later commentary, this section overviews dates' nutrients. In premodern times, when food was scarce more than plentiful, dates provided calories, a precious commodity in deserts bereft of other nourishment. French historian Delphine Roger emphasized that in this environment,

TABLE 14.2
Nutrient Range for Selected Fruits 100 g

Nutrient	Least	%DV	Most	%DV
Protein (g)	Apple, 0.3	N/A	Passion fruit, 2.6	N/A
Fat (g)	Most fruits, 0.1	N/A	Avocado, 19.5	N/A
Sugars (g)	Olives, 0	N/A	Bananas, 20.9	N/A
Fiber (g)	Watermelon, 0.1	N/A	Guava, 3.7	N/A
β-Carotene (mg)	Lemon, 7	N/A	Mangoes, 700	N/A
		Minerals		
K (mg)	Watermelon, 88	2.5	Dates, 696	19.9
Na (mg)	Peaches, 1	0.04	Honeydew, 32	1.3
		Vitamins		
B_9 (mcg)	Nectarine, 5	1.3	Blackberries, 25	6.3
C (mg)	Grapes, 3	5	Guava, 230	383.3

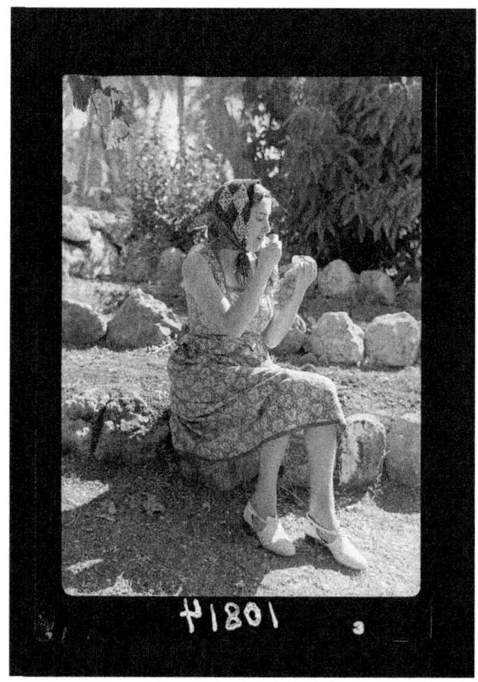

FIGURE 14.3 Grapes. (Photo courtesy of Library of Congress. https://www.loc.gov/pictures/item/2019710469/.)

dates were "sometimes the only food available."[42] As an energy packet, the fruit is 54 percent sugars by mass and easy to transport, according to *The Cambridge World History of Food* (*CWHF*), and easy to preserve, wrote American classicist Stephen Bertman (b. 1937).[43] *The CWHF* recommended it for potassium, iron, magnesium, and vitamins B_3 and B_6.[44]

Using the Medjool and Deglet Noor varieties as standard, the U.S. Department of Agriculture (USDA) and Table 14.3 list calories and nutrients in 100 grams.[45] The USDA calculates the Medjool date as 66.5 percent sugars by mass, a value that differs from the above figure. The USDA number is within American botanist Beryl Brintnall Simpson (b. 1942) and American botanist and science educator Molly Conner Ogorzaly's range of 60–70 percent sugars per date.[46]

TABLE 14.3
Nutrients in Dates 100 g

Nutrient	Date	%DV
Calories	277	N/A
Protein (g)	1.81	N/A
Fat (g)	0.15	N/A
Carbs (g)	74.97	N/A
Fiber (g)	6.7	N/A
	Minerals	
Ca (mg)	64	6.4
Fe (mg)	0.9	5
Mg (mg)	54	13.5
P (mg)	62	6.2
K (mg)	696	19.9
Na (mg)	1	0.04
Zn (mg)	0.44	2.9
Cu (mg)	0.36	18
Mn (mg)	0.3	15
Se (mcg)	3	4.3
	Vitamins	
A (IU)	149	3
B_1 (mg)	0.05	3.3
B_2 (mg)	0.06	3.5
B_3 (mg)	1.61	8.1
B_5 (mg)	0.81	8.1
B_6 (mg)	0.25	12.5
B_9 (mcg)	15	3.8
B_{12} (mcg)	0	0
C (mg)	0	0
D (IU)	0	0
E (mg)	0.05	0.3
K (mcg)	2.7	3.4

TABLE 14.4
Nutrients in Bananas 100 g

Nutrient	Banana	%DV
Calories	89	N/A
Protein (g)	1.09	N/A
Fat (g)	0.33	N/A
Carbs (g)	22.84	N/A
Fiber (g)	2.6	N/A
	Minerals	
Ca (mg)	5	0.5
Fe (mg)	0.26	1.4
Mg (mg)	27	6.8
P (mg)	22	2.2
K (mg)	358	10.2
Na (mg)	1	0.04
Zn (mg)	0.15	1
Cu (mg)	0.08	4
Mn (mg)	0.27	13.5
Se (mcg)	1	1.4
	Vitamins	
A (IU)	64	1.3
B_1 (mg)	0.03	2
B_2 (mg)	0.07	4.1
B_3 (mg)	0.67	3.4
B_5 (mg)	0.33	3.3
B_6 (mg)	0.37	18.5
B_9 (mcg)	20	5
B_{12} (mcg)	0	0
C (mg)	8.7	14.5
D (IU)	0	0
E (mg)	0.1	0.7
K (mcg)	0.5	0.6

The second fruit treated later is the banana. As noted, Gundry permitted consumption of only unripe bananas, though the USDA appears to list nutrients for ripe bananas, in Table 14.4, given 53.6 percent of carbohydrates from sugars.[47] Comparison of Tables 14.3 and 14.4 reveals that by mass dates have more potassium than bananas despite the latter's reputation as rich in it. Table 14.2 indicates that dates have the most potassium by mass among fruits. Besides potassium, dates, being dried, have more calories, protein, carbohydrates, fiber, calcium, iron, magnesium, phosphorus, zinc, copper, manganese, selenium, and vitamins A, B_1, B_3, B_5, and K than bananas by mass.

14.6 DATES

14.6.1 Dates, Humanity, and Domestication

Possibly the first domesticated fruit, dates are intertwined with the rise of civilization in southwestern Asia, a region earlier chapters mentioned as geographically imprecise.[48] Although colloquial use names it the Middle East, this label is unhelpful. If East means Asia, then Middle East should be Asia's midpoint. But no such location is meant because the Middle East includes the eastern

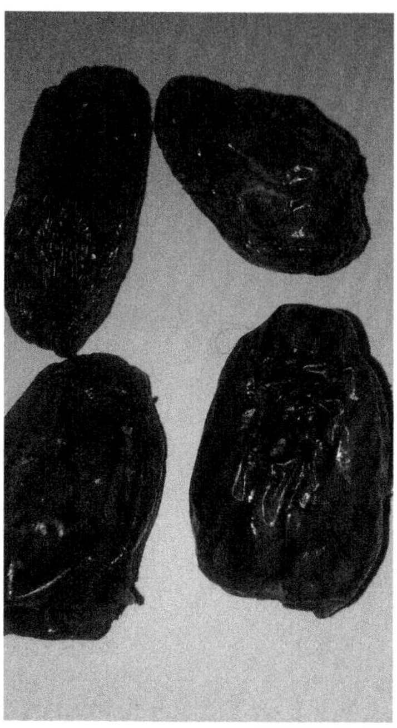

FIGURE 14.4 Dates. (Photo from author.)

Mediterranean basin, which is westernmost Asia rather than the middle. Moreover, the Middle East usually includes Egypt, which is mostly in northeastern Africa, and countries like Libya, which is wholly African, a practice that negates any notion of East as Asia.

Counter to this language, some archaeologists and historians refer to southwestern Asia as the Near East. This label makes sense if an onlooker insists that Europe is the frame of reference because southwestern Asia is just east of Europe. This book rejects Eurocentrism, believing instead that any attempt to define part of Asia should use Asia as the continent of reference. For this reason, Egypt and North Africa cannot be in the Middle East without decoupling the terms East and Asia.

If southwestern Asia is defined in terms of Asia, as seems sensible, Africa must be excluded because no part is in Asia except Egypt's Sinai Peninsula. From the peninsula, this book—looking east, southeast, and northeast—includes in southwestern Asia all of Arabia and Arab countries Jordan, Syria, and Iraq because they share a common history and ethnicity. From the Sinai Peninsula north to Syria is westernmost Asia, lands known as the Levant and included in this book's definition of southwestern Asia. From south to north, the Levant is the Sinai Peninsula, Israel, Lebanon, and Syria. To the east, Jordan is usually included in the Levant. Between Israel and Jordan is Palestine. Although journalists often include Turkey and Iran in the Middle East, and so in southwestern Asia, this book does not because Turkey has territory in Europe as well as in Asia and because Turkey and Iran are not Arab nations.

After Africa, southwestern Asia has the longest record of human habitation. Discussing our evolution, Chapter 3 indicated that *Homo erectus* was the first human to leave Africa, entering southwestern Asia around 1.8 million years ago. *H. erectus* fossils in what is today Georgia on the eastern shore of the Black Sea are about 1.7 million years old.[49] Georgia's colonization implies earlier habitation of southwestern Asia, from where *H. erectus* moved north and east. Chapter 3 overviewed these migrations.

After *H. erectus*, the first *Homo sapiens*—populations designated archaic—penetrated Asia perhaps 350,000 years ago.[50] Around 60,000 years ago, *Homo neanderthalensis* (Neanderthals or Neandertals) colonized westernmost Asia, occupying parts in what is today Israel.[51] Neanderthal fossils demonstrate that the species—whether distinct from *H. sapiens* cannot be decided here—moved as far east as Iraq. These remains suggest that Neanderthals inhabited all southwestern Asia. Simultaneously, anatomically modern peoples settled these lands, persisting into the present, whereas Neanderthals vanished about 28,000 years ago.[52]

As elsewhere, humans were latecomers to a region populated by plants and other animals. Among florae, the date palm arose at least 50 million years ago in Arabia and North Africa.[53] It may have originated from crosspollination between wild species *Phoenix reclinata* and *Phoenix sylvestris*.[54] French-Swiss botanist Alphonse Louis Pierre Pyrame de Candolle (1806–1893) believed that the tree's geographic range was greater before than after domestication.[55] Humans must have prized the palm, which tolerated intense heat, saline soils, and aridity, because it grew in deserts, where the climate supported few other resources. Before domestication, nomads in arid lands from India west throughout the Mediterranean likely ate wild dates.[56]

The tree's utility recommended it for domestication no later than 5000 BCE, making its edibles the earliest domesticate to satisfy the botanical definition of a fruit.[57] The oldest remnants of the domestic date palm, around 7,000 years old, came from what are today Kuwait and the United Arab Emirates.[58] Their geography suggests earliest domestication in lands northwest and south of the Persian Gulf. Arabian presses for extracting dibs (date syrup) are roughly 3,750 years old.[59] Arabian pastoralists took the palm north into the eastern Mediterranean, where it hybridized with the wild *Phoenix theophrasti*—native to Turkey and Greek island Crete—around 1000 BCE. These hybrids moved southwest into Egypt and west throughout North Africa. This chronology prioritizes domestication and cultivation in Arabia with later movements into the Levant, Egypt, and North Africa.

14.6.2 Dates, Arabs, and Bedouins

Their tenure in southwestern Asia involved dates, as noted, in the origin of Western civilization, which historians trace to Mesopotamia: lands between the Tigris and Euphrates Rivers in what are today Iraq and parts of Syria, Turkey, and Iran.[60] Before 3000 BCE, domesticated palms were common throughout this region.[61] Genesis, whose composition was probably incomplete until the sixth century BCE, connected Mesopotamia with human origins by tracing a river through Eden.[62]

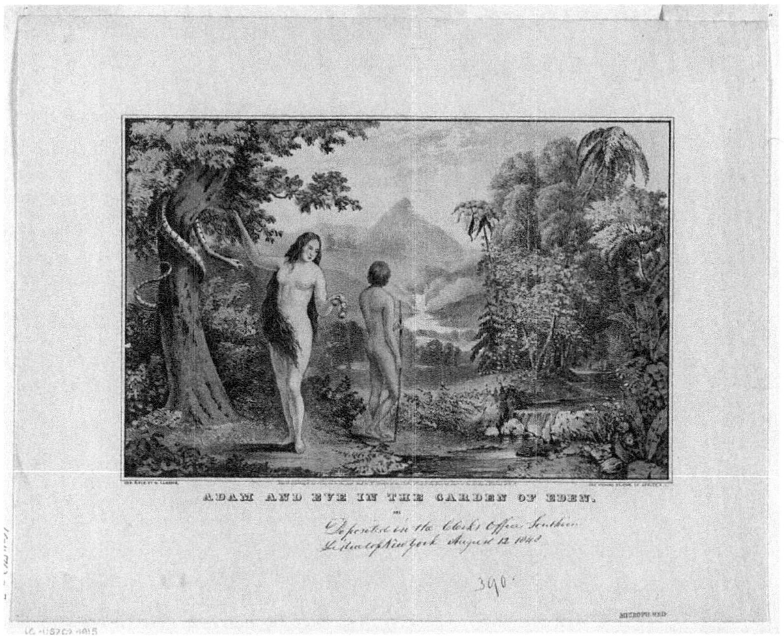

FIGURE 14.5 Eden. (Art courtesy of Library of Congress.)

Outside the garden, it divided into four branches, two being the Tigris and Euphrates.[63] Muslims anchored dates to this story, believing that their god Allah created the date palm from dust left after Adam's creation.[64] Whatever these accounts' historicity, Mesopotamia deserves the study it continues to receive.

The date palm's domestication in the sixth millennium BCE, already noted, coincided with gradual enlargement of the region's villages into the first cities between roughly 5800 and 3750 BCE.[65] Dates and other domesticates yielded the surpluses that freed urbanites from the drudgery of tending crops and livestock, allowing them to specialize in other pursuits. Historians credited them with inventing writing, establishing schools, enacting laws, advancing the study of astronomy, mathematics, engineering, and architecture, and building roads, bridges, canals, and aqueducts.[66]

Dates cannot receive inordinate credit for such lofty attainment, though they have long been prominent in Mesopotamia, Persia (now Iran), Egypt, Sudan, Arabia, Tunisia, Algeria, and Morocco.[67] Besides commoners, Mesopotamian royalty ate them, a fruitcake recipe specifying nine parts dates, three parts butter, one part each of raisins and cheese, and an unknown quantity of flour.[68] Delphine Roger described dates as "common everywhere" in Arabia, the Levant, Mesopotamia, Egypt, and North Africa from early times and the poor's staple.[69] In this capacity, the fruit was "bread of the desert" and "cake of the poor."[70] Without sucrose in ancient southwestern Asia and honey expensive, dates and date juice functioned as sweeteners. Roger, Simpson, and Ogorzaly traced Arabs' enthusiasm for dates to Bedouins—also referenced as Bedu, Qedarites, and Arabaa—who entered Arabia no later than 6000 BCE, established dates and dairy as primary sustenance, and designated the palm the "tree of life."[71] French author Maguelonne Toussaint-Samat (1926–2018) credited Egyptians with this language.[72] Over millennia, Bedouin and Arab reliance on dates and other plain fare changed little.

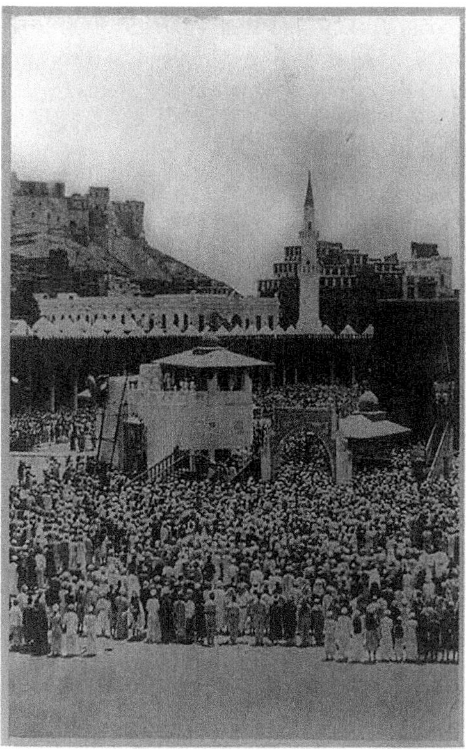

FIGURE 14.6 Mecca, Saudi Arabia, is the Prophet Muhammad's birthplace. (Photo courtesy of Library of Congress. https://www.loc.gov/pictures/item/2013646214/.)

Originating in the seventh century CE, Islam gave dates spiritual significance because the Prophet Muhammad (c. 570–632) named them among his favorite foods, often eating them to end a fast.[73] Muslims follow this practice, especially during the month Ramadan and the Hadj pilgrimage to Mecca, Saudi Arabia.[74] Muhammad's conception of dates as religious symbol may derive from ancient Sumerian and Babylonian veneration of date palms.[75] Dates' importance is also evident in the Arab belief that they have as many dietary and medicinal uses as the number of days per year.[76] Into the twentieth century, the fruit was one of four Arab and Bedouin principal foods, the others being unpasteurized milk, rice (*Oryza sativa*), and unleavened bread.[77] By 1980, Saudi Arabia had some 11 million date palms.[78] Southwestern Asia—including Saudi Arabia—and the Mediterranean have perhaps ten times this number.[79]

14.6.3 Arab and Bedouin Health

Health data came from an Arab settlement at Dor in what is today northwestern Israel's Haifa District. Dor's Arab skeletons—dating around 30 BCE—yielded an life expectancy at birth (e^0) for men of 32 years, compared with male e^0s for southwestern Asians of 30 years about 17,000 BCE and 34 years between roughly 7000 and 5800 BCE, and for Greek and Roman men of 39 years between about 336 BCE and 500 CE.[80] In all cases, women lived roughly 4 fewer years. Assuming an equal sex ratio for simplicity, overall e^0s should have been about 30 years for Dor's Arabs, 28 years for Southwestern Asians around 17,000 BCE and 32 years between around 7000 and 5800 BCE, and 37 years for Greeks and Romans between roughly 336 BCE and 500 CE.

Not all numbers need commentary, though Israeli anatomist Patricia Smith, Israeli archaeologist and anthropologist Ofer Bar-Yosef (1937–2020), and American anthropologist Andrew Sillen's e^0 of 37 years for Roman antiquity (c. 750 BCE–c. 500 CE) conflicts with American anthropologist and geneticist Kenneth M. Weiss' (b. 1941) calculation of 32 years and American classicists Roger Shaler Bagnall (b. 1947) and Bruce W. Frier's (b. 1943) computation of between 22 and 25 years for Roman Egypt during the first three centuries CE.[81] Bagnall and Frier's range came from Roman census records of roughly 300 Egyptians and, being the most comprehensive to date, is probably the best estimate of Roman e^0. Moreover, an e^0 between 22 and 25 years aligns with premodern e^0s referenced throughout this book. Even granting the upper bound of 25 years, Bagnall and Frier's estimate is still 12 years below Smith, Bar-Yosef, and Sillen's e^0 for ancient Rome. That is, Smith and coauthors overstated Roman e^0 by roughly 1.5 times.

The magnitude of this error applied to the other e^0s yields revised estimates in Table 14.5 of 18.7 years for southwestern Asians about 17,000 BCE and 21.3 years between 7000 and 5800 BCE and of 20 years for Arabs at Dor around 30 BCE. The differences among these numbers are small, and the Arab e^0 is exactly the mean between the other two. Reflecting on their e^0s, Smith, Bar-Yosef, and Sillen wrote that the "early Arab population from Dor represents a group in poor health with low life expectancy."[82] This opinion matches the fact that the revised Arab e^0 was under Bagnall and Frier's lower bound for Roman Egypt. The revised value was within American ecologist and limnologist Edward Smith Deevey Jr.'s (1914–1988) estimate that between Neanderthal

TABLE 14.5
Ancient e^0s (Years) by Source

Place	Dor, Israel	SW Asia	SW Asia	Greece and Rome
Time	c. 30 BCE	c. 17,000 BCE	c. 7000–c. 5800 BCE	c. 336 BCE–c. 500 CE
Smith, Bar-Yosef, and Sillen	30	28	32	37
Revised Smith, Bar-Yosef, and Sillen	20	18.7	21.3	24.7
Weiss	N/A	N/A	N/A	32
Bagnall and Frier	N/A	N/A	N/A	22–25

prehistory and 1900 CE, e^0 seldom departed over 5 years either way of 25 years.[83] Although Arab e^0 occupied the bottom of this range, and the bottom of Greek e^0 between roughly 1200 and 700 BCE, it may not have been abysmal enough on its own to warrant pessimism.[84]

Moreover, low e^0 may indicate high fertility more than poor health. Chapter 1 noted that e^0 may reveal more about births than deaths because birthrate tends to correlate inversely with e^0. As birthrate rises, the number of newborns grows. If newborn and infant mortality is constant, increase in the number of youths necessarily enlarges total juvenile deaths, dragging down e^0. That is, all else equal a fecund population exhibits lower e^0 than a barren one without being sicker.

Dor's fertility is unknown, though Smith, Bar-Yosef, and Sillen stated that on average Arab women weaned infants at 2.5 years.[85] This duration implies resumption of ovulation, and the possibility of conception, every 2.5 years. High infant mortality, however, suggests a shorter interval on average because death would have ended breastfeeding before weaning. For example, the Yanomami—examined in the next sections—had only 1.9 years on average between births when a newborn died in the first month.[86] Such fecundity, assuming no multiple births, would produce five newborns per decade, which must represent a woman's hypothetical maximum, again absent multiple offspring per litter.

A population seldom averages over eight births per woman, though individuals surpass as well as trail the mean.[87] For example, Anna Magdalena Bach (1701–1760), German composer Johann Sebastian Bach's (1685–1750) second wife, had thirteen children.[88] Dor's Arab women probably were less fertile. Recalling that these women lived about 4 fewer years than men on average, corrected female e^0 was 16.7 years. Even if menarche began early—around 13 years, for example—reproductive life averaged only 3 or 4 years. Supposing 4 years and a birth every second year, assumptions that are probably unrealistic, yields just two births per average woman. This exercise implies that low Arab e^0 did not result from high fertility. Moreover, if birthrate and e^0 were low, then Smith, Bar-Yosef, and Sillen may have been correct to doubt Arab vigor.

Although examination of modernity does not always illuminate the past, American anthropologist and archaeologist Henry Field (1902–1986) remarked in 1935 that Arab birthrates were low enough for contraception to have been widespread.[89] He computed that the mode of children per family was three. Table 14.6 shows that more families had no children (16.2 percent) or one (12.6 percent) than had five (11.8 percent). Low birthrate may also have resulted from late marriage, which most men delayed until after age 30 because of poor job prospects.

Stature supplied additional health information. Smith, Bar-Yosef, and Sillen assembled data from hunter-gatherers, agriculturists, and pastoralists, in Table 14.7. In the first camp were early Levantines, whose skeletons from Mount Carmel and Jebel Qafzel, Israel, are about 90,000–100,000 years old, and Natufians, whose culture existed between roughly 11,000 and 7000 BCE.[90] The second group contained occupants of Jericho in what is today the West Bank, of Byblos and Qaaqour, Lebanon, and of Sasa, Israel. The most important of these sites was Jericho because its skeletons spanned the entire Neolithic or New Stone Age (c. 7000–c. 5800 BCE), the Chalcolithic (c. 5800–c. 3750 BCE), the Bronze Age (c. 3750–c. 2900 BCE), and Hellenism (336–30 BCE). The third category was Arab pastoralists.

TABLE 14.6
% Arab Families with and without Children in 1928

Number of Children	% of Families
0	16.2
1	12.6
3	19.1
5	11.8

These different geographies and times produced dietary variations. The Levant's earliest inhabitants ate nuts, seeds, tubers, and game, notably deer (species in the family Cervidae), gazelles (*Gazella* species), aurochs (*Bos primigenius*), boars (*Sus scrofa*), onagers (*Equus hemionus*), mouflons (*Ovis orientalis*), and wild goats (*Capra aegagrus*).[91] As grasslands expanded around 12,000 BCE, humans concentrated on nuts and seeds.[92] About this time, wild emmer (*Triticum turgidum*) entered diets. Transition to farming during the Neolithic made barley (*Hordeum vulgare*) bread and gruel the staples.[93] As noted, dates and dairy fed Arab pastoralists.

The earliest inhabitants of the Levant furnished skeletons of three men from Mount Carmel and Jebel Qafzel, who averaged 180 centimeters (70.9 inches), and two women, who stood 166 centimeters (65.4 inches) on average.[94] These heights were tallest among all groups examined by Smith, Bar-Yosef, and Sillen and—if they were not artifacts of the small samples but instead typified the sites' populations—imply that the first southwestern Asians were healthiest. Comparison among these and later peoples is valid if, as American geneticist Juan L. Rodriguez-Flores and coauthors argued in 2016, genetic continuity characterized populations across time and if, as noted, the samples represented the larger populations.[95]

Next in the sequence were Natufians, whose skeletons included ten men averaging 167 centimeters (65.7 inches) and three women at 158 centimeters (62.2 inches) on average.[96] The earliest Neolithic residents of Jericho left remains of twenty-nine men at 167 centimeters on average and twenty-eight women at 157 centimeters (61.8 inches). Their immediate successors included skeletons of twenty-three men at 171 centimeters (67.3 inches) and eleven women at 158 centimeters.

As their names suggest, the Paleolithic or Old Stone Age (c. 70,000–c. 9000 BCE), Mesolithic or Middle Stone Age (c. 9000–c. 7000 BCE), and Neolithic Periods witnessed the development and use of stool tools and weapons. Transition from stone to the first metal implements and arms heralded a new period, the Chalcolithic, during which copper was the chief material. Chalcolithic Jericho furnished skeletons of four men at 170 centimeters (66.9 inches) and six women at 159 centimeters (62.6 inches).[97] Chalcolithic Byblos yielded remains of five men at 167 centimeters and four women at 152 centimeters (59.8 inches).

The combination of copper and tin created the alloy bronze, which gave its name to the Bronze Age. Bronze Age Qaaqour yielded skeletons of six men at 164 centimeters (64.6 inches) and four women at 154 centimeters (60.6 inches).[98] Bronze Age Sasa supplied remains of two men at 169 centimeters (66.5 inches) and three women at 156 centimeters (61.4 inches). Bronze Age Jericho had skeletons of ten men at 171 centimeters (67.3 inches) and six women at 154 centimeters (60.6 inches). Hellenistic Jericho provided remains of twelve men at 166 centimeters and twelve women at 152 centimeters. Northwest of Jericho, Dor furnished skeletons of seventeen Arab men at 169 centimeters and thirteen women at 156 centimeters.

If these numbers are taken at face value, the earliest peoples were tallest and healthiest. The roughly 80,000 or 90,000 years between them and the Natufians saw heights decrease some 10 centimeters (3.9 inches). Thereafter, stature fluctuated little. This description does not contrast

TABLE 14.7
Average Heights in Southwestern Asia

Period	Time	Men (cm)	Women (cm)
Mousterian	c. 100,000–c. 90,000 years ago	180	166
Natufian	c. 11,000–c. 7000 BCE	167	158
Neolithic	c. 7000–c. 5800 BCE	168.7	157.5
Chalcolithic	c. 5800–c. 3750 BCE	168.3	156.2
Bronze Age	c. 3750–c. 2900 BCE	168.4	154.5
Hellenism	336–30 BCE	166	152
Late Hellenism	c. 30 BCE	169	156

hunter-gatherers with farmers and stockmen because Mount Carmel and Jebel Qafzel's occupants and the Natufians hunted and collected food. That is, heights appear to have dropped between the first two groups of hunter-gatherers and stabilized during and after the transition to agriculture and animal husbandry, developments discussed in Chapter 3. As noted, the greatest temporal continuity came from Jericho, where from Neolithic to Bronze Age stature held roughly constant, though Bronze Age women were shorter than their predecessors. Women and men in Hellenic Jericho (336–30 BCE) were shortest among the city's denizens from roughly 7000 to 30 BCE, the decline being greater for women than men.

The problem with this approach is that it puts all statistics on an equal footing when, for example, Mount Carmel and Jebel Qafzel yielded just five skeletons, whereas Neolithic Jericho supplied ninety-one. The Chalcolithic was again data deficient, with ten skeletons from Jericho and nine from Byblos. The Bronze Age was little better, with ten skeletons from Qaaqour and five from Sasa. Only Bronze Age Jericho had sixteen skeletons. Rejection of samples with ten or fewer skeletons eliminates Mount Carmel, Jebel Qafzel, Byblos, Chalcolithic Jericho, Qaaqour, and Sasa. The Natufians yielded just three women, again too small a group for comfort. All that remains are Neolithic, Bronze Age, and Hellenic Jericho and Dor's Arabs. Men in Neolithic and Bronze Age Jericho were taller than Arab men, though Hellenic men were shorter. Arab women were taller than all Jericho women except those in the Neolithic. These comparisons reveal no obvious distinctions between Jericho agriculturists and stockmen on one hand and Arab pastoralists on the other.

These data's paucity contrasts with Field's measurements in the early twentieth century. Mean stature of 159 Arab men roughly 80 kilometers (49.7 miles) south of Baghdad, Iraq, examined in 1925 and 1926 was 169.6 centimeters (66.8 inches), an increase under half a percent over Dor's men.[99] Another 376 men measured in 1928 averaged 167.7 centimeters (66 inches), a decrease under 1 percent below Dor's men.[100] Thirty-eight Bedouins stood on average 168.3 centimeters (66.3 inches), again a diminution under 1 percent below Dor's men.[101] The fact that all Field's heights were within 1 percent of Dor's mean male stature implies continuity between ancient and modern Arab health.

Besides these comparisons, most Arab men in Field's study ranged between 162.6 centimeters (64 inches) and 172.7 centimeters (68 inches), though outliers populated both tails. For example, Field's colleague Scottish physician, anatomist, and anthropologist Arthur Keith (1866–1955) noted that "a very few tall people" stood at least 180.3 centimeters (71 inches).[102] Dor's Arabs averaged between 150 centimeters (59.1 inches) and 180 centimeters (70.9 inches).[103] These data are incomparable, however, because Smith, Bar-Yosef, and Sillen included all skeletons in their range, whereas Field and Keith omitted women and the tallest and shortest men and measured live men.

Crania provided no more certitude than Smith, Bar-Yosef, and Sillen's height data. Tables 14.8 and 14.9 show that half of Natufian children and 45 percent of adults had cribra orbitalia, a pathology defined in Chapter 1.[104] All Chalcolithic peoples and all Bronze Age children exhibited it. Sixty-three percent of Bronze Age adults displayed the malady. Sixty-two percent of Roman and Byzantine children and 64 percent of adults had the condition. Eighty-five percent of Arab children and 43 percent of adults had the affliction. Cribra orbitalia was least evident in Natufians, the only

TABLE 14.8
Cribra Orbitalia in Children

Period or People	Time	# of Crania Examined	# of Crania with CO	% of Crania with CO
Natufian	c. 11,000–c. 7000 BCE	2	1	50
Chalcolithic	c. 5800–c. 3750 BCE	4	4	100
Bronze Age	c. 3750–c. 2900 BCE	4	4	100
Rome and Byzantium	c. 750 BCE–1453 CE	21	13	62
Arab	c. 30 BCE	33	28	85

TABLE 14.9
Cribra Orbitalia in Adults

Period or People	Time	# of Crania Examined	# of Crania with CO	% of Crania with CO
Natufian	c. 11,000–c. 7000 BCE	11	5	45
Chalcolithic	c. 5800–c. 3750 BCE	2	2	100
Bronze Age	c. 3750–c. 2900 BCE	35	22	63
Rome and Byzantium	c. 750 BCE–1453 CE	36	23	64
Arab	c. 30 BCE	42	20	43

hunter-gatherers on the list. Nomadism likely prevented them from amassing the wastes that would have supported large populations of pathogens, parasites, rodents, and insects. With a lighter disease, parasite, rodent, and insect load than farmers, Natufians were healthier as measured by less cribra orbitalia. Being pastoralists, the Arabs likewise were more mobile than Chalcolithic, Bronze Age, Roman, and Byzantine farmers and stockmen and exhibited fewer cranial pathologies, at least as adults. Cribra orbitalia, therefore, likely arose from diseases, parasites, rodents, and insects and so revealed little about diets.

Examination of postcrania disclosed osteoporosis in under one-third of Bronze Age—but in 53 percent of Arab—women.[105] As is true of cribra orbitalia and many other maladies, more than one factor may have been involved. Chapter 2 discussed the roles of vitamin D, calcium, and other minerals in bone health. The body absorbs minerals only from foods but depends primarily on sunlight's ultraviolet radiation, this book emphasizes, for vitamin D. Israel's Science and Technology Directory ranks southwestern Asia among Earth's sunniest regions, though clothing blocks sunlight.[106] Beyond nourishment and sunlight, this book notes that exertion strengthens bones.

Consideration of these factors may implicate diet, especially dates, and lifestyle in Arab osteoporosis. On one hand, pastoralism must have made Arabs walk, a weight-bearing activity that should have fortified bones against osteoporosis. On the other hand, the tendency to cover much of the body, including the head, minimized sunlight absorption and consequent vitamin D synthesis. In 1935, Field likened Arab attire to a long nightgown covered by a robe that resembled academic regalia.[107] Only the feet were uncovered. Table 14.3 noted that dates lack vitamin D but have calcium, though not in abundance, and other minerals. Their nutrient profile disqualifies dates as protection against osteoporosis. Yet these Arabs also consumed dairy, notably camel, goat, or sheep's milk.[108] By volume, these three have more calcium than cow's milk.[109] Additionally, sheep's milk surpasses that from cows in vitamin D.[110] Iranian microbiologist Said Zibaee and coauthors identified vitamin D in camel's milk.[111] A 1984 study did not mention vitamin D in Saudi Arabian goats' milk.[112]

14.7 BANANAS

14.7.1 Bananas and the Yanomami

The perception that fruits function apart from the entrée applied to neither Arab date eaters nor the Yanomami, who occupy lands along the border between South America's Venezuela and Brazil. Chapter 3 acknowledged that anthropologists long debated when the first peoples entered the Americas. This book follows British anthropologists Christopher Brian Stringer (b. 1947) and Peter Andrews in estimating that these migrations happened about 15,000 years ago.[113] American anthropologist Kenneth Robert Good (b. 1942), however, asserted that the Yanomami's ancestors reached North America some 20,000 years ago and colonized lands near the Amazon River, which flows through what are today Peru, Bolivia, Venezuela, Colombia, Ecuador, and Brazil, roughly 5,000 years later.[114]

Within five degrees north of the equator, the Yanomami and their predecessors lived amid exceptional biodiversity.[115] Florae and faunae supplied numerous edibles, including insects, notably termites (species in the infraorder Isoptera) and larvae of several species, crabs (species in the infraorder Brachyura), fish, legumes, and nuts.[116] Hunters targeted peccaries (*Pecari tajacu* and *Tayassu pecari*) and tapirs (*Tapirus terrestris*), though these efforts seldom succeeded, causing Yanomami to crave meat. Fruits were likely important from an early date given their prevalence in tropical diets.[117]

Among fruits, Good mentioned "bananas and plantains"—which may have constituted two-thirds of diets—as the chief source of calories and nutrients.[118] *The CWHF* listed separate entries and scientific names for bananas (*Musa paradisiaca*) and plantains (*M.* × *paradisiaca*).[119] American geographer Judith Ann Carney (b. 1946) and independent scholar Richard Nicholas Rosomoff agreed that bananas and plantains, though close kin, differ.[120] American botanist Will C. McClatchey differentiated bananas from plantains by moisture, with bananas being around 83 percent water and plantains about 65 percent.[121] This criterion may be challenged given Chapter 9's discussion of fresh and dried acorns (*Quercus* species) and chestnuts (*Castanea* species), both of which remain the same nut irrespective of moisture. American food historian Linda Civitello differentiated bananas from plantains, asserting that the first may be eaten raw, whereas the second must be cooked.[122] Beryl Simpson, Molly Ogorzaly, and Brazilian horticulturist and ecologist Charles Roland Clement discarded the noun plantain, referring to the fruit as banana.[123] On the other hand, American anthropologists Michael D. Gurven and Hillard Seth Kaplan designated the fruit plantain.[124] This chapter follows Simpson, Ogorzaly, and Clement. Simpson and Ogorzaly favored the scientific name *M.* × *paradisiaca*, a designation retained in this book, whereas Clement used *Musa acuminata* and *M. acuminata* × *balbisiana*.[125]

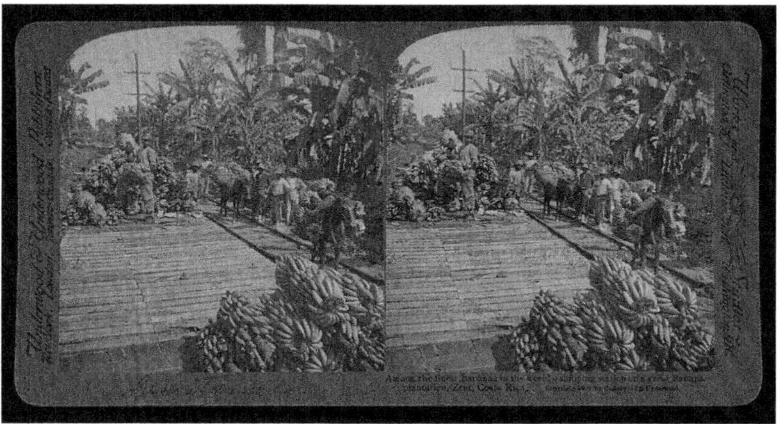

FIGURE 14.7 Bananas. (Photo courtesy of Library of Congress. https://www.loc.gov/pictures/item/2019634765/.)

These differences may reflect bananas' complex evolution. The fruit appears to have arisen in South Asia, Southeast Asia, and nearby Pacific islands.[126] This geography isolated species into discrete reproductive units distinct from neighboring populations. From this circumstance arose diploids (organisms with two sets of chromosomes per cell), triploids (three sets), and tetraploids (four sets).[127] The earliest fruits had many seeds and scant flesh, which made consumption laborious.[128] Humans selected for parthenocarpy (seedlessness) and large fruit. Cultivation of different types in adjacent areas in Southeast Asia and western Oceania led to hybrids through crosspollination.

From these lands, bananas spread east through Oceania, reaching Hawaii during the first millennium CE.[129] Simultaneously the fruit moved west to Madagascar and the African mainland. In contrast to these migrations, bananas were not commercially viable outside the humid tropics because temperatures must be above 20 degrees Celsius (68 degrees Fahrenheit) and rainfall not below 75 millimeters (3 inches) per month at least 8 months of the year.[130] Banana plants languish even in partial shade and at latitudes without intense sunshine. They tolerate a range of soils except those that are waterlogged.

Fifteenth-century Portugal planted bananas on the Atlantic Ocean's Canary Islands roughly 100 kilometers (62.1 miles) west of Morocco.[131] On them, slaves produced sugarcane (*Saccharum officinarum*) and bananas, permitting the Spanish to transfer all three to the Caribbean Islands by the early sixteenth century. Thereafter, Portugal introduced bananas to Brazil. The fruit's movement to the Yanomami is difficult to pinpoint. The peel decayed rapidly in the tropics, and the fruit left no seeds for possible preservation. American anthropologist John D. Early and Canadian sociologist John F. Peters implied that Yanomami acquired the banana during Europe's incursions into Brazil between the 1630s and around 1820.[132] Clement asserted that this acquisition was rapid, leading me to infer the seventeenth century as the probable period.[133]

Speedy adoption throughout the tropics is unsurprising because bananas required little labor to yield well. A perennial, the plant supplied food year-round in contrast to annuals, like wheat (*Triticum monococcum, Triticum dicoccon, Triticum aestivum,* and *Triticum durum*) or peas (*Pisum sativum*), grown in temperate locales. A banana plant lived at least 30 years, a lifetime for most premodern peoples.[134] Carney and Rosomoff quoted production above 224,170 kilograms per hectare (220,000 pounds per acre), tenfold the output of yams (*Dioscorea* species) and one hundredfold that of potatoes (*Solanum tuberosum*) per unit land.[135]

14.7.2 Yanomami Health

Prehistoric health is difficult to infer in the humid tropics because skeletons and other organic materials preserve poorly. Moreover, Chapter 1 mentioned that prehistory lacks the written records that scientists and scholars consult absent biofacts. In this situation, the impressions of Europeans who entered Amazonia (the Amazon rainforest) are necessary to paint images on a blank canvas. Chapter 6 noted that death attended Europeans' introduction of Old-World diseases into the Americas. The Yanomami and other South American natives suffered losses such that by 1800, pathogens had depopulated villages along the Amazon River's tributaries.[136] Despite this reversal, Early and Peters contended that overall Yanomami populations increased into the twentieth century because bananas provided the nutrients and calories to feed more mouths, because steel implements acquired from Europeans permitted cultivation of additional land, or because both factors interacted synergistically.[137] These circumstances increased birthrate and diminished mortality.

Summarizing Yanomami history after European contact, contagion eliminated vulnerable members in a population. The survivors had some immunities, which their offspring inherited such that later generations were less susceptible to the diseases that had killed so many in the initial epidemics. These postepidemic populations—benefitting from a novel food, a new technology, or both—grew beyond what had been possible without these innovations, recalibrating the equilibrium with their surroundings. These adjustments increased the land's carrying capacity.

Unable to reconstruct health from skeletons, anthropologists studied Yanomami in northern Brazil's Roraima state, an area few Europeans and their diseases penetrated before 1957.[138] Early and Peters compiled statistics about these indigenes, using data collected between 1930 and 1957 and between 1987 and 1995.[139] This research represents the best attempt to quantity health before and after European contact.

This section assumes that bananas' healthfulness is best gauged before contact in 1957 because only this period yielded information absent mortality from Old World diseases. Early and Peters estimated that Roraima's villages had ninety-six Yanomami in 1930, a population that grew to 120 in 1957.[140] The two calculated e^0 at 39.8 years over these 37 years.[141] Men lived on average 45.2 years, whereas women averaged 35.8 years.

These numbers are impressive for hunter-gather horticulturists with minimal technology, muscles rather than machines to accomplish tasks, and a subsistence economy. Chapter 3 noted that ten skeletons from Anatolia (Asia Minor or Asian Turkey)—a small sample—dating between roughly

540 and 30 BCE had an e^0 around 20 years.[142] An earlier section calculated an e^0 of 20 years for Dor's Arabs about 30 BCE. E^0 estimates for ancient Egypt ranged between 19 and 25 years.[143] Chapter 6 cited data from American anthropologist and osteologist Ann Lucy Wiener Stodder and coauthors that e^0 was 21.5 years at Hawikku near Zuni, New Mexico, between roughly 1425 and 1680 CE and 22.2 years at San Cristobal Pueblo in San Cristobal, New Mexico, between about 1350 and 1680.[144] Twenty-nine burials between 1829 and 1849 in a cemetery near Springfield, Illinois, yielded an e^0 of 18.4 years.[145] African Americans buried in Dallas, Texas' Freedman's Cemetery, between 1869 and 1907, had an e^0 of 21 years.[146] Those interred in southwestern Arkansas' Cedar Grove Cemetery between 1900 and 1915 yielded an e^0 of 19.3 years. Readers should be mindful that cemeteries overstate e^0 when families do not bury stillborns, newborns, or infants, or their fragile remains decay. As noted, Deevey summarized this pattern, writing that most premodern peoples died within 5 years of age 25.

Against the reality of life's brevity, Yanomami longevity nearly doubled what ancient Anatolians and Arabs achieved. Early and Peters stated that e^0 might have surpassed their calculation but for the fact that infanticide—especially against girls—truncated lives, at least partly explaining the gap between men and women.[147] This book indicates that premodern mortality tended to be high during infancy. Among Yanomami, Early and Peters believed that 17.7 percent of newborns died during life's first year between 1930 and 1957.[148] Survivors experienced lower mortality through age 10, after which deaths began to mount. Gurven and Kaplan computed a gradual increase in mortality at an additional 1 percent greater risk of death per year from ages 15 through 35.[149] Thereafter, mortality accelerated. Although no one reached age 70, forty did not mark life's end—as Chapters 1 and 3 documented throughout premodern times—because Early and Peters identified survivors into life's fifth, sixth, and seventh decades.[150]

Of the peoples examined in this book, only Tlatilco, Mexico's bean eaters—discussed in Chapter 8—from roughly 1600 BCE to 300 CE exhibited similar longevity with an e^0 of 37 years.[151] Chapter 8 argued that Tlatilco was an aberration because Teotihuacan, Mexico's bean consumers between about 300 BCE and 1 CE had an e^0 of 21 years.[152] The mean of these two is twenty-nine, an e^0 near Deevey's upper bound and almost 11 years below precontact Yanomami longevity.

Yanomami durability is difficult to explain and probably cannot be attributed wholly to bananas or another food. Note must be taken of infections, which caused only seventy of the 2,216 (3.2 percent) Yanomami deaths between 1930 and 1957.[153] In contrast, exposure to Old World diseases inflicted 3,632 of 5,556 (65.4 percent) deaths between 1958 and 1961. These numbers demonstrate that European intrusion shattered the equilibrium, achieved over millennia of natural selection, between the Yanomami and their surroundings, and that precontact longevity was an outcome of Yanomami adaptation to the environment. Yet this explanation is unhelpful if it requires the assumption that numerous other premodern peoples were maladapted to their surroundings. Belief in widespread maladaptation does not square with natural selection, which fits organisms to the environment rather than alienates them from it.

That said, humans create their environment by deciding what and how much to eat, when and how long to sleep, and whether to work in the garden or watch television, to bicycle or drive to the office, to take a brisk walk or light a cigarette, to drink water or whiskey, or to ponder any of innumerable lifestyles. This book emphasizes that choices have consequences. Turning to diet and nutrition, not all foods are equal. For example, Chapter 13 marshalled evidence that potatoes are far more nourishing than cassava (*Manihot esculenta*). Several other chapters described the dangers of sloth and the need for activity. This book believes that humans can choose to behave in ways that disrupt or reinforce the diet and lifestyle that millennia of hunting, fishing and gathering shaped them to pursue. This book argues that people erred in the twentieth century by buying cars and other labor-saving machines while continuing to eat many calories. Most evidence in this book derives from people who lived before 1900 and so resembled the Yanomami more than us. Because premodern peoples faced similar challenges, precontact Yanomami longevity remains peculiar in its excess.

Part of the explanation may lie in Yanomami seminomadism. Settlements were temporary and small.[154] In reconstructing Yanomami life, Early and Peters counted just eleven residents in Village A in 1930 and seventeen in 1957.[155] With thirty-three inhabitants in 1930, Village B contracted to twenty-one in 1957.[156] The largest precontact community, Village C, had fifty-two occupants in 1930 and eighty-two in 1957.[157] Movement every few years and sparseness limited aggregation of parasites, pathogens, rodents, and insects as evident in low mortality from contagion before 1957.

Mortality is only part of longevity. As mentioned, Chapter 1 indicated that e^0 may reveal more about births than deaths because birthrate tends to correlate inversely with e^0, a scenario that should apply to the Yanomami, who averaged about eight births per mother over a full reproductive life.[158] For example, ten Brazilian villages yielded 7.9 births per mother, and Venezuela's Yanomami averaged 8.1 pregnancies per woman. Comparison may be made with Greek and Roman antiquity, where the average woman who lived long enough to reach menopause had to birth between 4.5 and 6.5 children just to replace mortality's losses.[159] Even in this context, Yanomami fertility was high, implying that e^0 should have been low.

Given the incongruity of high fertility and high e^0, an onlooker might question e^0's accuracy. No records exist of Yanomami births and deaths before 1959.[160] Early and Peters reconstructed dates by questioning villagers, an approach that depended on memory and that yielded estimates.[161] Memory is fallible. Psychologists study the fabrication of false memories, though not all errors fall in this category. Despite honest efforts, people sometimes fail to recall the past as it happened.

When records are absent or poor, even people whose lives have received scrutiny cannot always be dated. For example, Jesus should have been born in 1 CE for the Gregorian Calendar to be accurate, but American diplomat, novelist, and historian Robin William Winks (1930–2003) and colleagues approximated his birth between 8 and 4 BCE.[162] Australian historian William Lewis Leadbetter (b. 1950) favored roughly 6 BCE as Jesus' birth year.[163] American historian of the Middle Ages Joseph Reese Strayer (1904–1987), German historian Hans Wilhelm Gatzke (1915–1987), and American theologians Kirk R. MacGregor and Jeffrey A. Trumbower put his birth around 4 BCE.[164] American historian of Europe John P. McKay (b. 1948) and coauthors estimated Jesus' birth at 3 BCE.[165] His death is no better attested, with McKay and colleagues specifying 29 CE, American theologian William Carl Placher (1948–2008) guessing "about" 30 CE, and Winks and coauthors stating "probably" in 29 or 30 CE.[166]

Ambiguity likewise surrounds Greek philosopher Plato, arguably the towering figure in Western thought. American classicist Matthew S. Santirocco gave his life dates as roughly 429–347 BCE, American attorney, author, and coeditor of Plato's complete dialogues Huntington Cairns (1904–1985) favored around 428–348 BCE, McKay and coauthors and British classicist William Henry Denham Rouse (1863–1950) chose 427–347 BCE, British chemist and historian William Hodson Brock (b. 1936) supplied the years 427–348 BCE, and Chicago, Illinois' Great Books Foundation supposed that Plato might have been born in 428 or 427 BCE and died in 348 or 347 BCE.[167]

Ages are sometimes exaggerated. For example, Genesis stated that Adam lived 930 years, Seth 912, Enosh 905, Kenan 910, Mahalalel 895, Jared 962, Methuselah 969, and Lamech 777.[168] In contrast, American poet, short story writer, and critic Edgar Allan Poe (1809–1849) falsified his birthdate to convince readers of his precocity in authoring poems at an untruthfully young age.[169]

Whatever Yanomami longevity, their health appears to have been at least as satisfactory as other premodern peoples in this book. Good health is incompatible with poor nutrition, implying that bananas, must have been nourishing. Early and Peters stated as much in writing of "adequate subsistence in spite of periodic shortages."[170] This judgment is unsurprising given bananas' provision of magnesium, potassium, manganese, and vitamins B_6 and C, noted in Table 14.4. To be sure, the fruit alone cannot meet all the body's needs, but humans never evolved to eat just one food. Moreover, the previous section mentioned bananas' high yields compared even with yams and potatoes. Chapter 13 described potatoes' value in supplying hungry Europeans badly needed nutrients and calories. Bananas appear to have functioned likewise throughout Old and New World tropics. Yanomami health leads this book, mindful that no single edible is perfect, to recommend bananas as wholesome.

NOTES

1 A. Stewart Truswell, "Fruit," in *Essentials of Human Nutrition*, 5th ed., ed. Jim Mann and A. Stewart Truswell (Oxford: Oxford University Press, 2017), 281.
2 Stanley J. Ulijaszek, Neil Mann, and Sarah Elton, *Evolving Human Nutrition: Implications for Public Health* (Cambridge, UK: Cambridge University Press, 2012), 32.
3 Loren Cordain, *The Paleo Diet: Lose Weight and Get Healthy by Eating the Foods You Were Designed to Eat*, rev. ed. (Hoboken, NJ: Wiley, 2011), 5.
4 Ulijanszek, Mann, and Elton, 30.
5 Ibid., 34.
6 Truswell, 281.
7 J. Patrick Henderson and Dellie Rex, *About Wine*, 2nd ed. (Cifton Park, NY: Delmar/Cengage Learning, 2012), 6.
8 Henry Hobhouse, *Seeds of Change: Six Plants That Transformed Mankind* (New York: Shoemaker and Hoard, 2005), 55.
9 Stephen Le, *100 Million Years of Food: What Our Ancestors Ate and Why It Matters Today* (New York: Picador, 2016), 18–19.
10 Steven R. Gundry, *The Plant Paradox: The Hidden Dangers in 'Healthy' Foods that Cause Disease and Weight Gain* (New York: Harper Wave, 2017), 10.
11 David Perlmutter, *Grain Brain: The Surprising Truth about Wheat, Carbs, and Sugar—Your Brain's Silent Killer*, rev. ed. (New York: Little, Brown Spark, 2018), 95.
12 Le, 19.
13 Lenka Kourimska and Anna Adamkova, "Nutritional and Sensory Qualities of Edible Insects," *NFS Journal* 4 (July 16, 2016): 22–26, https://www.researchgate.net/publication/305396814_Nutritional_and_sensory_quality_of_edible_insects.
14 Ulijaszek, Mann, and Elton, 30.
15 Modupe Ogunlesi, Wesley Okiei, Azeez Luqmon Adeyemi, Vincent Obakachi, Monisola Itohan Ikhile, and G. Nkenchor, "Vitamin C Contents of Tropical Vegetables and Foods Determined by Voltametric and Titrimetric Methods and Their Relevance to the Medicinal Uses of the Plants," *International Journal of Electrochemical Science* 5 (January 31, 2010): 105–115, https://www.researchgate.net/publication/313964413_Vitamin_C_contents_of_tropical_vegetables_and_foods_determines_by_voltammetric_and_titrimetric_methods_and_their_relevance_to_the_medicinal_uses_of_the_plants.
16 Le, 19–20.
17 Ulijaszek, Mann, and Elton, 31.
18 Ibid., 32.
19 Le, 18.
20 Ibid., 17–18.
21 Gundry, 10.
22 Ibid., 170–171.
23 "Top 20 Fruits and Vegetables Sold in the U.S.," *PMA*, 2019, accessed September 11, 2019, https://www.pma.com/content/articles/2017/05/top-20-fruits-and-vegetables-sold-in-the-us.
24 Gundry, 171.
25 "Top 20 Fruits and Vegetables Sold in the U.S."
26 "Candies, Mars Snackfood US, Skittles Original Bite Size Candies," *USDA FoodData Central*, April 1, 2019, accessed February 1, 2020, https://fdc.nal.usda.gov/fdc-app.html#/food-details/168843/nutrients;"Apples, Raw, with Skin (Includes Foods for USDA's Food Distribution Program)," April 1, 2019, accessed February 1, 2020, https://fdc.nal.usda.gov/fdc-app.html#/food-details/171688/nutrients.
27 Gen. 2:15 (New American Bible).
28 Gen. 2:16.
29 Gen. 3:1–2.
30 Gen. 2:17.
31 Gen. 3:7–11.
32 Gen. 3:16–24.
33 Truswell, 281.
34 Ibid.; T. Colin Campbell, *Whole: Rethinking the Science of Nutrition* (Dallas, TX: BenBella Books, 2013), 7.
35 Ibid., 282; "Grapefruit Juice and Some Drugs Don't Mix," *FDA*, July 18, 2017, accessed September 10, 2019, https://www.fda.gov/consumers/consumer-updates/grapefruit-juice-and-some-drugs-dont-mix.

36 Rodrigo Figueroa-Mendez and Selva Rivas-Arancibia, "Vitamin C in Health and Disease: Its Role in the Metabolism of Cells and Redox States in the Brain," *Frontiers in Physiology* 6 (December 23, 2015), https://www.ncbi.nlm.nih.gov/pmc/articles/PMC4688356.
37 Truswell, 281.
38 Ibid.
39 Ibid.; "Olives, Black," *USDA FoodData Central*, April 1, 2019, accessed January 26, 2020, https://fdc.nal.usda.gov/fdc-app.html#/food-details/343670/nutrients; "Nectarines, Raw," *USDA FoodData Central*, April 1, 2019, accessed January 26, 2020, https://fdc.nal.usda.gov/fdc-app.html#/food-details/169914/nutrients; "Blackberries, Raw," *USDA FoodData Central*, April 1, 2019, accessed January 26, 2020, https://fdc.nal.usda.gov/fdc-app.html#/food-details/173946/nutrients; Jessica Bruso, "What Fruit Has More Potassium than Bananas?" *SFGate*, last modified November 19, 2018, accessed January 26, 2020, https://healthyeating.sfgate.com/fruit-potassium-bananas-4738.html.
40 Truswell, 281–282.
41 Ibid., 282.
42 Delphine Roger, "The Middle East and South Asia," in *The Cambridge World History of Food*, vol. 2, ed. Kenneth F. Kiple and Kriemhild Conee Ornelas (Cambridge, UK: Cambridge University Press, 2000), 1141.
43 Ibid.; "Date," in *The Cambridge World History of Food*, vol. 2, ed. Kenneth F. Kiple and Kriemhild Conee Ornelas (Cambridge, UK: Cambridge University Press, 2000), 1767; Stephen Bertman, *Handbook to Life in Ancient Mesopotamia* (New York: Facts on File, 2003), 293.
44 "Date," 1768.
45 "Dates, Medjool," *USDA FoodData Central*, April 1, 2019, accessed February 16, 2020, https://fdc.nal.usda.gov/fdc-app.html#/food-details/168191/nutrients.
46 Beryl Brintnall Simpson and Molly Conner Ogorzaly, *Economic Botany: Plants in Our World*, 3rd ed. (Boston: McGraw Hill, 2001), 91.
47 "Bananas, Raw," USDA FoodData Central, April 1, 2019, accessed January 26, 2020, https://fdc.nal.usda.gov/fdc-app.html#/food-details/173944/nutrients.
48 Charles R. Clement, "Fruits," in *The Cultural History of Plants*, ed. Ghillean Prance and Mark Nesbitt (New York and London: Routledge, 2005), 83.
49 Clark Spencer Larsen, *Our Origins: Discovering Physical Anthropology* (New York and London: Norton, 2008), 315–316.
50 Ibid., 335.
51 Ibid., 342–343.
52 Ibid., 354, 361.
53 Tori Avey, "The History, Science, and Uses of Dates," *Tori's Kitchen*, 2010–2020, accessed February 16, 2020, https://toriavey.com/dates-history-science-uses; "Date," 1767.
54 Hans T. Beck, "Caffeine, Alcohol, and Sweeteners," in *The Cultural History of Plants*, ed. Ghillean Prance and Mark Nesbitt (New York and London: Routledge, 2005), 185.
55 Julia F. Morton, "Date," Purdue University, 1987, accessed February 16, 2020, https://hort.purdue.edu/newcrop/morton/date.html.
56 Simpson and Ogorzaly, 90.
57 "Date," 1767; Avey.
58 New York University, "History of North African Date Palm," *ScienceDaily*, January 14, 2019, accessed September 17, 2019, https://www.sciencedaily.com/releases/2019/01/190114161126.htm.
59 Clement, 83.
60 John P. McKay, Bennett D. Hill, John Buckler, Clare Haru Crowston, Merry E. Wiesner-Hanks, and Joe Perry, *Understanding Western Society: A Brief History* (Boston and New York: Bedford/St. Martin's, 2012), 8.
61 Clement, 83.
62 Gen. 2:10; Bertman, 2.
63 Gen. 2:14.
64 Simpson and Ogorzaly, 90–91.
65 Bertman, 55.
66 Ibid., 68–72, 185–210; McKay, Hill, Buckler, Crowston, Wiesner-Hanks, and Perry, 10–11; Don Nardo, *The Greenhaven Encyclopedia of Ancient Mesopotamia* (Detroit, MI: Thomson Gale, 2007), 44–45, 176–178.
67 Morton.
68 Bertman, 293.

69 Roger, 1145.
70 Avey.
71 Roger, 1141; Simpson and Ogorzaly, 91.
72 Maguelonne Toussaint-Samat, *A History of Food*, expanded ed., trans. Anthea Bell (Chichester, UK: Wiley-Blackwell, 2009), 608.
73 Roger, 1141.
74 Clement, 84.
75 "Date," 1767.
76 Ibid.
77 Henry Field, *Arabs of Central Iraq: Their History, Ethnology, and Physical Characters* (Chicago: Field Museum of Natural History, 1935), 89.
78 Morton.
79 Clement, 83.
80 Patricia Smith, Ofer Bar-Yosef, and Andrew Sillen, "Archaeological and Skeletal Evidence for Dietary Change during the Late Pleistocene/Early Holocene in the Levant," in *Paleopathology at the Origins of Agriculture*, ed. Mark Nathan Cohen and George J. Armelagos (Orlando, FL: Academic Press, 1984), 112, 120.
81 Kenneth M. Weiss, "Demographic Models for Anthropology," *American Antiquity* 38, no. 2 (April 1973): 48; Walter Scheidel, "Demography," in *The Cambridge Economic History of the Greco-Roman World*, ed. Walter Scheidel, Ian Morris, and Richard Saller (Cambridge, UK: Cambridge University Press, 2007), 38–39.
82 Smith, Bar-Yosef, and Sillen, 119.
83 Edward S. Deevey Jr., "The Human Population," *Scientific American* 203, no. 9 (September 1, 1960), 202.
84 Ibid.; Ian Morris, "Early Iron Age Greece," in *The Cambridge Economic History of the Greco-Roman World*, ed. Walter Scheidel, Ian Morris, and Richard Saller (Cambridge, UK: Cambridge University Press, 2007), 211, 216.
85 Smith, Bar-Yosef, and Sillen, 124.
86 John D. Early and John F. Peters, *The Xilixana Yanomami of the Amazon: History, Social Structure, and Population Dynamics* (Gainesville: University Press of Florida, 2000), 77.
87 Morris, 216.
88 Joseph Machlis, *The Enjoyment of Music: An Introduction to Perceptive Listening* (New York: Norton, 1955), 423.
89 Field, 430–431.
90 Smith, Bar-Yosef, and Sillen, 112; "What Does It Mean to Be Human?" Smithsonian Institution, last modified September 17, 2019, accessed September 23, 2019, http://humanorigins.si.edu/evidence/human-fossils/fossils/skh%C5%ABl-v; "What Does It Mean to Be Human?" Smithsonian Institution, last modified March 30, 2016, accessed September 23, 2019, http://humanorigins.si.edu/evidence/human-fossils/fossils/qafzeh-6; Ofer Bar-Yosef, "The Natufian Culture in the Levant, Threshold to the Origins of Agriculture," *Evolutionary Anthropology* (1998): 162, http://www.columbia.edu/itc/anthropology/v1007/baryo.pdf; Bertman, 55.
91 Naomi F. Miller and Wilma Wetterstrom, "The Beginnings of Agriculture: The Ancient near East and North Africa," in *The Cambridge World History of Food*, vol. 2, ed. Kenneth F. Kiple and Kriemhild Conee Ornelas (Cambridge, UK: Cambridge University Press, 2000), 1123.
92 Ibid., 1124.
93 Roger, 1141.
94 Smith, Bar-Yosef, and Sillen, 112.
95 Juan L. Rodriguez-Flores, Khalid Fakhro, Francisco Agosto-Perez, Monica D. Ramstetter, Leonardo Arbiza, Thomas L. Vincent, Amal Robay, Joel A. Malek, Karsten Suhre, Lotfi Chouchane, Ramin Badii, Ajayeb Al-Nabet Al-Marri, Charbel Abi Khalil, Mahmoud Zirie, Amin Jayyousi, Jacqueline Salit, Alon Keinan, Andrew G. Clark, Ronald G. Crystal, and Jason G. Mezey, "Indigenous Arabs Are Descendants of the Earliest Split from Ancient Eurasian Populations," *Genome Research* 26, no. 2 (February 2016): 151–162, https://www.ncbi.nlm.nih.gov/pmc/articles/PMC4728368.
96 Smith, Bar-Yosef, and Sillen, 112.
97 Ibid.
98 Ibid.
99 Field, 98.
100 Ibid., 444.

101 Ibid., 455.
102 Arthur Keith, "Arabs of Central Iraq: Introduction," in *Arabs of Central Iraq: Their History, Ethnology, and Physical Characters*, ed. Henry Field (Chicago: Field Museum of Natural History, 1935), 73.
103 Smith, Bar-Yosef, and Sillen, 112.
104 Ibid., 121.
105 Ibid., 120.
106 "Middle East Climate," Israel Science and Technology Directory, 1999–2018, accessed September 24, 2019, https://www.science.co.il/weather/middle-east-climate.
107 Field, 87.
108 Roger, 1141.
109 Lauren Panoff, "6 Surprising Benefits of Camel Milk (And 3 Downsides)," *Healthline*, June 27, 2019, accessed September 24, 2019, https://www.healthline.com/nutrition/camel-milk-benefits; Kate Morrison, "Goat Milk Versus Cow Milk: Which Is Healthier?" *The Spruce Eats*, last modified May 13, 2019, accessed September 24, 2019, https://www.thespruceeats.com/goats-milk-versus-cows-milk-3376918; "Why Sheep Milk Is Better for You than Cow or Goat Milk—Nutritional Benefits of Sheep Milk," *Woodlands Dairy*, April 26, 2017, accessed September 24, 2019, http://woodlandsdairy.co.uk/why-sheep-milk-is-better-for-you-than-cow-or-goat-milk-nutritional-benefits-of-sheep-milk.
110 "Why Sheep Milk Is Better for You than Cow or Goat Milk."
111 Said Zibaee, Syed Musa Al-Reza Hosseini, Mahdi Yousefi, Ali Taghipour, Mohammad Ali Kiani, and Mohammad Reza Noras, "Nutritional and Therapeutic Characteristics of Camel Milk in Children: A Systematic Review," *Electronic Physician* 7, no. 7 (November 2015): 1523–1528, https://www.ncbi.nlm.nih.gov/pmc/articles/PMC4700900.
112 W. N. Sawaya, J. K. Khalil, and A. F. Al-Shalhat, "Mineral and Vitamin Content of Goat's Milk," *Journal of the American Dietetic Association* 84, no. 4 (April 1984): 433–435.
113 Chris Stringer and Peter Andrews, *The Complete World of Human Evolution* (London: Thames and Hudson, 2005), 142.
114 Kenneth Good, "The Yanomami: Tropical Forest Dwellers of Venezuela and Brazil," in *Faces of the Rainforest: The Yanomami*, Valdir Cruz (New York: Powerhouse Books, 2002), 126.
115 Early and Peters, 4.
116 Good, 126–127.
117 Clement, 79.
118 Good, 126; Laura M. Rival, "Introduction: South America," in *The Cambridge Encyclopedia of Hunters and Gatherers*, ed. Richard B. Lee and Richard Daly (Cambridge, UK: Cambridge University Press, 2004), 80.
119 "Banana," in *The Cambridge World History of Food*, vol. 2, ed. Kenneth F. Kiple and Kriemhild Conee Ornelas (Cambridge, UK: Cambridge University Press, 2000), 1726; "Plantain," in *The Cambridge World History of Food*, vol. 2, ed. Kenneth F. Kiple and Kriemhild Conee Ornelas (Cambridge, UK: Cambridge University Press, 2000), 1836.
120 Judith A. Carney and Richard Nicholas Rosomoff, *In the Shadow of Slavery: Africa's Botanical Legacy in the Atlantic World* (Berkeley: University of California Press, 2009), 35.
121 Will C. McClatchey, "Bananas and Plantains," in *The Cambridge World History of Food*, vol. 1, ed. Kenneth F. Kiple and Kriemhild Conee Ornelas (Cambridge, UK: Cambridge University Press, 2000), 175.
122 Linda Civitello, *Cuisine and Culture: A History of Food and People*, 3rd ed. (Hoboken, NJ: Wiley, 2011), 130.
123 Simpson and Ogorzaly, 76; Clement, 80.
124 Michael Gurven and Hillard Kaplan, "Longevity among Hunter-Gatherers: A Cross-Cultural Examination," *Population and Development Review* 33, no. 2 (June 2007): 13, https://www.academia.edu/17979487/Longevity_Among_Hunter-_Gatherers_A_Cross-Cultural_Examination?auto=download.
125 Simpson and Ogorzaly, 92; Clement, 80.
126 "Banana," 1726; Clement, 80.
127 Clement; McClatchey, 177.
128 Carney and Rosomoff, 34.
129 Clement, 80.
130 McClatchey, 176.
131 Ibid., 178.
132 Early and Peters, 20.
133 Clement, 80.
134 Carney and Rosomoff, 35.

135 Ibid.
136 Early and Peters, 20.
137 Ibid., 21.
138 Ibid., 3.
139 Ibid., 7.
140 Ibid., 193.
141 Ibid., 199.
142 Muzaffer Suleyman Senyurek, "A Note on the Duration of Life of the Ancient Inhabitants of Anatolia," *American Journal of Physical Anthropology* 5, no. 1 (March 1947): 59.
143 Ann E. M. Liljas, "Old Age in Ancient Egypt," March 2, 2015, accessed January 18, 2019, https://blogs.ucl.ac.uk/researchers-in-museums/2015/03/02/old-age-in-ancient-egypt; Roger S. Bagnall and Bruce W. Frier, *The Demography of Roman Egypt* (Cambridge, UK and New York: Cambridge University Press, 2006), 109.
144 Ann L. W. Stodder, Debra L. Martin, Alan H. Goodman, and Daniel T. Reff, "Cultural Longevity and Biological Stress in the American Southwest," in *The Backbone of History: Health and Nutrition in the Western Hemisphere*, ed. Richard H. Steckel and Jerome C. Rose (Cambridge, UK: Cambridge University Press, 2002), 490–491.
145 Clark Spencer Larsen, *Skeletons in Our Closet: Revealing Our Past through Bioarchaeology* (Princeton, NJ and Oxford: Princeton University Press, 2000), 209, 212.
146 James M. Davidson, Jerome C. Rose, Myron P. Gutmann, Michael R. Haines, Keith Condon, and Cindy Condon, "The Quality of African-American Life in the Old Southwest near the Turn of the Twentieth Century," in *The Backbone of History: Health and Nutrition in the Western Hemisphere*, ed. Richard H. Steckel and Jerome C. Rose (Cambridge, UK: Cambridge University Press, 2002), 233.
147 Early and Peters, 200.
148 Ibid., 199.
149 Gurven and Kaplan, 24.
150 Early and Peters, 199.
151 Lourdes Marquez Morfin, Robert McCaa, Rebecca Storey, and Andres Del Angel, "Health and Nutrition in Pre-Hispanic Mesoamerica," in *The Backbone of History: Health and Nutrition in the Western Hemisphere*, ed. Richard H. Steckel and Jerome C. Rose (Cambridge, UK: Cambridge University Press, 2002), 310.
152 Ibid., 318–319.
153 Early and Peters, 201.
154 Ibid., 4.
155 Ibid., 103.
156 Ibid., 109.
157 Ibid., 127.
158 Ibid., 196–197.
159 Scheidel, 41.
160 Early and Peters, 73.
161 Ibid., 76–81.
162 Robin W. Winks, Crane Brinton, John B. Christopher, and Robert Lee Wolff, *A History of Civilization, vol. 1: Prehistory to 1715*, 7th ed. (Englewood Cliffs, NJ: Prentice Hall, 1988), 98.
163 Bill Leadbetter, "Jesus," in *Berkshire Encyclopedia of World History*, vol. 3, ed. William H. McNeill, Jerry H. Bentley, David Christian, David Levinson, J. R. McNeill, Heidi Roupp, and Judith Zinsser (Great Barrington, MA: Berkshire Publishing Group, 2005), 1054.
164 Joseph R. Strayer and Hans W. Gatzke, *The Mainstream of Civilization*, 3d ed. (New York: Harcourt Brace Jovanovich, 1979), 89; Kirk R. MacGregor, "Introduction: Christianity," in *World History Encyclopedia, Era 3: Classical Traditions, 1000 BCE–300 CE*, vol. 6, ed. William E. Mierse and Kevin M. McGeough (Santa Barbara, CA: ABC-CLIO, 2011), 570; Jeffrey Trumbower, "Life of Christ," in *World History Encyclopedia, Era 3: Classical Traditions, 1000 BCE–300 CE*, vol. 6, ed. William E. Mierse and Kevin M. McGeough (Santa Barbara, CA: ABC-CLIO, 2011), 571.
165 McKay, Hill, Buckler, Crowston, Wiesner-Hanks, and Perry, 157.
166 Ibid.; William C. Placher, *A History of Christian Theology: An Introduction* (Philadelphia: Westminster Press, 1983), 32; Winks, Brinton, Christopher, and Wolff, 98.
167 Matthew S. Santirocco, "Introduction: Discovering Plato," in *Great Dialogues of Plato: Complete Texts of The Republic, The Apology, Crito, Phaedo, Ion, Meno, Symposium*, trans. W. H. D. Rouse (New York: Signet Classics, 2008), viii; Huntington Cairns, "Introduction," in *Plato: The Collected Dialogues*

Including the Letters, ed. Edith Hamilton and Huntington Cairns (Princeton, NJ: Princeton University Press, 1961), xiii; McKay, Hill, Buckler, Crowston, Wiesner-Hanks, and Perry, 80; William H. Brock, *The History of Chemistry: A Very Short Introduction* (Oxford: Oxford University Press, 2016), 14; W. H. D. Rouse, "Preface," in *Great Dialogues of Plato*, trans. W. H. D. Rouse (New York and Scarborough, Ontario: New American Library, 1956), 8; Plato, *Apology, Crito*, trans. Benjamin Jowett (Chicago: Great Books Foundation, 1955), ii.

168 Gen. 5:5; Gen. 5:8; Gen. 5:11; Gen. 5:14; Gen. 5:17; Gen. 5:20; Gen. 5:27; Gen. 5:31.

169 Nina Baym, Francis Murphy, Ronald Gottesman, Hershel Parker, Laurence B. Holland, William H. Pritchard, and David Kalstone, *The Norton Anthology of American Literature*, 2d ed. (New York and London: Norton, 1986), 509.

170 Early and Peters, 21.

15 Vegetables

15.1 DEFINITION

15.1.1 Imprecision and Confusion

Vegetables' terminology frustrates the desire for precision. British archaeologist and botanist Jane Margaret Ewbank Renfrew and British botanist Helen Sanderson admitted that they are difficult to define.[1] Gardening book authors are silent on this matter. I retrieved three such books from my collection and four from an Ohio public library.[2] None of the seven, published between 1978 and 2018, defined the word "vegetable" or "vegetables," even though two—one of which claimed comprehensiveness—have glossaries.[3] This situation resembles an attempt to discuss triangles or another polygon absent geometric definitions. Curiously, National Gardening Association spokesperson and horticulturist Charlie Nardozzi defined "fruit" but not "vegetable" in *Vegetable Gardening for Dummies*, the opposite of what readers might expect from a book that purports to treat vegetables.[4] The analog would be a book about triangles that defines rectangles but not triangles. Under such circumstances, onlookers deserve no blame for bewilderment. Not only are they unable to define a triangle, but they may also conflate it with other polygons, creating a muddle in the process.

The foregoing implies that such confusion attends the word "vegetable," which has become a catchall for many types of plants just as an errant categorization of triangles might include several polygons. Imprecision afflicts even scientific treatment of vegetables. For example, Cornell University olericulturist Homer C. Thompson did not define them in the textbook *Vegetable Crops* but instead used the word "vegetable" or "vegetables" in three ways. First, he made "vegetables" a category in opposition to groupings of other crops.[5] This method might have permitted identification of vegetables by eliminating plants pigeonholed elsewhere. But elimination fails because Thompson included but did not define the classification "other crops." That this last category is unknown makes impossible vegetables' definition because any attempt to name specifics may be countered by the possibility that Thompson intended them as other. Second, he constructed different lists of vegetables. Table 4 included, but Table 5 omitted, artichokes (*Cynara scolymus*), broccoli (*Brassica oleracea var. italica*), collard (*Brassica oleracea var. viridis*) and dandelion (*Taraxacum officinale*) greens, eggplants (*Solanum melongena*), and muskmelons (*Cucumis melo*) as vegetables.[6] Table 4 excluded, but Table 5 included, brussels sprouts (*Brassica oleracea var. gemmifera*), okra (*Abelmoschus esculentus*), radishes (*Raphanus sativus*), and rutabagas (*Brassica napus*), also known as swedes. Table 4 divided corn (*Zea mays*) into yellow and white, whereas Table 5 specified only sweet corn. Table 4 included only beet (*Beta vulgaris*) roots, but Table 5 listed beet roots and leaves as separate categories. Third, Thompson multiplied ambiguities by listing five methods for classifying vegetables.[7] Favoring the fifth, he nonetheless admitted to following it only "in a general way."[8]

Perhaps wishing to avoid inconsistencies, American botanist Beryl Brintnall Simpson (b. 1942) and American botanist and science educator Molly Conner Ogorzaly never employed "vegetable" or "vegetables" as nouns in the textbook *Economic Botany* (2001). No chapter bears these terms as a title. The nearest they approached vegetables was a chapter on "foods from leaves, stems, and roots."[9] Even this formulation is unsatisfactory because the chapter included sugarcane (*Saccharum officinarum*), sugar beet (*Beta vulgaris ssp. vulgaris*), sorghum (*Sorghum bicolor*), dates (*Phoenix dactylifera*), sugar maple (*Acer saccharum*), and sucrose ($C_{12}H_{22}O_{11}$), none a vegetable.[10] Despite avoidance of "vegetable" as noun, Simpson and Ogorzaly used it as an adjective in opposition to the adjectives "animal" and "synthetic."[11] Such language makes vegetables plants, though failure to craft a narrow definition—or any definition in this case—leaves all florae as default members of this category.

15.1.2 Attempts to Define Vegetables

Unlike Thompson, Simpson, and Ogorzaly, American olericulturists Vincent E. Rubatzky and Mas Yamaguchi (d. 2019) attempted to define vegetables, considering them mostly herbaceous (nonwoody) plants, either domestic or wild, whose edible portions may be roots, tubers, stems, leaves, flowers, fruits, or seeds.[12] Vegetables usually contain ample water and may be cooked or raw.

This definition is concrete but broad. For example, inclusion of fruits from nonwoody plants seems to admit watermelon (*Citrullus lanatus*) as a vegetable, contradicting its conventional status as dessert fruit. Inclusion of seeds from nonwoody plants appears to make grains (cereals) vegetables, undermining the consensus since antiquity (c. 3000 BCE–c. 500 CE) that they form a separate category of edibles. Less controversial is inclusion of legume seeds because the public usually considers peas (*Pisum sativum*) and beans (*Phaseolus vulgaris, Phaseolus lunatus, Phaseolus acutifolius,* and *Phaseolus coccineus*), especially green beans (*P. vulgaris*), vegetables in the belief that anything green and edible qualifies. Less satisfactory is the opinion that wild plants may be vegetables because it undermines the conviction that vegetables are products of domestication. The stipulation that they may be cooked or raw appears to exclude the root cassava—which cannot be eaten raw because of toxins (see Chapter 13)—despite Rubatzky and Yamaguchi's insistence that edible roots are vegetables.

Equally perplexing is Renfrew and Sanderson's definition of a vegetable as an edible that tends not to be sweet, that accompanies savory foods such as fish, meat, cheese, or eggs, and that generally has little fat.[13] Besides these criteria, Renfrew and Sanderson excluded roots, tubers, nuts, seeds, and legumes and included tomatoes (*Solanum esculentum*) and cucumbers (*Cucumis sativus*). This definition's greatest defect is its subjectivity because the designation "sweet" depends on opinion. The parent who prizes fresh carrots (*Daucus carota ssp. sativus*) or beets for their sweetness may have children who abhor them as tasteless or worse. In this example, the adult's judgment eliminates both as vegetables, whereas the child's revulsion admits them. Renfrew and Sanderson excluded the two as vegetables, however, because they are roots despite public consensus to the contrary. Moreover, the criterion unsweet appears to exclude fresh, ripe tomatoes as vegetables even though Renfrew and Sanderson included them. Yet commercially raised tomatoes—picked green and exposed to ethylene gas (C_2H_4) to simulate ripeness—are unsweet. Depending on the method of cultivation, therefore, tomatoes are or are not vegetables despite having undergone no botanical change. In other words, the stipulation unsweet is too subjective and variable to define a vegetable.

Imprecision created an opportunity for the U.S. Supreme Court to define a vegetable as a precondition to deciding whether imported tomatoes should be subject to a tariff. In 1883, Congress assessed a tariff on imported vegetables but not fruits. Four years later, New York City grocer John Nix sued the city's federal agent for refusing to exempt imported tomatoes. Nix contended that the agent had erroneously classified them vegetables rather than fruits. Writing for the majority in 1893, associate justice Horace Gray (1828–1902) admitted that tomatoes satisfied the botanical definition of a fruit but held that the public convention of categorizing them as vegetables trumped this scientific understanding.[14] In articulating his opinion, Gray emphasized that vegetables were garden produce and were eaten with the main course rather than as dessert.

This opinion is unsatisfactory on three grounds. First, it did not resolve the issue of fruit versus vegetable. Despite Gray's ruling, Tennessee and Ohio list the tomato as their state fruit.[15] Second, an appeal to popular belief does not guarantee that the public can define fruits, vegetables, polygons, or anything else. Public opinion's murkiness is a poor substitute for scientific exactitude. Third, intentional or not, deference to the public condones slavery, racism, xenophobia, sexism, and homophobia wherever such deplorables are in the majority. If these practices and prejudices are evils, then they must be wrong irrespective of public sentiment and behavior. In the same

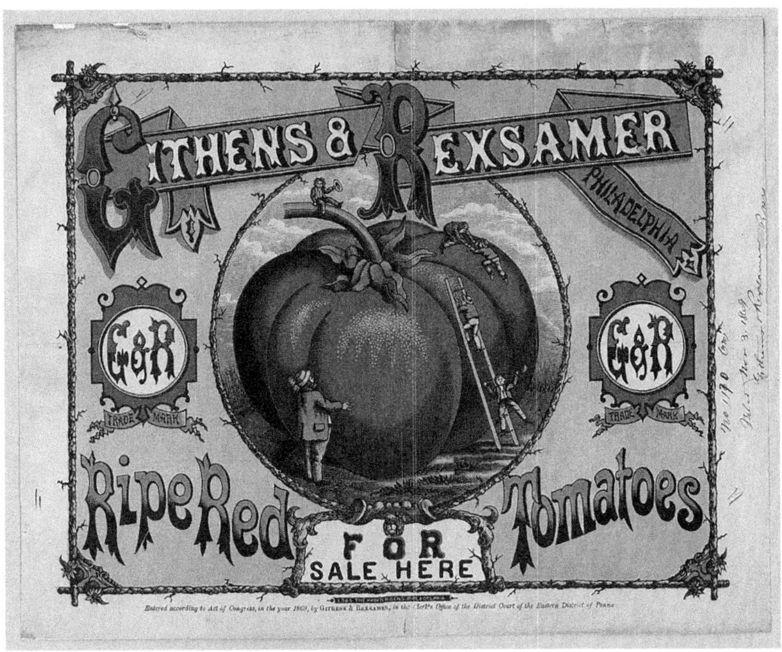

FIGURE 15.1 Tomato. (Art courtesy of Library of Congress. https://www.loc.gov/pictures/item/95509317/.)

manner, the definition of a vegetable, fruit, or any noun should be an absolute rather than an impulse. Because public opinion can change, it is relativistic. It seems perverse to erect a legal system on the principle that what is true today may be false tomorrow. The *Republic's* (c. 380 BCE) first pages exposed the weaknesses inherent in conflicting, changeable definitions of justice.[16] Its arguments should apply to vegetables.

The best definition of vegetable comes from New Zealand nutritionist and biochemist Meika Foster, who characterized it as any plant part except seed or fruit.[17] Vegetables may be roots, tubers, bulbs, stems, leaves, and flowers. Although her formulation is broad, it has the virtue of simplicity while eliminating fruits and seeds, which deserve to be independent categories but which the public tends to conflate with vegetables where tomatoes, peppers (*Capsicum annuum*), eggplants, okra, squashes (*Cucurbita* species), cucumbers, and legumes are concerned. Foster acknowledged but resisted the temptation to name tomatoes and mushrooms (*Agaricus bisporus* and other edible species) as vegetables. Indeed, mushrooms are fungi rather than plants.

Foster's definition includes above- and underground plant structures as vegetables. The large number of edibles that results from this breadth defies treatment in one chapter. This book combats inordinate scope by assigning roots sweet potato and cassava and tubers potato (*Solanum tuberosum*) and yams (*Dioscorea* species) to Chapter 13. This maneuver leaves as vegetables among subterranean edibles the genus *Allium* and taproots such as carrot, parsnip (*Pastinaca sativa*), turnip (*Brassica rapa ssp. rapa*), radish, beet, and rutabaga. Foster's rejection of seeds as vegetables accords with this book's allocation of legumes, nuts, and grains to Chapters 8, 9, and 12, respectively. Elimination of fruits as vegetables is correct, but assignment of all to Chapter 14 would again create a behemoth. For this reason, Chapter 14 treated only the staple fruits dates and bananas (*Musa × paradisiaca*). Foster's definition makes stems like asparagus (*Asparagus officinalis*); leaves such as spinach (*Spinacia oleracea*), lettuce (*Lactuca sativa*), cabbage (*Brassica oleracea var. capitata*), and swiss chard (*Beta vulgaris ssp. vulgaris*); and flower buds like broccoli vegetables. Celery (*Apium graveolens*) is classified as a stem or leaf structure known as the petiole depending on whom the reader consults.[18] This chapter categorizes no other plant parts as vegetables.

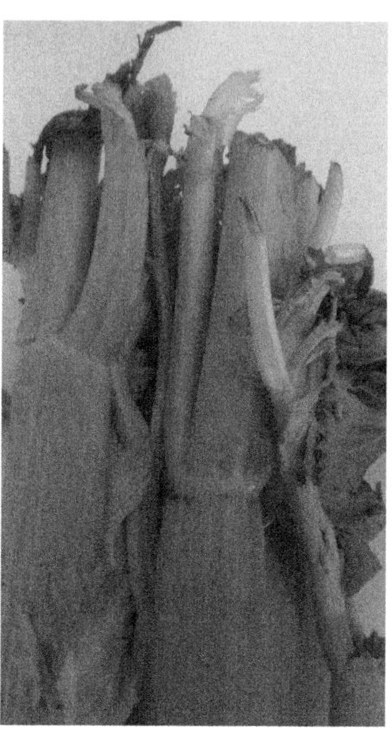

FIGURE 15.2 Celery. (Photo from author.)

15.2 NUTRITION AND HEALTH

15.2.1 A Reputation as Healthful

From the outset, this book acknowledged that controversies attend public and scientific discussions about diet, nutrition, and health. Chapter 1 described this book's method as an attempt to amass prehistoric and historic evidence about foods' health effects in response to these disagreements. For example, Chapter 4 tested the hypothesis—evident in the Paleo diet—that meat should be the dietary centerpiece. Chapters 10 and 11 marshalled data germane to the debate over carbohydrates and fat. Chapter 12 investigated grains in the context of attacks against them in general and against wheat and gluten specifically.

In contrast to these foods, vegetables bask in widespread praise. Rubatzky and Yamaguchi recommended them for fiber, minerals, and vitamins.[19] This appraisal has merit when vegetables are defined broadly enough to include legumes, roots, and tubers and when the number of leaves, stems, and flowers under consideration is broadened to include items that Americans seldom consume today. For example, lettuce is popular enough in the United States to have infiltrated fast food, but none of the five varieties listed in *World Vegetables* (1997) has over 0.7 grams of fiber per 100-gram serving.[20] By contrast, cassava leaves—eaten in the developing world's tropics but not in the United States—have 3.2 grams of fiber per 100 grams total.[21] Scarlet runner beans (*Phaseolus coccineus*)—defined here and in Chapter 8 as a legume rather than a vegetable—supply 12.2 grams of fiber per 100 grams total.[22]

15.2.2 Vitamins and Minerals in Vegetables

Renfrew and Sanderson amplified Rubatzky and Yamaguchi, lauding vegetables as frequently rich in B vitamins, C, and E and minerals iron and potassium.[23] For example, Table 15.1 shows that 100 grams of turnip greens have 4.7 percent of the U.S. Food and Drug Administration (FDA)'s daily value (DV) for vitamin B_1 (thiamine or thiamin), 5.9 percent for B_2 (riboflavin), 3 percent for B_3

TABLE 15.1
Nutrients in Turnip Greens and Turnips 100 g

Nutrient	Turnip Greens	%DV	Turnips	%DV
Calories	32	N/A	28	N/A
Protein (g)	1.5	N/A	0.9	N/A
Fat (g)	0.3	N/A	0.1	N/A
Carbs (g)	7.13	N/A	6.43	N/A
Fiber (g)	3.2	N/A	1.8	N/A
		Minerals		
Ca (mg)	190	19	30	3
Fe (mg)	1.1	6.1	0.3	1.7
Mg (mg)	31	7.8	11	2.8
P (mg)	42	4.2	27	2.7
K (mg)	296	8.5	191	5.5
Na (mg)	40	1.7	67	2.8
Zn (mg)	0.19	1.3	0.27	1.8
Cu (mg)	0.35	17.5	0.09	4.5
Mn (mg)	0.47	23.5	0.13	6.5
Se (mcg)	1.2	1.7	0.7	1
		Vitamins		
A (IU)	11,587	231.7	0	0
B_1 (mg)	0.07	4.7	0.04	2.7
B_2 (mg)	0.1	5.9	0.03	1.8
B_3 (mg)	0.6	3	0.4	2
B_5 (mg)	0.38	3.8	0.2	2
B_6 (mg)	0.26	13	0.09	4.5
B_9 (mcg)	194	48.5	15	3.8
B_{12} (mcg)	0	0	0	0
C (mg)	60	100	21	35
D (IU)	0	0	0	0
E (mg)	2.86	19.1	0.03	0.2
K (mcg)	251	313.8	0.1	0.1

(niacin or nicotinic acid), 3.8 percent for B_5 (pantothenic acid), 13 percent for B_6 (pyridoxine), 48.5 percent for B_9 (folate, folic acid, or pteroylmonoglutamic acid), no B_{12} (cobalamin), 100 percent for vitamin C, 19.1 percent for E, 313.8 percent for K, 19 percent for calcium, 8.5 percent for potassium, 17.5 percent for copper, and 23.5 percent for manganese.[24] By comparison, 100 grams of turnip taproot supply 2.7 percent of DV for vitamin B_1, 1.8 percent for B_2, 2 percent for B_3 and B_5, 4.5 percent for B_6, 3.8 percent for B_9, no B_{12}, 35 percent for vitamin C, under 0.5 percent for vitamins E and K, 3 percent for calcium, 1.7 percent for iron, 5.5 percent for potassium, 4.5 percent for copper, and 6.5 percent for manganese.[25]

15.3 RECOMMENDATIONS FOR VEGETABLE CONSUMPTION

The U.S. Department of Agriculture (USDA) provides volumetric guidelines for daily vegetable intake by age and sex, though volume does not readily convert to mass because leafy items are less dense than their alternatives and so occupy more space at constant mass. Conversely, when leafy and other vegetables occupy the same space, their masses differ. The USDA compensates for this complication by equating two cups of raw leafy vegetables with one cup of their raw or cooked nonleafy counterparts or with one cup of vegetable juice.[26] This equivalency translates into a recommendation of one cup of nonleafy and two cups of leafy vegetables for children ages 2 and 3. Allotments increase with age, peaking at three cups of nonleafy and six cups of leafy vegetables for men aged 19–50. Amounts are smaller for women. Quantities also diminish for men above 51 years, though the USDA omits recommendations for women over this age. Conversion of volume to mass yields recommendations of 160 grams of vegetables, leafy or not, for 2- and 3-year-olds and 480 grams for men aged 19–50.[27]

Nutrients vary by vegetable. Because all possibilities cannot be exhausted, a few examples in Table 15.2 must suffice.[28] With an eye on Roman preferences, discussed here and in later sections, 480 grams of celery—the amount for men aged 19–50—supply 67.2 calories, 7.68 grams of fiber, 14.26 grams of carbohydrates, 0.82 grams of fat, 3.31 grams of protein, 43.1 percent of DV for vitamin A (equivalents), 43.2 percent for B_9, 6.7 percent for B_1, 16.1 percent for B_2, 7.7 percent for B_3, 11.8 percent for B_5, 17.8 percent for B_6, 24.8 percent for C, 8.6 percent for E, 175.8 percent for K, 19.2 percent for calcium, 11.5 percent for phosphorus, 35.7 percent for potassium, 24.7 percent for manganese, 5.3 percent for iron, 16 percent for sodium, 8.4 percent for copper, and 13.2 percent for magnesium.[29] No other nutrient equals or exceeds 5 percent DV.

TABLE 15.2
Nutrients in Celery Collard Greens Mustard Greens and Kale 480 g

Nutrient	Celery	%DV	Collard Greens	%DV	Mustard Greens	%DV	Kale	%DV
Calories	67.2	N/A	153.6	N/A	129.6	N/A	168	N/A
Protein (g)	3.31	N/A	14.5	N/A	13.73	N/A	14.02	N/A
Fat (g)	0.82	N/A	2.93	N/A	2.02	N/A	7.15	N/A
Carbs (g)	14.26	N/A	26.02	N/A	22.42	N/A	21.22	N/A
Fiber (g)	7.68	N/A	19.2	N/A	15.36	N/A	19.68	N/A
				Minerals				
Ca (mg)	192	19.2	1,113.6	111.4	552	55.2	1,219.2	121.9
Fe (mg)	0.96	5.3	2.26	12.5	7.87	43.7	7.68	42.7
Mg (mg)	52.8	13.2	129.6	32.4	153.6	38.4	158.4	39.6
P (mg)	115.2	11.5	120	12	278.4	27.8	264	26.4
K (mg)	1248	35.7	1,022.4	29.2	1,843.2	52.7	1,670.4	47.4
Na (mg)	384	16	81.6	3.4	96	4	254.4	10.6
Zn (mg)	0.62	4.2	1	6.7	1.2	8	1.87	12.5
Cu (mg)	0.17	8.4	0.22	11	0.79	39.6	0.25	12.7
Mn (mg)	0.49	24.7	3.16	157.9	1.63	81.5	4.42	220.8
Se (mcg)	1.92	2.7	6.24	8.9	4.32	6.2	4.32	6.2
				Vitamins				
A (IU)	2,155.2	43.1	24,091.2	481.8	14,515.2	290.3	23,097.6	462
B_1 (mg)	0.1	6.7	0.26	17.3	0.38	25.6	0.54	36.2
B_2 (mg)	0.27	16.1	0.62	36.7	0.53	31.1	1.67	98
B_3 (mg)	1.54	7.7	3.56	17.8	3.84	19.2	5.66	28.3
B_5 (mg)	1.18	11.8	1.28	12.8	1	10	1.78	17.8
B_6 (mg)	0.36	17.8	0.79	39.6	0.86	43.2	0.71	35.3
B_9 (mcg)	172.8	43.2	619.2	154.8	57.6	14.4	297.6	74.4
B_{12} (mcg)	0	0	0	0	0	0	0	0
C (mg)	14.88	24.8	169.44	282.4	336	560	448.32	747.2
D (IU)	0	0	0	0	0	0	0	0
E (mg)	1.3	8.6	10.85	72.3	9.65	64.3	3.17	21.1
K (mcg)	140.64	175.8	2,098.08	2,622.6	1,236	1,545	1,870.08	2,337.6

15.4 VEGETABLES IN ANCIENT ROME

Historians mention cabbage as a Roman vegetable. Rubatzky and Yamaguchi itemized five: red, white or green, savoy, and two Chinese types.[30] But none was available in the ancient Mediterranean, where the climate was too warm for cabbage.[31] Moreover, *B. oleracea var. capitata*, arising only around the twelfth century CE, was unknown in antiquity.[32] The Romans ate what is usually termed "colewort" (*Brassica oleracea*), the ancestor of Europe's *Brassica* crops.[33] In this context, references to cabbage in Roman antiquity (c. 750 BCE–c. 500 CE) are unhelpful at best and confusing at worst. Readers should instead envision collard greens or kale (*Brassica oleracea var. sabellica*) as closest to colewort.[34]

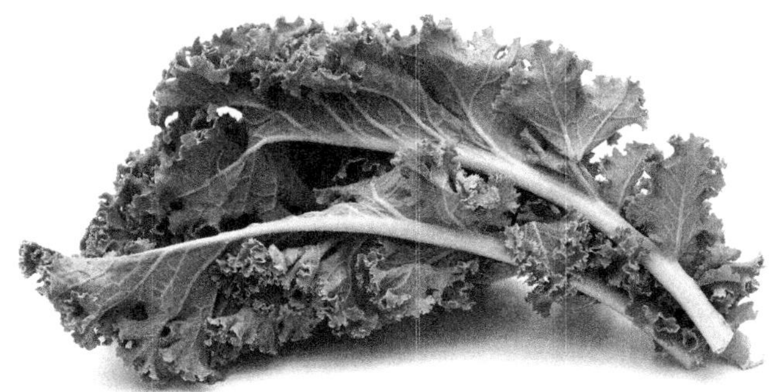

FIGURE 15.3 Kale. (Photo from Shutterstock.)

Four hundred eighty grams of collards, in Table 15.2, furnish 153.6 calories, 19.2 grams of fiber, 26.02 grams of carbohydrates, 2.93 grams of fat, 14.5 grams of protein, over the DV for vitamins A (equivalents), B_9, C, and K, calcium, and manganese, 17.3 percent for vitamin B_1, 36.7 percent for B_2, 17.8 percent for B_3, 12.8 percent for B_5, 39.6 percent for B_6, 72.3 percent for E, 12 percent for phosphorus, 29.2 percent for potassium, 32.4 percent for magnesium, 12.5 percent for iron, 11 percent for copper, 8.9 percent for selenium, and 6.7 percent for zinc.[35] No other nutrient equals or exceeds 5 percent DV.

Besides celery and colewort, Romans ate mustard greens (*Brassica juncea*).[36] Table 15.2 shows that 480 grams provide 129.6 calories, 15.36 grams of fiber, 22.42 grams of carbohydrates, 2.02 grams of fat, 13.73 grams of protein, above the DV for vitamins A (equivalents), C, and K, 25.6 percent for B_1, 31.1 percent for B_2, 19.2 percent for B_3, 10 percent for B_5, 43.2 percent for B_6, 14.4 percent for B_9, 64.3 percent for E, 55.2 percent for calcium, 27.8 percent for phosphorus, 52.7 percent for potassium, 38.4 percent for magnesium, 43.7 percent for iron, 39.6 percent for copper, 81.5 percent for manganese, 6.2 percent for selenium, and 8 percent for zinc.[37] No other nutrient equals or exceeds 5 percent DV.

15.5 VEGETABLES AS MORE POPULAR AMONG NUTRITIONISTS THAN PUBLIC

Vegetables' value was evident to American nutritionist Thomas Colin Campbell (b. 1934), who estimated that kale and spinach have roughly twice the protein per calorie as lean beef.[38] Beyond nutrients, he touted vegetables as flavorful, disputing the belief that wholesome foods "must be the most grim fare imaginable."[39] Appealing to "our dietary roots," Campbell asserted that evolution shaped us to prefer vegetables, fruits, and seeds like nuts, legumes, and whole grains.[40]

This praise has not enticed everyone. Students balked in 2011 when Los Angeles Unified School District in Los Angeles, California, offered more vegetables and fruits at lunch. Nearly two-fifths purchased no vegetables.[41] Of the remainder, 31 percent refused to taste them. Contrary to Los

Angeles, East Grand School District in Granby, Colorado, reported enthusiasm for kale chips and jicama (*Pachyrhizus erosus*) sticks.[42] Yet East Grand's success has not averted overall decline, as U.S. fresh vegetable consumption fell 10 percent between 2017 and 2018, reaching the lowest total in 19 years.[43]

This reality undermines Campbell's belief, first, that humans inherently favor vegetables, fruits, nuts, legumes, and whole grains. Chapters 3 and 4 traced humanity's quest for meat back millions of years. Such antiquity and persistence suggest peoples' preference for it. If this preference is innate, as its longevity implies, then evolution fashioned us to eat meat at least occasionally. Indeed, as incomes rise, consumers eat more meat. Second, legumes—discussed in Chapter 8—diminish in diets as income and meat intake increase. Third, the claim that people are partial toward whole grains contradicts preferences for soft, easily chewed and digested white flour and white rice, discussed in Chapter 12. To be fair, that chapter implicated refined grains in deficiency and chronic diseases, affirming nutritionists' condemnation of them. Nonetheless, Campbell overstated his case by equating the pursuits of flavor and wholesomeness, which sometimes conflict.

15.6 THE CONSENSUS TESTED IN HERCULANEUM

15.6.1 Suitability as Case Study

Flavor and preferences aside, if vegetables are as salubrious as experts claim, then past peoples who ate them should have been healthy. Like other qualities, health depends on context. Earlier chapters demonstrated that premodern peoples led difficult lives. Food was often scarce, and overwork, pathogens, parasites, rodents, and insects undermined vitality even when diet and nutrition were satisfactory. The issue is whether vegetables, like other foods, conferred benefits even when existence was precarious.

Chapters 4 and 10 mined evidence from the ancient Mediterranean to test the health effects of meat and olive (*Olea europaea*) oil, respectively. This chapter returns to the region, which archaeologists, anthropologists, historians, linguists, and other scientists and scholars have studied intensively for generations. The attraction lies partly in the quantity and quality of evidence about those who inhabited this area.

Interest in the Greek and Roman past, known as classical antiquity (c. 2000 BCE–c. 500 CE), appears to have languished during Europe's Middle Ages (c. 500–c. 1500 CE). Renaissance (c. 1350-c. 1600) intellectuals, however, came increasingly to study antiquity's material culture. Obvious targets of this movement were extant texts and ruins. Discoveries of artifacts intensified interest in antiquity. For example, British archaeologist Howard Carter (1874–1939) electrified the world in 1922 by unearthing Pharaoh Tutankhamun's (c. 1345–1327 BCE) tomb in the Valley of the Kings near Luxor, Egypt. Less dramatic has been the piecemeal rediscovery of Roman towns in the Bay of Naples, an area also termed the Gulf of Naples.

Among its features is Mount Vesuvius, which erupted in 79 CE, burying the towns Herculaneum and Pompeii in rock and ash.[44] Part of the tragedy lies in the likelihood that their inhabitants had no inkling that the volcano was active because it had not erupted since roughly 15,000 BCE.[45] Misfortune is also tied to the probability that those who died ignored Vesuvius' warnings. Although Roman lawyer and administrator Pliny the Younger (61–c.113 CE) reported an unusual cloud above the volcano around noon, August 24, the eruption must have begun earlier.[46] News spread immediately to his uncle, the naturalist Pliny the Elder (23–79), mentioned in earlier chapters. Before he could act, a servant delivered a letter from a friend, Rectina, too near the eruption to escape on her own. Hours must have elapsed from this letter's composition to its delivery to Pliny. During this time, escape from Herculaneum and Pompeii was possible for many people, if not for Rectina.

The eruption's gases asphyxiated some who stayed. Trying to rescue Rectina, Pliny the Elder was among the victims. Being nearer the volcano than Pompeii, Herculaneum experienced the initial shock; its residents likely perished first. Those not suffocated in the two towns died from the lava, its heat, or the fires the lava ignited. Rock and ash entombed the corpses.

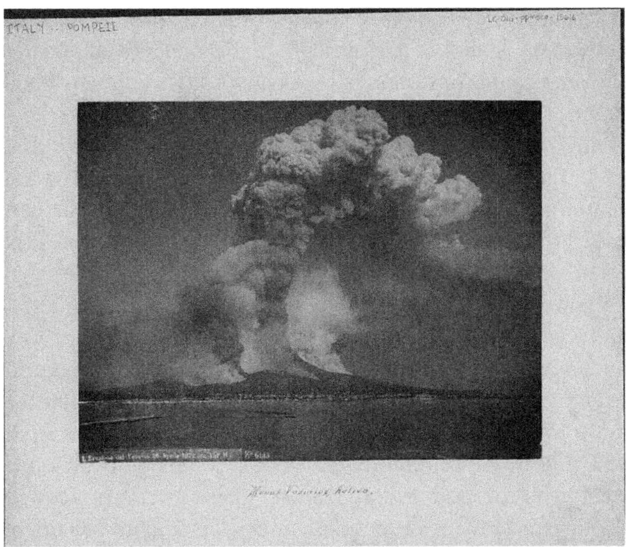

FIGURE 15.4 Mount Vesuvius. (Photo courtesy of Library of Congress. https://www.loc.gov/pictures/item/2008676737/.)

Because Pliny the Younger, encouraged by Roman historian Publius Cornelius Tacitus (56–120), wrote a detailed account of the eruption, Herculaneum and Pompeii were not forgotten.[47] Medieval Italians retained folk memories of both but could not pinpoint locations. These recollections' role in archaeology is unclear; the 1709 discovery of Herculaneum was the fortuitous outcome of an attempt to dig a well rather than the fruits of systematic excavation. Although Pompeii's excavation attracted greater attention, Herculaneum's unearthing permitted scientists and scholars to reconstruct inhabitants' diets with unusual precision.

15.6.2 Sources of Evidence

In this context, the grand discovery was the apartment complex *Insula Occidentalis II*, built during the reign of Emperor Augustus (63 BCE–14 CE) or Claudius (10 BCE–54 CE). Its two stories accommodated living quarters on the second floor and a bakery, a room that might have been a hotel or store, and a dye shop on the first. Both floors had several latrines whose shafts descended to a sewer roughly 80 meters (87.5 yards or 262.5 feet) below ground.[48] Absent running water, the sewer aggregated rather than removed wastes, preserving excrement and, to a lesser extent, urine. Because latrines were in or near a kitchen, they also accumulated debris from food preparation, including butchered bones. The uncertain date of construction leaves unknown how many years' deposits were in the sewer. British archaeologist Mark Robinson and Oxford University graduate student Erica Rowan supposed that workers emptied the sewer roughly every 20 years, but this too is unknown.[49] The important point is that the sewer had wastes when Vesuvius erupted, preserving them for identification and quantification. Chapter 1 described middens and coprolites' value in understanding and evaluating diets, nutrition, and health. As noted, this sewer was valuable because it had both trash and human wastes, an archaeological rarity.

Chapter 1 also cautioned that garbage and coprolites do not always accurately illuminate diets because bones are more durable than plants, exaggerating meat, poultry, and fish consumption. Persistence of shellfish's hard parts creates the same illusion. Bones and shells turned up not only in middens because some small fish bones and shell fragments were swallowed inadvertently during a meal. Passing through the digestive tract, they were defecated.

The foregoing does not exclude plants from the archeological record. Several factors affect persistence. First, by desiccating plants, aridity increases chances of preservation. Southwestern Asia,

Egypt, and North Africa supply such an environment, which may explain the antiquity of evidence for the regions' early invention or adoption of agriculture. Second, not all plant parts are equally susceptible to decay. For example, microbes cannot break down silica (silicon dioxide or SiO_2), which is common in plants wherever soils contain it. Plant structures with silica—like grain kernels' tough outer coat (the husk, hull, or chaff)—are known as phytoliths and may constitute the sole evidence for plant consumption in remote times. Third, cooking without enough oxygen prevents complete combustion. The remaining carbon persists through a process known as carbonization. Fourth, freezing temperatures retard decomposition. Fifth, waterlogging prevents aerobic but not anaerobic degradation. Sixth, where present, calcium (Ca^{2+}) cations and phosphate (PO_4^{3-}) anions may replace plant cells, a process known as mineralization. Calcium phosphate compounds endure longer than plants' organic molecules.

Covering Herculaneum with rock and ash, Vesuvius' eruption sealed the town. Ash even penetrated the sewer, preventing oxygen from entering and thereby arresting aerobic decomposition. As noted, lava ignited fires throughout the town, but the sewer's position underground protected it from heat. The latrines that led to the sewer and the sewer itself contained calcium and phosphate ions, which preserved the contents through mineralization. These circumstances permitted archaeologists, scientists, and historians to reconstruct first-century CE Roman diets in unusual detail.

Besides the sewer, some 350 skeletons examined by 2015 further illuminated diets. Teeth and bones revealed nutritional stresses defined in Chapter 1. In addition, bones' strontium, calcium, and zinc indicated the source of dietary protein. All three elements are metals on the Periodic Table, illustrated in Figure 2.9. In soils, they may be inorganic components of rocks. As rocks weather, these elements may ionize, in which state roots may absorb them. In this context, strontium deserves attention because it tends to exist in roughly equal proportions in plants and in soils in which they grow. That is, plants mirror soils in strontium content. Herbivores and omnivores acquire the element from plants, depositing it in bones but not muscles. Because muscles lack strontium, omnivores have less of the element than herbivores, and carnivores—eating no plants—have least. In bones, strontium replaces calcium such that strontium to calcium ratios correlate directly with plant, and inversely with meat, consumption. The third element, zinc, is in meat such that zinc amounts in bones correlate with meat intake. Herculaneum skeletons' excellent preservation, discussed below, permitted quantification of strontium, calcium, and zinc.

Like the sewer, Vesuvius' rock and ash preserved skeletons unexposed to the eruption's greatest heat with a fidelity rare in archeology. Entombed beneath 20 meters (21.9 yards or 65.6 feet) of debris, skeletons experienced constant temperature, humidity, and pH (a measure of acidity or alkalinity).[50] Together, sewer and skeletons formed a microcosm of Roman antiquity. Such circumstances lead this chapter to scrutinize first-century CE Herculaneum as among the best evidence of premodern diets, nutrition, and health.

The town, named after Greek god Heracles (Roman name Hercles or Hercules), indicates its origin as a Greek settlement. From its base in southeastern Europe, Greece began colonizing the Mediterranean in the eighth-century BCE.[51] Southern Italy was an early destination, with Greeks inhabiting what was a village of Oscan-speaking Italians around then.[52] Naming it Herculaneum, Greeks favored the area because its harbor in the Bay of Naples facilitated maritime trade. Likewise promoting commerce, Rome conquered the town about 310 BCE.[53] As elsewhere, Rome sought to maintain the stability conducive to trade rather than micromanage Herculaneum. Because Rome admired and copied Greek architecture, urban planning, and culture, it reinforced rather than remade the town's economy, appearance, and customs. As a relic, Herculaneum thus opens a window into the Greek, Roman, and Mediterranean worlds. Its lifeways and foodways reveal much about Mediterranean antiquity.

The foregoing does not pretend that Herculaneum can answer every question about its milieu. The spectacle of its destruction, a source of fascination, enhances and circumscribes the town's archaeological, anthropological, historical, demographic, and medical value. Vesuvius' engulfment turned the town into a kind of time capsule for which the moment of preservation can be pinpointed

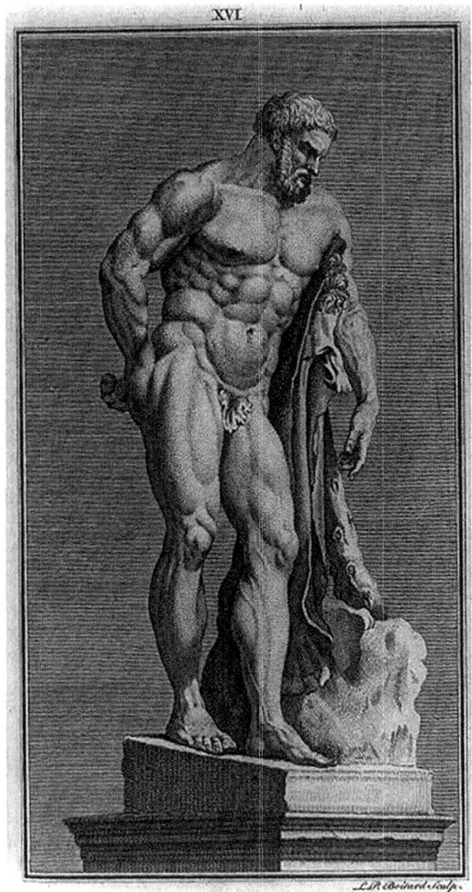

FIGURE 15.5 Hercules. (Photo courtesy of Library of Congress. https://www.loc.gov/pictures/item/89711289/.)

with unprecedented precision. On the other hand, demographers cannot hope to quantify life expectancy at birth (e^0) or at any age because everyone died prematurely. Absent this information, crucial evidence about residents' health cannot be retrieved.

15.6.3 Diets

Appreciation of Herculaneum's utility and limitations permits dispassionate investigation of diets, nutrition, and health to the extent that humans are capable of impartiality. In this inquiry, the sewer supplies more details about Herculaneum's diets than the skeletons and is our launchpad. As noted, the sewer best preserved foods' durable parts: bones, shells, and seed coats. Among the last are polyliths of vegetables and of fruits colloquially termed vegetables but which this book denies as such because these categories, as mentioned, do not overlap. Instructive is the fact that preservation is good enough to allow polyliths' tabulation. To be sure, this section supposes neither that the sewer preserved every seed, or even a sizable fraction, that entered nor that everything preserved has been identified. Nonetheless, no reason exists to suppose, for example, that lettuce seeds preserved better or worse than seeds from celery, from another vegetable, or from any other plant; counts might therefore indicate the place of each vegetable in diets relative to other foods even if the magnitude is unknown. This section acknowledges, however, that large seeds are easier to identify than small ones, introducing unintentional error into attempts to quantify Herculaneum diets.

A glance at the numbers downplays vegetables' dietary role. Researchers identified under eleven polyliths of seeds each from celery, colewort, and mustard.[54] Ambiguity shrouds the last two because of difficulty differentiating them. Additionally, seeds cannot pinpoint mustard's use because they are a spice, whereas leaves are a vegetable. Because only seeds were recovered, Herculaneum inhabitants may have used mustard as only a spice.

Expensiveness reserved spices for elites, making seeds' interpretation as vegetable or spice an economic and class issue. A picturesque location, beachfront Herculaneum was a resort where the rich went to socialize and frolic. Emperor Gaius Julius Caesar Germanicus (12–41 CE), known as Caligula, was among the fabulously wealthy who owned a villa there.[55] Even the merchants owned "luxuriously appointed" homes.[56]

Of the 139 skeletons they examined, American anthropologist and archaeologist Sara Louise Clark Bisel (1932–1996) and American editor Jane F. Bisel described four as "privileged."[57] At death, one woman wore "a lot of gold jewelry"—two rings, two bracelets, and earrings—and had coins in a bag.[58] Any laborer whose ring has caused blisters or callouses knows that it is more than jewelry when it advertises the wearer's ability to delegate work to inferiors rather than endure drudgery. A second woman had teeth with little wear, suggesting consumption of only refined foods.[59] Two of three adults scrutinized by the Bisels had robust bones, implying excellent nutrition throughout life.[60] They could afford food even when shortages increased prices. An 8-year-old girl wore a gold ring and a necklace of glass beads.[61]

The authors omitted whether these four were the only elites among the 139 or brevity limited coverage. These fortunate few had servants, slaves, and spacious quarters. One apartment, as large as some Herculaneum houses, had bronze—an alloy of copper and tin—and silver decorations.[62] Such elites afforded the spice pepper (*Piper nigrum*), represented by two peppercorns from the sewer.[63] Pepper was precious, arriving from southwestern India, a voyage that winds permitted once annually during the age of sail. Also imported were dates, represented by under eleven pits in the sewer.[64] Although Italy had date palms, they did not flower, necessitating importation from Syria, Palestine—now Israel and Palestine—and Egypt.[65] Besides pepper and dates, the wealthy bought pickles from Spain, ham from Gaul—now France and parts of Belgium, Germany, and Italy—pomegranates (*Punica granatum*) from Libya, and oysters (*Crassostrea* species) from Britain.[66]

The Bisels acknowledged "that the rich were few and that poor people and slaves vastly outnumbered them."[67] Chapter 4 furnished corroborating evidence for Egypt, which was part of the empire from 30 BCE to around 600 CE, and noted the chasm between haves and have nots, a recurrent theme in this book. As the wealthy's playground, Herculaneum had numerous commoners as servants and slaves. The town's furniture, also preserved by Vesuvius, evinced stratification. Of fifty wood samples examined in 1991, forty-six were silver fir (*Abies alba*) or maple (*Acer* species, likely *Acer pseudoplatanus*).[68] Noted for affordability, maple was attractive enough for those who wanted to appear stylish. The thirty-nine silver fir samples confirm the plebian origins of most residents. Roman authors omitted the wood as suitable for furniture, instead emphasizing its mundane uses in shipbuilding.[69] Grown throughout Italy, the tree was plentiful and may be thought the Model T rather than Rolls Royce of woods. By contrast, expensive woods—notably ebony (*Diospyros* species) and the coniferous *Callitris quadrivalvis*—were absent from the samples.[70] Both symbolized luxury, and ebony was popular in Egypt, a selling point given Roman reverence for Egyptian civilization and its trappings.

Herculaneum therefore had a nucleus of elites surrounded by many servants and slaves. The masses could not have afforded spices, leading this chapter to designate mustard, celery, and colewort seeds as evidence that most residents ate their vegetable equivalents: mustard, celery, and colewort leaves, which would have been less likely than seeds to persist as biofacts. Moreover, that leafy vegetables like colewort and lettuce were "common" in Roman diets suggests mustard greens' consumption.[71] That Romans ate colewort, earlier noted as most like collard greens or kale, strengthens the inference that they also consumed mustard greens. A worse showing comes from the sewer's carbonized plants, which have yet to yield identification of a single vegetable seed.[72]

Other foods appear to have been more prevalent than vegetables. For example, researchers counted at least 1,000 polyliths of fig (*Ficus carica*) seeds and eleven to 999 of seeds from apples (*Malus domestica*) or pears (*Pyrus* species), olives, broomcorn millet (*Panicum miliaceum*), foxtail millet (*Setaria italica*), grapes (*Vitis vinifera*), and opium poppy (*Papaver somniferum*).[73] The sewer yielded at least 1,000 carbonized olives and eleven to 999 carbonized grapes.[74] Bones from numerous fish species, chickens (*Gallus gallus domesticus*), pigs (*Sus scrofa domesticus*), and sheep (*Ovis aries*) and shells from mollusks (species in the phylum Mollusca), crabs (species in the infraorder Brachyura), and sea urchins (species in the class Echinoidea) have been identified. The apparent disparity between vegetables and other foods squares with belief that vegetables were minor in Roman diets.[75]

This opinion has four weaknesses. First, the attempt to quantify plant intake by tabulating seeds underreported vegetables because, as emphasized, they are not seeds. Seeds' exclusion leaves structures less likely to preserve. To put this reality another way, consumption of these plant parts leaves no seeds for possible preservation. For example, identification of under eleven celery seeds reveals little about the vegetable's place in Herculaneum diets because consumers ate the leaves and petiole not the seeds. Someone who consumed only celery ingested no seeds to defecate. In this light, identification of under eleven celery seeds must represent the proverbial tip of an iceberg, suggesting that celery intake—though hidden from view—was sizable.

This logic applies to seeds that people wanted to eat. For example, the sewer yielded under eleven polyliths of lentil (*Lens culinaris*) seeds, the same as for celery, colewort, or mustard. Whereas consumers did not want to ingest celery, colewort, or mustard seeds—unless mustard was a spice for the few wealthy—lentils were nothing but seeds where the consumer was concerned. Under such circumstances, lentils' consumption ensured that some seed coats—in this instance not above ten—preserved. If lentils were as plentiful in the sewer as accidental celery, colewort, and possibly mustard seeds, then celery, colewort, and mustard greens must have been larger parts of Herculaneum diets than lentils. That is, celery, colewort, and perhaps mustard greens must have been crucial to Roman diets given scholars' judgment that legumes were basic to ancient Mediterranean foodways.[76]

Second, seeds' use to gauge plants' dietary importance is most apt when species yield roughly the same number of seeds per edible. Such uniformity anticipates equal ratios of seeds preserved whenever two species constitute equal parts of diets. But this assumption is false. For example, readers should be unsurprised that fig seeds were numerous in the sewer because a single fig may have up to 1,600 seeds.[77] Preservation of even small proportions of the total defecated must have aggregated countless thousands over time. By contrast, a mustard plant has not over twenty seeds per pod.[78] This disparity may explain why fig seeds were more numerous in the sewer than mustard seeds. Alternatively, Herculaneum residents may have eaten more figs than mustard greens or seeds. A third possibility is that both factors combined to widen the divide between numbers of fig and mustard seeds retrieved.

Third, as noted, seeds are easier to identify when large than small. Size may explain identification of at least 1,000 carbonized olive pits.[79] Other medium to large seeds included lentils—both mineralized and carbonized—broad beans (*Vicia faba*), cherry or plum stones (both *Prunus* species), hazelnuts (*Corylus* species), walnuts (*Juglans regia*), cucumber or melon (both *Cucumis* species), foxtail and broomcorn millet, barley (*Hordeum vulgare*), einkorn (*Triticum monococcum*), emmer (*Triticum dicoccon*), and bread (*Triticum aestivum*) or durum (*Triticum durum*) wheat.[80] Numerous fig seeds, mentioned earlier, demonstrated that small seeds were retrievable. Researchers' use of 0.5-millimeter (0.02-inch) mesh aided their recovery.[81]

Fourth, attention on seeds omitted edibles that did not leave them. The sewer had no evidence of onion (*Allium cepa*) or garlic (*Allium sativum*)—which have long been propagated from bulbs more than from seeds—even though scholars agree that Romans ate both.[82] Farmers who wanted food harvested onions the first year, preventing flowering in these biennials. Garlic has been grown from cloves so long that it seldom flowers or produces viable seeds. Roman soldiers consumed garlic in the belief that it enhanced courage.[83] Greek and Roman physicians championed it as food and medicine.[84] Greek anatomist and author Galen (130–210 CE), physician to Roman emperor Marcus

Aurelius (121–180), counseled corpulent patients to lose weight by eating garlic and onion.[85] Of course, overweight and obesity concerned only the few whose wealth protected them from hunger and privation.

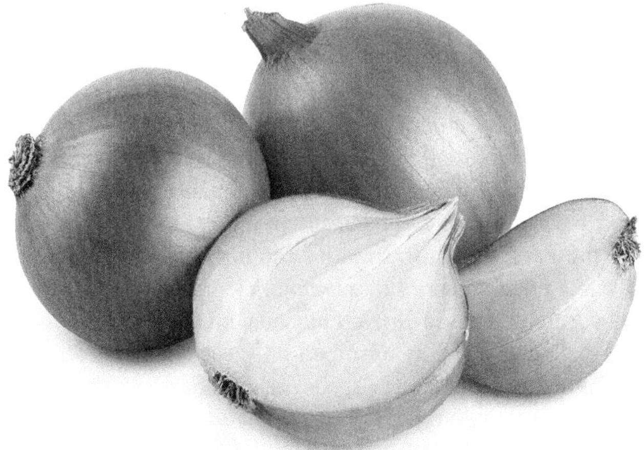

FIGURE 15.6 Onion. (Photo from Shutterstock.)

Reliance on seeds yielded a surprise for grains: carbonized foxtail millet, barley, einkorn, emmer, and bread or durum wheat numbered under eleven each.[86] Carbonized broomcorn millet was not found. Mineralized emmer kernels numbered under eleven.[87] Between eleven and 999 mineralized foxtail and broomcorn millet grains were counted. No other mineralized cereals were identified. Judging these numbers too small, Robinson and Rowan asserted that Herculaneum's inhabitants must have eaten bread made from flour absent chaff, just as would be expected of winnowed cereals.[88] Such flour would have left nothing to preserve in the sewer. They explained the greater number of millet kernels relative to other grains as the result of millets' consumption as porridge or gruel. Such fare fed the poor, who could not have afforded refined foods.

This explanation aside for a moment, the sewer yielded no more barley and wheat than vegetable seeds. This result, if not an artifact of cereals' preparation, challenges the orthodoxy that Romans ate primarily grains. For example, the Bisels pinpointed wheat as the "staple," with barley and millets as substitutes.[89] British classicist Peter David Arthur Garnsey (b. 1938) identified cereals as the ancient Mediterranean's only "truly ubiquitous" food.[90] American classicist John F. Donahue estimated that they gave Romans up to three quarters of calories.[91]

Against these judgments, the sewer's contents imply that Romans did not eat mostly grains, which bulked no larger in diets than vegetables. If cereals were central to ancient Rome, then so were vegetables. This view is adopted here because the poor, who were far more numerous than the wealthy, ate porridge or gruel as Robinson and Rowans stated and bread that kept the chaff because of coarse grinding.[92] The sewer must have preserved some of it, making seeds' tabulation an accurate gauge of grains' place in diets.

These considerations recommend Herculaneum as a test of vegetables' health effects. The skeletons, to which this chapter turns, best answer questions about vitality. Their strontium to calcium ratio is greater, but zinc content is less, than for modern Americans.[93] This result may appear puzzling because high strontium implies, but low zinc refutes, meat consumption. The sewer's numerous fish bones and aquatic shells resolve the quandary because seafood is rich in strontium but has less zinc than meat.[94] From these data, Sara and Jane Bisel concluded that the town's occupants derived much more protein from seafood than from meat or plants.[95] This insight appears to diminish legumes' place in the diet. Their dearth in the sewer confirms this likelihood. If Herculaneum's residents ate less bread and fewer legumes than has been supposed, and if most could not afford meat, then vegetables and fruits must have filled their bowls. Numerous fig seeds, already mentioned, support this view if their abundance accurately gauged figs' dietary prominence.

15.6.4 Health

In 79, Herculaneum had perhaps 4,000 denizens.[96] As noted, by 2015, researchers had studied 350 skeletons, though the most thorough treatment included only 139, about 3.5 percent of the population. Heterogeneous, these 139 complicate attempts to generalize about health. Heterogeneity is hardly unusual given that humans tend to exhibit diverse phenotypes, as is evident to anyone who has surveyed a street corner gathering. The Bisels ventured beyond phenotype to describe the town's "widely diverse genetic heritage."[97] "A great melting pot of peoples," Herculaneum displayed greater diversity than twenty-five Irish settlements separated in time and place.[98] On this foundation of biological variability, antiquity erected the stark economic and social stratification mentioned throughout this book.

This situation produced multiple outcomes. Atop the heap were four elites. A man and woman, both mentioned earlier and estimated to have been forty-six years old when Vesuvius truncated their lives, had thick bones from excellent nutrition throughout life. They apparently never missed a meal. Large muscles moved the man, whom Sara and Jane Bisel characterized as an athlete by avocation.[99] All muscles were big in contrast to laborers, whose exertions stressed only those necessary for work. He must have exercised, but not to exhaustion because his bones revealed no scars where tendons attached. Such signs of excessive wear identified laborers, servants, and slaves. In contrast, the man's hands were less developed. The Bisels suspected that he seldom wrote but rather dictated letters to servants. He must have delegated tasks because "Upper-class Romans took pride in doing no labor."[100] Additional evidence of nutrition came from his 172.4-centimeter (67.9-inch) frame, putting him over 3 centimeters (1.2 inches) above the average man in Herculaneum and in Hellenistic Greece (323–31 BCE).[101] At 157.2 centimeters (61.9 inches), the woman was 2.2 centimeters (0.9 inches) taller than her countrywomen and Greek women.[102]

The second privileged woman, estimated to have died at age 36, had "virtually perfect" teeth, with just the inception of a cavity in one molar.[103] The authors attributed this outcome to the absence of sucrose, discussed in Chapters 2 and 11, in Roman antiquity and to the likelihood that she ate only refined foods such as bakery breads rather than the poor's coarse fare. She too had large muscles from excellent nutrition and exercise or household tasks. Yet she had suffered anemia, probably during childhood, from dietary deficiency, parasites, or heredity. Chapter 1 characterized anemia as an adaptation to pathogens, parasites, or both because insufficient iron starved invaders. This woman might have had thalassemia as defense against malaria parasites in the genus *Plasmodium*.

The fourth elite was about eight at death.[104] Sex may be difficult to determine in children because bones—especially the pelvis—are immature, though the Bisels suspected that the youth was a girl. Her gold ring and necklace, mentioned earlier, identified her status. Unusual among the 139 skeletons, she had five cavities. Without sucrose, honey—which Chapters 2 and 11 also discussed and which the wealthy rather than the poor afforded—might have been the culprit. Although about the size of other Herculaneum children, she was 11 percent smaller than a modern sample her age from Denver, Colorado, implying that her nutrition trailed today's standards.[105]

Far below these few were antiquity's countless poor and infirm. One skeleton, likely of a slave girl around age 7 at death, exhibited an enlarged humerus where the deltoid (shoulder muscle) attached.[106] This hypertrophy betrayed strenuous exertions while so young, toil that must have been involuntary. Enamel hypoplasia, described in Chapter 1, indicated undernutrition, illness, or both between ages 4 and 6. Undernutrition is also evident in her having been smaller than three quarters of the above modern sample her age from Denver, Colorado.[107]

Another probable slave girl perished around age 14.[108] Her femur had flattened rather than rounded into a normal shape to provide width for enlarged quadriceps. The authors surmised that she had developed them from repeatedly climbing and descending steps in her masters' house to do chores or fetch items. Hypoplasias, especially on incisors and first molars, were sufficiently deep that the girl must have been so underfed that she lacked, or so ill that she could not absorb, calcium for about one month during childhood. The damage had necessitated two teeth's extraction only weeks before the eruption.

Examples need not be multiplied to convey the emotions these skeletons evoke. Rather than pathos, this section seeks patterns in the welter of details. But, as the particulars suggest, evidence does not point in one direction. An onlooker may infer health from femurs that were more robust among Herculaneum women than today's U.S. women and roughly equal among Herculaneum and American men.[109] Against these data, Herculaneum leg bones and pelvises were flatter—a phenomenon already mentioned as a response to exertions—than those of modern Americans. Flattening indicates that these ancients were more active than moderns, a fact emphasized throughout this book. Moreover, flattening is often an adaptation to undernutrition, which thins bones. Unable to bear weight in their normal shape—akin to a cylinder in long bones—they flatten to accommodate muscles. Herculaneum's thick femurs, however, demonstrated that undernutrition was not universal even though previous paragraphs referenced instances of it.

Beyond these considerations, the town's residents had better dental health than modern Americans. Whereas the typical American loses or suffers disease in 15.7 teeth during a lifetime, the Herculaneum mean was 3.4.[110] Some of the disparity may stem from Americans' longer lives, but, as noted, sucrose was unavailable to ancient Romans. Honey was mentioned as too expensive for the masses, though a previous example raised the possibility that the wealthy corrupted their teeth with it.

Vegetables may have reinforced the difference between antiquity and modernity. Low in sugars and fibrous, they required vigorous chewing when raw and bulky. The Bisels remarked that mastication strengthened jaws, aiding their development such that they were usually large enough for all teeth.[111] Absent this advantage, the modern mouth does not always have space for wisdom teeth. Moreover, abrasive foods like grains with chaff eroded enamel enough to scour away incipient caries. Finally, seafood, whose consumption was mentioned, supplied fluorine (F). As fluoride (F^-), the anion enhanced teeth's resistance to acids that otherwise penetrated enamel.

Returning to stature, Peter Garnsey assembled data from Herculaneum, Pompeii, and Poundbury, England. Overall, most men stood 162–170 centimeters (63.8–66.9 inches), whereas women were 152–157 centimeters (59.8–61.8 inches).[112] Near the top, Herculaneum men averaged 169.1 centimeters (66.6 inches). Women ranked slightly above the middle at 155.2 centimeters (61.1 inches). Both figures surpassed heights published in 1964 for Naples, Italy, where men averaged 164 centimeters (64.6 inches) and women 152.6 centimeters (60.1 inches).[113] Reluctant to credit nutrition, Garnsey supposed that the Bay of Naples was a healthier locale in antiquity than in the mid-twentieth century.[114]

Coming from an authority on Greek and Roman antiquity, this explanation deserves deference. It accords with British archeologist Andrew Frederic Wallace-Hadrill's (b. 1951) belief that Herculaneum's inhabitants were "notably healthy."[115] Greek geographer and historian Strabo (c. 64 BCE–c. 23 CE) wrote that Herculaneum benefited from winds that crossed the Mediterranean Sea from Libya in the south, making the town "a healthy place to stay."[116] This opinion encouraged the wealthy, as noted, to vacation at the seaside retreat.

Strabo's judgment appears to ignore premodernity's high mortality, a reality this book has repeatedly emphasized as a key health indictor. Aware of this problem, adults have many children in hopes that one or two survive to care for them in senescence. That is, ghastly mortality compels corresponding fecundity, without which populations cannot endure. Recalling American ecologist and limnologist Edward Smith Deevey Jr.'s (1914–1988) remark in earlier chapters that half of all children died before puberty, the combination of high fertility and mortality left many youths to bury upon death.[117]

But Herculaneum appears to have deviated from the norm because excavators found few juvenile skeletons.[118] This result may reflect the investigation's incompleteness given that the Bisels had just

139 skeletons to study, as noted, and Robinson and Rowan mentioned only 350 from a population of about 4,000. Perhaps the town's unexplored parts entomb most youths. Such an explanation, however, requires the unlikelihood that Herculaneum's residents segregated themselves by age before death and that researchers have yet to find the children. Paucity of juvenile remains must therefore indicate low birthrate. Examination of the pelvis in thirty-seven skeletons judged to have been women over age 15 yielded a mean 1.69 births per woman. The number is too small to sustain even populations without infant mortality. The eighteen skeletons identified as women over age 40 and so at or near menopause produced 1.81 births per woman on average, still too meager to perpetuate a population not beset by high mortality. Against these figures, the average woman who reached menopause had to birth between 4.5 and 6.5 children just to replace the losses from antiquity's mortality.[119] Population growth required still greater fertility.

Earlier chapters stated that nutrition affects fertility, though Chapter 1 articulated British demographers Edward Anthony Wrigley (b. 1931) and Roger Snowden Schofield's (1937–2019) opinion that the effects are small or nil at or above subsistence.[120] This perspective aside, adequate nutrients and calories appear to lower age of menarche. On the other hand, excessive leanness may impair ovulation, as discussed in Chapters 3 and 5, suggesting that some underfed Herculaneum women might have been unable to conceive. But this circumstance would not have characterized all women. Referencing the Pacific Northwest's Chinook, Chapter 1 noted that shortages prompted elites to take the poor's sustenance. This mechanism ensured ample food and fertility among Herculaneum's wealthy women even if it depressed pauper reproduction. Rather than undernutrition, Sara and Jane Bisel suggested that contraception, abortion, abstinence, and homosexuality reduced birthrates.[121]

Dearth of youth skeletons may also have stemmed from social and economic considerations if Herculaneum had numerous slaves. The estimate that around one-third of ancient Italians were slaves implies that Herculaneum had many unfree.[122] In such a society, buyers likely purchased slaves in their 20s, when labor output was greatest.[123] The few young slaves would have constituted a small population for Vesuvius to entomb.

These issues do not minimize diet and nutrition's health effects. For example, the Bisels proposed fish and vegetables as possible contributors to anemia, already noted in an elite woman.[124] Wallace-Hadrill blamed inadequate meat intake for the condition, which was severe enough to cause porotic hyperostosis, defined in Chapter 1.[125] Additionally, parasites and pathogens were factors because the Mediterranean climate supported organisms, now uncommon in the area, which had spread north from tropical Africa.[126] Anemia increased susceptibility to infections, which in turn may have caused or exacerbated hypoplasia.[127]

A previous paragraph introduced anemia in the form of thalassemia as defense against malaria. About forty species of *Anopheles* mosquitoes transmit *Plasmodium* parasites, with *Plasmodium falciparum* afflicting southern Italy.[128] Warm temperatures aid mosquitoes' development. Females lay eggs in water, preferring clean, still, small pools. Temporary bodies of water are best because they do not accumulate fish that eat eggs and larvae. These requirements favored mosquitoes and malaria from Rome south through the peninsula, especially as the region became marshier over time. Mosquitoes' proliferation during summers and autumns weakened laborers for the harvest, retarding southern Italy's economy and worsening food scarcity.[129] The resulting undernutrition diminished vitality.

The foregoing amplifies the fact that insects, parasites, rodents, and pathogens marred health. As another example, almost one-fifth of Herculaneum skeletons exhibited bone loss consistent with brucellosis.[130] Impure goat's milk likely transmitted the cause, *Brucella* bacteria. Roman author Aulus Cornelius Celsus (c. 25 BCE–c. 50 CE) wrote that dysentery—caused by *Shigella* bacteria or the parasite *Entamoeba histolytica*—killed children under age 10.[131] Skeletons revealed a form of treponematosis related to syphilis in Metapontum, a Greek settlement in southern Italy. The Mediterranean climate supported *Treponema* bacteria that caused the infections. Italy and other Mediterranean lands hosted sandflies (*Phlebotomus* species) that spread *Leishmania* parasites, the cause of leishmaniasis.[132] These scourges, especially malaria, reduced e^0 throughout the ancient

Mediterranean. Such misery implies that Herculaneum—and the Mediterranean in general—was less benign than Strabo, Garnsey, and Wallace-Hadrill suggested.

By contrast, mid-twentieth century Bay of Naples had a reputation for vigor. Enthusiastic reports led American physiologist Ancel Benjamin Keys (1904–2004), mentioned in Chapter 10, to visit Naples in 1954.[133] Touring hospitals, he found no admittances for heart disease and no history of it in the medical charts. Three years' research convinced him of Neapolitans' low cholesterol, normal blood pressure, and "nonexistent" heart disease.[134] Keys attributed these outcomes to vegetables, fruits, whole grains, and olive oil, the last discussed in Chapter 10. Fish, meat, and dairy were merely side dishes.

This regimen resembled Herculaneum diets, though seafood probably surpassed current intake given the sewer's numerous fish bones and shell fragments, noted earlier. Readers may recall that the Bisels posited seafood and vegetables as possible contributors to anemia, reinforcing the notion that the townspeople must have eaten much fish and shellfish. This difference aside, vegetables, fruits, whole grains, and olive oil united the Bay of Naples in antiquity and the mid-twentieth century.

Another health gauge was malaria's retreat. Officials reported over 15,000 Italian deaths from the malady annually through the nineteenth century.[135] Thereafter, symptoms and mortality diminished as antimalarial drug quinine ($C_{20}H_{24}N_2O_2$) became inexpensive.[136] Construction of well-insulated houses impeded *Anopheles* mosquitoes' entry. Swamp and marsh drainage, ongoing for centuries, reduced mosquito populations. Discovery of dichlorodiphenyltrichloroethane's (DDT) insecticidal properties in 1939 prompted its 1944 use against lice (*Pediculus humanus corporis, Pediculus humanus capitis,* and *Pthirus pubis*) in Naples and against mosquitoes throughout Italy and its islands.[137]

These considerations suggest, contrary to Garnsey's opinion, that the Bay of Naples was healthier in the mid-twentieth century than in antiquity. Yet Herculaneum's ancients were taller and so likely better nourished than 1960s' Neapolitans. As noted, diets were similar except for the likelihood of greater seafood intake in antiquity. If fish and shellfish were decisive, Herculaneum supplies evidence to augment Chapter 5's treatment of them. Data from Herculaneum and modern Naples imply that vegetables benefited health, though this chapter is unable to pinpoint their advantages.

NOTES

1 Jane M. Renfrew and Helen Sanderson, "Herbs and Vegetables," in *The Cultural History of Plants*, ed. Ghillean Prance and Mark Nesbitt (New York and London: Routledge, 2005), 112.

2 Dixie Dean Trainer, *Vegetable Gardening* (New York: Playmore, 1978); Suzanne Frutig Bales, *Vegetables* (New York: Prentice Hall Gardening, 1991); Peter McHoy, *Practical Gardening* (New York: Smithmark Publishers, 1994); Robert J. Dolezal, *Vegetable Gardening: Your Ultimate Guide* (Minnetonka, MN: Creative Publishing International, 2000); Charlie Nardozzi, *Vegetable Gardening for Dummies*, 2nd ed. (Hoboken, NJ: Wiley, 2009); Carol Klein, *Vegetable Gardening: The Complete Guide to Growing More Than 40 Popular Vegetables in Any Space* (London: i-5 Press, 2016); Clare Matthews, *Low-Maintenance Vegetable Gardening: Bumper Crops in Minutes a Day Using Raised Beds, Planning, and Plant Selection* (Mount Joy, PA: Companion House Books, 2018).

3 Matthews, 218–219; Klein, 218.

4 Nardozzi, 41.

5 Homer C. Thompson, *Vegetable Crops*, 3rd ed. (New York and London: McGraw-Hill, 1939), 2.

6 Ibid., 15–16.

7 Ibid., 18.

8 Ibid., 23.

9 Beryl Brintnall Simpson and Molly Conner Ogorzaly, *Economic Botany: Plants in Our World*, 3rd ed. (Boston: Houghton Mifflin, 2001), 155–191.

10 Ibid., 187–191.

11 Ibid., 355.

12 Vincent E. Rubatzky and Mas Yamaguchi, *World Vegetables: Principles, Production, and Nutritive Values*, 2nd ed. (New York: Chapman and Hall, 1997), 8, 829.

13 Renfrew and Sanderson, 112.
14 *Nix v. Hedden*, 149 U.S. 304 (1893).
15 Caitlin Dewey, "The Obscure Supreme Court Case That Decided Tomatoes Are Vegetables," *The Washington Post*, October 18, 2017, accessed June 17, 2019, https://www.washingtonpost.com/news/wonk/wp/2017/10/18/the-obscure-supreme-court-case-that-decided-tomatoes-are-vegetables/?utm_term=.bf9a37460dee.
16 Plato, *Republic*, in *Great Dialogues of Plato*, trans. W. H. D. Rouse (New York: New American Library, 1956), 128–165.
17 Meika Foster, "Vegetables," in *Essentials of Human Nutrition*, ed. Jim Mann and A. Stewart Truswell, 5th ed. (Oxford: Oxford University Press, 2017), 282.
18 Shaney Emerson and Michelle Risso, ed., "Edible Plant Parts," California Foundation for Agriculture in the Classroom, September 2013, accessed July 24, 2019, http://agritech.tnau.ac.in/horticulture/Ediple%20Plant%20Parts.pdf, 17; "Plant Parts," Missouri Botanical Garden, 2009, accessed July 24, 2019, http://www.mbgnet.net/bioplants/parts.html.
19 Rubatzky and Yamaguchi, 6.
20 Ibid., 806.
21 Ibid., 812.
22 Ibid., 813.
23 Renfrew and Sanderson, 113.
24 Rubatzky and Yamaguchi, 808; "Turnip Greens, Raw," *USDA FoodData Central*, April 1, 2019, accessed January 26, 2020, https://fdc.nal.usda.gov/fdc-app.html#/food-details/170061/nutrients; "Turnips, Raw," *USDA FoodData Central*, April 1, 2019, accessed January 26, 2020, https://fdc.nal.usda.gov/fdc-app.html#/food-details/170465/nutrients; "FDA Vitamins and Minerals Chart," *FDA*, accessed April 24, 2019, https://www.accessdata.fda.gov/scripts/interactivenutritionfactslabel/factsheets/vitamin_and_mineral_chart.pdf.
25 Rubatzky and Yamaguchi, 808; "Turnips, Raw;" "FDA Vitamins and Minerals Chart."
26 "What Foods Are in the Vegetable Group?" *USDA*, last modified January 3, 2018, accessed June 30, 2019, https://www.choosemyplate.gov/vegetables.
27 Ibid.; Alina Petre, "How Many Servings of Vegetables Should You Eat Per Day?" *Healthline*, November 26, 2017, accessed June 30, 2019, https://www.healthline.com/nutrition/servings-of-vegetables-per-day.
28 Rubatzky and Yamaguchi, 803; "FDA Vitamins and Minerals Chart;" "Celery, Raw," *USDA FoodData Central*, April 1, 2019, accessed January 26, 2020, https://fdc.nal.usda.gov/fdc-app.html#/food-details/169988/nutrients; "Collards, Raw," *USDA FoodData Central*, April 1, 2019, accessed January 26, 2020, https://fdc.nal.usda.gov/fdc-app.html#/food-details/342053/nutrients; "Collards, Raw," *USDA FoodData Central*, April 1, 2019, accessed January 26, 2020, https://fdc.nal.usda.gov/fdc-app.html#/food-details/170406/nutrients; "Mustard Greens, Raw," *USDA FoodData Central*, April 1, 2019, accessed January 26, 2020, https://fdc.nal.usda.gov/fdc-app.html#/food-details/169256/nutrients; "Mustard Greens, Frozen, Unprepared," *USDA FoodData Central*, April 1, 2019, accessed January 26, 2020, https://fdc.nal.usda.gov/fdc-app.html#/food-details/169258/nutrients; "Kale, Raw," *USDA FoodData Central*, April 1, 2019, accessed January 26, 2020, https://fdc.nal.usda.gov/fdc-app.html#/food-details/168421/nutrients.
29 Rubatzky and Yamaguchi, 803; "Celery, Raw;" "FDA Vitamins and Minerals Chart."
30 Rubatzky and Yamaguchi, 807.
31 "Of Cabbages and Celts," Texas A & M Agri Life Extension, accessed July 2, 2019, https://aggie-horticulture.tamu.edu/archives/parsons/publications/vegetabletravelers/cabbage.html.
32 J. G. Vaughan and C. A. Geissler, *The New Oxford Book of Food Plants: A Guide to the Fruit, Vegetables, Herbs and Spices of the World*, rev. ed. (Oxford: Oxford University Press, 1997), 166.
33 "The Medieval Garden Enclosed," The Metropolitan Museum of Art, 2000–2011, accessed July 2, 2019, http://blog.metmuseum.org/cloistersgardens/2010/10/22/colewort-and-kale.
34 Vaughan and Geissler, 166.
35 Rubatzky and Yamaguchi, 807; "Collards, Cooked, Boiled, Drained, without Salt," *USDA FoodData Central*, April 1, 2019, accessed February 17, 2020, https://fdc.nal.usda.gov/fdc-app.html#/food-details/170407/nutrients; "FDA Vitamins and Minerals Chart."
36 Mark Robinson and Erica Rowan, "Roman Food Remains in Archaeology and the Contents of a Roman Sewer at Herculaneum," in *A Companion to Food in the Ancient World*, ed. John Wilkins and Robin Nadeau (Chichester, UK: Wiley Blackwell, 2015), 109.
37 "Mustard Greens, Raw;" "FDA Vitamins and Minerals Chart."
38 T. Colin Campbell, *Whole: Rethinking the Science of Nutrition* (Dallas, TX: BenBella Books, 2013), 31.

39 Ibid., 7.
40 Ibid.
41 Mark Wheeler, "Love at First Bite? Not for L.A. School Kids and Their Vegetables," *UCLA Newsroom*, May 24, 2014, accessed July 3, 2019, http://newsroom.ucla.edu/releases/love-at-first-bite.
42 Heidi Stimac, "Creative Marketing Sparks Salad Bar Popularity," *Salad Bars to Schools*, 2019, accessed July 3, 2019, http://www.saladbars2schools.org/2019/02/creative-marketing-sparks-salad-bar-popularity.
43 Broderick Parr, Jennifer K. Bond, and Travis Minor, "Vegetables and Pulses Outlook," *USDA Economic Research Service*, May 6, 2019, accessed July 3, 2019, https://www.ers.usda.gov/webdocs/publications/93033/vgs-362.pdf?v=1958.8, 1, 3.
44 Michael Kerrigan, *Ancient Rome and the Roman Empire* (London: Dorling Kindersley, 2001), 39.
45 Haraldur Sigurdsson, "Mount Vesuvius before the Disaster," in *The Natural History of Pompeii*, ed. Wilhelmina Feemster Jashemski and Frederick G. Meyer (Cambridge, UK: Cambridge University Press, 2002), 30.
46 Haraldur Sigurdsson and Steven Carey, "The Eruption of Vesuvius in A.D. 79," in *The Natural History of Pompeii*, ed. Wilhelmina Feemster Jashemski and Frederick G. Meyer (Cambridge, UK: Cambridge University Press, 2002), 38, 47.
47 Ibid., 38.
48 Robinson and Rowan, 107.
49 Ibid.
50 Sara C. Bisel and Jane F. Bisel, "Health and Nutrition at Herculaneum: An Examination of Human Skeletal Remains," in *The Natural History of Pompeii*, ed. Wilhelmina Feemster Jashemski and Frederick G. Meyer (Cambridge, UK: Cambridge University Press, 2002), 451.
51 John P. McKay, Bennett D. Hill, John Buckler, Clare Haru Crowston, Merry E. Wiesner-Hanks, and Joe Perry, *Understanding Western Society: A Brief History* (Boston and New York: Bedford/St. Martin's 2012), 62.
52 Andrew Wallace-Hadrill, *Herculaneum: Past and Future* (London: Frances Lincoln Publishers, 2011), 91, 93.
53 Michael Grant, *Cities of Vesuvius: Pompeii and Herculaneum* (London: Phoenix Press, 2005), 7.
54 Robinson and Rowan, 109.
55 Joanne Berry, *The Complete Pompeii* (London: Thames and Hudson, 2007), 89.
56 Kerrigan, 39.
57 Bisel and Bisel, 460–463.
58 Ibid., 461.
59 Ibid., 463.
60 Ibid., 461.
61 Ibid., 463.
62 Robinson and Rowan, 114.
63 Ibid.
64 Ibid., 110.
65 Ibid., 114.
66 Bisel and Bisel, 458.
67 Ibid., 460.
68 Stephan T. A. M. Mols, "Identification of the Wood Used in the Furniture at Herculaneum," in *The Natural History of Pompeii*, ed. Wilhelmina Feemster Jashemski and Frederick G. Meyer (Cambridge, UK: Cambridge University Press, 2002), 228.
69 Ibid., 226.
70 Ibid., 228.
71 Carroll Moulton, ed., *Ancient Greece and Rome: An Encyclopedia for Students*, vol. 2 (New York: Charles Scribner's Sons, 1998), 73.
72 Robinson and Rowan, 110.
73 Ibid., 109.
74 Ibid., 110.
75 Moulton, 73.
76 Peter Garnsey, *Food and Society in Classical Antiquity*. Cambridge, UK: Cambridge University Press, 1999), 15.
77 "Fig," Purdue University, July 11, 2019, accessed July 11, 2019, https://hort.purdue.edu/newcrop/morton/fig.html.

78 The Editors of Encyclopaedia Britannica, "Mustard: Plant, Vegetable, and Condiment," *Encyclopaedia* Britannica, last modified January 10, 2020, accessed January 17, 2020, https://www.britannica.com/plant/mustard.
79 Robinson and Rowan, 110.
80 Ibid., 109–110.
81 Ibid., 107.
82 Moulton, 73.
83 Ibid., 74.
84 John Wilkins, "Medical Literature, Diet, and Health," in *A Companion to Food in the Ancient World*, ed. John Wilkins and Robin Nadeau (Chichester, UK: Wiley Blackwell, 2015), 65.
85 Ibid., 66.
86 Robinson and Rowan, 110.
87 Ibid., 109.
88 Ibid., 109–110.
89 Bisel and Bisel, 458.
90 Garnsey, 14.
91 John F. Donahue, "Roman Dining," in *A Companion to Food in the Ancient World*, ed. John Wilkins and Robin Nadeau (Chichester, UK: Wiley Blackwell, 2015), 254.
92 Bisel and Bisel, 458.
93 Ibid.
94 Ibid.; Robinson and Rowan, 111.
95 Bisel and Bisel.
96 Berry, 89.
97 Bisel and Bisel, 454.
98 Ibid., 454–455.
99 Ibid., 461.
100 Ibid.
101 Ibid., 455, 461.
102 Ibid.
103 Ibid., 463.
104 Ibid.
105 Ibid., 456, 463.
106 Ibid., 464.
107 Ibid., 456, 464.
108 Ibid., 464–465.
109 Ibid., 455–456.
110 Ibid., 455.
111 Ibid.
112 Garnsey, 58.
113 Ibid.; Bisel and Bisel, 455.
114 Garnsey, 58.
115 Wallace-Hadrill, 129.
116 Ibid., 89.
117 Edward S. Deevey Jr., "The Human Population," *Scientific American* 203, no 9 (September 1, 1960), 202.
118 Bisel and Bisel, 453.
119 Walter Scheidel, "Demography," in *The Cambridge Economic History of the Greco-Roman World*, ed. Walter Scheidel, Ian Morris, and Richard Saller (Cambridge, UK: Cambridge University Press, 2007), 41.
120 E. A. Wrigley and R. S. Schofield, *The Population History of England, 1541–1871: A Reconstruction* (Cambridge, UK: Cambridge University Press, 1989), 309.
121 Bisel and Bisel, 453.
122 Alex Butterworth and Ray Laurence, *Pompeii: The Living City* (New York: St. Martin's Press, 2005), 65.
123 Wallace-Hadrill, 129.
124 Bisel and Bisel, 458.
125 Wallace-Hadrill, 130.

126 Robert Sallares, "Ecology," in *The Cambridge Economic History of the Greco-Roman World*, ed. Walter Scheidel, Ian Morris, and Richard Saller (Cambridge, UK: Cambridge University Press, 2007), 35.
127 Bisel and Bisel, 458.
128 "Mosquito Malaria Vectors," *Malaria Atlas Project*, 2020, accessed January 18, 2020, https://malariaatlas.org/mosquito-malaria-vectors; Sallares, 34.
129 Sallares, 36.
130 Ibid., 34.
131 Ibid.
132 Ibid., 35.
133 Ivan Oransky, "Ancel Keys," *The Lancet* 364, no. 9452 (December 18, 2004): 2174.
134 Ibid.
135 Piero Bevilacqua, "The Distinctive Character of Italian Environmental History," in *Nature and History in Modern Italy*, ed. Marco Armiero and Marcus Hall (Athens: Ohio University Press, 2010), 16–17.
136 Ibid., 17; Marcus Hall, "Environmental Imperialism in Sardinia: Pesticides and Politics in the Struggle against Malaria," in *Nature and History in Modern Italy*, ed. Marco Armiero and Marcus Hall (Athens: Ohio University Press, 2010), 71.
137 Hall, 70–72; John H. Perkins, *Insects, Experts, and the Insecticide Crisis: The Quest for New Pest Management Strategies* (New York and London: Plenum Press, 1982), 6, 10.

16 Conclusion

16.1 DIET AND CIVILIZATION

German composer Wilhelm Richard Wagner (1813–1883) sought to make opera—which he designated "music drama"—a vehicle for unifying all art.[1] The desire for totality also undergirded the Annales school of history, named after the French journal *Annales d'histoire economique et sociale* (*Annals of History, Economics, and Society*) founded in 1929. This brand of history aimed to create a "science of man" that attempted to understand the gamut of human experiences.[2]

This book cannot hope to scale such lofty heights, though it affirms the necessity of subsuming history within the natural sciences. Such an ambition begins by acknowledging that humans are organisms circumscribed by their biology. Scientists seek to understand that biology, noted Chapter 2, in terms of chemistry and physics. In this light, nothing is more elemental to understanding ourselves than identifying what we have eaten during prehistory and history and evaluating these foods' health effects. Such an approach to the past is total in embracing foods as products of the environment, as parts of the biota, as outcomes of natural and artificial selection, and as packages of biochemicals. Little contemplation is needed to see humans in these terms such that study of diet, nutrition, and health becomes central to apprehending patterns in civilizations' development and dissolution. In this way, diet, nutrition, and health shaped the tempo and configuration of prehistory and history.

For example, the Middle Ages (c. 500–c. 1500 CE) evinced foods' ability to shape societies. Once conceived as a bleak interlude in Europe between Roman antiquity (c. 750 BCE–c. 500 CE) and the Renaissance (c. 1350–c. 1600), the Middle Ages are now known for the interplay between

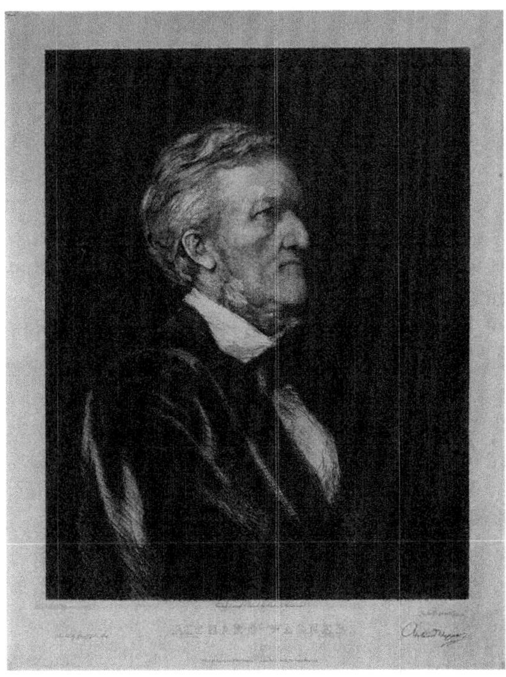

FIGURE 16.1 Richard Wagner. (Photo courtesy of Library of Congress. https://www.loc.gov/pictures/item/2004667976/.)

advancement and tragedy. The Medieval Warm Period, discussed in Chapters 6, 8, and 9, between the ninth and thirteenth centuries lengthened the growing season 3 or 4 weeks yearly.[3] Harvests enlarged, and crops failed less often in northern Europe. Viticulturists benefited from the warmth by moving grapes (*Vitis vinifera*) north into Britain and into higher latitudes in what are today France and Germany. Seventh-century converts to Islam, Arabs moved west throughout the Mediterranean, fattening and selectively breeding sheep (*Ovis aries*) in Spain and Portugal and introducing sugarcane (*Saccharum officinarum*), rice (*Oryza sativa*), and citrus trees (*Citrus* species) wherever climate permitted cultivation. Christian monks settled Europe's hinterlands, clearing forests to make model farms.

Populations grew with increases in food production. Surpluses enlarged cities, where occupants specialized in tasks besides farming. Urbanities traded throughout Europe and Asia and founded universities, which stimulated interest in many disciplines, including mathematics and the natural sciences. Scholarship in these fields fueled advances in astronomy, physics, and medicine celebrated as the Scientific Revolution. Translations of Greek philosopher Aristotle's (384–322 BCE) treatises invigorated the study of classical civilization and laid a foundation for the Renaissance. Looking outward, Europe launched the Crusades in the late eleventh century. Expansionism took Europeans south to South Africa's Cape of Good Hope in 1488, west to the Americas in 1492, and east to India in 1498.

This dynamism, predicated on reliable food production, faltered in the early fourteenth century, when cold rains damaged crops. The climate's deterioration made hunger ubiquitous as populations that had grown during the warm interlude were now too large to feed. Scarcity increased vulnerability to diseases, and the Black Death (1347–1351), mentioned in Chapters 1, 3, and 8, killed around one-third of Europeans.[4] Antisemitism worsened as gentiles blamed Jews for these deaths. Unable to prevent catastrophe, the Catholic Church suffered a leadership crisis, having two popes between 1378 and 1409 and three between 1409 and 1417.[5] Beginning in the 1320s in Flanders—today northern Belgium—and intensifying in 1358 in France and in 1381 in England, peasants revolted against oppressive taxes and tithes.[6] Macabre art and literature vanquished optimism as images of skeletons defined a worldview.[7]

16.2 DIET, NUTRITION, HEALTH, AND SLIMNESS

The Black Death underscored the connection between undernutrition and susceptibility to contagion, a reality that beset humans when they formed permanent settlements. The link between diet and health was evident at medicine's beginnings. Chapter 1 mentioned that Greek physician and medicine's putative founder Hippocrates (c. 460–c. 375 BCE) is thought to have prioritized the identification and consumption of healthful foods, though the texts attributed to him were written by several doctors.[8] In this tradition was Greek physician, anatomist, and author Galen (130–210 CE), introduced in Chapter 2, whose sensible dietary advice deserves to be better known.

The partnership among medicine, diet, nutrition, and health changed over time. American neurologist David Perlmutter (b. 1954), introduced in Chapter 1, characterized medical school as training in diagnosing and treating ailments, usually with drugs.[9] Such an orientation deemphasized investigation of the linkages among diet, nutrition, and health. Swedish family physician Andreas Eenfeldt (b. 1972) wrote in 2014 that medical curricula devoted roughly 2 weeks to diet and nutrition but years to pharmacology and surgery.[10] At the same time, as the specialist in a white coat lost prominence as the sole arbiter of diet and nutrition, their investigation grew into public phenomena suitable for journalistic and lay treatment. Chapter 1 noted the appeal of popular books on these subjects and the potential to enrich publishers and authors.

Interest in diet and nutrition is not merely concerned with health but derives its greatest motivation by conflating vitality, sexiness, slimness, and youthfulness as though these attributes always align. When food is scarce, societies tend to prize the full figure as index of prosperity.[11] On the other hand, when food is abundant—as it is today—the svelte figure reigns supreme. Such thinking prevails in a society that venerates celebrities and rates actresses by their appearance in a bikini. Preoccupation with appearance may be an outcome of evolution. Compared with our closest relatives—the chimpanzee (*Pan troglodytes*), bonobo (*Pan paniscus*), and gorilla (*Gorilla gorilla* and *Gorilla beringei*)—humans are virtually hairless. The fewer the clothes, the easier becomes evaluation of a body that cannot hide adipose.

Under these circumstances, people who understand that no literal fountain of youth exists nonetheless seek youth's proxy in a trim physique. Diet and nutrition writers exploit this desire by equating health and slenderness. Although his focus was more exercise than diet, American author and runner James Fuller Fixx (1932–1984) targeted readers' fear of looking "slightly puffy around the waist."[12] He quoted African American ultramarathoner Ted Corbitt's (1919–2007) warning that "When people tell you how good you look, you can be sure you're not fit. If you don't look gaunt, you're out of shape."[13] American nutritionist and exercise physiologist Loren Cordain (b. 1950) entitled his 2002 book *The Paleo Diet: Lose Weight and Get Healthy by Eating the Foods You Were Designed to Eat*. In 2011, American cardiologist William Davis (b. 1957) published *Wheat Belly: Lose the Wheat, Lose the Weight, and Find Your Path Back to Health*. The next year's expanded edition was *Lose the Wheat, Lose the Weight!: Banish Your Wheat Belly, Feel Better Than Ever, and Turbocharge Your Health*. Both are part confession, with Davis admitting embarrassment, dissatisfaction, and puzzlement at having gained some 13.6 kilograms (30 pounds) of abdominal fat over the years and become diabetic despite jogging daily and watching his diet.[14] Eenfeldt titled his 2014 offering *Low Carb, High Fat Food Revolution: Advice and Recipes to Improve Your Health and Reduce Your Weight*. In the first paragraph of *The Plant Paradox: The Hidden Dangers in "Healthy" Foods that Cause Disease and Weight Gain* (2017), American cardiac surgeon Steven R. Gundry wrote that his hypertension, headaches, arthritis, high cholesterol, and insulin resistance vanished after he lost 31.8 kilograms (70 pounds).[15] In the 2018 edition of *Grain Brain*, Perlmutter excerpted testimonial from a woman who adopted his regimen, reporting that the "weight just flew off me and I felt so much better."[16] An August 2019 Google search of the words "health weight loss" generated roughly 632 million results. "Weight loss" alone found almost 1.7 billion websites.

Pursuit of youthfulness and vigor through weight reduction has become an obsession. In the 1980s, American actor Billy Crystal (b. 1948) spoofed the preoccupation with appearance, vanity, insincerity, superficiality, and the trappings of celebrity on the television program *Saturday Night Live*, repeatedly remarking that "It is better to look good than to feel good."[17] Dawning in the twentieth century, the age of television held potential to expose everyone to scrutiny. The adage that the camera adds 4.5 kilograms (10 pounds) expresses the fear of being objectified in a way that permits others to disparage our appearance. The only remedy is to be forever slender, even at the cost of perpetual hunger and suppression of cravings.

Rooted in our biology, hunger and cravings are unsurprising responses to privation. This book emphasizes that premodern peoples lived amid food scarcity more than abundance. Chapter 10 quoted Cretans' post–World War II plight in the lament that "We are hungry most of the time."[18] Chapter 3 noted that dearth rewarded individuals who easily accumulated adipose during plentitude and husbanded it during shortages. That is, an environment with variable resources and frequent shortages selected for survival people whose descendants today look soft and round in a bikini or speedo. The modern revulsion against this appearance is at the core a repudiation of the implacable realities that guided our evolution. Reality's denial makes weight loss and maintenance all the harder while it divorces notions of body shape from the habits that promote health.

None of the foregoing seeks to devalue efforts at weight control. This book acknowledges that overweight and obesity, and the diseases they cause or exacerbate, persist wherever food is plentiful. Beyond statistics about liposuction and longevity, these problems mar quality of life in ways difficult to summarize because they are so pervasive. Humans endure much suffering, but ridicule over appearance is unbearable when it fuels a psychology of inferiority.

These reflections aside, vitality and slimness are not synonyms. United Kingdom (UK) pharmacologist Paul Clayton and historian Judith D. Rowbotham (b. 1952), both introduced in Chapter 1, stated that overweight and obesity were unknown among nineteenth-century laborers.[19] This observation appears valid for most premodern humans; yet this book documents how ill these trim people often were.

16.3 FACTORS THAT GOVERN HEALTH

But misery was not universal. Previous chapters identified instances of vigor and posited factors, including diet, that enhanced it. Interest in diet and nutrition, Chapter 1 remarked, led me to test numerous foods' health effects in prehistory and history. Few emerged from this study as universals, as items worthy of every diet. In this category, Chapter 13 amassed evidence that the potato (*Solanum tuberosum*) approximates a perfect food as nearly as may be possible. This book recommends it above meat as the foundation of a hearty meal, though animal products may merit inclusion as side dishes. Examined in Chapter 8, peas (*Pisum sativum*) sustained medieval peasants, beans (*Phaseolus vulgaris*) nourished prehistoric Mexicans, and peas, peanuts (*Arachis hypogaea*), and beans may have made African slaves better nourished than free whites. Chapter 9 indicated that acorn (*Quercus* species) eaters were unusual among premodern peoples in displaying few skeletal and dental pathologies besides caries. Chapter 14 identified bananas as a probable factor in Yanomami health and longevity. On the other hand, Chapter 12 faulted corn (*Zea mays*) for anemia, pellagra, and kwashiorkor. Chapter 13 implicated cassava (*Manihot esculenta*) in goiter, cognitive impairment, and paralysis. Earlier chapters and a later paragraph emphasize, however, that foods' utility depends largely on context.

Even the best diet and nutrition do not alone invigorate the body. Although I did not begin this investigation to study activity's health effects, evidence of its benefits recurred frequently enough to compel the conclusion that vitality requires physical labor, exercise, exertion, activity, or whatever language an onlooker wishes to employ. For example, Chapter 4 identified activity as common to Paraguay's Ache and Great Plains Indians. Both were far healthier than Chapter 4's Egyptian elites, whose sloth caused heart disease. All three ate meat, eliminating it as explanation for divergent outcomes. Absent dietary differences, exertion among Ache and Plains Indians and indolence among Egypt's wealthy offer the best explanation for health disparities.

Other research corroborates my emphasis on activity. American nutritionist Thomas Colin Campbell (b. 1934) and his son American physician and marathoner Thomas M. Campbell II calculated that rural Chinese had seventeen times fewer deaths from heart disease than Americans in the 1970s.[20] Cholesterol was lower, and cancers were less frequent in China than in the United States.[21] Although they scrutinized dietary contrasts between rural China and the United States, the Campbells observed that Chinese were more active than Americans.[22] Manual labor was ubiquitous in China's countryside. Even Chinese office workers were more vigorous than Americans because they bicycled rather than drove wherever they went.

In a similar vein, American anthropologist Stephen Le, introduced in Chapter 1, upheld prehistoric hunter-gatherers as paragons, asserting that on an average day, men walked 14.5 kilometers (9 miles) and women 9.7 kilometers (6 miles).[23] Without a citation, these numbers may be speculation, though Le used them to claim paradoxically that our ancestors expended no more energy than we do today. He seems to have undermined this statement by estimating that Americans now average just 4 kilometers (2.5 miles) by foot, allotting the balance of the day to "sitting, driving, and watching nearly 5 hours of television."[24] Even were an average defensible, it would provide almost no real information given diverse habitats, some requiring enormous efforts to extract food, others far less, and the rest between the extremes. Nonetheless, this book notes that preagricultural peoples' use as models of what moderns should eat and do appeals to anthropologists and some scientists and physicians.

Examination of hunter-gatherers confirms strenuousness that appears to contradict Le's assertion that they metabolized no more calories than we do now. The hunt took Amerindians in the Great Basin—today Nevada, most of Oregon and Utah, and parts of Wyoming, Idaho, and California—up to

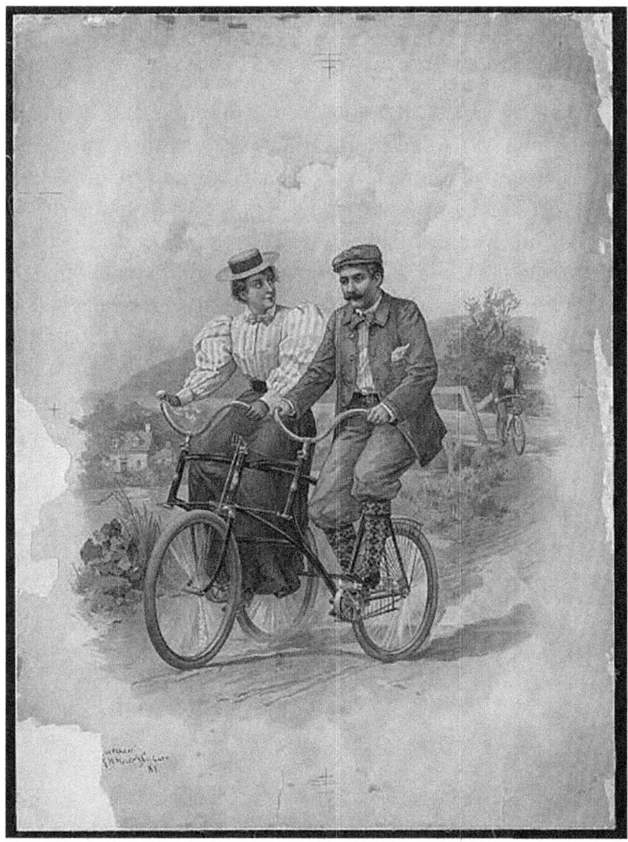

FIGURE 16.2 Bicycles. (Photo courtesy of Library of Congress. https://www.loc.gov/pictures/item/2018756236/.)

96.6 kilometers (sixty miles) from camp.[25] American anthropologist Clark Spencer Larsen (b. 1952), introduced in Chapter 2, characterized their lives as "rigorous and demanding," writing that "These people were subjecting their legs to very heavy physical activity, compared to other populations."[26] Their skeletons revealed osteoarthritis in 77 percent of adults and in everyone over age 30.[27] The condition, uncommon in modern Americans, evinced intense exertions.[28] Great Basin Amerindians' robust bones, having supported strong muscles, indicated activity and adequate nourishment.[29] Even those with light bones, signaling undernutrition, were energetic.[30] Prolonged walking, often over rough terrain, strengthened lightweight bones. Despite inhabiting a harsh environment, they were healthy.[31] At the risk of belaboring the obvious, such evidence implies that exertion must accompany nutrition to confer maximum vigor and that indolence weakens even satisfactorily nourished bodies.

On the other hand, excessive labor appears to be no better than torpor. Chapters 6, 8, and 15 emphasized that overwork enervated slaves, increased illnesses' frequency and severity, and truncated lives. Although governments may boast of having ended slavery, overwork and exploitation persist. Farm and factory labor remains arduous wherever it requires muscles rather than machines. The argument may be advanced that many governments do little to prevent businesses from extracting maximum exertions from employees while paying scant wages. As a landscaper, I had a supervisor who lamented the ubiquity of exhausting, filthy jobs, their meager pay, and the difficulty finding people to perform them.

Connected to activity is sun exposure, another topic I did not intend to examine. Yet it could not be ignored because hunting, gathering, fishing, farming, and livestock raising occurred outdoors. Plains Indians' bones grew stout, as noted, with the body's manufacture of vitamin D from sunlight.

Conversely, Chapter 7 noted rickets in French peasants who wore too much clothing and a hat, preventing vitamin D synthesis.

These incidents were not isolated examples. As early as the fifth century BCE, Greek historian Herodotus (c. 480–c. 425 BCE) called attention to sunshine's benefits and deprivation's dangers.[32] Examining remains from those who died in a sixth-century battle between Persia (now Iran) and Egypt, he noticed that Egyptian skulls were thicker and sturdier than their Persian counterparts. Herodotus explained the difference by referencing Egyptians' practice of shaving the head and thereby exposing it to the sun, whereas Persians wore turbans. In the second century CE, Greek physician Soranus of Ephesus (98–138) described rickets' symptoms, which Galen blamed on the habit of spending too much time indoors.[33] In 2014, Eenfeldt warned against sunlight's avoidance, comparing Swedes who languished indoors to Gollum, the pale, gaunt creature in British author and scholar John Ronald Reuel (J. R. R.) Tolkien's (1892–1973) novels *The Hobbit* (1937) and *The Lord of the Rings* (1954–1955).[34]

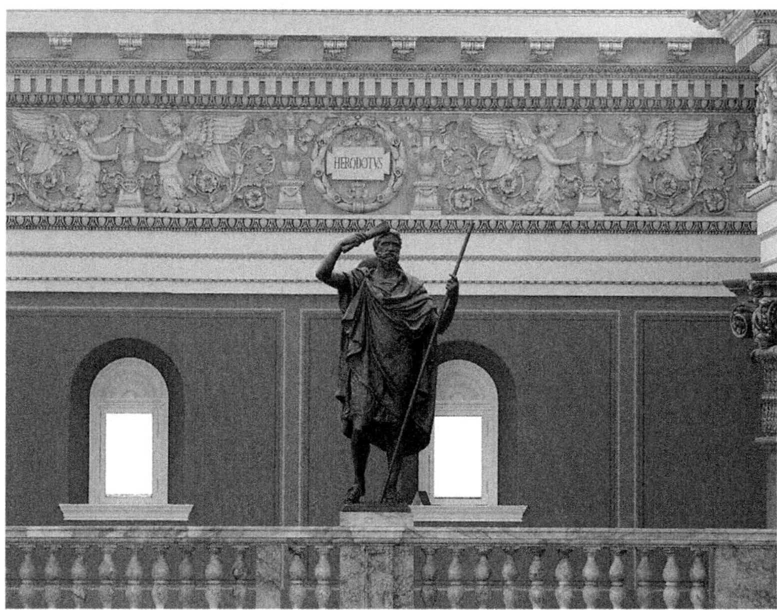

FIGURE 16.3 Herodotus. (Photo courtesy of Library of Congress. https://www.loc.gov/pictures/item/2007684411/.)

16.4 DIET DEPENDS ON CONTEXT

Previous chapters and an earlier section stated that circumstances should influence food choices. This book has repeated, perhaps ad nauseam, that after millennia of depending on muscles to accomplish tasks, people now rely on machines powered by fossil fuels. The pedestrian or cyclist is rare on roads, whether desolate or, more often, clogged with cars. Tempers flare when drivers compete for parking spots nearest a destination because no one wants to take one stride more than necessary. Elevators are full and stairwells empty. This book argues that inactivity spiked in the 1920s with the automobile's adoption. Although his timing ignores this development, Larsen wrote that "one of the most profound lifestyle changes to occur in recent memory is the growing sedentism of late twentieth-century Americans, resulting in unprecedented levels of obesity."[35]

Activity at its nadir, people should restrict calories. This dictum minimizes consumption of marbled meats, peanuts, most nuts, vegetable oils, most dairy products, sweets, and kindred items. The result is unsatisfactory because peanuts, for example, have many nutrients, as Chapter 8 detailed.

Chapters 4 and 7 noted that meat and dairy, respectively, are full of protein, vitamins, and minerals; they should be avoided not because they are inherently unhealthy—quite the opposite—but because too many people are too inert to splurge on caloric fare.

Instead, inactivity demands foods that have many nutrients but few calories. The criticism that potatoes, for example, are fattening is untrue. Chapter 13 noted that 100 grams have just seventy-seven calories, a bargain given ample nourishment. Many vegetables, treated in Chapter 15, furnish few calories and abundant nourishment. Lean meats, fish, shellfish, and poultry may be eaten in small quantities. On the other hand, the sugar sucrose ($C_{12}H_{22}O_{11}$), discussed in Chapters 2 and 11, has nothing but carbohydrates and should be avoided. Vegetable oils—discussed in Chapter 10—butter, ghee, and other fats should be used sparingly. This appeal to a spartan existence is too severe to convince anyone of its virtues. Indeed, austerity for its own sake may not be a virtue. Foods are not just nutrient packages because people derive pleasure—arguably a virtue in its own right—from those that are especially tasty. Someone who dislikes broccoli (*Brassica oleracea var. italica*), for instance, will resent the command to eat it. For example, forty-first U.S. President George Herbert Walker Bush (1924–2018) remarked in 1990 that "I do not like broccoli.... And I haven't liked it since I was a little kid and my mother made me eat it. And I'm President of the United States, and I'm not going to eat any more broccoli!"[36]

This problem resists easy solution. The high-fat, meaty diet that appealed to Icelandic-Canadian explorer Vilhjalmur Stefansson (1879–1962), introduced in Chapter 5, suited the Inuit because they lived strenuous lives. Similarly, a 1968 study reported that British railroads fed each laborer 0.9 kilograms (2 pounds) of meat daily.[37] Plentiful nourishment and exertion made him "about as strong as he would ever be."[38] In the machine age, hard labor is uncommon except under compulsion, mandating that physically-taxed workers eat like the Inuit, Plains Indians, Ache, and railroad gangs during their heyday. The first three hunted and fished diverse species in contrast to the modern dependence on beef, pork, and chicken. Beyond this trio, as late as 1921 American home economist Helen Woodard Atwater (1876–1947) reported mutton and game in U.S. rural diets.[39] This book urges a return to such variety. Meat, fish, peanuts, peas, and beans are excellent choices to sustain arduous work because they combine calories and nutrients.

But Chapters 4 and 5 demonstrated that Plains Indian, Ache, and Inuit health diminished as they became sedentary and ate white flour, canned goods, and other undesirables. Although regrettable, calorie counting's arithmetic mandates equality between energy intake and expenditure. Acknowledging reality, this book rejects the fantasy of pretending that people may eat mostly what they want so long as they avoid a single food or group of foods, once thought wholesome, but now unmasked as sinister. Such thinking is wishful, dishonest, and does nothing but worsens confusion about the relationship among diet, nutrition, and health. Rather than deception, readers deserve to know that health is not a commodity that can be purchased at discount. It requires work, discipline, and sometimes self-denial. Even the best efforts guarantee nothing because disease may incapacitate those who do everything right. Life's risks cannot be eliminated. The best we can do is strive to minimize them, to maximize health, and to endure what fate delivers. Greek historian and philosopher Arrian of Nicomedia (c. 92–c. 175 CE) attributed to his teacher stoic philosopher Epictetus (c. 60–c. 138) the doctrine that "We must make the best of those things that are in our power, and take the rest as nature gives it."[40]

NOTES

1 Joseph Machlis, *The Enjoyment of Music: An Introduction to Perceptive Listening* (New York: Norton, 1955), 226.
2 John Day, "Foreword," in *The Peasants of Languedoc*, Emmanuel Le Roy Ladurie, trans. John Day (Urbana: University of Illinois Press, 1974), xi.
3 Richard H. Steckel, *Health and Nutrition in the Preindustrial Era: Insights from a Millennium of Average Heights in Northern Europe* (Cambridge, MA: National Bureau of Economic Research, 2001), 18.

4 John P. McKay, Bennett D. Hill, John Buckler, Clare Haru Crowston, Merry E. Wiesner-Hanks, and Joe Perry, *Understanding Western Society: A Brief History* (Boston and New York: Bedford/St. Martin's, 2012), 324.
5 Ibid., 335–338.
6 Ibid., 340–341.
7 Robin W. Winks, Crane Brinton, John B. Christopher, and Robert Lee Wolff, *A History of Civilization*, vol. 1: Prehistory to 1715, 7th ed. (Englewood Cliffs, NJ: Prentice Hall, 1988), 257–259.
8 John Wilkins, "Medical Literature, Diet, and Health," in *A Companion to Food in the Ancient World*, ed. John Wilkins and Robin Nadeau (Oxford: Wiley Blackwell, 2015), 60.
9 David Perlmutter, *Grain Brain: The Surprising Truth about Wheat, Carbs, and Sugar—Your Brain's Silent Killers*, rev. ed. (New York: Little, Brown Spark, 2018), 33.
10 Andreas Eenfeldt, *Low Carb, High Fat Food Revolution: Advice and Recipes to Improve Your Health and Reduce Your Weight* (New York: Skyhorse Publishing, 2014), 186.
11 Leslie Sue Lieberman, "Obesity," in *The Cambridge World History of Food*, vol. 1, ed. Kenneth F. Kiple and Kriemhild Conee Ornelas (Cambridge, UK: Cambridge University Press, 2000), 1068–1069.
12 James F. Fixx, *The Complete Book of Running* (New York: Random House, 1977), 75.
13 Ibid.
14 William Davis, *Wheat Belly: Lose the Wheat, Lose the Weight, and Find Your Path Back to Health* (Emmaus, PA: Rodale, 2011), 8; William Davis, *Lose the Wheat, Lose the Weight!: Banish Your Wheat Belly, Feel Better Than Ever, and Turbocharge Your Health*, expanded ed. (Emmaus, PA: Rodale, 2012), 8.
15 Steven R. Gundry, *The Plant Paradox: The Hidden Dangers in "Healthy" Food that Cause Disease and Weight Gain* (New York: Harper Wave, 2017), ix.
16 Perlmutter, 41.
17 "Fernando's Hideaway," *SNL Transcripts Tonight*, October 8, 2018, accessed August 31, 2019, https://snltranscripts.jt.org/84/84dfernando.phtml.
18 Leland G. Allbaugh, *Crete: A Case Study of an Underdeveloped Area* (Princeton, NJ: Princeton University Press, 1953), 105.
19 Paul Clayton and Judith Rowbotham, "How the Mid-Victorians Worked, Ate and Died," *International Journal of Environmental Research and Public Health* 6, no. 3, March 2009, https://www.ncbi.nlm.nih.gov/pmc/articles/PMC2672390.
20 T. Colin Campbell and Thomas M. Campbell, *The China Study*, rev. ed. (Dallas, TX: BenBella Books, 2016), 69.
21 Ibid., 61, 68.
22 Ibid., 89–90.
23 Stephen Le, *100 Million Years of Food: What Our Ancestors Ate and Why It Matters Today* (New York: Picador, 2016), 4.
24 Ibid., 4–5.
25 Clark Spencer Larsen, *Skeletons in Our Closet: Revealing Our Past through Bioarchaeology* (Princeton, NJ and Oxford, UK: Princeton University Press, 2000), 56.
26 Ibid., 47, 55–56.
27 Ibid., 46.
28 Ibid., 24.
29 Ibid., 21.
30 Ibid., 55.
31 Ibid., 21, 45.
32 Elmer Verner McCollum, *A History of Nutrition: The Sequence of Ideas in Nutrition Investigations* (Boston: Houghton Mifflin, 1957), 266.
33 Peter Garnsey, *Food and Society in Classical Antiquity* (Cambridge, UK: Cambridge University Press, 1999), 47.
34 Eenfeldt, 245.
35 Larsen, 222.
36 Maureen Dowd, "'I'm President,' So No More Broccoli," *New York Times*, March 23, 1990, accessed September 3, 2019, https://www.nytimes.com/1990/03/23/us/i-m-president-so-no-more-broccoli.html.
37 Garnsey, 44.
38 Ibid.
39 Helen W. Atwater, "Food for Farm Families," in *U.S. Department of Agriculture Yearbook, 1920*, ed. L. C. Everard (Washington: GPO, 1921), 476.
40 Epictetus, *Discourses: Selections*, trans. P. E. Matheson (Chicago: Great Books Foundation, 1955), 5.

Bibliography

"1 in 5 Obese Adults Satisfied with Body Weight." Centraal Bureau voor de Statistiek. September 25, 2018. Accessed June 16, 2019. https://www.cbs.nl/en-gb/news/2018/37/1-in-5-obese-adults-satisfied-with-body-weight.

"About Us." Bunker Hill Cheese. 1935–2019. Accessed March 14, 2019. https://bunkerhillcheese.com/about-us-en-2.html.

"About Us." Fox's Pizza Den. Accessed March 14, 2019. http://www.foxspizza.com/locations/oh/millersburg/millersburg-oh-119/index.html.

Abuye, C., U. Kelbessa, and S. Wolde-Gebriel. "Health Effects of Cassava Consumption in South Ethiopia." *East African Medical Journal* 75, no. 3 (February 28, 1998): 166–170. http://europepmc.org/article/med/9640816.

"Ache." *Cengage*. Last modified January 13, 2020. Accessed February 10, 2020. https://www.encyclopedia.com/places/latin-america-and-caribbean/south-american-political-geography/ache.

"Achievements in Public Health, 1900–1999: Healthier Mothers and Babies." CDC. October 1, 1999. Accessed February 10, 2019. https://www.cdc.gov/mmwr/preview/mmwrhtml/mm4838a2.htm.

"Acorn." In *The Cambridge World History of Food*. Vol. 2, ed. Kenneth F. Kiple and Kriemhild Conee Ornelas, 1714. Cambridge, UK: Cambridge University Press, 2000.

"Action on Salt." Wolfson Institute of Preventive Medicine. Accessed February 27, 2019. http://www.actiononsalt.org.uk/salthealth/salt-and-ethnic-minorities.

Adams, Cecil. "Does Thinking Hard Burn More Calories?" *Washington City Paper*. December 7, 2012. Accessed January 17, 2019. https://www.washingtoncitypaper.com/columns/straight-dope/article/13043347/straight-dope-does-thinking-hard-burn-more-calories.

Ajibola, Abdulwahid, Joseph P. Chamunorwa, and Kennedy H. Erlwanger. "Nutraceutical Values of Natural Honey and Its Contribution to Health and Wealth." *Nutrition and Metabolism* 9 (June 20, 2012). https://www.ncbi.nlm.nih.gov/pmc/articles/PMC3583289.

Akinpelu, A. O., L. E. F. Amamgbo, A. O. Olojede, and A. S. Oyekale. "Health Implications of Cassava Production and Consumption." *Journal of Agriculture and Social Research* 11, no. 1 (2011): 118–125. https://www.ajol.info/index.php/jasr/article/view/73684/64364.

Albala, Ken. *Beans: A History*. Oxford and New York: Berg, 2007.

———. *Nuts: A Global History*. London: Reaktion Books, 2014.

Alireza, Mariam. "Legumes: The Poor Man's Protein." *Arab News*. December 8, 2004. Accessed April 27, 2019. http://www.arabnews.com/node/259264.

Allaby, Michael. *Oceans: A Scientific History of Oceans and Marine Life*. New York: Facts on File, 2009.

Allbaugh, Leland G. *Crete: A Case Study of an Underdeveloped Area*. Princeton, NJ: Princeton University Press, 1953.

Allem, Antonio C. "The Origins and Taxonomy of Cassava." In *Cassava: Biology, Production and Utilization*, ed. R. J. Hillocks, J. M. Thresh, and A. C. Bellotti, 1–16. Wallingford, UK and New York: CABI Publishing, 2002.

Allman-Farinelli, Margaret. "Nuts and Seeds." In *Essentials of Human Nutrition*, ed. Jim Mann and A. Stewart Truswell, 279–280. 5th ed. Oxford, UK: Oxford University Press, 2017.

"Amish Studies." *The Young Center*. Accessed March 14, 2019. https://groups.etown.edu/amishstudies.

"Ancient Humans Arrived in South America in Multiple Waves." *Science Daily*. February 24, 2017. Accessed February 9, 2019. https://www.sciencedaily.com/releases/2017/02/170224121748.htm.

Andersen, S., E. Boeskov, and P. Laurberg. "Ethnic Differences in Bone Mineral Density between Inuit and Caucasians in North Greenland Are Caused by Differences in Body Size." *Journal of Clinical Densitometry* 8, no. 4 (Winter 2005): 409–414.

Angel, J. Lawrence. "Health as a Crucial Factor in the Changes from Hunting to Developed Farming in the Eastern Mediterranean." In *Paleopathology at the Origins of Agriculture*, ed. Mark Nathan Cohen and George J. Armelagos, 51–73. Orlando, FL: Academic Press, 1984.

"Anthropometric Reference Data for Children and Adults: United States, 2007–2012." *Vital and Health Statistics*. October 2012. Accessed February 8, 2019. https://www.cdc.gov/nchs/data/series/sr_11/sr11_252.pdf.

Araki, Kadya. "Why All Humans Need to Eat Meat for Health." Accessed January 26, 2019. https://breakingmuscle.com/healthy-eating/why-all-humans-need-to-eat-meat-for-health.

Arbuckle, Dani. "What Is the Average Adult Male Height and Weight?" *Livestrong*. 2019. Accessed February 8, 2019. https://www.livestrong.com/article/289265-what-is-the-average-adult-male-height.

"Arctic Char." Government of Northwest Territories. October 2016. Accessed March 4, 2019. https://www.hss.gov.nt.ca/sites/hss/files/resources/contaminants-fact-sheets-arctic-char.pdf.

"Arctic Ocean Diversity." *Census of Marine Life*. Accessed February 23, 2019. http://www.arcodiv.org/Fish.html.

Ardrey, Robert. *African Genesis: A Personal Investigation into the Animal Origins and Nature of Man*. New York: Atheneum, 1970.

"AreWeGettingEnoughVitaminsandNutrients?"CDC.LastmodifiedMarch2,2016.AccessedJune1,2019.https://blogs.cdc.gov/yourhealthyourenvironment/2016/03/02/are-we-getting-enough-vitamins-and-nutrients.

Aristotle. *Nicomachean Ethics*, trans. Martin Oswald. Upper Saddle River, NJ: Prentice Hall, 1999.

Armelagos, George J. "Paleopathology." In *History of Physical Anthropology*. Vol. 2: M-Z, ed. Frank Spencer, 790–796. New York and London: Garland Publishing, 1997.

Arnarson, Atli. "20 Foods That Are High in Vitamin E." *Healthline*. May 24, 2017. Accessed May 11, 2019. https://www.healthline.com/nutrition/foods-high-in-vitamin-e.

———. "20 Foods That Are High in Vitamin K." *Healthline*. September 6, 2017. Accessed June 29, 2019. https://www.healthline.com/nutrition/foods-high-in-vitamin-k.

———. "Beef 101: Nutrition Facts and Health Effects." *Healthline*. March 30, 2015. Accessed January 26, 2019. https://www.healthline.com/nutrition/foods/beef.

———. "Butter 101: Nutrition Facts and Health Effects." *Healthline*. November 3, 2014. Accessed March 13, 2019. https://www.healthline.com/nutrition/foods/butter.

———. "Pork 101: Nutrition Facts and Health Effects." *Healthline*. April 1, 2015. Accessed January 26, 2019. https://www.healthline.com/nutrition/foods/pork.

———. "Wheat 101: Nutrition Facts and Health Effects." *Healthline*. February 25, 2015. Accessed March 13, 2019. https://www.healthline.com/nutrition/foods/wheat.

Asch, Michael, and Shirleen Smith. "Slavey Dene." In *The Cambridge Encyclopedia of Hunters and Gatherers*, ed. Richard B. Lee and Richard Daly, 46–50. Cambridge, UK: Cambridge University Press, 2004.

Askham, Gemma. "There's a Reason Why Having a Low Body Fat Percentage Isn't Always Healthy." *Women's Health*. August 24, 2018. Accessed February 25, 2019. https://www.womenshealthmag.com/uk/health/female-health/a708160/body-fat-percentage-women.

Atack, Jeremy, and Peter Passell. *A New Economic View of American History: From Colonial Times to 1940*. 2nd ed. New York and London: Norton, 1994.

Atkins, P. J. "The Pasteurization of England: The Science, Culture and Health Implications of Food Processing, 1900–1950." *Academia*. Accessed March 22, 2019. https://www.academia.edu/3161171/The_pasteurization_of_England_the_science_culture_and_health_implications_of_food_processing_1900-1950.

Atkins, Robert C. *Dr. Atkins' Diet Revolution: The High Calorie Way to Stay Thin Forever*. New York: McKay, 1972.

"Attractions, Shops and Artisans." *Ohio Amish Country Map and Visitors' Guide, 2019*.

Atwater, Helen W. "Food for Farm Families." In *U.S. Department of Agriculture Yearbook, 1920*, ed. L. C. Everard, 471–484. Washington: GPO, 1921.

Aubrey, Allison. "More Salt, Fewer Whole Grains: USDA Eases School Lunch Nutrition Rules." *National Public Radio*. December 7, 2018. Accessed January 18, 2020. https://www.npr.org/sections/the-salt/2018/12/07/674533555/more-salt-in-school-lunch-fewer-whole-grains-usda-eases-school-lunch-rules.

Avey, Tori. "Christopher Columbus—Foods of the New World." *Tori's Kitchen*. October 8, 2012. Accessed March 20, 2019. https://toriavey.com/history-kitchen/what-christopher-columbus-discovered-foods-of-the-new-world.

———. "The History, Science, and Uses of Dates." *Tori's Kitchen*. 2010–2020, accessed February 16, 2020. https://toriavey.com/dates-history-science-uses.

Babal, Ken. *Seafood Sense: The Truth about Seafood Nutrition and Safety*. Laguna Beach, CA: Basic Health Publications, 2005.

Bacon, David. *In the Fields of the North*. Berkeley: University of California Press, 2016.

Bagnall, Roger S., and Bruce W. Frier. *The Demography of Roman Egypt*. Cambridge, UK and New York: Cambridge University Press, 2006.

Bahn, Andrew. "Water, Electrolytes, and Acid-Base Balance." In *Essentials of Human Nutrition*, ed. Jim Mann and A. Stewart Truswell, 113–130. 5th ed. Oxford: Oxford University Press, 2017.

Bahuchet, Serge. "Aka Pygmies." In *The Cambridge Encyclopedia of Hunters and Gatherers*, ed. Richard B. Lee and Richard Daly, 190–194. Cambridge, UK: Cambridge University Press, 2004.

Bailey, Diane. *How the Automobile Changed History*. Minneapolis, MN: ABDO Publishing, 2016.

Baldwin, James. "From the Fire Next Time." In *The Norton Anthology of American Literature*. 2nd ed. Nina Baym, Francis Murphy, Ronald Gottesman, Hershel Parker, Laurence B. Holland, William H. Pritchard, and David Kalstone, 2372–2386. New York and London: Norton, 1986.

Bales, Suzanne Frutig. *Vegetables*. New York: Prentice Hall Gardening, 1991.

Balibar, Francoise. *Einstein: Decoding the Universe*, trans. David J. Baker and Dorie B. Baker. New York: Harry N. Abrams, 2001.

Balikci, Asen. "The Netsilik Eskimos: Adaptive Processes." In *Man the Hunter*, ed. Richard B. Lee and Irven DeVore, 78–82. Chicago: Aldine, 1968.

"Banana." In *The Cambridge World History of Food*. Vol. 2, ed. Kenneth F. Kiple and Kriemhild Conee Ornelas, 1726. Cambridge, UK: Cambridge University Press, 2000.

Barclay, Eliza. "A Nation of Meat Eaters: See How It All Adds Up." *NPR*. June 27, 2012. Accessed January 26, 2019. https://www.npr.org/sections/thesalt/2012/06/27/155527365/visualizing-a-nation-of-meat-eaters.

Barber, Nigel. "Do Humans Need Meat?" *Psychology Today*. October 12, 2016. Accessed January 24, 2019. https://www.psychologytoday.com/us/blog/the-human-beast/201610/do-humans-need-meat.

Barber, Shelley, ed. *The Prendergast Letters: Correspondence from Famine-Era Ireland, 1840–1850*. Amherst and Boston: University of Massachusetts Press, 2006.

Barksdale, J. Allen. "American Bison." In *The Cambridge World History of Food*. Vol. 1, ed. Kenneth F. Kiple and Kriemhild Conee Ornelas, 450–455. Cambridge, UK: Cambridge University Press, 2000.

Barras, Colin. "How Humanity First Killed the Dodo, Then Lost It as Well." April 9, 2016. Accessed August, 4, 2019. http://www.bbc.com/earth/story/20160408-how-humanity-first-killed-the-dodo-then-lost-it-as-well.

Barrett, James H., Alison M. Locker, and Callum M. Roberts. "The Origins of Intensive Marine Fishing in Medieval Europe: the English Evidence." *Proceedings of the Royal Society* 271, no. 1556 (December 7, 2004): 2417–2421. https://royalsocietypublishing.org/doi/abs/10.1098/rspb.2004.2885.

Bartoletti, Susan Campbell. *Black Potatoes: The Story of the Great Irish Famine, 1845–1850*. Boston: Houghton Mifflin, 2001.

Bartolini, Giorgio, and Raffaella Petruccelli. *Classification, Origin, Diffusion and History of the Olive*. Rome: Food and Agriculture Organization of the United Nations, 2002.

Bar-Yosef, Ofer. "Eat What Is There: Hunting and Gathering in the World of the Neanderthals and Their Neighbors." *International Journal of Osteoarchaeology* 14, no. 3–4 (May 2004): 333–342.

———. "The Natufian Culture in the Levant, Threshold to the Origins of Agriculture." *Evolutionary Anthropology* (1998): 159–177. http://www.columbia.edu/itc/anthropology/v1007/baryo.pdf.

Baym, Nina, Francis Murphy, Ronald Gottesman, Hershel Parker, Laurence B. Holland, William H. Pritchard, and David Kalstone. *The Norton Anthology of American Literature*. 2nd ed. New York and London: Norton, 1986.

"Bean Nutrition Overview." The Bean Institute. 2019. Accessed April 27, 2019. http://beaninstitute.com/bean-nutrition-overview.

"Beans." In *The Cambridge World History of Food*. Vol. 2, ed. Kenneth F. Kiple and Kriemhild Conee Ornelas, 1728–1730. Cambridge, UK: Cambridge University Press, 2000.

Beck, Hans T. "Caffeine, Alcohol, and Sweeteners." In *The Cultural History of Plants*, ed. Ghillean Prance and Mark Nesbitt, 173–190. New York and London: Routledge, 2005.

Beck, Lane Anderson. "The Influence of Preservation on Observability of Pathology: A Case Study from Pecos." In *Pecos Pueblo Revisited: The Biological and Social Context*, ed. Michele E. Morgan, 71–78. Cambridge, MA: Peabody Museum of Archaeology and Ethnology, Harvard University, 2010.

"Beef. It's What's for Dinner." Cattlemen's Beef Board and National Cattlemen's Beef Association. 2019. Accessed January 25, 2019. https://www.beefitswhatsfordinner.com.

Bellwood, Peter. "Archaeology of Southeast Asian Hunters and Gatherers." In *The Cambridge Encyclopedia of Hunters and Gatherers*, ed. Richard B. Lee and Richard Daly, 284–288. Cambridge, UK: Cambridge University Press, 1999.

Berkheiser, Kaitlyn. "9 Healthy Foods That Are Rich in Iodine." *Healthline*. February 2, 2018. Accessed June 2, 2019. https://www.healthline.com/nutrition/iodine-rich-foods.

Bernard, R. J. "Peasant Diet in Eighteenth-Century Gevaudan." In *European Diet from Pre-Industrial to Modern Times*, ed. Elborg Forster and Robert Forster, 19–46. New York: Harper Torchbooks, 1975.

Berry, Joanne. *The Complete Pompeii*. London: Thames and Hudson, 2007.

Bertman, Stephen. *Handbook to Life in Ancient Mesopotamia*. New York: Facts on File, 2003.

Betts, H. S. *Chestnut*. Washington, DC: U.S. Department of Agriculture, 1945.

Bevilacqua, Piero. "The Distinctive Character of Italian Environmental History." In *Nature and History in Modern Italy*, ed. Marco Armiero and Marcus Hall, 15–32. Athens: Ohio University Press, 2010.

Bhanoo, Sindya N. "Life Span of Early Man Same as Neanderthals'." *New York Times*. January 10, 2011. Accessed January 18, 2019. https://www.nytimes.com/2011/01/11/science/11obneanderthal.html.

Biello, David. "Climate Change Future Suggested by Looking Back 4 Million Years." *Scientific American*. April 3, 2013. Accessed January 17, 2019. https://blogs.scientificamerican.com/observations/climate-change-future-suggested-by-looking-back-4-million-years.

Biraben, Jean Noel. "Pasteur, Pasteurization, and Medicine." In *The Decline of Mortality in Europe*, ed. R. Schofield, D. Reher, and A. Bideau, 220–232. Oxford: Clarendon Press, 1991.

Bird-David, Nurit. "Introduction: South Asia." In *The Cambridge Encyclopedia of Hunters and Gatherers*, ed. Richard B. Lee and Richard Daly, 231–237. Cambridge, UK: Cambridge University Press, 2004.

Bisel, Sara C., and Jane F. Bisel. "Health and Nutrition at Herculaneum: An Examination of Human Skeletal Remains." In *The Natural History of Pompeii*, ed. Wilhelmina Feemster Jashemski and Frederick G. Meyer, 451–475. Cambridge, UK: Cambridge University Press, 2002.

"Bison vs. Beef—Which Red Meat Reigns Supreme?" *Onnit Labs*. August 24, 2016. Accessed February 7, 2019. www.onnit.com/academy/bison-vs-beef.

Bisson, Wilfred J. "Sixteenth-Century Demographic Catastrophes in Peru." In *World History Encyclopedia. Vol 11. Era 6: The First Global Age, 1450–1770*, ed. Alfred J. Andrea, Carolyn Neel, Dane A. Morrison, Alexander Mikaberidze, D. Harland Hagler, Jeffrey M. Diamond, and Monique Vallance, 48–50. Santa Barbara, CA: ABC-CLIO, 2011.

Biswas, Soutik. "How ChurCchill 'Starved' India." *BBC*. October 28, 2010. Accessed March 6, 2019. http://www.bbc.co.uk/blogs/thereporters/soutikbiswas/2010/10/how_churchill_starved_india.html.

Bjarnadottir, Adda. "Olives 101: Nutrition Facts and Health Benefits." *Healthline*. May 21, 2019. Accessed May 23, 2019. https://www.healthline.com/nutrition/foods/olives.

Blanning, Tim. *Frederick the Great: King of Prussia*. New York: Random House, 2016.

Blench, Roger, and Kevin C. MacDonald. "Chickens." In *The Cambridge World History of Food*. Vol. 1, ed. Kenneth F. Kiple and Kriemhild Conee Ornelas, 496–499. Cambridge, UK: Cambridge University Press, 2000.

Bloom, Olivia. "The Great Taste of Amish Country." *Ohio's Amish Country*, Winter 2018, 22–23.

Borushek, Allan. *The CalorieKing Calorie, Fat, and Carbohydrate Counter*. Huntington Beach, CA: Family Health Publications, 2019.

Boserup, Ester. "The Impact of Scarcity and Plenty on Development." *Journal of Interdisciplinary History* 14, no. 2 (Autumn 1983): 383–407.

Bowen, J. E., and D. L. Anderson. "Sugar-Cane Cropping Systems." In *Field Crop Ecosystems*, ed. C. J. Pearson, 143–165. Amsterdam: Elsevier, 1992.

Bower, Bruce. "Orangutans Use Simple Tools to Catch Fish." *Wired*. April 18, 2011. Accessed February 14, 2019. https://www.wired.com/2011/04/orangutan-tools-fishing.

Bowman, Bradley L. "Middle East, Relations with (Except Israel)." In *Postwar America: An Encyclopedia of Social, Political, Cultural, and Economic History*. Vol. 3, ed. James Ciment, 854–862. Armonk, NY: Sharpe Reference, 2007.

Bradford, Alina. "What Is Gluten?" *Live Science*. November 18, 2017. Accessed October 2, 2019. https://www.livescience.com/53265-what-is-gluten.html.

"Brain Size and Cultural Evolution." Accessed January 17, 2019. http://www.bradshawfoundation.com/origins/australopithecus_afarensis.php.

Braudel, Fernand. *Capitalism and Material Life, 1400–1800*, trans. Miriam Kochan. New York: Harper Colophon Books, 1973.

Braund, David. "Food among Greeks of the Black Sea: The Challenging Diet of Olbia." In *A Companion to Food in the Ancient World*, ed. John Wilkins and Robin Nadeau, 296–308. Malden, MA: Wiley Blackwell, 2015.

Bray, George A., Samara Joy Nielsen, and Barry M. Popkin. "Consumption of High-Fructose Corn Syrup in Beverages May Play a Role in the Epidemic of Obesity." *American Journal of Clinical Nutrition* 79, no. 4 (April 2004): 537–543. https://academic.oup.com/ajcn/article/79/4/537/4690128.

Brewer, Sarah. *Nutrition: A Beginner's Guide*. London: Oneworld, 2013.

Brier, Bob, and Hoyt Hobbs. *Ancient Egypt: Everyday Life in the Land of the Nile*. New York: Sterling, 2009.

Briggs, Jean L. "Sadlermiut Inuit." *The Canadian Encyclopedia*. March 1, 2012. Last modified March 4, 2015. Accessed February 24, 2019. https://www.thecanadianencyclopedia.ca/en/article/sadlermiut-inuit.

Brinkley, Alan. *American History: A Survey*. 2 vols. 9th ed. New York: McGraw-Hill, 1995.

Brock, William H. *The History of Chemistry: A Very Short Introduction*. Oxford: Oxford University Press, 2016.

Brouns, Fred J. P. H., Vincent J. van Buul, and Peter R. Shewry. "Does Wheat Make Us Fat and Sick?" *Journal of Cereal Science* 58, no. 2 (September 2013): 209–215. https://www.sciencedirect.com/science/article/pii/S0733521013000969#!.

Brown, Heather. "Good Question: Why Isn't Seafood Considered Meat?" CBS Minnesota. March 13, 2014. Accessed January 24, 2019. https://minnesota.cbslocal.com/2014/03/13/good-question-why-isnt-seafood-considered-meat.

Brown, Sanborn C. "Thompson, Benjamin (Count Rumford)." In *Dictionary of Scientific Biography*. Vol 13, ed. Charles Coulston Gillispie, 350–352. New York: Charles Scribner's Sons, 1981.

Brown, William H., Christopher S. Foote, and Brent L. Iverson. *Organic Chemistry*. 4th ed. Belmont, CA: Thomson Brooks/Cole, 2005.

Brumbaugh, Robert S. *The Philosophers of Greece*. Albany: State University of New York Press, 1981.

Brush, Mark. "Lake Erie Has 2% of the Water in the Great Lakes, but 50% of the Fish." *Michigan Radio*. November 5, 2013. Accessed February 14, 2019. http://www.michiganradio.org/post/lake-erie-has-2-water-great-lakes-50-fish.

Brush, Stephen G. *The History of Modern Science: A Guide to the Second Scientific Revolution, 1800–1950*. Ames: Iowa State University Press, 1988.

Bruso, Jessica. "What Fruit Has More Potassium than Bananas?" *SFGate*. Last modified November 19, 2018. Accessed January 26, 2020. https://healthyeating.sfgate.com/fruit-potassium-bananas-4738.html.

Bubel, Shawn. "Plant and Animal Domestication in the Ancient Near East." In *World History Encyclopedia. Vol 2. Era 1: Beginnings of Human Society*, ed. Mark Aldenderfer, 133–135. Santa Barbara, CA: ABC-CLIO, 2011.

Bunn, Henry T. "Meat Made Us Human." In *Evolution of the Human Diet: The Known, the Unknown, and the Unknowable*, ed. Peter S. Ungar, 191–211. Oxford and New York: Oxford University Press, 2007.

Burch, Ernest S. Jr., and Yvon Csonka. "The Caribou Inuit." In *The Cambridge Encyclopedia of Hunters and Gatherers*, ed. Richard B. Lee and Richard Daly, 56–60. Cambridge, UK: Cambridge University Press, 2004.

Burgan, Michael. *George Washington Carver: Scientist, Inventor, and Teacher*. Minneapolis, MN: Compass Point Books, 2007.

Burnett, John. *Plenty and Want: A Social History of Diet in England from 1815 to the Present Day*. London: Scolar Press, 1979.

Busch, Sandi. "Does the Skin of a Potato Really Have All the Vitamins?" *SF Gate*. November 27, 2018. Accessed October 14, 2019. https://healthyeating.sfgate.com/skin-potato-really-vitamins-5378.html.

Butt, C. M., and N. Salem Jr. "Fish and Fish Oil for the Aging Brain." In *Fish and Fish Oil in Health and Disease Prevention*, ed. Susan K. Raatz and Douglas M. Bibus, 143–158. Amsterdam: Academic Press, 2016.

Butterworth, Alex, and Ray Laurence. *Pompeii: The Living City*. New York: St. Martin's Press, 2005.

"C3, C4 and CAM Plants." *Biology Dictionary*. 2018. Accessed January 28, 2019. https://biologydictionary.net/c3-c4-cam-plants.

"Of Cabbages and Celts." *Texas A & M Agri Life Extension*. Accessed July 2, 2019. https://aggie-horticulture.tamu.edu/archives/parsons/publications/vegetabletravelers/cabbage.html.

Cairns, Huntington. "Introduction." In *Plato: The Collected Dialogues Including the Letters*, ed. Edith Hamilton and Huntington Cairns, xiii–xxv. Princeton, NJ: Princeton University Press, 1961.

"Calcium & pH." *Cheese Science Toolkit*. 2019. Accessed November 16, 2019. https://www.cheesescience.org/calcium.html.

Calder, Daniel. "Insect Harvesting: Edible Flies and Fly Larvae (Maggots) Pack a Nutritional Punch." *The Dietician's Guide to Eating Bugs*. 2018. Accessed March 13, 2019. https://www.secretsofsurvival.com/survival/insect-harvesting-flies.html.

Callaway, Ewen. "Seafood Gave Us the Edge on the Neanderthals." *New Scientist* (August 12, 2009). http://www.newscientist.com/article/dn17595-seafood-gave-us-the-edge-on-neanderthals.

"Calories Burned in 30 Minutes for People of Three Different Weights." *Harvard Medical School*. July 2004. Last modified August 13, 2018. Accessed May 30, 2019. https://www.health.harvard.edu/diet-and-weight-loss/calories-burned-in-30-minutes-of-leisure-and-routine-activities.

Campbell, T. Colin. *Whole: Rethinking the Science of Nutrition*. Dallas, TX: BenBella Books, 2013.

Campbell, T. Colin, and Thomas M. Campbell II. *The China Study*. Rev. ed. Dallas, TX: BenBella Books, 2016.

———. "'The Plant Paradox' by Steven Gundry MD—A Commentary." Center for Nutrition Studies. August 23, 2017. Accessed January 26, 2019. https://nutritionstudies.org/the-plant-paradox-by-steven-grundy-md-commentary.

Campisi, Jessica, and Brandon Griggs. "Nearly 100 Bodies Found at a Texas Construction Site Were Probably Black People Forced into Labor—after Slavery Ended." July 19, 2018. Accessed January 18, 2019. https://www.cnn.com/2018/07/18/us/bodies-found-construction-site-slavery-trnd/index.html.

Cannon, Aubrey. "Archaeology of North American Hunters and Gatherers." In *The Cambridge Encyclopedia of Hunters and Gatherers*, ed. Richard B. Lee and Richard Daly, 31–35. Cambridge, UK: Cambridge University Press, 2004.

Cantrell II, Phillip A. "Beer and Ale." In *The Cambridge World History of Food*. Vol. 1, ed. Kenneth F. Kiple and Kriemhild Conee Ornelas, 619–625. Cambridge, UK: Cambridge University Press, 2000.

Cardell, Nicholas Scott, and Mark Myron Hopkins. "The Effect of Milk Intolerance on the Consumption of Milk by Slaves in 1860." *Journal of Interdisciplinary History* 8, no. 3 (Winter 1978): 507–513.

Carney, Judith A., and Richard Nicholas Rosomoff. *In the Shadow of Slavery: Africa's Botanical Legacy in the Atlantic World*. Berkeley: University of California Press, 2009.

Carpenter, Kenneth J. "The History of Enthusiasm for Protein." *Journal of Nutrition* 116, no. 7 (July 1986): 1364–1370.

———. *The History of Scurvy and Vitamin C*. Cambridge, UK: Cambridge University Press, 1986.

Carr, Anitra C., and Balz Frei. "Toward a New Recommended Dietary Allowance for Vitamin C Based on Antioxidant and Health Effects in Humans." *The American Journal of Clinical Nutrition* 69, no. 6 (June 1, 1999): 1086–1107.

Carrington, Damian. "Insects Could Be the Key to Meeting Food Needs of Growing Global Population." *The Guardian*. July 31, 2010. Accessed January 16, 2019. https://www.theguardian.com/environment/2010/aug/01/insects-food-emissions.

Caseau, Beatrice. "Byzantium." In *A Companion to Food in the Ancient World*, ed. John Wilkins and Robin Nadeau, 365–376. Chichester, UK: Wiley Blackwell, 2015.

"Cassava's Link to Iodine Deficiency Requires Further Study." *Modern Ghana*. January 17, 2009. Accessed March 22, 2019. https://www.modernghana.com/news/198981/cassavas-link-to-iodine-deficiency-requires-further-study.html.

Casson, Lionel. *Everyday Life in Ancient Egypt*. Rev. ed. Baltimore and London: Johns Hopkins University Press, 2001.

Cato, Marcus Porcius. *On Agriculture*, trans. William Davis Hooper. Cambridge, MA: Harvard University Press, 1979.

Ceresa, Marco. "Milk and National Identity in China." In *Food and Identity in the Ancient World*, ed. Cristiano Grottanelli and Lucio Milano, 1–13. Padova: Sargon, 2004.

Chaline, Eric. *Fifty Animals that Changed the Course of History*. New York: Firefly Books, 2011.

Chambers, Mortimer, Raymond Grew, David Herlihy, Theodore K. Rabb, and Isser Woloch. *The Western Experience*. 2 vols. 4th ed. New York: Knopf, 1987.

Chandezon, Christophe. "Animals, Meat, and Alimentary By-Products: Patterns of Production." In *A Companion to Food in the Ancient World*, ed. John Wilkins and Robin Nadeau, 133–146. Chichester, UK: Wiley Blackwell, 2015.

Chang, Te-Tzu. "Rice." In *The Cambridge World History of Food*. Vol. 1, ed. Kenneth F. Kiple and Kriemhild Conee Ornelas, 132–149. Cambridge, UK: Cambridge University Press, 2000.

Chase, Robin. "Does Everyone in America Own a Car?" U.S. Department of State. March 2010. Accessed April 17, 2019. https://static.america.gov/uploads/sites/8/2016/04/You-Asked-Series_Does-Everyone-in-America-Own-a-Car_English_Lo-Res_508.pdf.

Chauhan, Parth. "Early Food Producers in the Indus Valley." In *World History Encyclopedia. Vol 2. Era 1: Beginnings of Human Society*, ed. Mark Aldenderfer, 138–140. Santa Barbara, CA: ABC-CLIO, 2011.

Cheng, Te-k'un. *The World of the Chinese: A Struggle for Human Unity*. Hong Kong: Chinese University Press, 1980.

"Chestnut Production." *World Mapper*. 2019. Accessed August 17, 2019. https://worldmapper.org/maps/chestnut-production–2016.

Childs, Veronica, and Laura Childs. *The Complete Low Carb, High Fat, No Hunger Diet: A User Manual for Our KetoHybrid Diet Constructed from the Best Practices of Low Carb, Ketogenic, & Paleo-Inspired Diets*. Delhi: Hula Books, 2014.

"Choose Sensibly." U.S. Department of Health and Human Services. Accessed June 1, 2019. https://health.gov/dietaryguidelines/dga2000/document/choose.htm.

Chung-Lee, Tan, and Elizabeth Schmermund. *Finland*. New York: Cavendish Square, 2017.

Ciarfella, A. T., L. J. Sivoli, and E. E. Perez. "Food Products Developed Using Cassava Roots and Its Derivatives: A Review." In *Cassava: Production, Nutritional Properties and Health Effects*, ed. Francis P. Molinari, 161–176. New York: Nova Publishers, 2014.

Ciciora, Phil. "Study: Surge in Obesity Correlates with Increased Automobile Usage." *Illinois News Bureau*. May 11, 2011. Accessed April 2, 2019. https://news.illinois.edu/view/6367/205328.

Civitello, Linda. *Cuisine and Culture: A History of Food and People*. 3rd ed. Hoboken, NJ: Wiley, 2011.

Clampitt, Cynthia. *Midwest Maize: How Corn Shaped the U.S. Heartland.* Urbana: University of Illinois Press, 2015.

Clark, Geri. *Finland: Enchantment of the World.* North Mankato, MN: Scholastic, 2019.

Clayton, Paul, and Judith Rowbotham. "How the Mid-Victorians Worked, Ate and Died." *International Journal of Environmental Research and Public Health* 6, no. 3 (March 2009): 1235–1253. https://www.ncbi.nlm.nih.gov/pmc/articles/PMC2672390.

Clement, Charles R. "Fruits." In *The Cultural History of Plants*, ed. Ghillean Prance and Mark Nesbitt, 77–96. New York and London: Routledge, 2005.

Coffman, Elesha. "What Is the Origin of the Christian Fish Symbol?" *Christianity Today*, 2019. Accessed February 26, 2019. https://www.christianitytoday.com/history/2008/august/what-is-origin-of-christian-fish-symbol.html.

Cohen, Mark Nathan. *The Food Crisis in Prehistory: Overpopulation and the Origins of Agriculture.* New Haven and London: Yale University Press, 1977.

———. *Health and the Rise of Civilization.* New Haven, CT and London: Yale University Press, 1989.

———. "History, Diet, and Hunter-Gatherers." In *The Cambridge World History of Food.* Vol. 1, ed. Kenneth F. Kiple and Kriemhild Conee Ornelas, 63–71. Cambridge, UK: Cambridge University Press, 2000.

Collins, Nathan. "Are Peanuts the Answer to Preventing Malnutrition in Africa?" February 10, 2016. Accessed July 2, 2019. https://psmag.com/social-justice/is-preventing-malnutrition-in-africa-as-easy-as-peanuts.

Compton, John S. *Human Origins: How Diet, Climate and Landscape Shaped Us.* Cape Town, South Africa: Earthspun Books, 2016.

Conroy, Glenn C. *Reconstructing Human Origins: A Modern Synthesis.* New York and London: Norton, 1997.

Cook, Rob. "Top 10 Largest Crops in the World." January 21, 2019. Accessed January 22, 2019. http://beef2live.com/story-top-10-largest-crops-world-0-142257.

Cordain, Loren. *The Paleo Diet: Lose Weight and Get Healthy by Eating the Foods You Were Designed to Eat.* Rev. ed. Hoboken, NJ: Wiley, 2011.

"Corn—October Grain of the Month." Whole Grains Council. Accessed April 12, 2019. https://wholegrainscouncil.org/whole-grains-101/easy-ways-enjoy-whole-grains/grain-month-calendar/corn-%E2%80%93-october-grain-month.

Cornford, F. M. *Before and After Socrates.* Cambridge, UK: Cambridge University Press, 1932.

"Countries Who Drink the Most Milk." *World Atlas.* 2019. Accessed March 17, 2019. https://www.worldatlas.com/articles/countries-who-drink-the-most-milk.html.

Coursey, D. G. *Yams: An Account of the Nature, Origins, Cultivation and Utilisation of the Useful Members of the Dioscoreaceae.* London: Longmans, 1967.

Cousteau, Jacques. *The Ocean World.* New York: Bradale Press/Harry N. Abrams, 1985.

"Cowpeas Facts and Health Benefits." *Health Benefits Times.* Accessed April 27, 2019. https://www.healthbenefitstimes.com/cowpeas.

Crampton, Liz. "USDA Changes Obama-Era School Lunch Rules, Citing 'Flexibility.'" *Politico.* January 17, 2020. Accessed January 18, 2020. https://www.politico.com/news/2020/01/17/school-lunch-rule-changes-100578.

"Cream—Types of Cream and Their Uses." *The Epicentre.* Accessed March 9, 2019. http://theepicentre.com/ingredient/cream-types-of-cream-and-their-uses.

Cummings, John, and Jim Mann. "Carbohydrates." In *Essentials of Human Nutrition*, ed. Jim Mann and A. Stewart Truswell, 13–39. 5th ed. Oxford: Oxford University Press, 2017.

Cumo, Christopher. *Science and Technology in 20th Century American Life.* Westport, CT and London: Greenwood Press, 2007.

"Current World Population." *Worldometers.* Accessed August 20, 2019. https://www.worldometers.info/world-population.

Currier, Russell W., and John A. Widness. "A Brief History of Milk Hygiene and Its Impact on Infant Mortality from 1875 to 1925 and Implications for Today: A Review." *Journal of Food Protection* 81, no. 10 (October 2018): 1713–1722. https://jfoodprotection.org/doi/full/10.4315/0362-028X.JFP–18–186.

Curtis, Kimberly M. "Du Bois, W. E. B." In *Encyclopedia of African American History.* Vol. 3, ed. Leslie M. Alexander and Walter C. Rucker, 746–748. Santa Barbara, CA: ABC-CLIO, 2010.

Cwiertka, Katarzyna J., and Akiko Moriya. "Fermented Soyfoods in South Korea: The Industrialization of Tradition." In *The World of Soy*, ed. Christine M. Du Bois, Chee-Beng Tan, and Sidney W. Mintz, 161–181. Urbana: University of Illinois Press, 2008.

Daley, Cynthia A., Amber Abbott, Patrick S. Doyle, Glenn A. Nader, and Stephanie Larson. "A Review of Fatty Acid Profiles and Antioxidant Content in Grass-Fed and Grain-Fed Beef." *Nutrition Journal* 9 (March 10, 2010), https://www.ncbi.nlm.nih.gov/pmc/articles/PMC2846864.

Daly, Richard. "Witsuwit'en and Gitxsau of the Western Cordillera." In *The Cambridge Encyclopedia of Hunters and Gatherers*, ed. Richard B. Lee and Richard Daly, 71–76. Cambridge, UK: Cambridge University Press, 2004.

Damas, David. "The Copper Eskimo." In *Hunters and Gatherers Today: A Socioeconomic Study of Eleven Such Cultures in the Twentieth Century*, ed. M. G. Bicchieri, 3–50. Prospect Heights, IL: Waveland Press, 1972.

Damron, W. Stephen. *Introduction to Animal Science: Global, Biological, Social, and Industry Perspectives*. 3rd ed. Upper Saddle River, NJ and Columbus, OH: Pearson/Prentice Hall, 2006.

Daniels, Patricia, Trisha Gura, Susan Tyler Hitchcock, Lisa Stein, and John Thompson. *The Body: A Complete User's Guide*. Rev. ed. Washington, DC: National Geographic, 2014.

Darmadi-Blackberry, Irene, Mark L. Wahlqvist, Antigone Kouris-Blazos, Bertil Steen, Widjaja Lukito, Yoshimitsu Horie, and Kazuyo Horie. "Legumes: The Most Important Dietary Predictor of Survival in Older People of Different Ethnicities." *Asia Pacific Journal of Clinical Nutrition* 13, no. 2 (2004): 217–220.

Dart, Raymond A. "The Predatory Transition from Ape to Man." *International Anthropological and Linguistic Review* 1, no. 4 (1953). http://www.users.miamioh.edu/erlichrd/350website/classrel/dart.html.

Darwin, Charles. *The Descent of Man, and Selection in Relation to Sex*. London: Penguin Books, 2004.

Da-shun, Guo. "Lower Xiajiadian Culture." In *The Archaeology of Northeast China: Beyond the Great Wall*, ed. Sarah Milledge Nelson, 147–181. London and New York: Routledge, 1995.

"Date." In *The Cambridge World History of Food*. Vol. 2, ed. Kenneth F. Kiple and Kriemhild Conee Ornelas, 1767–1768. Cambridge, UK: Cambridge University Press, 2000.

Davidson, Alan. "Europeans' Wary Encounter with Tomatoes, Potatoes, and Other New World Foods." In *Chilies to Chocolate: Food the Americas Gave the World*, ed. Nelson Foster and Linda S. Cordell, 1–14. Tucson and London: University of Arizona Press, 1992.

Davidson, James M., Jerome C. Rose, Myron P. Gutmann, Michael R. Haines, Keith Condon, and Cindy Condon. "The Quality of African-American Life in the Old Southwest Near the Turn of the Twentieth Century." In *The Backbone of History: Health and Nutrition in the Western Hemisphere*, ed. Richard H. Steckel and Jerome C. Rose, 226–277. Cambridge, UK: Cambridge University Press, 2002.

Davis, William. *Lose the Wheat, Lose the Weight!: Banish Your Wheat Belly, Feel Better than Ever, and Turbocharge Your Health*. Expanded ed. Emmaus, PA: Rodale, 2012.

———. *Wheat Belly: Lose the Wheat, Lose the Weight, and Find Your Path Back to Health*. Emmaus, PA: Rodale, 2011.

Day, John. "Forward." In *The Peasants of Languedoc*, Emmanuel Le Roy Ladurie, trans. John Day, ix–xii. Urbana: University of Illinois Press, 1974.

Decker, Fred. "Butter Fat vs. Milk Fat." *SFGate*. Last modified November 19, 2018. Accessed March 9, 2019. https://healthyeating.sfgate.com/butter-fat-vs-milk-fat-11424.html.

Deevey, Edward S. Jr. "The Human Population." *Scientific American* 203, no. 9 (September 1, 1960): 195–205.

De Foilart, Gene R. "Chapter 9: Western Attitudes toward Insects as Food: Europe, the United States, Canada." In *The Human Use of Insects as a Food Resource: A Bibliographic Account in Progress*. Last modified September 29, 2002. Accessed March 13, 2019. http://labs.russell.wisc.edu/insectsasfood/files/2012/09/Book_Chapter_9.pdf.

Delange, F., C. Thilly, P. Bourdoux, P. Hennart, P. Courtois, and A. M. Ermans. "Influence of Dietary Goitrogens during Pregnancy in Humans on Thyroid Function of the Newborn." In *Nutritional Factors Involved in the Goitrogenic Action of Cassava*, ed. F. Delange, F. B. Iteke, and A. M. Ermans, 40–50. Ottawa: International Development Research Centre, 1982.

Dethloff, Henry C. *A History of the American Rice Industry, 1685–1985*. College Station: Texas A & M University Press, 1988.

Dewey, Caitlin. "The Obscure Supreme Court Case That Decided Tomatoes Are Vegetables." *The Washington Post*, October 18, 2017. Accessed June 17, 2019. https://www.washingtonpost.com/news/wonk/wp/2017/10/18/the-obscure-supreme-court-case-that-decided-tomatoes-are-vegetables/?utm_term=.bf9a37460dee.

Diamond, Jared. "The Worst Mistake in the History of the Human Race." *Discover*, May 1, 1999. Accessed July 21, 2019. http://discovermagazine.com/1987/may/02-the-worst-mistake-in-the-history-of-the-human-race.

Dickel, David N., Peter D. Schulz, and Henry M. McHenry. "Central California: Prehistoric Subsistence Changes and Health." In *Paleopathology at the Origins of Agriculture*, ed. Mark Nathan Cohen and George J. Armelagos, 439–461. Orlando, FL: Academic Press, 1984.

Diffendal, R. F. Jr. *Great Plains Geology*. Lincoln and London: University of Nebraska Press, 2017.

Diller, Jesse D. *Chestnut Blight*. Washington, DC: U.S. Department of Agriculture, 1965.

Dillon, Conor. "Obese? Not Us! Why the Netherlands Is Becoming the Skinniest EU Country." *Deutsche Welle*. September 6, 2015. Accessed June 16, 2019. https://www.dw.com/en/obese-not-us-why-the-netherlands-is-becoming-the-skinniest-eu-country/a-18503808.

"Dining." *Ohio Amish Country Map and Visitors' Guide, 2019.*

Dixon, John A. "Consumption." In *The Cassava Economy of Java*, ed. Walter P. Falcon, William O. Jones, Scott R. Pearson, John A. Dixon, Gerald C. Nelson, Frederick C. Roche, and Laurian J. Unnevehr, 63–90. Stanford, CA: Stanford University Press, 1984.

Dizikes, Peter. "New Study Shows Rich, Poor Have Huge Mortality Gap in U.S." *MIT News*. April 11, 2016. http://news.mit.edu/2016/study-rich-poor-huge-mortality-gap-us-0411.

"Does Ghee Expire?" *The Times of India*. Last modified August 21, 2019. Accessed November 12, 2019. https://timesofindia.indiatimes.com/life-style/health-fitness/photo-stories/does-ghee-expire/photostory/60308368.cms.

Dolezal, Robert J. *Vegetable Gardening: Your Ultimate Guide*. Minnetonka, MN: Creating Publishing International, 2000.

Dolman, Claude E. "Spallanzani, Lazzaro." In *Dictionary of Scientific Biography*. Vol. 12, ed. Charles Coulston Gillispie, 553–567. New York: Charles Scribner's Sons, 1981.

Domett, Kathryn M. *Health in Late Prehistoric Thailand*. Oxford: Archaeopress, 2001.

Domett, Kathryn M., and Nancy Tayles. "Human Biology from the Bronze Age to the Iron Age in the Mun River Valley of Northeast Thailand." In *Bioarchaeology of Southeast Asia*, ed. Marc Oxenham and Nancy Tayles, 220–240. Cambridge, UK: Cambridge University Press, 2006.

Donahue, John F. "Roman Dining." In *A Companion to Food in the Ancient World*, ed. John Wilkins and Robin Nadeau, 253–264. Chichester, UK: Wiley Blackwell, 2015.

Donaldson, Blake F. *Strong Medicine*. Garden City, NY: Doubleday, 1962.

Donnelly, James S. Jr. *The Great Irish Potato Famine*. Gloucestershire: Sutton Publishing, 2001.

Dowd, Maureen. "'I'm President,' So No More Broccoli." *New York Times*, March 23, 1990. Accessed September 3, 2019. https://www.nytimes.com/1990/03/23/us/i-m-president-so-no-more-broccoli.html.

Drewnowski, Adam, and Victoria Warren-Mears. "Role of Taste and Appetite in Body Weight Regulation." in *Nutrition in the Prevention and Treatment of Disease*, ed. Ann M. Coulston, Cheryl L. Rock, and Elaine R. Monsen, 539–548. San Diego: Academic Press, 2001.

Drummond, J. C., and Anne Wilbraham. *The Englishman's Food: A History of Five Centuries of English Diet*. Rev. ed. London: Pimlico, 1991.

Dubisch, Jill. "Low Country Fevers: Cultural Adaptations to Malaria in Antebellum South Carolina." *Social Science and Medicine* 21, no. 6 (February 1985): 641–649.

Du Bois, Christine M. "Social Context and Diet: Changing Soy Production and Consumption in the United States." In *The World of Soy*, ed. Christine M. Du Bois, Chee-Beng Tan, and Sidney W. Mintz, 208–233. Urbana: University of Illinois Press, 2008.

———. *The Story of Soy*. London: Reaktion Books, 2018.

Dubour, Darna L., and Richard L. Bender. "Nutrition Transitions: A View from Anthropology." In *Nutritional Anthropology: Biocultural Perspectives on Food and Nutrition*. 2nd. ed., ed. Darna L. Dufour, Alan H. Goodman, and Gretel H. Pelto, 372–382. New York and Oxford: Oxford University Press, 2013.

Duignan, Brian, ed. *Economics and Economic Systems*. New York: Britannica, 2013.

Dunn, Frederick L. "Beriberi." In *The Cambridge World History of Food*. Vol. 1, ed. Kenneth F. Kiple and Kriemhild Conee Ornelas, 914–919. Cambridge, UK: Cambridge University Press, 2000.

Dunn, Richard S. *Sugar and Slaves: The Rise of the Planter Class in the English West Indies, 1624–1713*. Chapel Hill: University of North Carolina Press, 1972.

Dupont, Jacqueline L. "Essential Fatty Acids." In *The Cambridge World History of Food*. Vol. 1, ed. Kenneth F. Kiple and Kriemhild Conee Ornelas, 876–882. Cambridge, UK: Cambridge University Press, 2000.

Durham, Sharon. "Nuts for Calories!" Last modified March 22, 2018. Accessed January 23, 2019. https://www.ars.usda.gov/news-events/news/research-news/2018/nuts-for-calories.

Early, John D., and John F. Peters. *The Xilixana Yanomami of the Amazon: History, Social Structure, and Population Dynamics*. Gainesville: University Press of Florida, 2000.

"Early Modern Humans Consumed More Plants than Neanderthals But Ate Very Little Fish." *Phys.org*. August 8, 2017. Accessed February 14, 2019. https://phys.org/news/2017-08-early-modern-humans-consumed-neanderthals.html.

Eaton, Louise, and Kara Rogers, ed. *Examining Basic Chemical Molecules*. New York: Britannica, 2018.

Eaton, S. Boyd, and Melvin Konner. "Paleolithic Nutrition: A Consideration of Its Nature and Current Implications." In *Nutritional Anthropology: Biocultural Perspectives on Food and Nutrition*. 2nd ed., ed. Darna L. Dufour, Alan H. Goodman, and Gretel H. Pelto, 51–59. New York and Oxford: Oxford University Press, 2013.

Eaton, S. Boyd, and Stanley B. Eaton III. "Hunter-Gatherers and Human Health." In *The Cambridge Encyclopedia of Hunters and Gatherers*, ed. Richard B. Lee and Richard Daly, 449–456. Cambridge, UK: Cambridge University Press, 2004.

Echenberg, Myron. *Africa in the Time of Cholera: A History of Pandemics from 1817 to the Present.* Cambridge, UK: Cambridge University Press, 2011.

"Economy GDP Per Capita in 1900: Countries Compared." *Nation Master.* 2003–2019. Accessed February 10, 2019. https://www.nationmaster.com/country-info/stats/Economy/GDP-per-capita-in-1900.

Eder, James F. "The Batak of Palawan Island, the Philippines." In *The Cambridge Encyclopedia of Hunters and Gatherers*, ed. Richard B. Lee and Richard Daly, 294–297. Cambridge, UK: Cambridge University Press, 2004.

The Editors. "Introduction." In *The Cambridge World History of Food.* Vol. 1, ed. Kenneth F. Kiple and Kriemhild Conee Ornelas, 1–10. Cambridge, UK: Cambridge University Press, 2000.

The Editors of Encyclopaedia Britannica. "Mustard: Plant, Vegetable, and Condiment." *Encyclopaedia Britannica.* Last modified January 10, 2020. Accessed January 17, 2020. https://www.britannica.com/plant/mustard.

Eenfeldt, Andreas. *Low Carb, High Fat Food Revolution: Advice and Recipes to Improve Your Health and Reduce Your Weight*, trans. Viktoria Lindback. New York: Skyhorse Publishing, 2014.

"Egyptian Mummies." Smithsonian Institution. Accessed January 31, 2019. www.si.edu/spotlight/ancient-egypt/mummies.

Ellis, Hattie. *Sweetness and Light: The Mysterious History of the Honeybee.* New York: Harmony Books, 2004.

Emerson, Shaney, and Michelle Risso, ed. "Edible Plant Parts." California Foundation for Agriculture in the Classroom. September 2013. Accessed July 24, 2019. http://agritech.tnau.ac.in/horticulture/Ediple%20Plant%20Parts.pdf.

Engels, Frederick. "Preface." In *Communist Manifesto*, Karl Marx and Friedrich Engels, trans. Samuel Moore, 1–6. Chicago: Great Books Foundation, 1955.

Epictetus. *Discourses: Selections*, trans. P. E. Matheson. Chicago: Great Books Foundation, 1955.

Erlichson, Herman. "Mechanics and Thermodynamics." In *History of Modern Science and Mathematics.* Vol 3, ed. Brian S. Baigrie, 160–183. New York: Charles Scribner's Sons, 2002.

Eschbach, Karl. "Longevity." In *Encyclopedia of Health & Aging*, ed. Kyriakos S. Markides, 330–332. Los Angeles: SAGE Reference, 2007.

Essig, Frederick B. *Plant Life: A Brief History.* Oxford: Oxford University Press, 2015.

Estes, E. A. "Marketing Sweetpotatoes in the United States: A Serious Challenge for Small-to-Moderate Volume Growers." In *The Sweetpotato*, ed. Gad Loebenstein and George Thottappilly, 269–283. Dordrecht: Springer, 2009.

Eyres, Laurence. "Fats and Oils." In *Essentials of Human Nutrition*, ed. Jim Mann and A. Stewart Truswell, 292–296. 5th ed. Oxford: Oxford University Press, 2017.

Ezzo, Joseph A. *Human Adaptation at Grasshopper Pueblo, Arizona.* Ann Arbor, MI: International Monographs in Prehistory, 1993.

"The Facts about Bleach." *Clorox.* 2015. Accessed March 23, 2019. http://factsaboutbleach.com/clorox_history.html.

Fagan, Brian. *Fishing: How the Sea Fed Civilization.* New Haven, CT and London: Yale University Press, 2017.

———. *The Great Warming: Climate Change and the Rise and Fall of Civilizations.* New York: Bloomsbury Press, 2008.

"FAQs: 100% OJ and Sugar." Florida Department of Citrus. Accessed May 22, 2019. https://www.floridacitrus.org/newsroom/citrus-411/100-juice-and-sugar/faqs-100-oj-and-sugar.

Farb, Peter. *Ecology.* New York: Time, 1963.

Farvin, K. H. Sabeena, A. Surendraraj, and Charlotte Jacobsen. "Composition and Health Benefits of Potato Peel." In *Potatoes: Production, Consumption and Health Benefits*, ed. Claudio Caprara, 195–228. New York: Nova Science Publishers, 2012.

"Fashion History Timeline, 1790–1799." State University of New York. 2020. Accessed March 9, 2020. https://fashionhistory.fitnyc.edu/1790–1799.

"Fat: What You Need to Know." Cleveland Clinic. November 28, 2014. Accessed June 1, 2019. https://my.clevelandclinic.org/health/articles/11208-fat-what-you-need-to-know.

"Fat to Fit: How Finland Did It." *The Guardian*, January 15, 2005. Accessed March 17, 2019. https://www.theguardian.com/befit/story/0,15652,1385645,00.html.

Fauve-Chamoux, Antoinette. "Chestnuts." In *The Cambridge World History of Food.* Vol. 1, ed. Kenneth F. Kiple and Kriemhild Conee Ornelas, 359–364. Cambridge, UK: Cambridge University Press, 2000.

"FDA Vitamins and Minerals Chart." *FDA*. Accessed April 24, 2019. https://www.accessdata.fda.gov/scripts/interactivenutritionfactslabel/factsheets/vitamin_and_mineral_chart.pdf.

Feit, Harvey A. "James Bay Cree." In *The Cambridge Encyclopedia of Hunters and Gatherers*, ed. Richard B. Lee and Richard Daly, 41–45. Cambridge, UK: Cambridge University Press, 2004.

Fernandes, L. C. "Fish Intake and Strength in the Elderly." In *Fish and Fish Oil in Health and Disease Prevention*, ed. Susan K. Raatz and Douglas M. Bibus, 137–142. Amsterdam: Academic Press, 2016.

"Fernando's Hideaway." *SNL Transcripts Tonight*. October 8, 2018. Accessed August 31, 2019. https://snltranscripts.jt.org/84/84dfernando.phtml.

Ferris, Marcie Cohen. *The Edible South: The Power of Food and the Making of an American Region*. Chapel Hill: University of North Carolina Press, 2014.

Field, Henry. *Arabs of Central Iraq: Their Habits, Ethnology, and Physical Characteristics*. Chicago: Field Museum of Natural History, 1935.

"Fig." Purdue University. July 11, 2019. Accessed July 11, 2019. https://hort.purdue.edu/newcrop/morton/fig.html.

Figueroa-Mendez, Rodrigo, and Selva Rivas-Arancibia. "Vitamin C in Health and Disease: Its Role in the Metabolism of Cells and Redox States in the Brain." *Frontiers in Physiology* 6 (December 23, 2015). https://www.ncbi.nlm.nih.gov/pmc/articles/PMC4688356.

Fixx, James F. *The Complete Book of Running*. New York: Random House, 1977.

Flandrin, Jean-Louis. "Introduction: The Early Modern Period." In *Food: A Culinary History from Antiquity to the Present*, Jean-Louis Flandrin and Massimo Montanari, trans. Clarissa Botsford, Arthur Goldhammer, Charles Lambert, Frances M. Lopez-Morillas, and Sylvia Stevens, 349–373. New York: Columbia University Press, 1999.

Floud, Roderick. "Medicine and the Decline of Mortality: Indicators of Nutritional Status." In *The Decline of Mortality in Europe*, ed. R. Schofield, D. Reher, and A. Bideau, 146–157. Oxford: Clarendon Press, 1991.

Floud, Roderick, Kenneth Wachter, and Annabel Gregory. *Height, Health and History: Nutritional Status in the United Kingdom, 1750–1980*. Cambridge, UK: Cambridge University Press, 1990.

Fogel, Robert William. *The Escape from Hunger and Premature Death, 1700–2100: Europe, America, and the Third World*. Cambridge, UK: Cambridge University Press, 2004.

———. "Nutrition and the Decline in Mortality Since 1700: Some Preliminary Findings." In *Long-Term Factors in American Economic Growth*, ed. Stanley L. Engerman and Robert E. Gallman, 439–556. Chicago: University of Chicago Press, 1985.

Fogel, Robert William, and Stanley L. Engerman. *Time on the Cross: The Economics of American Negro Slavery*. New York and London: Norton, 1995.

Fogel, Robert William, Stanley L. Engerman, Roderick Floud, Gerald Friedman, Robert A. Margo, Kenneth Sokoloff, Richard H. Steckel, T. James Trussell, Georgia Villaflor, and Kenneth W. Wachter. "Secular Changes in American and British Stature and Nutrition." *Journal of Interdisciplinary History* 14, no. 2 (Autumn 1983): 445–481.

Food and Agriculture Organization. *The State of World Fisheries and Aquaculture*. Rome: Food and Agriculture Organization of the United Nations, 2018.

"Food Stores." *Ohio Amish Country Map and Visitors' Guide, 2019.*

Foster, Meika. "Vegetables." In *Essentials of Human Nutrition*, ed. Jim Mann and A. Stewart Truswell, 282–284. 5th ed. Oxford: Oxford University Press, 2017.

Freeman, Joshua, Nelson Lichtenstein, Stephen Brier, David Bensman, Susan Porter Brundage, Bret Eynon, Bruce Levine, and Bryan Palmer. *Who Built America?: Working People and the Nation's Economy, Politics, Culture, and Society*. 2 vols. New York: Pantheon Books, 1992.

Freinkel, Susan. *American Chestnut: The Life, Death, and Rebirth of a Perfect Tree*. Berkeley: University of California Press, 2007.

Friborg, Jeppe T., and Mads Melbye. "Cancer Patterns in Inuit Populations." *Lancet Oncology* 9, no. 9 (September 1, 2008): 892–900.

Fussell, Betty. *The Story of Corn*. New York: Knopf, 1992.

Galinat, Walton C. "Maize: Gift from America's First Peoples." In *Chilis to Chocolate: Food the Americas Gave the World*, ed. Nelson Foster and Linda S. Cordell, 47–60. Tucson and London: University of Arizona Press, 1992.

Gallacci, Caroline. "Driven to Extinction—The North American Fur Trade." In *World History Encyclopedia. Vol 11. Era 6: The First Global Age, 1450–1770*, ed. Alfred J. Andrea, Carolyn Neel, Dane A. Morrison, Alexander Mikaberidze, D. Harland Hagler, Jeffrey M. Diamond, and Monique Vallance, 63–65. Santa Barbara, CA: ABC-CLIO, 2011.

Galloway, J. H. "Sugar." In *The Cambridge World History of Food*. Vol. 1, ed. Kenneth F. Kiple and Kriemhild Conee Ornelas, 437–449. Cambridge, UK: Cambridge University Press, 2000.

Gander, Kashmira. "Japan's High Life Expectancy Linked to Diet, Study Finds." *Independent*. March 28, 2016. Accessed February 16, 2019. https://www.independent.co.uk/life-style/health-and-families/health-news/high-life-expectancy-in-japan-partly-down-to-diet-carbohydrates-vegetables-fruit-fish-meat-a6956011.html.

Garden-Robinson, Julie, and Krystle McNeal. "All about Beans: Nutrition, Health Benefits, Preparation and Use in Menus." North Dakota State University. February 2018. Accessed April 27, 2019. https://www.ag.ndsu.edu/publications/food-nutrition/all-about-beans-nutrition-health-benefits-preparation-and-use-in-menus#section-0.

Garnsey, Peter. *Food and Society in Classical Antiquity*. Cambridge, UK: Cambridge University Press, 1999.

Gartside D. F., and I. R. Kirkegaard. "A History of Fishing." *UNESCO*. Accessed December 7, 2019. https://www.eolss.net/sample-chapters/C10/E5-01A-03-00.pdf.

"Gateway to Dairy Production and Products." Food and Agriculture Organization of the United Nations. 2019. Accessed March 13, 2019. http://www.fao.org/dairy-production-products/products/milk-composition/en.

Geison, Gerald L. "Pasteur, Louis." In *Dictionary of Scientific Biography*. Vol. 10, ed. Charles Coulston Gillispie, 350–416. New York: Charles Scribner's Sons, 1981.

Germer, Renate. *Mummies: Life after Death in Ancient Egypt*. Munich and New York: Prestel, 1997.

Giesey, Ralph E. "Rules of Inheritance and Strategies of Mobility in Prerevolutionary France." *American Historical Review* 82, no. 2 (April 1977): 271–289.

Gifford, Edward Winslow. "Californian Anthropometry." In *University of California Publications in American Archaeology and Ethnology*, ed. A. L. Kroeber and Robert H. Lowie, 217–390. Berkeley: University of California Press, 1965.

"Global Meat Production and Consumption Continue to Rise." Worldwatch Institute. Last modified January 26, 2019. Accessed January 26, 2019. http://www.worldwatch.org/global-meat-production-and-consumption-continue-rise.

Glowacki, Donna M. *Living and Leaving: A Social History of Regional Depopulation in Thirteenth-Century Mesa Verde*. Tucson: University of Arizona Press, 2015.

Godber, J. Samuel. "Nutritional Value of Muscle Foods." In *Muscle Foods: Meat, Poultry, and Seafood Technology*, ed. Donald M. Kinsman, Anthony W. Kotula, and Burdette C. Breidenstein, 430–455. New York and London: Chapman and Hall, 1994.

Golson, Jack. "The Making of the New Guinea Highlands." in *The Melanesian Environment*, ed. John H. Winslow, 45–56. Canberra: Australian National University Press, 1977.

Gonzales, Doreen. *The Huge Pacific Ocean*. Berkeley Heights, NJ: Enslow, 2013.

Good, Kenneth. "The Yanomami: Tropical Forest Dwellers of Venezuela and Brazil." In *Faces of the Rainforest: The Yanomami*, ed. Valdir Cruz, 126–130. New York: PowerHouse Books, 2002.

Goodman, Alan H., and Debra L. Martin. "Reconstructing Health Profiles from Skeletal Remains." In *The Backbone of History: Health and Nutrition in the Western Hemisphere*, ed. Richard H. Steckel and Jerome C. Rose, 11–60. Cambridge, UK: Cambridge University Press, 2002.

Gould, Stephen Jay. *Eight Little Piggies: Reflections in Natural History*. New York and London: Norton, 1993.

———. *Hen's Teeth and Horse's Toes: Further Reflections in Natural History*. New York and London: Norton, 1983.

———. *The Panda's Thumb: More Reflections in Natural History*. New York and London: Norton, 1980.

"Grain: World Markets and Trade." U.S. Department of Agriculture. December 11, 2018. Last modified December 21, 2018. Accessed January 23, 2019. https://www.fas.usda.gov/data/grain-world-markets-and-trade.

"GrainsCompared2017_SR28." Whole Grains Council. Accessed April 14, 2019. https://wholegrainscouncil.org/whole-grains-101/health-studies-health-benefits/compare-nutrients-various-grains.

Granados, Jose A. Tapia, and Ana V. Diez Roux. "Life and Death during the Great Depression." *Proceedings of the National Academy of Sciences* 106, no. 41 (October 13, 2009): 17290–17295. https://www.ncbi.nlm.nih.gov/pmc/articles/PMC2765209.

Grant, Michael. *Cities of Vesuvius: Pompeii and Herculaneum*. London: Phoenix Press, 2005.

"Grapefruit Juice and Some Drugs Don't Mix." *FDA*. July 18, 2017. Accessed September 10, 2019. https://www.fda.gov/consumers/consumer-updates/grapefruit-juice-and-some-drugs-dont-mix.

Gratzer, Walter. *Terrors of the Table: The Curious History of Nutrition*. Oxford and New York: Oxford University Press, 2005.

Green, Elise. "Exporting Obesity: Micronesia as a Microcosm." Center for Strategic and International Studies. 2019. Accessed June 13, 2019. https://www.csis.org/npfp/exporting-obesity-micronesia-microcosm.

Green, Stephanie. *Optimum Nutrition*. New York: Alpha, 2015.

Gremillion, Kristen J. *Ancestral Appetites: Food in Prehistory*. New York: Cambridge University Press, 2011.

Griffin, Andrew. "Eva Ekblad: The Woman Who Brought Potatoes, Flour and Alcohol to the People." *Independent*. July 10, 2017. Accessed January 4, 2020. https://www.independent.co.uk/news/science/eva-ekblad-potato-flour-alcohol-potatoes-google-doodle-swedish-scientist-starch-a7832911.html.

Griffiths, J. Gwyn. "Hecataeus and Herodotus on 'a Gift of the River'." *Journal of Near Eastern Studies* 25, no. 1 (January 1966): 57–61.

Gudger, E. W. "Fishing with Spider's Webs." *Scientific American Supplement* 87, no. 2253 (March 8, 1919): 149–150.

Guggenheim, Karl Y. *Nutrition and Nutritional Diseases: The Evolution of Concepts*. Lexington, MA and Toronto: D. C. Health, 1981.

Gundry, Steven R. *The Plant Paradox: The Hidden Dangers in 'Healthy' Foods that Cause Disease and Weight Gain*. New York: Harper Wave, 2017.

Gurven, Michael, and Hillard Kaplan. "Longevity among Hunter-Gatherers: A Cross-Cultural Examination." *Population and Development Review* 33, no. 2 (June 2007): 1–73. https://www.academia.edu/17979487/Longevity_Among_Hunter-_Gatherers_A_Cross-Cultural_Examination?auto=download.

Haines, Michael R. and Richard H. Steckel, eds. *A Population History of North America*. Cambridge, UK and New York: Cambridge University Press, 2000.

Hales, Craig M., Margaret D. Carroll, Cheryl D. Fryar, and Cynthia L. Ogden. "Prevalence of Obesity among Adults and Youth: United States, 2015–2016." *NCHS Data Brief*. U.S. Department of Health and Human Services. October 2017. Accessed February 13, 2020. https://www.cdc.gov/nchs/data/databriefs/db288.pdf.

Hall, Marcus. "Environmental Imperialism in Sardinia: Pesticides and Politics in the Struggle against Malaria." In *Nature and History in Modern Italy*, ed. Marco Armiero and Marcus Hall, 70–88. Athens: Ohio University Press, 2010.

Hammons, R. O. "The Origin and History of the Groundnut." In *The Groundnut Crop: A Scientific Basis for Improvement*, ed. J. Smartt, 24–42. London: Chapman and Hall, 1994.

Hand, Carol. *The Evolution of Birds*. Minneapolis, MN: Essential Library, 2019.

———. *The Evolution of Fish*. Minneapolis, MN: ABDO Publishing, 2019.

Handler, Jerome S., and Robert S. Corruccini. "Plantation Slave Life in Barbados: A Physical Anthropological Analysis." *Journal of Interdisciplinary History* 14, no. 1 (Summer 1983): 65–90.

Hansen, J. D. L. "Protein-Energy Malnutrition." In *The Cambridge World History of Food*. Vol. 1, ed. Kenneth F. Kiple and Kriemhild Conee Ornelas, 977–988. Cambridge, UK: Cambridge University Press, 2000.

Hardy, Bruce L., and Marie-Helene Moncel. "Neanderthal Use of Fish, Mammals, Birds, Starchy Plants and Wood 125–250,000 Years Ago." *Plos One* 6, no. 8 (August 24, 2011). http://doi.org/10.1371/journal.pone.0023768

Harlan, Jack R. *Crops and Man*. 2nd ed. Madison, WI: American Society of Agronomy, Crop Science Society of America, 1992.

Harper, Alfred E. "Recommended Dietary Allowances and Dietary Guidance." In *The Cambridge World History of Food*. Vol. 2, ed. Kenneth F. Kiple and Kriemhild Conee Ornelas, 1606–1621. Cambridge, UK: Cambridge University Press, 2000.

Harrington, John. "From Bahrain to Qatar: These Are the 25 Richest Countries in the World." *USA Today*, November 28, 2018. Accessed May 29, 2019. https://www.usatoday.com/story/money/2018/11/28/richest-countries-world-2018-top-25/38429481.

Harris, Bernard. "Height and Nutrition." In *The Cambridge World History of Food*. Vol. 2, ed. Kenneth F. Kiple and Kriemhild Conee Ornelas, 1427–1438. Cambridge, UK: Cambridge University Press, 2000.

Harris, David R. "Origins and Spread of Agriculture." In *The Cultural History of Plants*, ed. Ghillean Prance and Mark Nesbitt, 13–26. New York and London: Routledge, 2005.

Haslam, D. "Weight Management in Obesity—Past and Present." *International Journal of Clinical Practice* 70, no. 3 (February 26, 2016): 206–217. https://www.ncbi.nlm.nih.gov/pmc/articles/PMC4832440.

Hathaway, Milicent L. "Trends in Heights and Weights." In *Yearbook of Agriculture, 1959*, ed. Alfred Stefferud, 181–185. Washington, DC: GPO, 1959. https://naldc.nal.usda.gov/download/IND43861419/PDF.

Haytowitz, David B., and Ruth H. Matthews. *Composition of Foods: Legume and Legume Products: Raw, Processed, Prepared*. Washington, DC: USDA, 1986.

"Healthiest Countries 2019." *World Population Review*. Accessed March 18, 2019. http://worldpopulationreview.com/countries/healthiest-countries.

Heini's. Millersburg, OH.

Heizer, Robert F., and Carol Treanor. "Observations on Physical Strength of Some Western Indians and 'Old American' Whites." In *Two Papers on the Physical Anthropology of California Indians*, 47–57. Berkeley, CA: Archaeological Research Facility, 1974.

Hellemans, Alexander. "What Did Ancient Egyptians Really Eat?" *Inside Science*. May 8, 2014. Accessed January 27, 2019. https://www.insidescience.org/news/what-did-ancient-egyptians-really-eat.

Helm, June. "The Dogrib Indians." In *Hunters and Gatherers Today: A Socioeconomic Study of Eleven Such Cultures in the Twentieth Century*, ed. M. G. Bicchieri, 51–89. Prospect Heights, IL: Waveland Press, 1972.

Helm, June, and Thomas D. Andrews. "Tlicho (Dogrib)." *The Canadian Encyclopedia*. August 6, 2009. Last modified March 4, 2015. Accessed February 21, 2019. https://www.thecanadianencyclopedia.ca/en/article/tlicho-dogrib.

Patrick, Henderson, J., and Dellie Rex. *About Wine*. 2nd ed. Cifton Park, NY: Delmar/Cengage Learning, 2012.

Hennart, P., P. Bourdoux, R. Lagasse, C. Thilly, G. Putzeys, P. Courtois, H. L. Vis, Y. Yunga, P. Seghers, and F. Delange. "Epidemiology of Goitre and Malnutrition and Dietary Supplies of Iodine, Thiocyanate, and Proteins in Bas Zaire, Kivu, and Ubangi." In *Nutritional Factors Involved in the Goitrogenic Action of Cassava*, ed. F. Delange, F. B. Iteke, and A. M. Ermans, 25–33. Ottawa: International Development Research Centre, 1982.

Hennessy, Kathryn, ed. *Smithsonian Natural History: The Ultimate Visual Guide to Everything on Earth*. New York: DK, 2010.

Herzberg, Guillaume, and Raoul Perrot. "Paleopathologie de 31 Cranes Egyptiens Momifies du Museum d'Histoire Naturelle de Lyon." *Paleobios* 1, no. 1–2 (1983): 91–108.

Hewings-Martin, Yella. "Does Magnesium Hold the Key to Vitamin D Benefits?" *Medical News Today*. December 30, 2018, accessed October 11, 2019. https://www.medicalnewstoday.com/articles/324022.php.

Hewitt, Nancy A., and Steven F. Lawson. *Exploring American Histories: A Brief Survey with Sources*. Boston and New York: Bedford/St. Martin's, 2013.

Higgins, Rosanne L., Michael R. Haines, Lorena Walsh, and Joyce E. Sirianni. "The Poor in the Mid-Nineteenth-Century Northeastern United States: Evidence from the Monroe County Almshouse, Rochester, New York." In *The Backbone of History: Health and Nutrition in the Western Hemisphere*, ed. Richard H. Steckel and Jerome C. Rose, 162–184. Cambridge, UK: Cambridge University Press, 2002.

Hill Kim, and A. Magdalena Hurtado. *Ache Life History: The Ecology of and Demography of a Foraging People*. New York: Aldine, 1996.

———. "The Ache of Paraguay." In *The Cambridge Encyclopedia of Hunters and Gatherers*, ed. Richard B. Lee and Richard Daly, 92–96. Cambridge, UK: Cambridge University Press, 2004.

Hillocks, Rory J. "Cassava in Africa." In *Cassava: Biology, Production and Utilization*, ed. R. J. Hillocks, J. M. Thresh, and A.C. Bellotti, 41–54. Wallingford, UK and New York: CABI Publishing 2002.

Hines, Nick. "Americans Eat Enough Burgers to Circle the Earth 32 Times Every Year." *Vinepair*. April 12, 2017. Accessed January 25, 2019. https://vinepair.com/cocktail-chatter/how-many-burgers-americans-eat-per-year.

"The History of Guggisberg Cheese." *Guggisberg Cheese*. 2019. Accessed March 14, 2019. https://www.babyswiss.com/history.

"History of the Potato." *Klondike Brands*. 2019. Accessed March 27, 2019. http://www.klondikebrands.com/potato-history.

Ho, Ping-ti. "The Introduction of American Food Plants into China." *American Anthropologist* 57, no. 2 (April 1955): 191–201. https://anthrosource.onlinelibrary.wiley.com/doi/pdf/10.1525/aa.1955.57.2.02a00020.

Hobbs, Thomas. *Leviathan*. Oxford: Oxford University Press, 1996.

Hobhouse, Henry. *Seeds of Change: Six Plants that Transformed Mankind*. New York: Shoemaker and Hoard, 2005.

Hoffman, Richard, and Mariette Gerber. *The Mediterranean Diet: Health and Science*. West Sussex, UK: Wiley-Blackwell, 2012.

Hofman, Jack L., and Russell W. Graham. "The Paleo-Indian Cultures of the Great Plains." In *Archaeology on the Great Plains*, ed. W. Raymond Wood, 87–139. Lawrence: University Press of Kansas, 1998.

Holmes, Thom. *Early Humans: The Pleistocene and Holocene Epochs*. New York: Chelsea House, 2009.

Holum, John R. *Organic and Biological Chemistry*. New York: Wiley, 1996.

"Hominid Species." *Talk Origins*. Last modified April 30, 2010. Accessed January 17, 2019. http://www.talkorigins.org/faqs/homs/species.html.

"*Homo habilis.*" Smithsonian National Museum of Natural History. Last modified August 24, 2018. Accessed January 17, 2019. http://humanorigins.si.edu/evidence/human-fossils/species/homo-habilis.

"*Homo rudolfensis.*" Smithsonian National Museum of Natural History. Last modified August 24, 2018. Accessed January 17, 2019. http://humanorigins.si.edu/evidence/human-fossils/species/homo-rudolfensis.

Hooton, Earnest Albert. *The Indians of Pecos Pueblo: A Study of Their Skeletal Remains.* New Haven, CT: Yale University Press, 1930.

Hopkins, F. Gowland. "Feeding Experiments Illustrating the Importance of Accessory Factors in Normal Dietaries." *Journal of Physiology* 44, no. 5–6 (July 15, 1912): 425–460.

"How Far Could an English War Bow Shoot?" *History Stack Exchange.* Accessed September 19, 2019. https://history.stackexchange.com/questions/8022/how-far-could-an-english-war-bow-shoot.

Howell, F. Clark. *Early Man.* New York: Time-Life Books, 1965.

Hufton, Olwen. "Social Conflict and the Grain Supply in Eighteenth-Century France." *Journal of Interdisciplinary History* 14, no. 2 (Autumn 1983): 303–331.

Hughes, Meredith Sayles. *Glorious Grasses: The Grains.* Minneapolis, MN: Lerner Publications, 1999.

———. *Spill the Beans and Pass the Peanuts: Legumes.* Minneapolis, MN: Lerner Publications, 1999.

Hughes, Meredith Sayles, and Tom Hughes. *Buried Treasure: Roots and Tubers.* Minneapolis, MN: Lerner Publications, 1998.

Hughes, R. E. "Scurvy." In *The Cambridge World History of Food.* Vol. 1, ed. Kenneth F. Kiple and Kriemhild Conee Ornelas, 988–1000. Cambridge, UK: Cambridge University Press, 2000.

———. "Vitamin C." In *The Cambridge World History of Food.* Vol. 1, ed. Kenneth F. Kiple and Kriemhild Conee Ornelas, 754–763. Cambridge, UK: Cambridge University Press, 2000.

Hurst, Charles E., and Daniel L. McConnell. *An Amish Paradox: Diversity and Change in the World's Largest Amish Community.* Baltimore: Johns Hopkins University Press, 2010.

Hymowitz, Theodore. "Soybeans: The Success Story." In *Advances in New Crops: Proceedings of the First National Symposium New Crops, Research, Development, Economics, Indianapolis, Indiana, October 23–26, 1988*, ed. Jules Janick and James E. Simon, 159–163. Portland, OR: Timber Press, 1990.

Hymowitz, Theodore, and Jack R. Harlan. "Introduction of the Soybean to North America by Samuel Bowen in 1765." *Economic Botany* 37, no. 4 (October 1983): 371–379.

Iannelli, Vincent. "What Is the Average Height for an Adult Woman?" *Verywellfit.com.* Last modified October 25, 2018. Accessed February 8, 2019. https://www.verywellfit.com/average-height-for-a-woman-statistics-2632136.

The Illustrated Encyclopedia of Fruits, Vegetables, and Herbs. New York: Chartwell Books, 2017.

"Improving America's Diet and Health: From Recommendations to Action." *National Academy of Sciences.* 1991. Accessed June 2, 2019. https://www.ncbi.nlm.nih.gov/books/NBK235267.

"Indigenous Peoples in Greenland." *IWGIA.* Accessed February 21, 2019. https://www.iwgia.org/en/greenland.

Infante, Benito, and Omar Garcia. "Cassava Bread (Casabe) in Venezuela: Some Nutritional Considerations." In *Cassava: Production, Nutritional Properties and Health Effects*, ed. Francis P. Molinari, 115–138. New York: Nova Publishers, 2014.

"International Year of the Potato." *FAO.* 2008. Accessed March 10, 2020. http://www.fao.org/potato-2008/en/potato/origins.html.

"Introduction." In *On Agriculture*, Marcus Porcius Cato, trans. William Davis Hooper and Harrison Boyd Ash. Cambridge, MA: Harvard University Press, 1967.

"Is Clarified Butter Healthy?" *Nutritious Life.* Accessed March 9, 2019. https://nutritiouslife.com/eat-empowered/clarified-butter-healthy.

Ishige, Naomichi. "Japan." In *The Cambridge World History of Food.* Vol. 2, ed. Kenneth F. Kiple and Kriemhild Conee Ornelas, 1175–1183. Cambridge, UK: Cambridge University Press, 2000.

Jackson, Alan A., and A. Stewart Truswell. "Protein." In *Essentials of Human Nutrition*, ed. Jim Mann and A. Stewart Truswell, 60–81. 5th ed. Oxford: Oxford University Press, 2017.

Jacobs, Bonnie F., John D. Kingston, and Louis L. Jacobs. "The Origin of Grass-Dominated Ecosystems." *Annals of the Missouri Botanical Garden* 86, no. 2 (Spring 1999): 590–643.

Jacobson, Andrew B. "Age of Industrialization and Agro-industry." In *The Cultural History of Plants*, ed. Ghillean Prance and Mark Nesbitt, 357–376. New York and London: Routledge, 2005.

Jacobson v. Massachusetts. 197 U.S. 11 (1905).

Jahns, L. "Fish Intake in the United States." In *Fish and Fish Oil in Health and Disease Prevention*, ed. Susan K. Raatz and Douglas M. Bibus, 1–11. Amsterdam: Elsevier, 2016.

"Japan, Basic Statistics." CGIAR. Ricepedia: The Online Authority on Rice. Accessed March 30, 2019. http://ricepedia.org/japan.

Jarcho, Saul. ed. *Human Palaeopathology*, ed. Saul Jarcho. New Haven, CT and London: Yale University Press, 1966.

Jarow, Gail. *Red Madness: How a Medical Mystery Changed What We Eat*. Honesdale, PA: Calkins Creek, 2014.

Jenike, Mark R. "Nutritional Ecology: Diet, Physical Activity and Body Size." In *Hunter-Gatherers: An Interdisciplinary Perspective*, ed. Catherine Panter-Brick, Robert H. Layton, and Peter Rowley-Conwy, 205–238. Cambridge, UK: Cambridge University Press, 2001.

Johansson, S. Ryan, and Douglas Owsley. "Welfare History on the Great Plains: Mortality and Skeletal Health, 1650 to 1900." In *The Backbone of History: Health and Nutrition in the Western Hemisphere*, ed. Richard H. Steckel and Jerome C. Rose, 524–560. Cambridge, UK: Cambridge University Press, 2002.

Johnson, Rachel K., Lawrence J. Appel, Michael Brands, Barbara V. Howard, Michael Lefevre, Robert H. Lustig, Frank Sacks, Lyn M. Steffen, and Judith Wylie-Rosett. "Dietary Sugar Intake and Cardiovascular Health." *Circulation* 120, no. 11 (September 15, 2009). https://www.ahajournals.org/doi/10.1161/CIRCULATIONAHA.109.192627

Johnson, Sylvia A. *Tomatoes, Potatoes, Corn, and Beans: How the Foods of the Americas Changed Eating around the World*. New York: Atheneum Books, 1997.

Johnston, Richard F. "Pigeons." In *The Cambridge World History of Food*. Vol. 1, ed. Kenneth F. Kiple and Kriemhild Conee Ornelas, 561–565. Cambridge, UK: Cambridge University Press, 2000.

Jones, Glenville. "Vitamin D." In *The Cambridge World History of Food*. Vol. 1, ed. Kenneth F. Kiple and Kriemhild Conee Ornelas, 763–768. Cambridge, UK: Cambridge University Press, 2000.

Jongman, Willem M. "The Early Roman Empire: Consumption." In *The Cambridge Economic History of the Greco-Roman World*, ed. Walter Scheidel, Ian Morris, and Richard P. Saller, 592–618. Cambridge, UK: Cambridge University Press, 2007.

Jurmain, Robert, Lynn Kilgore, Wenda Trevathan, and Russell L. Ciochon. *Introduction to Physical Anthropology*. 2013–2014 ed. Belmont, CA: Wadsworth Cengage Learning, 2014.

Justo, Graca, Eloy Macchiute de Oliveira, and Claudia Jurberg. "Functional Foods and Cancer on Pinterest and PubMed: Myths and Science." *Future Science OA* 4, no. 9 (August 9, 2018). https://www.ncbi.nlm.nih.gov/pmc/articles/PMC6225095.

Kalland, Arne, and Jon Pedersen. "Famine and Population in Fukuoka Domain during the Tokugawa Period." *Journal of Japanese Studies* 10, no. 1 (Winter 1984): 31–72.

Kaplan, Lawrence. "Beans, Peas, and Lentils." In *The Cambridge World History of Food*. Vol. 1, ed. Kenneth F. Kiple and Kriemhild Conee Ornelas, 271–281. Cambridge, UK: Cambridge University Press, 2000.

———. "Legumes in the History of Human Nutrition." In *The World of Soy*, ed. Christine M. Du Bois, Chee-Beng Tan, and Sidney W. Mintz, 27–44. Urbana: University of Illinois Press, 2008.

Kaplan, Lawrence, and Lucille N. Kaplan. "Beans of the Americas." In *Chilies to Chocolate: Food the Americas Gave the World*, ed. Nelson Foster and Linda S. Cordell, 61–80. Tucson and London: University of Arizona Press, 1992.

Karasch, Mary. "Manioc." In *The Cambridge World History of Food*. Vol. 1, ed. Kenneth F. Kiple and Kriemhild Conee Ornelas, 181–187. Cambridge, UK: Cambridge University Press, 2000.

Kawasaki, Yohei, Yu Tanaka, Keisuke Katsura, Larry C. Purcell, and Tatsuhiko Shiraiwa. "Yield and Dry Matter Productivity of Japanese and U.S. Soybean Cultivars." *Plant Production Science* 19, no. 2 (2016): 257–266. https://www.tandfonline.com/doi/full/10.1080/1343943X.2015.1133235.

Keith, Arthur. "Arabs of Central Iraq: Introduction." *Arabs of Central Iraq: Their Habits, Ethnology, and Physical Characteristics*, ed. Henry Field, 11–76. Chicago: Field Museum of Natural History, 1935.

Kellner, Corina M., Margaret Schoeninger, Katherine A. Spielmann, and Katherine Moore. "Stable Isotope Data Show Temporal Stability in Diet at Pecos Pueblo and Diet Variation among Southwest Pueblos." In *Pecos Pueblo Revisited: The Biological and Social Context*, ed. Michele E. Morgan, 79–92. Cambridge, MA: Peabody Museum of Archaeology and Ethnology, Harvard University, 2010.

Kellogg, Elizabeth A. "Evolutionary History of the Grasses." *Plant Physiology*, March 2001. Accessed March 4, 2020. http://www.plantphysiol.org/content/125/3/1198#ref-21.

Kemp, Barry, Anna Stevens, Gretchen R. Dabbs, Melissa Zabecki, and Jerome C. Rose. "Life, Death and beyond in Akhenaten's Egypt: Excavating the South Tombs Cemetery at Amarna." *Antiquity* 87, no. 335 (March 1, 2013): 64–78.

Kent, Susan. "Iron Deficiency and Anemia of Chronic Diseases." In *The Cambridge World History of Food*. Vol. 1, ed. Kenneth F. Kiple and Kriemhild Conee Ornelas, 919–939. Cambridge, UK: Cambridge University Press, 2000.

Kerrigan, Michael. *Ancient Rome and the Roman Empire*. London: Dorling Kindersley, 2001.

Keys, Ancel. *Seven Countries: A Multivariate Analysis of Death and Coronary Heart Disease*. Cambridge, MA and London: Harvard University Press, 1980.

Killgrove, Kristina. "Ancient DNA Explains How Chickens Got to the Americas." *Forbes*, November 23, 2017. Accessed August 3, 2019. https://www.forbes.com/sites/kristinakillgrove/2017/11/23/ancient-dna-explains-how-chickens-got-to-the-americas/#613e395256db.

———. "Potatoes Were Not Just a Symbol of the Elite in Ancient Peru, Archaeologists Find." *Forbes*, November 2, 2018. Accessed March 26, 2019. https://www.forbes.com/sites/kristinakillgrove/2018/11/02/potatoes-were-not-just-a-symbol-of-the-elite-in-ancient-peru-archaeologists-find/#4c16f90d1877.

Kim, John M. "Nutrition and the Decline of Mortality." In *The Cambridge World History of Food*. Vol. 2, ed. Kenneth F. Kiple and Kriemhild Conee Ornelas, 1381–1389. Cambridge, UK: Cambridge University Press, 2000.

King, Christopher A., and Lynette Norr. "Paleodietary Change among Pre-State Metal Age Societies in Northeast Thailand: A Study Using Stable Isotopes." In *Bioarchaeology of Southeast Asia*, ed. Marc Oxenham and Nancy Tayles, 241–262. Cambridge, UK: Cambridge University Press, 2006.

Kinyuru, J. N., G. M. Kenji, S. N. Muhoho, and M. Ayieko. "Nutritional Potential of Longhorn Grasshopper (Ruspolia differens) Consumed in Siaya District, Kenya." *Journal of Agriculture, Science and Technology* (November 2009). Accessed July 11, 2019. https://www.researchgate.net/publication/268186085_Nutritional_potential_of_longhorn_grasshopper_Ruspolia_differens_consumed_in_Siaya_District_Kenya.

Kiple, Kenneth F. "The Question of Paleolithic Nutrition and Modern Health: From the End to the Beginning." In *The Cambridge World History of Food*. Vol. 2, ed. Kenneth F. Kiple and Kriemhild Conee Ornelas, 1704–1709. Cambridge, UK: Cambridge University Press, 2000.

Kaplan, Lawrence, and Virginia H. Kiple. "Deficiency Diseases in the Caribbean." In *Caribbean Slavery in the Atlantic World: A Student Reader*, ed. Verene A. Shepherd and Hilary McD. Beckles, 785–794. Princeton, NJ: Markus Wiener Publishers, 2000.

Kaplan, Lawrence, and Virginia Himmelsteib King. *Another Dimension to the Black Diaspora: Diet, Disease, and Racism*. Cambridge: Cambridge University Press, 1981.

Klein, Carol. *Vegetable Gardening: The Complete Guide to Growing More Than 40 Popular Vegetables in Any Space*. London: i-5 Press, 2016.

Knowles, John H. "The Responsibility of the Individual." *Daedalus* 106, no. 1 (Winter 1977): 57–80.

Kolata, Gina. "In Struggle with Weight, Taft Used a Modern Diet." *New York Times*, October 14, 2013. Accessed March 29, 2019. https://www.nytimes.com/2013/10/15/health/in-struggle-with-weight-william-howard-taft-used-a-modern-diet.html.

Kolonel, Laurence N. "Nutrition and Prostate Cancer." In *Nutrition in the Prevention and Treatment of Disease*, ed. Ann M. Coulston, Cheryl L. Rock, and Elaine R. Monsen, 373–386. San Diego: Academic Press, 2001.

Komlos, John, and Marek Brabec. "The Evolution of BMI Values of US Adults: 1882–1986." *Vox*. August 31, 2010. Accessed March 18, 2019. https://voxeu.org/article/100-years-us-obesity.

Kopke, Nikola C. G. "Regional Differences and Temporal Development of Nutritional Status in Europe from the 8th Century B.C. until the 18th Century A.D." PhD diss., Universitat Tubingen, 2008.

Kourimska, Lenka, and Anna Adamkova. "Nutritional and Sensory Qualities of Edible Insects." *NSF Journal* 4 (July 16, 2016): 22–26. https://www.researchgate.net/publication/305396814_Nutritional_and_sensory_quality_of_edible_insects.

Kragh, Helge S. *Conceptions of Cosmos: From Myths to the Accelerating University: A History of Cosmology*. Oxford: Oxford University Press, 2007.

Kratz, Corinne A. "The Okiek of Kenya." In *The Cambridge Encyclopedia of Hunters and Gatherers*, ed. Richard B. Lee and Richard Daly, 220–224. Cambridge, UK: Cambridge University Press, 2004.

Kubala, Jillian. "Is Peanut Oil Healthy? The Surprising Truth." *Healthline*. November 10, 2017. Accessed May 31, 2019. https://www.healthline.com/nutrition/is-peanut-oil-healthy#section2.

Kuhn, Steven L., and Mary C. Stiner. "The Antiquity of Hunter-Gatherers." In *Hunter-Gatherers: An Interdisciplinary Perspective*, ed. Catherine Panter-Brick, Robert H. Layton, and Peter Rowley-Conwy, 99–142. Cambridge, UK and New York: Cambridge University Press, 2001.

Kuhn, Thomas S. *The Structure of Scientific Revolutions*. 4th ed. Chicago and London: University of Chicago Press, 2012.

Kumar, Rajesh, Hui-Ju Tsai, Xiumei Hong, Xin Liu, Guoying Wang, Colleen Pearson, Katherin Ortiz, Melanie Fu, Jacqueline A. Pongracic, Howard Bauchner, and Xiobin Wang. "Race, Ancestry, and Development of Food-Allergen Sensitization in Early Childhood." *Pediatrics* 128, no. 4 (October 2011): 821–829. https://www.ncbi.nlm.nih.gov/pmc/articles/PMC3182844.

Kurlansky, Mark. *Milk!: A 10,000-Year Food Fracas.* New York: Bloomsbury Publishing, 2018.

Kuster, Hansjorg. "Rye." In *The Cambridge World History of Food.* Vol. 1, ed. Kenneth F. Kiple and Kriemhild Conee Ornelas, 149–152. Cambridge, UK: Cambridge University Press, 2000.

LaFranchi, Howard. "From Famine to Food Basket: How Bangladesh Became a Model for Reducing Hunger." *Christian Science Monitor.* June 17, 2015. Accessed January 19, 2019. https://www.csmonitor.com/USA/Foreign-Policy/2015/0617/From-famine-to-food-basket-how-Bangladesh-became-a-model-for-reducing-hunger.

"Lake Okeechobee Fishing Records Catch." Accessed February 14, 2019. https://lakeokeechobeebassfishing.com/fish-records.

Lamour, Joseph. "Americans Eat on Average almost 300 Eggs a Year." *Kitchn.* March 1, 2019. Accessed August 2, 2019. https://www.thekitchn.com/americans-eat-on-average-almost-300-eggs-a-year-267411.

Lanza, Fabrizia. *Olive: A Global History.* London: Reaktion Books, 2011.

Larsen, Clark Spencer. "Dietary Reconstruction and Nutritional Assessment of Past Peoples: The Bioanthropological Record." In *The Cambridge World History of Food.* Vol. 1, ed. Kenneth F. Kiple and Kriemhild Conee Ornelas, 13–34. Cambridge, UK: Cambridge University Press, 2000.

———. *Our Origins: Discovering Physical Anthropology.* New York and London: Norton, 2008.

———. *Skeletons in Our Closet: Revealing Our Past through Bioarchaeology.* Princeton, NJ and Oxford, UK: Princeton University Press, 2000.

Laszlo, Pierre. *Citrus: A History.* Chicago and London: University of Chicago Press, 2008.

Lawler, Andrew. *Why Did the Chicken Cross the World?: The Epic Saga of the Bird that Powers Civilization.* New York: Atria Books, 2014.

Laws, Bill. *Fifty Plants that Changed the Course of History.* Buffalo, NY and Richmond Hill, Ontario: Firefly Books, 2015.

Le, Stephen. *100 Million Years of Food: What Our Ancestors Ate and Why It Matters Today.* New York: Picador, 2016.

Leadbetter, Bill. "Jesus." In *Berkshire Encyclopedia of World History.* Vol. 3, ed. William H. McNeill, Jerry H. Bentley, David Christian, David Levinson, J. R. McNeill, Heidi Roupp, and Judith Zinsser, 1054–1056. Great Barrington, MA: Berkshire Publishing Group, 2005.

Lean, Mike, and Emilie Combet. *Barasi's Human Nutrition: A Health Perspective.* 3rd ed. Boca Raton, FL: CRC Press, 2017.

"Lecture on Soybeans and Their Products." Accessed April 27, 2019. https://www.chefshalhoub.com/Soybeanlecture.htm.

"Legumes." In *The Cambridge World History of Food.* Vol. 2, ed. Kenneth F. Kiple and Kriemhild Conee Ornelas, 1799–1800. Cambridge, UK: Cambridge University Press, 2000.

le Play, Frederic. *Les ouvriers europeens.* 2 vols. Tours, France: A. Mame, 1879.

Le Roy Ladurie, Emmanuel. *The Peasants of Languedoc*, trans. John Day. Urbana: University of Illinois Press, 1974.

Levine, Susan. *School Lunch Politics: The Surprising History of America's Favorite Welfare Program.* Princeton, NJ and Oxford, UK: Princeton University Press, 2008.

Lewis, Nancy Davis. "The Pacific Islands." In *The Cambridge World History of Food.* Vol. 2, ed. Kenneth F. Kiple and Kriemhild Conee Ornelas, 1351–1366. Cambridge, UK: Cambridge University Press, 2000.

Li, Peng-Gao, and Tai-Hua Mu. "Sweet Potato: Health Benefits, Production and Utilization in China." In *Potatoes: Production, Consumption and Health Benefits*, ed. Claudio Caprara, 147–172. New York: Nova Science Publishers, 2012.

Lieberman, Leslie Sue. "Obesity." In *The Cambridge World History of Food.* Vol. 1, ed. Kenneth F. Kiple and Kriemhild Conee Ornelas, 1062–1077. Cambridge, UK: Cambridge University Press, 2000.

"Life Expectancy at Birth (Male and Female), 1971–2017." Centre for Health Protection. Last modified January 11, 2019. Accessed January 20, 2019. https://www.chp.gov.hk/en/statistics/data/10/27/111.html.

Lila, Mary Ann. "Anthocyanins and Human Health: An In Vitro Investigative Approach." *Journal of Biomedicine and Biotechnology* 2004, no. 5 (December 1, 2004): 306–313. https://www.ncbi.nlm.nih.gov/pmc/articles/PMC1082894.

Liljas, Ann E. M. "Old Age in Ancient Egypt." March 2, 2015. Accessed January 18, 2019. https://blogs.ucl.ac.uk/researchers-in-museums/2015/03/02/old-age-in-ancient-egypt.

Lindsey, Joe. "One in Three Americans Rides a Bike." *Bicycling* magazine, March 3, 2015. Accessed June 16, 2019. https://www.bicycling.com/news/a20010688/cycling-advocacy-1.

Link, Rachael. "Antioxidant-Loaded Purple Potatoes: The Healthy, Versatile Carb." *Dr. Axe.* August 29, 2019. Accessed January 25, 2020. https://draxe.com/nutrition/purple-potatoes.

Linkov, Faina, Barbara Stadterman, and Emanuela Taioli. "Fish Consumption and Cancer: Summary of Evidence." In *Fish Consumption and Health*, ed. George P. Gagne and Richard H. Medrano, 117–134. New York: Nova Science Publishers, 2009.

Liu, KeShun. *Soybeans: Chemistry, Technology, and Utilization*. New York: Chapman and Hall, 1997.

"Live Stock, 1920." In *Yearbook of Agriculture, 1920*, ed. L. C. Everard, 701–760. Washington, DC: GPO, 1921.

Lloyd, Christopher. *Absolutely Everything!: A History of Earth, Dinosaurs, Rulers, Robots and Other Things too Numerous to Mention*. Tonbridge, UK: What on Earth Books, 2018.

Loebenstein, Gad. "Origin, Distribution and Economic Importance." In The Sweetpotato, ed. Gad Loebenstein and George Thottappilly, 9–12. Dordrecht: Springer, 2009.

Long, Lucy M. *Honey: A Global History*. London: Reaktion Books, 2017.

Louie, Jimmy. "Breads and Cereals." In *Essentials of Human Nutrition*, ed. Jim Mann and A. Stewart Truswell, 273–276. 5th ed. Oxford, UK: Oxford University Press, 2017.

"Lowest Calorie Foods." *Health Assist*. 2006–2017. Accessed October 2, 2019. http://www.healthassist.net/food/calories-chart.shtml.

Lucassen, Leo. "Total Population Europe, 1500–1900 (Millions)." *Research Gate*. Accessed March 27, 2019. https://www.researchgate.net/figure/2-Total-population-Europe-1500-1900-millions_tbl35_47723061.

Luff, Rosemary. "Ducks." In *The Cambridge World History of Food*. Vol. 1, ed. Kenneth F. Kiple and Kriemhild Conee Ornelas, 517–524. Cambridge, UK: Cambridge University Press, 2000.

Lunn, Peter G. "Nutrition, Immunity and Infection." In *The Decline of Mortality in Europe*, ed. R. Schofield, D. Reher, and A. Bideau, 131–145. Oxford: Clarendon Press, 1991.

Maalouf, Naim. "How Much Calcium Is Too Much?" UT Southwestern Medical Center. February 2, 2015. Accessed March 15, 2019. https://utswmed.org/medblog/calcium.

MacDougall, Pauleena. "Virgin Soil Epidemics in North America." In *World History Encyclopedia. Vol 11. Era 6: The First Global Age, 1450–1770*, ed. Alfred J. Andrea, Carolyn Neel, Dane A. Morrison, Alexander Mikaberidze, D. Harland Hagler, Jeffrey M. Diamond, and Monique Vallance, 104–106. Santa Barbara, CA: ABC-CLIO, 2011.

Macfarlane, Alan. "The Three Major Famines of Japanese History." 2002. Accessed March 29, 2019. http://www.alanmacfarlane.com/savage/A-JAPFAM.PDF.

MacGregor, Kirk R. "Introduction: Christianity." In *World History Encyclopedia, Era 3: Classical Traditions, 1000 BCE–300 CE*. Vol. 6, ed. William E. Mierse and Kevin M. McGeough, 570–571. Santa Barbara, CA: ABC-CLIO, 2011.

Machlis, Joseph. *The Enjoyment of Music: An Introduction to Perceptive Listening*. New York: Norton, 1955.

Mackay, Alan L. *A Dictionary of Scientific Quotations*. Bristol, UK and Philadelphia: Institute of Physics Publishing, 1991.

Maczulak, Anne. *The Smart Guide to Nutrition*. 2nd ed. Norman, OK: Smart Guide Publications, 2014.

Magner, Lois N. "Korea." In *The Cambridge World History of Food*. Vol. 2, ed. Kenneth F. Kiple and Kriemhild Conee Ornelas, 1183–1192. Cambridge, UK: Cambridge University Press, 2000.

Malihot, Jose. "The Innu of Quebec and Labrador." In *The Cambridge Encyclopedia of Hunters and Gatherers*, ed. Richard B. Lee and Richard Daly, 51–55. Cambridge, UK: Cambridge University Press, 2004.

"Malnutrition in Children—UNICEF Data." UNICEF. May 2018. Accessed January 19, 2019. https://data.unicef.org/topic/nutrition/malnutrition/#.

Malthus, Thomas. *An Essay on the Principle of Population*. Amherst, New York: Prometheus Books, 1998.

Mangelsdorf, Paul C. *Corn: Its Origin, Evolution, and Improvement*. Cambridge, MA: Harvard University Press, 1974.

"Manioc." In *The Cambridge World History of Food*. Vol. 2, ed. Kenneth F. Kiple and Kriemhild Conee Ornelas, 1810. Cambridge, UK: Cambridge University Press, 2000.

Mann, Charles C. "How the Potato Changed the World." *Smithsonian Magazine*, November 2011. Accessed February 27, 2020. https://www.smithsonianmag.com/history/how-the-potato-changed-the-world-108470605.

Mann, Jim, and Rachael McLean, "Cardiovascular Diseases." In *Essentials of Human Nutrition*. 5th ed., ed. Jim Mann and A. Stewart Truswell, 381–407. Oxford: Oxford University Press, 2017.

Mannion, A. M. "Plant Cultivation and Animal Use in the Nile Valley." In *World History Encyclopedia. Vol 2. Era 1: Beginnings of Human Society*, ed. Mark Aldenderfer, 135–137. Santa Barbara, CA: ABC-CLIO, 2011.

Mara, Wil. *Inside the Oil Industry*. Minneapolis, MN: ABDO, 2017.

Marden, Kerriann. "Human Burials of Chaco Canyon: New Developments in Cultural Interpretations through Skeletal Analysis." In *Chaco Revisited: New Research on the Prehistory of Chaco Canyon, New Mexico*, ed. Carrie C. Heitman and Stephen Plog, 162–186. Tucson: University of Arizona Press, 2015.

Marie, Joanne. "Foods Containing Sucrose." *Livestrong*. Accessed May 21, 2019. https://www.livestrong.com/article/142823-foods-containing-sucrose.

Marrin, Albert. *Black Gold: The Story of Oil in Our Lives*. New York: Knopf, 2012.

Marx, Karl, and Friedrich Engels. *Communist Manifesto*, trans. Samuel Moore. Chicago: Great Books Foundation, 1955.

Mason, Sarah. "Acornutopia?: Determining the Role of Acorns in Past Human Subsistence." In *Food in Antiquity*, ed. John Wilkins, David Harvey, and Mike Dobson, 12–24. Exeter, UK: University of Exeter Press, 1995.

Matsuyama, Toshio. "Nut Gathering and Processing Methods in Traditional Japanese Villages." In *Affluent Foragers: Pacific Coasts East and West*, ed. Shuzo Koyama and David Hurst Thomas, 117–140. Osaka, Japan: National Museum of Ethnology, 1979.

Matthews, Clare. *Low-Maintenance Vegetable Gardening: Bumper Crops in Minutes a Day Using Raised Beds, Planning, and Plant Selection*. Mount Joy, PA: Companion House Books, 2018.

Matthews, Ruth H., ed. *Legumes: Chemistry, Technology, and Human Nutrition*. New York and Basel: Marcel Dekker, 1989.

Mayer, Jorge. "The Golden Rice Project." 2005–2018. Accessed January 18, 2019. http://www.goldenrice.org/Content4-Info/info.php.

Mayne, Susan T. "Nutrition and Lung Cancer." In *Nutrition in the Prevention and Treatment of Disease*, ed. Ann M. Coulston, Cheryl L. Rock, and Elaine R. Monsen, 387–396. San Diego: Academic Press, 2001.

Mayr, Ernst. *The Growth of Biological Thought: Diversity, Evolution, and Inheritance*. Cambridge, MA and London: Belknap Press of Harvard University Press, 1982.

McAlpin, Michelle B. "Famines, Epidemics, and Population Growth: The Case of India." *Journal of Interdisciplinary History* 14, no. 2 (Autumn 1983): 351–366.

McCaa, Robert. "Paleodemography of the Americas: From Ancient Times to Colonialism and Beyond." In *The Backbone of History: Health and Nutrition in the Western Hemisphere*, ed. Richard H. Steckel and Jerome C. Rose, 94–124. Cambridge, UK: Cambridge University Press, 2002.

McCallum, Linsay, Stefanie Lip, and Sandosh Padmanabhan. "The Hidden Hand of Chloride in Hypertension." *Pflugers Archiv* 467, no. 3 (January 27, 2015): 595–603.

McClatchey, Will C. "Bananas and Plantains." In *The Cambridge World History of Food*. Vol. 1, ed. Kenneth F. Kiple and Kriemhild Conee Ornelas, 175–181. Cambridge, UK: Cambridge University Press, 2000.

McCollum, Elmer Verner. *A History of Nutrition: The Sequence of Ideas in Nutrition Investigations*. Boston: Houghton Mifflin, 1957.

McCorriston, Joy. "Barley." In *The Cambridge Encyclopedia of Food*. Vol. 1, ed. Kenneth F. Kiple and Kriemhild Conee Ornelas, 81–89. Cambridge, UK: Cambridge University Press, 2000.

———. "Wheat." In *The Cambridge World History of Food*. Vol. 1, ed. Kenneth F. Kiple and Kriemhild Conee Ornelas, 158–174. Cambridge, UK: Cambridge University Press, 2000.

McGreger, April. *Sweet Potatoes*. Chapel Hill: University of North Carolina Press, 2014.

McHoy, Peter. *Practical Gardening*. New York: Smithmark Publishers, 1994.

McKay, John P., Bennett D. Hill, John Buckler, Clare Haru Crowston, Merry E. Wiesner-Hanks, and Joe Perry. *Understanding Western Civilization: A Brief History*. Boston and New York: Bedford/St. Martin's, 2012.

McKeown, Thomas. "Food, Infection, and Population." *Journal of Interdisciplinary History* 14, no. 2 (Autumn 1983): 227–247.

McNeill, William H. "How the Potato Changed the World's History." *Social Research* 66, no. 1 (Spring 1999): 67–82.

———. "The Introduction of the Potato into Ireland." *Journal of Modern History* 21, no. 3 (September 1949): 218–222.

"Meat, Poultry, Fish, and Shellfish CIDs." *USDA*. Accessed January 24, 2019. https://www.ams.usda.gov/grades-standards/cid/meat.

"Meat Science." *Elsevier*. 2019. Accessed January 24, 2019. https://www.journals.elsevier.com/meat-science.

"The Medieval Garden Enclosed." *The Metropolitan Museum of Art*, 2000–2011. Accessed July 2, 2019. http://blog.metmuseum.org/cloistersgardens/2010/10/22/colewort-and-kale.

Meltzer, Milton. *The Amazing Potato: A Story in which the Incas, Conquistadors, Marie Antoinette, Thomas Jefferson, Wars, Famines, Immigrants, and French Fries All Play a Part*. New York: HarperCollins, 1992.

Merriam, C. Hart. "The Acorn, A Possibly Neglected Source of Food." *National Geographic Magazine* 34, no. 1 (August 1918): 129–137.

Mertz, Barbara. *Red Land, Black Land: Daily Life in Ancient Egypt*. New York: William Morrow, 1978.

Messer, Ellen. "Maize." In *The Cambridge World History of Food*. Vol. 1, ed. Kenneth F. Kiple and Kriemhild Conee Ornelas, 97–112. Cambridge, UK: Cambridge University Press, 2000.

———. "Potatoes (White)." In *The Cambridge World History of Food*. Vol. 1, ed. Kenneth F. Kiple and Kriemhild Conee Ornelas, 187–201. Cambridge, UK: Cambridge University Press, 2000.

Messina, Mark J. "Soyfoods: Their Role in Disease Prevention and Treatment." In *Soybeans: Chemistry, Technology, and Utilization*, ed. KeShun Liu, 442–477. New York: Chapman and Hall, 1997.

"Metabolism." Victoria State Government. 2018. Accessed August 26, 2019. https://www.betterhealth.vic.gov.au/health/conditionsandtreatments/metabolism.

"Micronutrient Deficiencies." World Health Organization. Accessed January 1, 2020. https://www.who.int/nutrition/topics/idd/en.

Midant-Reynes, Beatrix. *The Prehistory of Egypt: From the First Egyptians to the First Pharaohs*, trans. Ian Shaw. Oxford, UK and Malden, MA: Blackwell, 2000.

"Middle East Climate." *Israel Science and Technology Directory*. 1999–2018. Accessed September 24, 2019. https://www.science.co.il/weather/middle-east-climate.

Miller, Naomi F., and Wilma Wetterstrom. "The Beginnings of Agriculture: The Ancient Near East and North Africa." In *The Cambridge World History of Food*. Vol. 2, ed. Kenneth F. Kiple and Kriemhild Conee Ornelas, 1123–1139. Cambridge, UK: Cambridge University Press, 2000.

Minogue, Sara. "Changes in Arctic Diet Put Inuit at Risk for Rickets." *The Globe and Mail*. June 8, 2007. Last modified April 25, 2018. Accessed March 4, 2019. https://www.theglobeandmail.com/life/changes-in-arctic-diet-put-inuit-at-risk-for-rickets/article20404517.

Mintz, Sidney W. "Fermented Beans and Western Taste." In *The World of S*oy, ed. Christine M. Du Bois, Chee-Beng Tan, and Sidney W. Mintz, 56–73. Urbana and Chicago: University of Illinois Press, 2008.

"Miscellaneous Agricultural Statistics." In *Yearbook of* Agriculture, 1920, ed. L. C. Everard, 803–840. Washington, DC: GPO, 1921.

Misra, Tanvi. "Global Car, Motorcycle, and Bike Ownership, in 1 Infographic." *CityLab*. April 17, 2015. Accessed April 17, 2019. https://www.citylab.com/transportation/2015/04/global-car-motorcycle-and-bike-ownership-in-1-infographic/390777.

Mitchell, Braxton D., Woei-Jyh Lee, Magdalena I. Tolea, Kelsey Shields, Zahra Ashktorab, Laurence S. Magder, Kathleen A. Ryan, Toni I. Pollin, Patrick F. McArdle, Alan R. Shuldiner, and Alejandro A. Schaffer. "Living the Good Life? Mortality and Hospital Utilization Patterns in the Old Order Amish." *Plos One* 7, no. 12 (December 19, 2012). https://journals.plos.org/plosone/article?id=10.1371/journal.pone.0051560.

Mitchell, Nia, Vicki Catenacci, Holly R. Wyatt, and James O. Hill. "Obesity: Overview of an Epidemic." *Psychiatric Clinics of North America* 34, no. 4 (December 2011): 717–732. https://www.ncbi.nlm.nih.gov/pmc/articles/PMC3228640.

Mols, Stephan T. A. M. "Identification of the Woods in the Furniture at Herculaneum." In *The Natural History of Pompeii*, ed. Wilhelmina Feemster Jashemski and Frederick G. Meyer, 225–234. Cambridge, UK: Cambridge University Press, 2002.

Moore, Paul H., Andrew H. Paterson, and Thomas Tew. "Sugarcane: The Crop, the Plant, and Domestication." In *Sugarcane: Physiology, Biochemistry, and Functional Biology*, ed. Paul H. Moore and Frederik C. Botha, 1–17. Ames, IA: Wiley Blackwell, 2014.

Moore, Ruth. *Evolution*. Rev. ed. New York: Time-Life Books, 1968.

"More Sugar!—The Causes of the Rise in British Sugar Consumption." *Chocolate Class*. March 11, 2019. Accessed January 31, 2020. https://chocolateclass.wordpress.com/2019/03/11/more-sugar-the-causes-of-the-rise-in-british-sugar-consumption.

Morfin, Lourdes Marquez, Robert McCaa, Rebecca Storey, and Andres Del Angel. "Health and Nutrition in Pre-Hispanic Mesoamerica." In *The Backbone of History: Health and Nutrition in the Western Hemisphere*, ed. Richard H. Steckel and Jerome C. Rose, 307–338. Cambridge, UK: Cambridge University Press, 2002.

Morgan, Michele E. "Conclusion." In *Pecos Pueblo Revisited: The Biological and Social Context*, ed. Michele E. Morgan, 161–167. Cambridge, MA: Peabody Museum of Archaeology and Ethnology, Harvard University, 2010.

Morris, Ian. "Early Iron Age Greece." In *The Cambridge Economic History of the Greco-Roman World*, ed. Walter Scheidel, Ian Morris, and Richard Saller, 211–241. Cambridge, UK: Cambridge University Press, 2007.

Morrison, Kate. "Goat Milk Versus Cow Milk: Which Is Healthier?" *The Spruce Eats*. Last modified May 13, 2019. Accessed September 24, 2019. https://www.thespruceeats.com/goats-milk-versus-cows-milk-3376918.

Morton, Julia F. "Date." Purdue University. 1987. Accessed February 16, 2020. https://hort.purdue.edu/newcrop/morton/date.html.

"Mosquito Malaria Vectors." *Malaria Atlas Project*. 2020. Accessed January 18, 2020. https://malariaatlas.org/mosquito-malaria-vectors.

Moulton, Carroll, ed. *Ancient Greece and Rome: An Encyclopedia for Students*. 2 vols. New York: Charles Scribner's Sons, 1998.

Mueller, Tom. *Extra Virginity: The Sublime and Scandalous World of Olive Oil*. New York and London: Norton, 2012.

"Mystery of Yemen Cholera Epidemic Solved." *Science Daily*. January 2, 2019. Accessed January 23, 2019. https://www.sciencedaily.com/releases/2019/01/190102140745.htm.

Nair, Rathish, and Arun Maseeh. "Vitamin D: The 'Sunshine' Vitamin." *Journal of Pharmacology and Pharmacotherapeutics* 3, no. 2 (April-June 2012): 118–126. https://www.ncbi.nlm.nih.gov/pmc/articles/PMC3356951.

Nardo, Don. *The Greenhaven Encyclopedia of Ancient Mesopotamia*. Detroit: Thomson Gale, 2007.

———. *Life in Ancient Egypt*. San Diego: Reference Point Press, 2015.

Nardozzi, Charlie. *Vegetable Gardening for Dummies*. 2d ed. Hoboken, NJ: Wiley, 2009.

Nash, Colin E. "Aquatic Animals." In *The Cambridge World History of Food*. Vol. 1, ed. Kenneth F. Kiple and Kriemhild Conee Ornelas, 456–467. Cambridge, UK: Cambridge University Press, 2000.

Nash, Gary B., Julie Roy Jeffrey, John R. Howe, Peter J. Frederick, Allen F. Davis, Allan M. Winkler. *The American People: Creating a Nation and a Soc*iety. 2 vols. 2nd ed. New York: HarperCollins, 1990.

Neel, James V. "Diabetes Mellitus: A 'Thrifty' Genotype Rendered Detrimental by Progress?" *American Journal of Human Genetics* 14, no. 4 (December 1962): 353–362.

Nelson, Joseph S. "Fish." *The Canadian Encyclopedia*. October 25, 2010. Last modified March 4, 2015. Accessed February 23, 2019. https://www.thecanadianencyclopedia.ca/en/article/fishes.

Nelson, Sarah M. "Conclusion." In *The Archaeology of Northeast China: Beyond the Great Wall*, ed. Sarah Milledge Nelson, 251–254. London and New York: Routledge, 1995.

Nemet-Nejat, Karen Rhea. *Daily Life in Ancient Mesopotamia*. Westport, CT and London: Greenwood Press, 1998.

Nesbitt, Mark. "Grains." In *The Cultural History of Plants*, ed. Ghillean Prance and Mark Nesbitt, 45–60. New York and London: Routledge, 2005.

"New CDC Report: More than 100 Million Americans Have Diabetes or Prediabetes." *CDC*. Last modified July 18, 2017. Accessed January 23, 2019. https://www.cdc.gov/media/releases/2017/p0718-diabetes-report.html.

"New Link between Heart Disease and Red Meat: New Understanding of Cardiovascular Health Benefits of Vegan, Vegetarian Diets." *Science Daily*. April 7, 2013. Accessed January 31, 2019. https://www.sciencedaily.com/releases/2013/04/130407133320.htm.

New York University. "History of North African Date Palm." *Science Daily*. January 14, 2019. Accessed September 17, 2019. https://www.sciencedaily.com/releases/2019/01/190114161126.htm.

Newby, P. K. *Food and Nutrition: What Everyone Needs to Know*. New York: Oxford University Press, 2018.

Nhassico, Dulce, Humberto Muquingue, Julie Cliff, Arnaldo Cumbana, and J. Howard Bradbury. "Rising African Cassava Production, Diseases Due to High Cyanide Intake and Control Measures." *Journal of the Science of Food and Agriculture* 88 (2008): 2043–2049. https://biology-assets.anu.edu.au/hosted_sites/CCDN/papers/PAPCYREV.pdf.

Nietzsche, Friedrich. *The Birth of Tragedy*, trans. Douglas Smith. Oxford and New York: Oxford University Press, 2000.

———. *On the Genealogy of Morals*, trans. Walter Kaufmann and R. J. Hollingdale. New York: Vintage Books, 1969.

Nieves, J. J. "Cuba: An Overweight Country." *Havana Times*. May 6, 2015. Accessed July 5, 2019. https://havanatimes.org/features/cuba-an-overweight-country.

Nix v. Hedden. 149 U.S. 304 (1893).

Nock, Catherine J., Craig M. Hardner, Juan D. Montenagro, Ainnatul A. Ahmad Termizi, Satomi Hayashi, Julia Playford, David Edwards, and Jacqueline Batley. "Wild Origins of Macadamia Domestication Identified through Intraspecific Chloroplast Genome Sequencing." *Frontiers in Plant Science* (March 21, 2019). https://www.frontiersin.org/articles/10.3389/fpls.2019.00334/full.

Nolt, Steven M. *A History of the Amish*, rev. ed. Intercourse, PA: Good Books, 2003.

Nunn, Nathan, and Nancy Qian. "The Potato's Contribution to Population and Urbanization: Evidence from a Historical Experiment." *Quarterly Journal of Economics* 126, no. 2 (May 2011): 593–650. https://academic.oup.com/qje/article/126/2/593/1868756.

"The Nutrients—Deficiencies, Surfeits, and Food-Related Disorders." In *The Cambridge World History of Food*. Vol. 1, ed. Kenneth F. Kiple and Kriemhild Conee Ornelas, 739. Cambridge, UK: Cambridge University Press, 2000.

"Obesity Definition." Harvard University, 2019. Accessed April 13, 2019. https://www.hsph.harvard.edu/obesity-prevention-source/obesity-definition.

"Obesity and Overweight." World Health Organization. February 16, 2018. Accessed April 13, 2019. https://www.who.int/news-room/fact-sheets/detail/obesity-and-overweight.

"Obesity Update 2017." OECD. Accessed July 5, 2019. https://www.oecd.org/els/health-systems/Obesity-Update-2017.pdf.

O'Brien, Patricia J. "Sweet Potatoes and Yams." In *The Cambridge World History of Food*. Vol. 1, ed. Kenneth F. Kiple and Kriemhild Conee Ornelas, 207–218. Cambridge, UK: Cambridge University Press, 2000.

O'Connor, Kaori. *Pineapple: A Global History*. London: Reaktion Books, 2013.

O Grada, Cormac. *Ireland before and after the Famine: Explorations in Economic History, 1800–1925*. Manchester and New York: Manchester University Press, 1988.

———. "The Population of Ireland, 1700–1900: A Survey." *Annales de Demographie Historique* (1979): 281–299. https://www.persee.fr/doc/adh_0066-2062_1979_num_1979_1_1425.

O'Grady, Kathleen. "Early Puberty for Girls. The New 'Normal' and Why We Need to Be Concerned." *Canadian Women's Health Network*. Fall-Winter 2008–2009. Accessed February 10, 2019. www.cwhn.ca/en/node/39365.

Ogunji, Johnny O. "Fish Consumption: A Paradox of Good Health." In *Fish Consumption and Health*, ed. George P. Gagne and Richard H. Medrano, 77–91. New York: Nova Science Publishers, 2009.

Ogunlesi, Modupe, Wesley Okiei, Azeez Luqmon Adeyemi, Vincent Obakachi, Monisola Itohan Ikhile, and G. Nkenchor. "Vitamin C Contents of Tropical Vegetables and Foods Determined by Voltametric and Titrimetric Methods and Their Relevance to the Medicinal Uses of the Plants." *International Journal of Electrochemical Science* 5 (January 31, 2010): 105–115. https://www.researchgate.net/publication/313964413_Vitamin_C_contents_of_tropical_vegetables_and_foods_determines_by_voltammetric_and_titrimetric_methods_and_their_relevance_to_the_medicinal_uses_of_the_plants.

O'Keefe, Sean Francis. "An Overview of Oils and Fats, with a Special Emphasis on Olive Oil." In *The Cambridge World History of Food*. Vol. 1, ed. Kenneth F. Kiple and Kriemhild Conee Ornelas, 375–388. Cambridge, UK: Cambridge University Press, 2000.

The Oldest Code of Laws in the World: The Code of Laws Promulgated by Hammurabi, King of Babylon, B.C. 2285–2242, trans. C. H. W. Johns. Union, NJ: Lawbook Exchange, 2000.

Olsen, Stanley J. "Turkeys." In *The Cambridge World History of Food*. Vol. 1, ed. Kenneth F. Kiple and Kriemhild Conee Ornelas, 578–583. Cambridge, UK: Cambridge University Press, 2000.

Olson, Miles. "11 Edible Bugs and How to Eat Them." *Mother Earth News*. May 30, 2013. Accessed March 13, 2019. https://www.motherearthnews.com/real-food/edible-bugs-zebz1305znsp.

Ommanney, F. D. *The Fishes*. New York: Time, 1964.

O'Neill, Joseph R. *The Irish Potato Famine*. Edina, MN: ABDO Publishing, 2009.

Onwueme, I. C. "Cassava in Asia and the Pacific." In *Cassava: Biology, Production and Utilization*, ed. R. J. Hillocks, J. M. Thresh, and A.C. Bellotti, 55–65. Wallingford, UK and New York: CABI Publishing 2002.

Oransky, Ivan. "Ancel Keys." *The Lancet* 364, no. 9452 (December 18, 2004): 2174.

O'Riordan, Tomas. "The Introduction of the Potato into Ireland." *History Ireland: Ireland's History Magazine*, 2019. Accessed March 27, 2019. https://www.historyireland.com/early-modern-history-1500-1700/the-introduction-of-the-potato-into-ireland.

Ortner, Donald J., and Gretchen Theobald. "Paleopathological Evidence of Malnutrition." In *The Cambridge World History of Food*. Vol. 1, ed. Kenneth F. Kiple and Kriemhild Conee Ornelas, 34–44. Cambridge, UK: Cambridge University Press, 2000.

Osler, Tom. *Serious Runner's Handbook: Answers to Hundreds of Your Running Questions*. Mountain View, CA: World Publications, 1978.

O'Sullivan, James. "Demystifying Finnish Dairy Food." *This Is Finland*. March 2015. Accessed March 17, 2019. https://finland.fi/life-society/demystifying-finnish-dairy-food.

"Overweight and Obesity." World Health Organization. February 16, 2018. Accessed July 8, 2019. https://www.who.int/news-room/fact-sheets/detail/obesity-and-overweight.

Owen, James. "Egyptian Princess Mummy Had Oldest Known Heart Disease." *National Geographic News*. April 15, 2011. Accessed February 5, 2019. https://news.nationalgeographic.com/news/2011/04/110415-ancient-egypt-mummies-princess-heart-disease-health-science.

Oxenham, Marc, Nguyen Lan Cuong, and Nguyen Kim Thuy. "The Oral Health Consequences of the Adoption and Intensification of Agriculture in Southeast Asia." In *Bioarchaeology of Southeast Asia*, ed. Marc Oxenham and Nancy Tayles, 263–289. Cambridge, UK: Cambridge University Press, 2006.

Ozeki, Erino. "Fermented Soybean Products and Japanese Standard Taste." In *The World of Soy*, ed. Christine M. Du Bois, Chee-Beng Tan, and Sidney W. Mintz, 144–160. Urbana: University of Illinois Press, 2008.

Pajonas, S. J. "How Sweet Potatoes Saved Japan." April 12, 2016. Accessed March 29, 2019. https://www.spajonas.com/2016/04/12/how-sweet-potatoes-saved-japan.

Panoff, Lauren. "6 Surprising Benefits of Camel Milk (And 3 Downsides)." *Healthline*. June 27, 2019. Accessed September 24, 2019. https://www.healthline.com/nutrition/camel-milk-benefits.

Panter-Brick, Catherine, Robert H. Layton, and Peter Rowley-Conwy, eds. *Hunter-Gatherers: An Interdisciplinary Perspective*. Cambridge, UK: Cambridge University Press, 2001.

Pappas, Stephanie. "Ancient 'Brain Food' Helped Humans Get Smart." *Live Science*. June 3, 2010. Accessed February 14, 2019. https://www.livescience.com/10664-ancient-brain-food-helped-humans-smart.html.

———. "Once-Green Sahara Hosted Early African Dairy Farms." *Live Science*. June 20, 2012. Accessed March 12, 2019. https://www.livescience.com/21070-green-sahara-hosted-african-dairy-farms.html.

"*Paranthropus boisei*." Smithsonian National Museum of Natural History. Last modified August 24, 2018. Accessed October 16, 2019. http://humanorigins.si.edu/evidence/human-fossils/species/paranthropus-boisei.

Paravattil, Blossom. "Fast Food Facts: Calories and Fat." National Center for Health Research. 2019. Accessed May 30, 2019. http://www.center4research.org/fast-food-facts-calories-and-fat.

Parcell, Joe, Yasutomo Kojima, Alice Roach, and Wayne Cain. "Global Edible Vegetable Oil Market Trends." *Biomedical Journal of Scientific and Technical Research* 2, no. 1 (January 22, 2018): 2282–2291. https://biomedres.us/pdfs/BJSTR.MS.ID.000680.pdf.

Parker, Matthew. *The Sugar Barons: Family, Corruption, Empire, and War in the West Indies*. New York: Walker, 2011.

Parr, Broderick, Jennifer K. Bond, and Travis Minor. "Vegetables and Pulses Outlook." USDA Economic Research Service. May 6, 2019. Accessed July 3, 2019. https://www.ers.usda.gov/webdocs/publications/93033/vgs-362.pdf?v=1958.8.

Parrott, Zach. "Indigenous Peoples in Canada." *The Canadian Encyclopedia*. March 13, 2007. Last modified October 12, 2018. Accessed February 21, 2019. https://www.thecanadianencyclopedia.ca/en/article/aboriginal-people.

Parsons, Russ. *How to Pick a Peach: The Search for Flavor from Farm to Table*. Boston and New York: Houghton Mifflin, 2007.

"Part I: Determining What Our Ancestors Ate." In *The Cambridge World History of Food*. Vol. 1, ed. Kenneth F. Kiple and Kriemhild Conee Ornelas, 11. Cambridge, UK: Cambridge University Press, 2000.

"Peanut Butter May Help Overcome Malnutrition in Developing World." *Voice of America*. October 29, 2009. Accessed July 2, 2019. https://www.voanews.com/archive/peanut-butter-may-help-overcome-malnutrition-developing-world-2002-03-20.

Pearman, Georgina. "Nuts, Seeds, and Pulses." In *The Cultural History of Plants*, ed. Ghillean Prance and Mark Nesbitt, 133–152. New York and London: Routledge, 2005.

Peden, Alex. "An Introduction to the Marine Fish of British Columbia." *Electronic Atlas of the Wildlife of British Columbia*. 2018. Accessed February 23, 2019. http://ibis.geog.ubc.ca/biodiversity/efauna/IntroductiontotheMarineFishofBritishColumbia.html.

Pedersen, Stephanie. *Roots: The Complete Guide to the Underground Superfood*. New York: Sterling, 2017.

Pellett, Peter L. "Energy and Protein Metabolism." In *The Cambridge World History of Food*. Vol. 1, ed. Kenneth F. Kiple and Kriemhild Conee Ornelas, 888–913. Cambridge, UK: Cambridge University Press, 2000.

Pelto, Gretel H., and Pertti J. Pelto. "Diet and Delocalization: Dietary Changes Since 1750." *Journal of Interdisciplinary History* 14, no. 2 (Autumn 1983): 507–528.

"Per Capita Consumption of High Fructose Corn Syrup in the United States from 2000 to 2017 (in Pounds)." *Statista*. 2019. Accessed June 12, 2019. https://www.statista.com/statistics/328893/per-capita-consumption-of-high-fructose-corn-syrup-in-the-us.

Percival, John. *The Great Famine: Ireland's Potato Famine, 1845–51*. New York: Viewer Books, 1995.

Perkins, John H. *Insects, Experts, and the Insecticide Crisis: The Quest for New Pest Management Strategies*. New York: Plenum Press, 1982.

Perlmutter, David. "The #1 Reason to Avoid Orange Juice." Accessed May 22, 2019. https://www.drperlmutter.com/avoid-orange-juice.

———. *Grain Brain: The Surprising Truth about Wheat, Carbs, and Sugar—Your Brain's Silent Killers*. Rev. ed. New York: Little, Brown Spark, 2018.

Peterson, David M., and J. Paul Murphy. "Oat." In *The Cambridge World History of Food*. Vol. 1, ed. Kenneth F. Kiple and Kriemhild Conee Ornelas, 121–132. Cambridge, UK: Cambridge University Press, 2000.

Petre, Alina. "9 Impressive Health Benefits of Barley." *Healthline*. September 18, 2018. Accessed March 13, 2019. https://www.healthline.com/nutrition/barley-benefits.

———. "How Many Servings of Vegetables Should You Eat Per Day?" *Healthline*. November 26, 2017. Accessed June 30, 2019. https://www.healthline.com/nutrition/servings-of-vegetables-per-day.

Pfeiffer, Kelly. *Superfood Weeknight Meals: Healthy, Delicious Dinners Ready in 30 Minutes or Less*. Beverly, MA: Quarto Publishing Group, 2017.

Phillips, Delisa L., Jerome C. Rose, and Willem M. van Haarlem. "Bioarchaeology of Tell Ibrahim Awad." *Egypt and the Levant* 19 (December 2009): 157–210.

Pierotti, Raymond. "Diseases, Animal." In *Berkshire Encyclopedia of World History*. Vol. 2, ed. William H. McNeill, Jerry H. Bentley, David Christian, David Levinson, J. R. McNeill, Heidi Roupp, and Judith P. Zinsser, 551–558. Great Barrington, MA: Berkshire Publishing Group, 2005.

Pilcher, Jeffrey M. *Food in World History*. New York and London: Routledge, 2006.

Pinola, Melanie. "The Best Cheeses to Eat If You're Lactose Intolerant." *Life Hacker*. April 15, 2014. Accessed March 8, 2019. https://lifehacker.com/the-best-cheeses-to-eat-if-youre-lactose-intolerant–1563386663.

Pitofsky, Marina. "What Countries Have the Longest Life Expectancies?" *USA Today*, July 27, 2018. Last modified August 5, 2018. Accessed April 6, 2019. https://www.usatoday.com/story/news/2018/07/27/life-expectancies-2018-japan-switzerland-spain/848675002.

Pitsavos, Christos, Christina-Maria Kastorini, and Christodoulos Stefanadis. "Fish Consumption and Health." In *Fish Consumption and Health*, ed. George P. Gagne and Richard H. Medrano, 1–35. New York: Nova Science Publishers, 2009.

Pitts, Martin. "'Celtic' Food: Perspectives from Britain." In *A Companion to Food in the Ancient World*, ed. John Wilkins and Robin Nadeau, 326–334. Malden, MA: Wiley Blackwell, 2015.

Placher, William C. *A History of Christian Theology: An Introduction*. Philadelphia: Westminster Press, 1983.

"Plant Parts." Missouri Botanical Garden. 2009. Accessed July 24, 2019. http://www.mbgnet.net/bioplants/parts.html.

"Plantain." In *The Cambridge World History of Food*. Vol. 2, ed. Kenneth F. Kiple and Kriemhild Conee Ornelas, 1836. Cambridge, UK: Cambridge University Press, 2000.

"Plants for a Future." 1996–2012. Accessed January 16, 2019. https://pfaf.org/user/edibleuses.aspx.

Plato. *Apology, Crito*, trans. Benjamin Jowett. Chicago: Great Books Foundation, 1955.

———. *Phaedo*. In *Great Dialogues of Plato*, trans. W. H. D. Rouse, 460–521. New York and Scarborough, Ontario: New American Library, 1956.

———. *The Republic*. In *Great Dialogues of Plato*, trans. W. H. D. Rouse, 118–422. New York and Scarborough, Ontario: New American Library, 1956.

Pliny. *Natural History*, trans. H. Rackman. 10 vols. Cambridge, MA: Harvard University Press, 1949.

Pobiner, Briana. "Meat-Eating among the Earliest Humans." *American Scientist* 104, no. 2 (March–April 2016). https://www.americanscientist.org/article/meat-eating-among-the-earliest-humans.

Pocock, Gillian, Christopher D. Richards, and David A. Richards. *Human Physiology*. 5th ed. Oxford: Oxford University Press, 2018.

Pollan, Michael. *In Defense of Food: An Eater's Manifesto*. New York: Penguin Press, 2008.

———. *The Omnivore's Dilemma: A Natural History of Four Meals*. New York: Penguin Press, 2006.

"Ponca History." Ponca Tribe of Indians of Oklahoma. 2018. Accessed February 7, 2019. http://ponca.com/ponca-history.

"Poorer Girls over Twice as Likely to Start Period by 11." Economic and Social Research Council. October 12, 2016. Accessed February 10, 2019. https://esrc.ukri.org/news-events-and-publications/news/news-items/poorer-girls-over-twice-as-likely-to-start-period-by–11.

"The Poorest Countries in the World." *FocusEconomics*. November 19, 2018. Accessed May 29, 2019. https://www.focus-economics.com/blog/the-poorest-countries-in-the-world.

Pope, Geoffrey G. "Asian Paleoanthropology." In *History of Physical Anthropology: An Encyclopedia*. Vol. 1: A-L, ed. Frank Spencer, 127–133. New York and London: Garland Publishing, 1997.

Postma, Johannes. *The Atlantic Slave Trade*. Westport, CT and London: Greenwood Press, 2003.

"The Potato Sector." *PotatoPro*. Accessed January 4, 2020. https://www.potatopro.com/russian-federation/potato-statistics.

Potts, Annie. *Chicken*. London: Reaktion Books, 2012.

Powell, Albrecht. "Amish Origin, Beliefs, and Lifestyle." *Trip Savvy*. Last modified December 26, 2018. Accessed March 15, 2019. https://www.tripsavvy.com/guide-to-the-amish-lifestyle-2707217.

Powell, Joseph F. *The First Americans: Race, Evolution, and the Origin of Native Americans*. Cambridge, UK: Cambridge University Press, 2005.

Prantl, Maria. "Diocletian's Edict on Maximum Prices of 301 AD. A Fragment Found in Aigeira." *historia.scribere* 3 (2011): 359–398. https://webapp.uibk.ac.at/ojs/index.php/historiascribere/article/viewFile/208/105.

Price, Annie. "Improve Your Waistline and Heart Health with Rye Flour." *Dr. Axe*. April 2, 2016. Accessed March 13, 2019. https://draxe.com/rye-flour.

Prince, Joseph M., and Richard H. Steckel. *Tallest in the World: Native Americans of the Great Plains in the Nineteenth Century*. Cambridge, MA: National Bureau of Economic Research, 1998.

Probst, A. H., and Robert W. Judd. "Origin, United States History and Development, and World Distribution." In *Soybeans: Improvement, Production, and Uses*, ed. Billy E. Caldwell, Robert W. Howell, Robert W. Judd, and Herbert W. Johnson, 1–15. Madison, WI: American Society of Agronomy, 1973.

Pryor, J. Luke, and Deanna M. Dempsey. "Should Sodium (Via Foods, Salt Tablets, or Pickle Juice) Be Consumed prior to or during Endurance Activities for the Prevention of Exertional Heat Illness?" In *Quick Questions in Heat-Related Illness and Hydration: Expert Advice in Sports Medicine*, ed. Rebecca M. Lopez and Eric L. Sauers, 171–176. Thorofare, NJ: Slack, 2015.

Pullen, Caroline. "Xanthan Gum—Is This Food Additive, Healthy or Harmful?" *Healthline*. May 27, 2017. Accessed April 18, 2019. https://www.healthline.com/nutrition/xanthan-gum.

Quammen, David. *The Song of the Dodo: Island Biogeography in an Age of Extinctions*. New York: Scribner, 1996.

Rakita, Gordon F. M., and Rafael Cruz. "Organization of Production at Paquime." In *Ancient Paquime and the Casas Grandes World*, ed. Paul E. Minnis and Michael E. Whalen, 58–82. Tucson: University of Arizona Press, 2015.

Rasmussen, Knud. *The Netsilik Eskimos: Social Life and Spiritual Culture*. Copenhagen: Gyldendal, 1931.

Rathbun, Ted A., and Richard H. Steckel. "The Health of Slaves and Free Blacks in the East." In *The Backbone of History: Health and Nutrition in the Western Hemisphere*, ed. Richard H. Steckel and Jerome C. Rose, 208–225. Cambridge, UK: Cambridge University Press, 2002.

Reader, John. *Man on Earth*. Austin: University of Texas Press, 1988.

———. *Potato: A History of the Propitious Esculent*. New Haven, CT: Yale University Press, 2009.

Redd, Nola Taylor. "How Fast Does Light Travel? The Speed of Light." *Space*. March 7, 2018. Accessed December 12, 2019. https://www.space.com/15830-light-speed.html.

Reinagel, Monica. "Can You Be Overweight and Still Be Healthy?" *Scientific American*, July 31, 2013. Accessed April 13, 2019. https://www.scientificamerican.com/article/can-you-be-overweight-still-be-healthy.

Reitz, Elizabeth J. "Temperate and Arctic North America to 1492." In *The Cambridge World History of Food*. Vol. 2, ed. Kenneth F. Kiple and Kriemhild Conee Ornelas, 1288–1304. Cambridge, UK: Cambridge University Press, 2000.

Relethford, John. *The Human Species: An Introduction to Biological Anthropology*. Mountain View, CA: Mayfield Publishing, 1990.

Renaud, S., and A. Nordoy, "'Small is Beautiful': Alpha-Linolenic Acid and Eicosapentaenoic Acid in Man." *The Lancet* 321, no. 8334 (May 21, 1983): 1169.

Renfrew, Jane M., and Helen Sanderson. "Herbs and Vegetables." In *The Cultural History of Plants*, ed. Ghillean Prance and Mark Nesbitt, 97–132. New York and London: Routledge, 2005.

Requena, Miguel. "Socialism, Roast Beef, and Apple Pie: Werner Sombart on Socialism a Hundred Years Later." *Sociologica* 2–3 (May–December 2009): 1–16. http://citeseerx.ist.psu.edu/viewdoc/download?doi=10.1.1.882.2203&rep=rep1&type=pdf.

Rice, Stanley A. *Encyclopedia of Evolution*. New York: Facts on File, 2007.

Riley, Danny. "Walk on the Wild Side: Bach and Buxtehude." *Bachtrack*. April 23, 2017. Accessed March 9, 2019. https://bachtrack.com/feature-at-home-guide-bach-buxtehude-lubeck-arnstadt-august–2017.

Riley, James C. *Low Income, Social Growth, and Good Health: A History of Twelve Countries*. Berkeley: University of California Press, 2008.

Ristaino, Jean Beagle, and Donald H. Pfister. "'What a Painfully Interesting Subject': Charles Darwin's Studies of Potato Late Blight." *BioScience* 66, no. 12 (December 2016): 1035–1045. https://academic.oup.com/bioscience/article/66/12/1035/2646818.

Rival, Laura M. "Introduction: South America." In *The Cambridge Encyclopedia of Hunters and Gatherers*, ed. Richard B. Lee and Richard Daly, 77–85. Cambridge, UK: Cambridge University Press, 2004.

Roberts, Alice. *Evolution: The Human Story*. 2nd ed. New York: DK Publishing, 2018.

Robertson, Ruairi. "Omega 3-6-9 Fatty Acids: A Complete Overview." *Healthline*. January 15, 2017. Accessed May 31, 2019. https://www.healthline.com/nutrition/omega-3-6-9-overview.

Robinson, Mark, and Erica Rowan. "Roman Food Remains in Archaeology and the Contents of a Roman Sewer at Herculaneum." In *A Companion to Food in the Ancient World*, ed. John Wilkins and Robin Nadeau, 105–115. Chichester, UK: Wiley Blackwell, 2015.

Rock, Cheryl L., and Wendy Demark-Wahnefried. "Nutrition and Breast Cancer." In *Nutrition in the Prevention and Treatment of Disease*, ed. Ann M. Coulston, Cheryl L. Rock, and Elaine R. Monsen, 337–356. San Diego: Academic Press, 2001.

Rodriguez-Flores, Juan L., Khalid Fakhro, Francisco Agosto-Perez, Monica D. Ramstetter, Leonardo Arbiza, Thomas L. Vincent, Amal Robay, Joel A. Malek, Karsten Suhre, Lotfi Chouchane, Ramin Badii, Ajayeb Al-Nabet Al-Marri, Charbel Abi Khalil, Mahmoud Zirie, Amin Jayyousi, Jacqueline Salit, Alon Keinan, Andrew G. Clark, Ronald G. Crystal, and Jason G. Mezey. "Indigenous Arabs Are Descendants of the Earliest Split from Ancient Eurasian Populations." *Genome Research* 26, no. 2 (February 2016): 151–162. https://www.ncbi.nlm.nih.gov/pmc/articles/PMC4728368.

Roe, Daphne A., and Stephen V. Beck. "Pellagra." In *The Cambridge World History of Food*. Vol. 1, ed. Kenneth F. Kiple and Kriemhild Conee Ornelas, 960–967. Cambridge, UK: Cambridge University Press, 2000.

Roger, Delphine. "The Middle East and South Asia." In *The Cambridge World History of Food*. Vol. 2, ed. Kenneth F. Kiple and Kriemhild Conee Ornelas, 1140–1151. Cambridge, UK: Cambridge University Press, 2000.

Rogers, Edward S. "The Mistassini Cree." In *Hunters and Gatherers Today: A Socioeconomic Study of Eleven Such Cultures in the Twentieth Century*, ed. M. G. Bicchieri, 3–50. Prospect Heights, IL: Waveland Press, 1972.

Rogers, Sarah. "Rickets, Vitamin D Deficiency Still Plague Inuit Children." *Nunatsiaq News*. April 7, 2015. Accessed March 4, 2019. https://nunatsiaq.com/stories/article/65674vitamin_d_deficiency_rickets_still_plagues_inuit_children.

Romano, James F. *Daily Life of the Ancient Egyptians*. Pittsburgh: Carnegie Museum of Natural History, 1990.

Rooney, Anne. *The History of Medicine*. New York: Rosen Publishing, 2013.

Roosevelt, Anna C. "Archaeology of South American Hunters and Gatherers." In *The Cambridge Encyclopedia of Hunters and Gatherers*, ed. Richard B. Lee and Richard Daly, 86–91. Cambridge, UK and New York: Cambridge University Press, 2004.

Roosevelt, Theodore. "The Strenuous Life." Speech before the Hamilton Club. April 10, 1899. Accessed February 10, 2019. https://en.wikisource.org/wiki/The_Strenuous_Life.

Root, Waverley, and Richard de Rochemont. *Eating in America: A History*. Hopewell, NJ: Ecco Press, 1995.

Rose, Jerome C., and Melissa Zabecki. "The Commoners of Tell el-Amarna." In *Beyond the Horizon: Studies in Egyptian Art, Archaeology, and History in Honour of Barry J. Kemp*. Vol 2, ed. Salima Ikram and Aidan Dodson, 408–422. Cairo: Supreme Council of Antiquities, 2009.

Rougier, Helene, Isabelle Crevecoeur, Cedric Beauval, Cosimo Posth, Damien Flas, Christoph WiBing, Anja Furtwangler, Mietje Germonpre, Asier Gomez-Olivencia, Patrick Semal, Johannes van der Plicht, Herve Bocherens, and Johannes Krause. "Neandertal Cannibalism and Neandertal Bones Used as Tools in Northern Europe." *Scientific Reports* 6 (July 6, 2016). https://www.nature.com/articles/srep29005.

Rouse, W. H. D. "Preface." In *Great Dialogues of Plato*, trans. W. H. D. Rouse, 7–9. New York and Scarborough, Ontario: New American Library, 1956.

Rubatzky, Vincent E., and Mas Yamaguchi. *World Vegetables: Principles, Production, and Nutritive Values*. 2nd ed. New York: Chapman and Hall, 1997.

Rubel, William. *Bread: A Global History*. London: Reaktion Books, 2011.

The Rule of St. Benedict, trans. Anthony C. Meisel and M. L. del Mastro. New York: Doubleday, 1975.

Runtastic Team. "11 Incredible Running Records that Will Knock Your Socks off." *Runtastic*. May 17, 2015. Accessed September 19, 2019. https://www.runtastic.com/blog/en/11-incredible-running-records-that-will-knock-your-socks-off.

Sabbahy, Lisa. "A Decade of Advances in the Paleopathology of the Ancient Egyptians." In *Egyptian Bioarchaeology: Humans, Animals, and the Environment*, ed. Salima Ikram, Jessica Kaiser, and Roxie Walker, 113–119. Leiden: Sidestone Press, 2015.

Sabban, Francoise. "China." In *The Cambridge World History of Food*. Vol. 2, trans. Elborg Forster, ed. Kenneth F. Kiple and Kriemhild Conee Ornelas, 1165–1175. Cambridge, UK: Cambridge University Press, 2000.

Sahrhage, Dietrich, and Johannes Lundbeck. *A History of Fishing*. Berlin: Springer-Verlag, 1992.

Salaman, Redcliffe N. *The History and Social Influence of the Potato*. Rev. ed. Cambridge, UK and New York: Cambridge University Press, 1985.

Sallares, Robert. "Ecology." In *The Cambridge Economic History of the Greco-Roman World*, ed. Walter Scheidel, Ian Morris, and Richard Saller, 13–37. Cambridge, UK: Cambridge University Press, 2007.

Sandberg, Lars G., and Richard H. Steckel. "Soldier, Soldier, What Made You Grow So Tall?: A Study of Height, Health and Nutrition in Sweden, 1720–1881." *Economy and History* 23, no. 2 (1980): 91–105.

Sander, Gordon F. "An Offer Finns Can't Refuse? Helsinki Woos Car Owners to Give up Their Autos." *Christian Science Monitor*, June 23, 2017. Accessed March 17, 2019. https://www.csmonitor.com/World/Europe/2017/0623/An-offer-Finns-can-t-refuse-Helsinki-woos-car-owners-to-give-up-their-autos.

Sanderson, Helen. "Roots and Tubers." In *The Cultural History of Plants*, ed. Ghillean Prance and Mark Nesbitt, 61–76. New York and London: Routledge, 2005.

Sandle, Tim. "Pharaohs and Mummies: Diseases of Ancient Egypt and Modern Approaches." *Journal of Infectious Diseases and Preventative Medicine* 1, no. 4 (2013): 1–2. https://www.longdom.org/open-access/pharaohs-and-mummies-diseases-of-ancient-egypt-and-modern-approaches-2329-8731.1000e110.pdf.

Sansone, Leslie. "Calorie Burn Per Mile?" *Walk at Home*. Accessed October 8, 2019. https://walkathome.com/calorie-burn-per-mile.

Santirocco, Matthew S. "Introduction: Discovering Plato." In *Great Dialogues of Plato: Complete Texts of The Republic, The Apology, Crito, Phaedo, Ion, Meno, Symposium*, trans. W. H. D. Rouse, vii–xxi. New York: Signet Classics, 2008.

Sardesai, Vishwanath. *Introduction to Clinical Nutrition*. 3rd ed. Boca Raton, FL: CRC Press, 2012.

Saunders, Shelley R., Ann Herring, Larry Sawchuk, Gerry Boyce, Rob Hoppa, and Susan Klepp. "The Health of the Middle Class: The St. Thomas' Anglican Church Cemetery Project." In *The Backbone of History: Health and Nutrition in the Western Hemisphere*, ed. Richard H. Steckel and Jerome C. Rose, 130–161. Cambridge, UK: Cambridge University Press, 2002.

Sawaya, W. N., J. K. Khalil, and A. F. Al-Shalhat. "Mineral and Vitamin Content of Goat's Milk." *Journal of the American Dietetic Association* 84, no. 4 (April 1984): 433–435.

Scanes, Colin. *Fundamentals of Animal Science*. Clifton Park, NY: Delmar Cengage Learning, 2011.

Schadewaldt, H. "Hellriegel, Hermann." In *Dictionary of Scientific Biography*. Vol. 6, ed. Charles Coulston Gillispie, 237–238. New York: Charles Scribner's Sons, 1981.

Scheidel, Walter. *Death on the Nile: Disease and the Demography of Roman Egypt*. Leiden: Brill, 2001.

———. "Demography." In *The Cambridge Economic History of the Greco-Roman World*, ed. Walter Scheidel, Ian Morris, and Richard Saller, 38–86. Cambridge, UK: Cambridge University Press, 2007.

Schmid, Alexandra, and Barbara Walther. "Natural Vitamin D Content in Animal Products." *Advances in Nutrition* 4, no. 4 (July 2013): 453–462. https://www.ncbi.nlm.nih.gov/pmc/articles/PMC3941824.

"School Milk." *FAO*. 2019. Accessed March 14, 2019. http://www.fao.org/economic/est/est-commodities/dairy/school-milk/en.

Schumann, Gail L., and Cleora J. D'Arcy. *Hungry Planet: Stories of Plant Diseases*. St. Paul, MN: American Phytopathological Society, 2012.

Seely, Stephen. "The Cardiovascular System, Coronary Artery Disease, and Calcium: A Hypothesis." In *The Cambridge World History of Food*. Vol. 1, ed. Kenneth F. Kiple and Kriemhild Conee Ornelas, 1109–1120. Cambridge, UK: Cambridge University Press, 2000.

Semba, Richard D. "The Discovery of the Vitamins." *International Journal of Vitamin and Nutrition Research* 82, no. 5 (October 2012): 310–315.

Senyurek, Muzaffer Suleyman. "A Note on the Duration of Life of the Ancient Inhabitants of Anatolia." *American Journal of Physical Anthropology* 5, no. 1 (March 1947): 55–66.

Shamin A. N., and A. I. Volodarsky. "Kirchhof, Konstantin Sigizmundovich." In *Dictionary of Scientific Biography*. Vol. 7, ed. Charles Coulston Gillispie, 378–379. New York: Charles Scribner's Sons, 1981.

Shewry, Peter R., and Sandra Hey. "Do "Ancient" Wheat Species Differ from Modern Bread Wheat in Their Contents of Bioactive Components?" *Journal of Cereal Science* 65 (September 2015): 236–243. https://www.sciencedirect.com/science/article/pii/S073352101530045X.

Shmerling, Robert H. "Ditch the Gluten, Improve Your Health?" *Harvard Medical School*. May 2015. Last modified April 12, 2017. Accessed April 18, 2019. https://www.health.harvard.edu/staying-healthy/ditch-the-gluten-improve-your-health.

———. "Fertility and Diet: Is There a Connection?" *Harvard Health Publishing*. May 31, 2018. Accessed February 7, 2019. https://www.health.harvard.edu/blog/fertility-and-diet-is-there-a-connection-2018053113949.

Short, Larry. "Disaster Response in 5 Hot Spots around the World." *World Vision*. Last modified August 17, 2011. Accessed January 19, 2019. https://www.worldvision.org/blog/disaster-response-hot-spots.

Sidharta, Myra. "Soyfoods in Indonesia." In *The World of Soy*, ed. Christine M. Du Bois, Chee-Beng Tan, and Sidney W. Mintz, 195–207. Urbana and Chicago: University of Illinois Press, 2008.

Sigurdsson, Haraldur. "Mount Vesuvius before the Disaster." In *The Natural History of Pompeii*, ed. Wilhelmina Feemster Jashemski and Frederick G. Meyer, 29–36. Cambridge, UK: Cambridge University Press, 2002.

Sigurdsson, Haraldur, and Steven Carey. "The Eruption of Vesuvius in A.D. 79." In *The Natural History of Pompeii*, ed. Wilhelmina Feemster Jashemski and Frederick G. Meyer, 37–64. Cambridge, UK: Cambridge University Press, 2002.

Silverstein, Alvin, and Virginia Silverstein. *Beans: All about Them*. Englewood Cliffs, NJ: Prentice-Hall, 1975.

Simoons, Frederick J. *Food in China: A Cultural and Historical Inquiry*. Boca Raton, FL: CRC Press, 1991.

Simopoulos, Artemis P. "Evolutionary Aspects of the Dietary Omega-6/Omega-3 Fatty Acid Ratio: Medical Implications." In *Evolutionary Thinking in Medicine: From Research to Policy and Practice*, ed. Alexandra Alvergne, Crispin Jenkinson, Charlotte Faurie, 119–136. Switzerland: Springer, 2016.

———. "An Increase in the Omega-6/Omega-3 Fatty Acid Ratio Increases the Risk for Obesity." *Nutrients* 8, no. 3 (March 2016): 128. https://www.ncbi.nlm.nih.gov/pmc/articles/PMC4808858.

Simopoulos, Artemis P, and Jo Robinson. *The Omega Diet: The Lifesaving Nutritional Program Based on the Diet of the Island of Crete*. New York: Harper, 1999.

Simpson, Beryl Brintnall, and Molly Conner Ogorzaly. *Economic Botany: Plants in Our World*. 3rd ed. Boston: McGraw Hill, 2001.

"Singapore: Seafood Report 2017." *USDA*. November 10, 2017. Accessed February 16, 2019. https://www.fas.usda.gov/data/singapore-seafood-report-2017.

"Sir Frederick Hopkins." The Nobel Prize Organisation. 2019. Accessed May 17, 2019. https://www.nobelprize.org/prizes/medicine/1929/hopkins/facts.

Skeaff, C. Murray, and Jim Mann. "Lipids." In *Essentials of Human Nutrition*, ed. Jim Mann and A. Stewart Truswell, 40–59. 5th ed. Oxford: Oxford University Press, 2017.

Skeaff, Sheila., and Christine D. Thomson. "Iodine." In *Essentials of Human Nutrition*, ed. Jim Mann and A. Stewart Truswell, 172–178. 5th ed. Oxford: Oxford University Press, 2017.

Slanker, Ted. "Omega-3 Fatty Acids." Slanker Grass-Fed Meat. 2000–2019. Accessed February 7, 2019. https://www.texasgrassfedbeef.com/grass-fed-meat-education/omega-3-fatty-acids.

Slattery, Martha L., and Bette J. Caan. "Nutrition and Colon Cancer." In *Nutrition in the Prevention and Treatment of Disease*, ed. Ann M. Coulston, Cheryl L. Rock, and Elaine R. Monsen, 357–372. San Diego: Academic Press, 2001.

Small, Ernest. *North American Cornucopia: Top 100 Indigenous Food Plants*. Boca Raton, FL: CRC Press, 2014.

Small, Meredith F. "Mummy Reveals Egyptian Queen Was Fat, Balding and Bearded." *Live Science*. July 6, 2007. Accessed February 5, 2019. https://www.livescience.com/7336-mummy-reveals-egyptian-queen-fat-balding-bearded.html.

Smith, Andrew F. "From Garum to Ketchup. A Spicy Tale of Two Fish Sauces." In *Food in the Arts: Proceedings of the Oxford Symposium on Food and Cookery, 1997*, ed. Harlan Walker, 299–306. Devon, UK: Prospect Books, 1998.

———. *Peanuts: The Illustrious History of the Goober Pea*. Urbana and Chicago: University of Illinois Press, 2002.

———. *Sugar: A Global History*. London: Reaktion Books, 2015.

Smith, C. Wayne. *Crop Production: Evolution, History, and Technology*. New York: Wiley, 1995.

Smith, Hayden Ros. "Rich Swamps and Rice Grounds: The Specialization of Inland Rice Culture in the South Carolina Lowcountry, 1670–1861." Ph.D. diss., University of Georgia, 2012.

Smith, Patricia, Ofer Bar-Yosef, and Andrew Sillen. "Archaeological and Skeletal Evidence for Dietary Change during the Late Pleistocene/Early Holocene in the Levant." In *Paleopathology at the Origins of Agriculture*, ed. Mark Nathan Cohen and George J. Armelagos, 101–136. Orlando, FL: Academic Press, 1984.

Smith, T. P., S. Stoddard, M. Shankle, and J. Schultheis. "Sweetpotato Production in the United States." In *The Sweetpotato*, ed. Gad Loebenstein and George Thottappilly, 287–323. Dordrecht: Springer, 2009.

Snow, Meredith, and Steven A. LeBlanc. "A Biological Perspective on Chacoan Identity." In *Chaco Revisited: New Research on the Prehistory of Chaco Canyon, New Mexico*, ed. Carrie C. Heitman and Stephen Plog, 187–214. Tucson: University of Arizona Press, 2015.

Sobolik, Kristin D. "Dietary Reconstruction as Seen in Coprolites." In *The Cambridge World History of Food*. Vol. 1, ed. Kenneth F. Kiple and Kriemhild Conee Ornelas, 44–51. Cambridge, UK: Cambridge University Press, 2000.

Sokolov, Raymond. "Culture and Obesity." *Social Research* 66, no. 1 (Spring 1999): 31–36.

Soliman, Ashraf, Vincenzo De Sanctis, and Rania Elalaily. "Nutrition and Pubertal Development." *Indian Journal of Endocrinology and Metabolism* 18 (November 2014). https://www.ncbi.nlm.nih.gov/pmc/articles/PMC4266867.

Sonneborn, Liz. *California Indians.* Chicago: Heinemann Library, 2012.

Sorosiak, Thomas. "Soybean." In *The Cambridge World History of Food.* Vol. 1, ed. Kenneth F. Kiple and Kriemhild Conee Ornelas, 422–427. Cambridge, UK: Cambridge University Press, 2000.

Spallholz, Julian E., L. Mallory Boylan, and Judy A. Driskell. *Nutrition: Chemistry and Biology.* 2d ed. Boca Raton, FL: CRC Press, 1999.

Spencer, Frank. "Hrdlicka, Ales." In *History of Physical Anthropology.* Vol. 1: A-L, ed. Frank Spencer, 503–505. New York and London: Garland Publishing, 1997.

Spencer, Herta. "Calcium." In *The Cambridge World History of Food.* Vol. 1, ed. Kenneth F. Kiple and Kriemhild Conee Ornelas, 785–797. Cambridge, UK: Cambridge University Press, 2000.

Spiegel, Alison. "You Won't Believe How Hard It Is to Find Peanut Butter in These Countries." *Huffington Post,* April 9, 2014. Accessed March 31, 2019. https://www.huffpost.com/entry/peanut-butter_n_5105203.

Stadelman, William J. "Chicken Eggs." In *The Cambridge World History of Food.* Vol. 1, ed. Kenneth F. Kiple and Kriemhild Conee Ornelas, 499–508. Cambridge, UK: Cambridge University Press, 2000.

Stanford, Craig. "The Predatory Behavior and Ecology of Wild Chimpanzees." Accessed January 17, 2019. https://www-bcf.usc.edu/~stanford/chimphunt.html.

"State and Famine in the Sahel Region in the 20th Century." Accessed January 19, 2019. http://www.msu.ac.zw/elearning/material/1180596897state%20and%20famine%20in%20the%20sahel%20region.doc.

Staub, Jack. *The Illustrated Book of Edible Plants.* Layton, UT: Gibbs Smith, 2017.

Staum, Martin S. "Marggraf, Andreas Sigismund." In *Dictionary of Scientific Biography.* Vol. 9, ed. Charles Coulston Gillispie, 104–107. New York: Charles Scribner's Sons, 1981.

Steckel, Richard H. "Birth Weights and Infant Mortality among American Slaves." *Explorations in Economic History* 23, no. 2 (April 1986): 173–198.

———. *Health and Nutrition in the Preindustrial Era: Insights from a Millennium of Average Heights in Northern Europe.* Cambridge, MA: National Bureau of Economic Research, 2001.

Steckel, Richard H., and Jerome C. Rose. "Introduction." In *The Backbone of History: Health and Nutrition in the Western Hemisphere,* ed. Richard H. Steckel and Jerome C. Rose, 3–8. Cambridge, UK: Cambridge University Press, 2002.

———. "Patterns of Health in the Western Hemisphere." In *The Backbone of History: Health and Nutrition in the Western Hemisphere,* ed. Richard H. Steckel and Jerome C. Rose, 563–579. Cambridge, UK: Cambridge University Press, 2002.

Steckel, Richard H., Clark Spencer Larsen, and Phillip L. Walker. "Skeletal Health in the Western Hemisphere from 4000 BC to the Present." *Evolutionary Anthropology* 11, no. 4 (August 13, 2002): 142–155.

Steckel, Richard H., Paul W. Sciulli, and Jerome C. Rose. "A Health Index from Skeletal Remains." In *The Backbone of History: Health and Nutrition in the Western Hemisphere,* ed. Richard H. Steckel and Jerome C. Rose, 61–93. Cambridge, UK: Cambridge University Press, 2002.

Stimac, Heidi. "Creative Marketing Sparks Salad Bar Popularity." *Salad Bars to Schools.* 2019. Accessed July 3, 2019. http://www.saladbars2schools.org/2019/02/creative-marketing-sparks-salad-bar-popularity.

Stodder, Ann L. W., Debra L. Martin, Alan H. Goodman, and Daniel T. Reff. "Cultural Longevity and Biological Stress in the American Southwest." In *The Backbone of History: Health and Nutrition in the Western Hemisphere,* ed. Richard H. Steckel and Jerome C. Rose, 481–505. Cambridge, UK: Cambridge University Press, 2002.

Storey, Rebecca, Lourdes Marquez Morfin, and Vernon Smith. "Social Disruption and the Maya Civilization of Mesoamerica: A Study of Health and Economy of the Last Thousand Years." In *The Backbone of History: Health and Nutrition in the Western Hemisphere,* ed. Richard H. Steckel and Jerome C. Rose, 283–306. Cambridge, UK: Cambridge University Press, 2002.

Story, Colleen, Kristeen Cherney, and Rachel Nall. "The History of Heart Disease." *Healthline.* July 9, 2018. Accessed February 5, 2019. https://www.healthline.com/health/heart-disease/history.

Strawbridge, Holly. "Going Gluten-Free Just Because? Here's What You Need to Know." *Harvard Medical School.* February 20, 2013. Last modified January 18, 2018. Accessed April 18, 2019. https://www.health.harvard.edu/blog/going-gluten-free-just-because-heres-what-you-need-to-know-201302205916.

Strayer, Joseph R., and Hans W. Gatzke. *The Mainstream of Civilization.* 3rd ed. New York: Harcourt Brace Jovanovich, 1979.

Stringer, Chris, and Peter Andrews, *The Complete World of Human Evolution.* London: Thames and Hudson, 2005.

Stroud, G. D. FAO Ministry of Agriculture. Fisheries and Food. Torry Advisory Note No. 57. 2001. Accessed November 3, 2019. http://www.fao.org/3/x5933e/x5933e01.htm#TopOfPage.

"Study Finds Nearly Quarter of German Population Obese." Xinhua. May 19, 2017. Accessed April 17, 2019. http://www.xinhuanet.com//english/2017-05/19/c_136296081.htm.

"Sugar Consumption in the U.S. Diet between 1822 and 2005." Accessed January 12, 2020. http://onlinestatbook.com/2/case_studies/sugar.html.

"The Sugar Timeline." Hippocrates Health Institute. September 9, 2016. Accessed May 26, 2019. https://hippocratesinst.org/the-sugar-timeline.

"Sugarcane." In *The Cambridge World History of Food*. Vol. 2, ed. Kenneth F. Kiple and Kriemhild Conee Ornelas, 1859–1860. Cambridge, UK: Cambridge University Press, 2000.

Sun, Lena H. "Flu Broke Records for Deaths, Illnesses in 2017–2018, New CDC Numbers Show." *Washington Post*, September 27, 2018. Accessed April 18, 2019. https://www.washingtonpost.com/national/health-science/last-years-flu-broke-records-for-deaths-and-illnesses-new-cdc-numbers-show/2018/09/26/97cb43fc-c0ed-11e8-90c9-23f963eea204_story.html?noredirect=on&utm_term=.7b7839dfdccc.

"Sustainable Development Goals." UN Press Release. June 21, 2017. Accessed June 1, 2019. https://www.un.org/en/development/desa/population/events/pdf/other/21/21June_FINAL%20PRESS%20RELEASE_WPP17.pdf.

Suttles, Wayne. "Coping with Abundance: Subsistence on the Northwest Coast." In *Man the Hunter*, ed. Richard B. Lee and Irven DeVore, 56–68. Chicago: Aldine, 1968.

"Sweet Potato." In *The Cambridge World History of Food*. Vol. 2, ed. Kenneth F. Kiple and Kriemhild Conee Ornelas, 1863. Cambridge, UK: Cambridge University Press, 2000.

Szalay, Jessie. "Lemons: Health Benefits and Nutrition Facts." *Live Science*. April 23, 2018. Accessed February 27, 2019. https://www.livescience.com/54282-lemon-nutrition.html.

Tabler, Dave. "Old Order Amish." *Appalachian History*. November 21, 2017. Accessed March 15, 2019. http://www.appalachianhistory.net/2017/11/old-order-amish.html.

Tacitus. *The Germania*. In *The Agricola and the Germania*, trans. H. Mattingly and S. A. Handford, 101–141. London: Penguin Books, 1970.

Tallet, Pierre. "Food in Ancient Egypt." In *A Companion to Food in the Ancient World*, ed. John Wilkins and Robin Nadeau, 319–325. Chichester, UK: Wiley Blackwell, 2015.

Tan, Chee-Beng. "Tofu and Related Products in Chinese Foodways." In *The World of Soy*, ed. Christine M. Du Bois, Chee-Beng Tan, and Sidney W. Mintz, 99–120. Urbana and Chicago: University of Illinois Press, 2008.

Tanner, Thomas Hawkes. *The Practice of Medicine*. 5th ed. Philadelphia: Lindsay and Blakiston, 1866.

Taubes, Gary. *The Case against Sugar*. New York: Knopf, 2016.

———. *Good Calories, Bad Calories: Challenging the Conventional Wisdom on Diet, Weight Control, and Disease*. New York: Knopf, 2008.

———. *Why We Get Fat and What to Do about It*. New York: Knopf, 2011.

"Ten Health Benefits of Sugarcane Juice." *The Daily Observer*. September 28, 2015. Accessed May 22, 2019. https://antiguaobserver.com/ten-health-benefits-of-sugarcane-juice.

Teutenberg, H. J. "The General Relationship between Diet and Industrialization." In *European Diet from Pre-Industrial to Modern Times*, ed. Elborg Forster and Robert Forster, 61–109. New York: Harper Torchbooks, 1975.

Than, Ker. "First Proof Gorillas Eat Monkeys?: Mammal DNA in Gorilla Feces Hints the Big Apes Might Eat Meat After All." *National Geographic*. March 7, 2010. Accessed January 16, 2019. https://news.nationalgeographic.com/news/2010/03/100305-first-proof-gorillas-eat-monkeys-mammals-feces-dna.

Thernstrom, Stephan. *A History of the American People*. 2 vols. 2nd ed. San Diego, CA: Harcourt Brace Jovanovich, 1989.

Thomas, Frederic, Francois Renaud, Eric Benefice, Thierry de Meeus, and Jean-Francois Guegan. "International Variability of Ages at Menarche and Menopause: Patterns and Main Determinants." *Human Biology* 73, no. 2 (April 2001): 271–290.

"Thompson, Benjamin." In *World Book's Biographical Encyclopedia of Scientists*, 139. Vol 7. Chicago: World Book, 2003.

Thompson, Homer C. *Vegetable Crops*. 3rd ed. New York and London: McGraw-Hill, 1939.

Thompson, R. C., A. H. Allam, G. P. Lombardi, L. S. Wann, M. L. Sutherland, J. D. Sutherland, M. A. Soliman, B. Frohlich, D. T. Mininberg, J. M. Monge, C. M. Vallodolid, S. L. Cox, G. Abd el-Maksoud, I. Badr, M. I. Miyamoto, A. el-Halim Nur el-Din, J. Narula, C. E. Finch, and G. S. Thomas. "Atherosclerosis across 4000 Years of Human History: The Horus Study of Four Ancient Populations." *Lancet* 381 (April 6, 2013). https://www.ncbi.nlm.nih.gov/pubmed/23489753.

Thottappilly, George. "Introductory Remarks." In *The Sweetpotato*, ed. Gad Loebenstein and George Thottappilly, 3–7. Dordrecht: Springer, 2009.

Thurnham, David I. "*Vitamin A and Carotenoids*." In *Essentials of Human Nutrition*, ed. Jim Mann and A. Stewart Truswell, 191–209. 5th ed. Oxford: Oxford University Press, 2017.

"Time for More Vitamin D." *Harvard Medical School*. September 2008. Accessed November 16, 2019. https://www.health.harvard.edu/staying-healthy/time-for-more-vitamin-d.

"Top 20 Fruits and Vegetables Sold in the U.S." *PMA*. 2019. Accessed September 11, 2019. https://www.pma.com/content/articles/2017/05/top-20-fruits-and-vegetables-sold-in-the-us.

Toussaint-Samat, Maguelonne. *A History of Food*. Expanded ed., trans. Anthea Bell. Chichester, UK: Wiley-Blackwell, 2009.

Touzeau, Alexandra, Romain Amiot, Janne Blichert-Toft, Jean-Pierre Flandrois, Francois Fourel, Vincent Grossi, Francois Martineau, Pascale Richardin, and Christophe Lecuyer. "Diet of Ancient Egyptians Inferred from Stable Isotope Systematics." *Journal of Archaeological Science* 46, no. 1 (June 2014): 114–124.

Train, John. *The Olive Tree of Civilization*. Easthampton, MA and Woodbridge, UK: Antique Collectors' Club, 2004.

Trainer, Dixie Dean. *Vegetable Gardening*. New York: Playmore, 1978.

"Trans Fat." U.S. Department of Health and Human Services. Last modified May 18, 2018. Accessed January 23, 2019. https://www.fda.gov/food/ucm292278.htm.

Trinkaus, Erik. "Late Pleistocene Adult Mortality Patterns and Modern Human Establishment." *Proceedings of the National Academy of Sciences* 108, no. 4 (January 25, 2011): 1267–1271. https://www.pnas.org/content/108/4/1267.

Trumbower, Jeffrey. "Life of Christ." In *World History Encyclopedia, Era 3: Classical Traditions, 1000 BCE–300 CE*. Vol. 6, ed. William E. Mierse and Kevin M. McGeough, 571–572. Santa Barbara, CA: ABC-CLIO, 2011.

Trussell, James, and Richard H. Steckel. "The Age of Slaves at Menarche and Their First Birth." *Journal of Interdisciplinary History* 8, no. 3 (Winter 1978): 477–505.

Truswell, A. Stewart. "Fruit." In *Essentials of Human Nutrition*, ed. Jim Mann and A. Stewart Truswell, 281–282. 5th ed. Oxford: Oxford University Press, 2017.

Truswell, A. Stewart, and Jim Mann, "Introduction." In *Essentials of Human Nutrition*, ed. Jim Mann and A. Stewart Truswell, 3–10. 5th ed. Oxford: Oxford University Press, 2017.

Tsutsui, Sakio, Yoshihiko Shiga, and Tetsuo Mikami. "Japanese Sweetpotatoes: Production, Cultivars, and Possible Ancestry." *Notulae Botanicae Horti Agrobotanici Cluj-Napoca* 44, no. 1 (June 2016): 1–5. https://www.notulaebotanicae.ro/index.php/nbha/article/view/10400/7869.

Tucker, Aimee. "Succotash." *Yankee magazine*, July 28, 2015. Accessed April 1, 2019. https://newengland.com/yankee-magazine/food/succotash-recipe-with-a-history.

Turner, Grahame. "The Silverback Gorilla's Diet." *Sciencing*. Last updated April 5, 2018. Accessed January 16, 2019. https://sciencing.com/silverback-gorillas-diet-6548298.html.

Ubelaker, Douglas H., and Linda A. Newson. "Patterns of Health and Nutrition in Prehistoric and Historic Ecuador." In *The Backbone of History: Health and Nutrition in the Western Hemisphere*, ed. Richard H. Steckel and Jerome C. Rose, 343–375. Cambridge, UK: Cambridge University Press, 2002.

Ulijaszek, Stanley, Neil Mann, and Sarah Elton. *Evolving Human Nutrition: Implications for Public Health*. New York: Cambridge University Press, 2012.

"United States Amish and Pennsylvania Dutch." Food in Every Country. 2019. Accessed March 14, 2019. http://www.foodbycountry.com/Spain-to-Zimbabwe-Cumulative-Index/United-States-Amish-and-Pennsylvania-Dutch.html.

U.S. Const. Amend. XIII.

USDA FoodData Central. 2019. https://fdc.nal.usda.gov.

Vallin, Jacques. "Mortality in Europe from 1720 to 1914: Long-Term Trends and Changes in Patterns by Age and Sex." In *The Decline of Mortality in Europe*, ed. R. Schofield, D. Reher, and A. Bideau, 38–67. Oxford: Clarendon Press, 1991.

Vallois, Henri V. "The Social Life of Early Man: The Evidence of Skeletons." In *Social Life of Early Man*, ed. Sherwood L. Washburn, 214–235. Chicago: Aldine, 1961.

van Dusen, Allison, and Ana Patricia Ferrey. "World's Healthiest Countries." April 8, 2008. Accessed March 18, 2019. https://www.forbes.com/2008/04/07/health-world-countries-forbeslife-cx_avd_0408health_slide.html?thisspeed=25000#168589b943c5.

van Heerden, Philippus D. R., Gillian Eggleston, and Robin A. Donaldson. "Ripening and Postharvest Deterioration." In *Sugarcane: Physiology, Biochemistry, and Functional Biology*, ed. Paul H. Moore and Frederik C. Botha, 55–84. Ames, IA: Wiley Blackwell, 2014.

van Huis, Arnold, Joost Van Itterbeeck, Harmke Klunder, Esther Mertens, Afton Halloran, Giulia Muir, and Paul Vantomme. *Edible Insects: Future Prospects for Food and Feed Security*. Rome, Italy: Food and Agriculture Organization of the United Nations, 2013.

van Otterloo, Anneke H. "The Low Countries." In *The Cambridge World History of Food*. Vol. 2, ed. Kenneth F. Kiple and Kriemhild Conee Ornelas, 1232–1240. Cambridge, UK: Cambridge University Press, 2000.

van Straten, Michael, and Barbara Griggs. *SuperFoods: Nutrient-Dense Foods to Protect Your Health*. London: DK, 2006.

Vanderpas, J., M. Vanderpas-Rivera, P. Bourdoux, M. Dramaix, R. Lagasse, P. Seghers, F. Delange, A. M. Ermans, and C. Thilly. "Breast Feeding, Thiocyanate Metabolism, and Thyroid Function in Young Infants in Severe Endemic Goitre." In *Nutritional Factors Involved in the Goitrogenic Action of Cassava*, ed. F. Delange, F. B. Iteke, and A. M. Ermans, 59–64. Ottawa: International Development Research Centre, 1982.

Vartabedian, Ralph. "One-Car Family? That's So 1959." *Los Angeles Times*, February 14, 2007. Accessed April 1, 2019. https://www.latimes.com/archives/la-xpm-2007-feb-14-hy-wheels14-story.html.

Vaughan, J. G., and C. A. Geissler. *The New Oxford Book of Food Plants: A Guide to the Fruit, Vegetables, Herbs and Spices of the World*. Rev. ed. Oxford: Oxford University Press, 1997.

Venn, Bernard. "Legumes." In *Essential of Human Nutrition*, ed. Jim Mann and A. Stewart Truswell, 277–279. 5th ed. Oxford: Oxford University Press, 2017.

Viegas, Jennifer. "Fat Jolly Monks Had Painful Secrets." *ABC*. July 26, 2004. Accessed March 28, 2019. http://www.abc.net.au/science/news/health/HealthRepublish_1161819.htm.

"Vitamin D Fact Sheet for Health Professionals." NIH Office of Dietary Supplements. Last modified November 9, 2018. Accessed January 23, 2019. https://ods.od.nih.gov/factsheets/VitaminD-HealthProfessional.

"Vitamin E Fact Sheet for Consumers." NIH Office of Dietary Supplements. Last modified May 9, 2016. Accessed April 24, 2019. https://ods.od.nih.gov/factsheets/VitaminE-Consumer.

"Vitamin E Fact Sheet for Health Professionals." NIH Office of Dietary Supplements. Last modified August 17, 2018. Accessed January 23, 2019. https://ods.od.nih.gov/factsheets/VitaminE-HealthProfessional.

"Vitamin K Fact Sheet for Health Professionals." NIH Office of Dietary Supplements. Last modified September 26, 2018. Accessed June 1, 2019. https://ods.od.nih.gov/factsheets/VitaminK-HealthProfessional/#h2.

Vivian, R. Gwinn, and Adam S. Watson. "Reevaluating and Modeling Agricultural Potential in the Chaco Core." In *Chaco Revisited: New Research on the Prehistory of Chaco Canyon, New Mexico*, ed. Carrie C. Heitman and Stephen Plog, 30–65. Tucson: University of Arizona Press, 2015.

von Reden, Sitta. "Classical Greece: Consumption." In *The Cambridge Economic History of the Greco-Roman World*, ed. Walter Scheidel, Ian Morris, and Richard P. Saller, 385–406. Cambridge, UK: Cambridge University Press, 2007.

Wade, Lizzie. "Traces of Some of South America's Earliest People Found under Ancient Dirt Pyramid." *ScienceMag*. American Association for the Advancement of Science. May 24, 2017. Accessed February 9, 2019. https://www.sciencemag.org/news/2017/05/traces-some-south-america-s-earliest-people-found-under-ancient-dirt-pyramid?r3f_986=https://www.google.com.

Walker, Phillip L., and Russell Thornton. "Health, Nutrition, and Demographic Change in Native California." In *The Backbone of History: Health and Nutrition in the Western Hemisphere*, ed. Richard H. Steckel and Jerome C. Rose, 506–523. Cambridge, UK: Cambridge University Press, 2002.

Wallace-Hadrill, Andrew. *Herculaneum: Past and Future*. London: Frances Lincoln Publishers, 2011.

Ware, Megan. "Health Benefits and Sources of Vitamin K." *Medical News Today*. Last modified January 22, 2018. Accessed January 23, 2019. https://www.medicalnewstoday.com/articles/219867.php.

Warman, Arturo. *Corn and Capitalism: How a Botanical Bastard Grew to Global Dominance*, trans. Nancy L. Westrate. Chapel Hill and London: University of North Carolina Press, 2003.

Warner, Deborah Jean. *Sweet Stuff: An American History of Sweeteners from Sugar to Sucralose*. Washington, DC: Smithsonian Institution, 2011.

Watts, Timothy J. "'The Indians…Are Its Riches'—Depopulation in the Caribbean and Mesoamerica after 1492." In *World History Encyclopedia. Vol 11. Era 6: The First Global Age, 1450–1770*, ed. Alfred J. Andrea, Carolyn Neel, Dane A. Morrison, Alexander Mikaberidze, D. Harland Hagler, Jeffrey M. Diamond, and Monique Vallance, 99–102. Santa Barbara, CA: ABC-CLIO, 2011.

———. "Smallpox and Slavery—Demographic Catastrophe within the Americas." In *World History Encyclopedia. Vol 11. Era 6: The First Global Age, 1450–1770*, ed. Alfred J. Andrea, Carolyn Neel, Dane A. Morrison, Alexander Mikaberidze, D. Harland Hagler, Jeffrey M. Diamond, and Monique Vallance, 106–108. Santa Barbara, CA: ABC-CLIO, 2011.

———. "The Taino Suffer Smallpox." In *World History Encyclopedia. Vol 11.* Era 6: The First Global Age, 1450–1770, ed. Alfred J. Andrea, Carolyn Neel, Dane A. Morrison, Alexander Mikaberidze, D. Harland Hagler, Jeffrey M. Diamond, and Monique Vallance, 100. Santa Barbara, CA: ABC-CLIO, 2011.

Weil, Andrew. "Forward." In *The Okinawa Program: How the World's Longest-Lived People Achieve Everlasting Health—And How You Can Too*, ed. Bradley J. Willcox, D. Craig Willcox, and Makoto Suzuki, ix–x. New York: Three Rivers Press, 2001.

Weinberger, Margaret J. "Pica." In *The Cambridge World History of Food*. Vol. 1, ed. Kenneth F. Kiple and Kriemhild Conee Ornelas, 967–977. Cambridge, UK: Cambridge University Press, 2000.

Weisensee, Katherine E., and Richard L. Jantz. "Rethinking Hooton: A Reexamination of the Pecos Cranial and Postcranial Data Using Recent Methods." In *Pecos Pueblo Revisited: The Biological and Social Context*, ed. Michele E. Morgan, 43–56. Cambridge, MA: Peabody Museum of Archaeology and Ethnology, Harvard University, 2010.

Weiss, Kenneth M. "Demographic Models for Anthropology." *American Antiquity* 38, no. 2 (April 1973): 1–186.

Weissmann, Jordan. "How Kim Jong Il Starved North Korea." *The Atlantic*. December 20, 2011. Accessed January 19, 2019. https://www.theatlantic.com/business/archive/2011/12/how-kim-jong-il-starved-north-korea/250244.

"Welcome." *Ohio Amish Country Map and Visitors' Guide, 2019.*

Welsh, Jennifer. "Mozart's Death Was Written in the Key of (Vitamin) D." *Live Science*. July 6, 2011. Accessed February 2, 2019. https://www.livescience.com/14925-mozart-death-vitamin.html.

Westerbeek, Thijs. "Geert Bruggeman—Maggots: The Perfect Protein Source." *Youris.com*. European Research Media Center. April 1, 2014. Accessed March 13, 2019. http://www.youris.com/bioeconomy/interviews/geert-bruggeman--maggots-the-perfect-protein-source.kl.

"What Are Pulses?" American Pulse Association, Pulse Canada, and USA Dry Pea and Lentil Council. Accessed April 21, 2019. https://pulses.org/nap/what-are-pulses.

"What Do Amish Eat?" Amish America. Accessed March 14, 2019. http://amishamerica.com/what-do-amish-eat.

"What Does It Mean to Be Human?" Smithsonian Institution. Last modified March 30, 2016. Accessed September 23, 2019. http://humanorigins.si.edu/evidence/human-fossils/fossils/qafzeh-6.

"What Does It Mean to Be Human?" Smithsonian Institution. Last modified September 17, 2019. Accessed September 23, 2019. http://humanorigins.si.edu/evidence/human-fossils/fossils/skh%C5%ABl-v.

"What Foods Are in the Vegetable Group?" USDA. Last modified January 3, 2018. Accessed June 30, 2019. https://www.choosemyplate.gov/vegetables.

"What Is Ornish Diet?" U.S. News and World Report. 2018. Accessed January 22, 2019. https://health.usnews.com/best-diet/ornish-diet.

"What's Lacking?" Einkorn.com. 2015. Accessed April 19, 2019. https://www.einkorn.com/whats-lacking.

"Wheat in the World." CGIAR. 2017. Accessed April 25, 2019. https://wheat.org/wheat-in-the-world.

Wheeler, Mark. "Love at First Bite? Not for L.A. School Kids and Their Vegetables." *UCLA Newsroom*. May 24, 2014. Accessed July 3, 2019. http://newsroom.ucla.edu/releases/love-at-first-bite.

"When to Visit Ohio's Amish Country." *Touring Ohio*. 2019. Accessed March 14, 2019. http://touringohio.com/ohio-amish.html.

White, K. D. *Roman Farming*. Ithaca, NY: Cornell University Press, 1970.

"White Potato." In *The Cambridge World History of Food*. Vol. 2, ed. Kenneth F. Kiple and Kriemhild Conee Ornelas, 1878–1880. Cambridge, UK: Cambridge University Press, 2000.

"Wholesale and Retail Prices for Chicken, Beef, and Pork." National Chicken Council. March 25, 2019. Accessed August 1, 2019. https://www.nationalchickencouncil.org/about-the-industry/statistics/wholesale-and-retail-prices-for-chicken-beef-and-pork.

Whorton, James C. "Vegetarianism." In *The Cambridge World History of Food*. Vol. 2, ed. Kenneth F. Kiple and Kriemhild Conee Ornelas, 1553–1564. Cambridge, UK: Cambridge University Press, 2000.

"Why Sheep Milk Is Better for You than Cow or Goat Milk—Nutritional Benefits of Sheep Milk." *Woodlands Dairy*. April 26, 2017. Accessed September 24, 2019. http://woodlandsdairy.co.uk/why-sheep-milk-is-better-for-you-than-cow-or-goat-milk-nutritional-benefits-of-sheep-milk.

Wilcox, Robert W., and Alexander Mikaberidze. "Introduction: Demographic Changes." In *World History Encyclopedia. Vol 11. Era 6: The First Global Age, 1450–1770*, ed. Alfred J. Andrea, Carolyn Neel, Dane A. Morrison, Alexander Mikaberidze, D. Harland Hagler, Jeffrey M. Diamond, and Monique Vallance, 87–89. Santa Barbara, CA: ABC-CLIO, 2011.

Wiley, Andrea S. *Re-Imagining Milk*. New York and London: Routledge, 2011.

Wilkins, John. "Medical Literature, Diet, and Health." In *A Companion to Food in the Ancient World*, ed. John Wilkins and Robin Nadeau, 59–66. Chichester, UK: Wiley Blackwell, 2015.

Willcox, Bradley J., D. Craig Willcox, and Makoto Suzuki. *The Okinawa Program: How the World's Longest-Lived People Achieve Everlasting Health—And How You Can Too*. New York: Three Rivers Press, 2001.

Williams, Geoff. "The Heavy Price of Losing Weight." *U.S. News and World Report*. January 2, 2013. Accessed January 28, 2019. https://money.usnews.com/money/personal-finance/articles/2013/01/02/the-heavy-price-of-losing-weight

Williams, J. R., J. M. Roseland, Q. V. Nguyen, J. C. Howe, K. Y. Patterson, P. R. Pehrsson, and L. D. Thompson. "Nutrient Composition and Retention in Whole Turkeys with and without Added Solution." *Poultry Science* 96, no. 10 (October 2017): 3586–3592. https://www.sciencedirect.com/science/article/pii/S003257911931572X?via%3Dihub.

Wilson, C. Anne. *Food and Drink in Britain: From the Stone Age to the 19th Century*. Chicago: Academy Chicago Publishers, 1973.

Wilson, Cameron. "Rethinking Indigenous Australia's Agricultural Past." *Bush Telegraph*. May 15, 2014. Accessed January 23, 2019. https://www.abc.net.au/radionational/programs/archived/bushtelegraph/rethinking-indigenous-australias-agricultural-past/5452454.

Wing, Elizabeth S. "Animals Used for Food in the Past: As Seen by Their Remains Excavated from Archaeological Sites." In *The Cambridge World History of Food*. Vol. 1, ed. Kenneth F. Kiple and Kriemhild Conee Ornelas, 51–58. Cambridge, UK: Cambridge University Press, 2000.

Winks, Robin W., Crane Brinton, John B. Christopher, Robert Lee Wolff. *A History of Civilization*. 2 vols. 7th ed. Englewood Cliffs, NJ: Prentice Hall, 1988.

Wise, Janae. "Okinawan Diet: How Much Sweet Potatoes Do Okinawans Really Eat? (Part 2)." *The Okinawan Diet*. 2016. Accessed March 28, 2019. http://bring-joy.com/2016/07/31/okinawan-diet-sweet-potatoes.

Wishart, David J. *An Unspeakable Sadness: The Dispossession of the Nebraska Indians*. Lincoln: University of Nebraska Press, 1994.

Wolf, George. "Vitamin A." In *The Cambridge World History of Food*. Vol. 1, ed. Kenneth F. Kiple and Kriemhild Conee Ornelas, 741–750. Cambridge, UK: Cambridge University Press, 2000.

Wood, Bernard. *Human Evolution: A Very Short Introduction*. Oxford: Oxford University Press, 2005.

Wood, Jessie I. "Three Billion Dollars a Year." In *Plant Diseases: The Yearbook of Agriculture, 1953*, ed. Alfred Stefferud, 1–9. Washington, DC: GPO, 1953.

Woodham-Smith, Cecil. "The Great Hunger: Ireland, 1845–1849." In *European Diet from Pre-Industrial to Modern Times*, ed. Elborg Forster and Robert Forster, 1–18. New York: Harper Torchbooks, 1975.

———. *The Great Hunger: Ireland, 1845–1849*. New York: Harper and Row, 1962.

Woodruff, Sandra. *Secrets of Good-Carb/Low-Carb Living*. New York: Avery, 2004.

Woolfe, Jennifer A. *Sweet Potato: An Untapped Food Resource*. Cambridge, UK and New York: Cambridge University Press, 1992.

Worl, Rosita. "Inupiat Arctic Whalers." In *The Cambridge Encyclopedia of Hunters and Gatherers*, ed. Richard B. Lee and Richard Daly, 61–65. Cambridge, UK and New York: Cambridge University Press, 2004.

World Atlas. United States: Hammond Publications, 1999.

"The World: Life Expectancy (2018)." *geoba.se*. 2019. Accessed January 26, 2019. http://www.geoba.se/population.php?pc=world&type=015&year=2018&st=country&asde=&page=1.

World Vision Staff. "East Africa Hunger, Famine: Facts, FAQs, and How to Help." *World Vision*. Last modified July 10, 2018. Accessed January 19, 2019. https://www.worldvision.org/hunger-news-stories/east-africa-hunger-famine-facts.

Wrigley, E. A., and R. S. Schofield. *The Population History of England, 1541–1871: A Reconstruction*. Cambridge, UK: Cambridge University Press, 1989.

Yafa, Stephen. *Big Cotton: How a Humble Fiber Created Fortunes, Wrecked Civilizations, and Put America on the Map*. New York: Viking, 2005.

———. *Grain of Truth: The Real Case for and against Wheat and Gluten*. New York: Avery, 2015.

"Yam Facts and Figures." Accessed April 4, 2019. https://www.integratedbreeding.net/attachment/1376/Yam%20Brief.pdf.

Yeoman, Barry. "Why the Passenger Pigeon Went Extinct." *Audubon*, May–June 2104. Accessed August 4, 2019. https://www.audubon.org/magazine/may-june-2014/why-passenger-pigeon-went-extinct.

Yirka, Bob. "Neanderthal Home Made of Mammoth Bones Discovered in Ukraine." *Phys.org*. December 19, 2011. Accessed January 17, 2019. https://phys.org/news/2011-12-neanderthal-home-mammoth-bones-ukraine.html.

Yomtov, Nel. *Ancient Egypt*. New York: Scholastic, 2013.

Young, Arthur. *Tours in Ireland: 1776–1779*. 2 vols., ed. A. W. Hutton. London: George Bell and Sons, 1892.

Zelman, Kathleen M. "The Truth about Beer." *WebMD*. 2014. Accessed November 16, 2019. https://www.webmd.com/food-recipes/features/truth-about-beer.

Zeratsky, Katherine. "Nutrition and Healthy Eating." *Mayo Clinic*. May 3, 2019. Accessed June 1, 2019. https://www.mayoclinic.org/healthy-lifestyle/nutrition-and-healthy-eating/expert-answers/fat-grams/faq-20058496.

Zhang, Sarah. "Rice Was First Grown at Least 9,400 Years Ago." *The Atlantic*, May 29, 2017. Accessed April 3, 2019. https://www.theatlantic.com/science/archive/2017/05/rice-domestication/528288.

Zhang, Xue, Casey M. Owens, and M. Wes Schilling. "Meat: The Edible Flesh from Mammals Only or Does It Include Poultry, Fish, and Seafood?" *Animal Frontiers* 7, no. 4 (October 1, 2017): 12–18.

Zhen-hua, Liu. "Recent Neolithic Discoveries in Jilin Province." In *The Archaeology of Northeast China: Beyond the Great Wall*, ed. Sarah Milledge Nelson, 89–117. London and New York: Routledge, 1995.

Zibaee, Said, Syed Musa Al-Reza Hosseini, Mahdi Yousefi, Ali Taghipour, Mohammad Ali Kiani, and Mohammad Reza Noras. "Nutritional and Therapeutic Characteristics of Camel Milk in Children: A Systematic Review." *Electronic Physician* 7, no. 7 (November 2015): 1523–1528. https://www.ncbi.nlm.nih.gov/pmc/articles/PMC4700900.

Zielinski, Sarah. "Man Cannot Live on Rice and Beans Alone (But Many Do)." *NPR*. May 3, 2012. Accessed June 23, 2019. https://www.npr.org/sections/thesalt/2012/05/03/151932410/man-cannot-live-on-rice-and-beans-alone-but-many-do.

Zimmer, Carl. *Smithsonian Intimate Guide to Human Origins*. Washington, DC: Smithsonian Books, 2005.

Zioupos, P. A. Williams, G. Christodoulou, and R. Giles. "Determining 'Age at Death' for Forensic Purposes Using Human Bone by a Laboratory-Based Biochemical Analytical Method." *Journal of the Mechanical Behavior of Biomedical Materials* 33 (May 2014): 109–123. https://dspace.lib.cranfield.ac.uk/bitstream/handle/1826/9951/Determining_%27age_at_death%27_for_forensic_purposes-2014.pdf?sequence=3&isAllowed=y.

Index

For Product Safety Concerns and Information please contact our EU representative GPSR@taylorandfrancis.com Taylor & Francis Verlag GmbH, Kaufingerstraße 24, 80331 München, Germany

Printed and bound by CPI Group (UK) Ltd, Croydon, CR0 4YY
01/05/2025
01858539-0001